Systemic Lupus Erythematosus

Systemic Lupus Erythematosus

Edited by Carrie Kane

hayle medical

New York

Hayle Medical,
750 Third Avenue, 9ᵗʰ Floor,
New York, NY 10017, USA

Visit us on the World Wide Web at:
www.haylemedical.com

© Hayle Medical, 2020

ISBN: 978-1-63241-868-5

Trademark Notice: Registered trademark of products or corporate names are used only for explanation and identification without intent to infringe.

Cataloging-in-Publication Data

Systemic lupus erythematosus / edited by Carrie Kane.
p. cm.
Includes bibliographical references and index.
ISBN 978-1-63241-868-5
1. Systemic lupus erythematosus. 2. Autoimmune diseases. 3. Skin--Diseases. I. Kane, Carrie.
RC924.5.L85 S97 2020
616.772--dc23

Table of Contents

Preface.. IX

Chapter 1   **Anti-CD22/CD20 Bispecific Antibody with Enhanced Trogocytosis for Treatment
of Lupus**...1
Edmund A. Rossi, Chien-Hsing Chang and David M. Goldenberg

Chapter 2   **Interleukin-17 Expression Positively Correlates with Disease Severity of Lupus
Nephritis by Increasing Anti-Double-Stranded DNA Antibody Production in
a Lupus Model Induced by Activated Lymphocyte Derived DNA**.............................9
Zhenke Wen, Lin Xu, Wei Xu, Zhinan Yin, Xiaoming Gao and Sidong Xiong

Chapter 3   **Gene–Gene and Gene-Sex Epistatic Interactions of *MiR146a*, *IRF5*, *IKZF1*,
ETS1 and *IL21* in Systemic Lupus Erythematosus** 19
Rui-Xue Leng, Wei Wang, Han Cen, Mo Zhou, Chen-Chen Feng, Yan Zhu,
Xiao-Ke Yang, Mei Yang, Yu Zhai, Bao-Zhu Li, Xiao-Song Wang, Rui Li,
Gui-Mei Chen, Hong Chen, Hai- Feng Pan and Dong-Qing Ye

Chapter 4   **Platelet Activation and Anti-Phospholipid Antibodies Collaborate in
the Activation of the Complement System on Platelets in Systemic Lupus
Erythematosus**..25
Christian Lood, Helena Tydén, Birgitta Gullstrand, Gunnar Sturfelt,
Andreas Jönsen, Lennart Truedsson and Anders A. Bengtsson

Chapter 5   **Lipid Anti-Lipid Antibody Responses Correlate with Disease Activity in
Systemic Lupus Erythematosus**...35
Vojislav Jovanović, Nurhuda Abdul Aziz, Yan Ting Lim, Amanda Ng Ai Poh,
Sherlynn Jin Hui Chan, Eliza Ho Xin Pei, Fei Chuin Lew, Guanghou Shui,
Andrew M. Jenner, Li Bowen, Eoin F. McKinney, Paul A. Lyons,
Michael D. Kemeny, Kenneth G. C. Smith, Markus R. Wenk and Paul A. MacAry

Chapter 6   **Association of Increased Frequencies of *HLA-DPB1*05:01* with the Presence of
Anti-Ro/SS-A and Anti-La/SS-B Antibodies in Japanese Rheumatoid Arthritis and
Systemic Lupus Erythematosus Patients** 44
Hiroshi Furukawa, Shomi Oka, Kota Shimada, Shoji Sugii, Atsushi Hashimoto,
Akiko Komiya, Naoshi Fukui, Tatsuo Nagai, Shunsei Hirohata, Keigo Setoguchi,
Akira Okamoto, Noriyuki Chiba, Eiichi Suematsu, Taiichiro Miyashita,
Kiyoshi Migita, Akiko Suda, Shouhei Nagaoka, Naoyuki Tsuchiya and
Shigeto Tohma

Chapter 7   **The Tolerogenic Peptide, hCDR1, Down-Regulates the Expression of
Interferon-α in Murine and Human Systemic Lupus Erythematosus** 52
Zev Sthoeger, Heidy Zinger, Amir Sharabi, Ilan Asher and Edna Mozes

Chapter 8   **The Clinical Significance of Vitamin D in Systemic Lupus Erythematosus**........................... 60
Rajalingham Sakthiswary and Azman Ali Raymond

Chapter 9   **Evidence of New Risk Genetic Factor to Systemic Lupus
Erythematosus: The *UBASH3A* Gene** 66
Lina-Marcela Diaz-Gallo, Elena Sánchez, Norberto Ortego-Centeno,
Jose Mario Sabio, Francisco J. García-Hernández, Enrique de Ramón,
Miguel A. González-Gay, Torsten Witte, Hans-Joachim Anders,
María F. Gonzá lez-Escribano and Javier Martin

Chapter 10   **Metabolic Alterations and Increased Liver mTOR Expression Precede
the Development of Autoimmune Disease in a Murine Model of Lupus
Erythematosus** 71
Laia Vilà, Núria Roglans, Miguel Baena, Emma Barroso, Marta Alegret,
Manuel Merlos and Juan C. Laguna

Chapter 11   **Construct and Criterion Validity of the Euro Qol-5D in Patients with Systemic
Lupus Erythematosus** 83
Su-li Wang, Bin Wu, Li-an Zhu, Lin Leng, Richard Bucala and Liang-jing Lu

Chapter 12   **Galectin-9 Ameliorates Clinical Severity of MRL/lpr Lupus-Prone Mice by
Inducing Plasma Cell Apoptosis Independently of Tim-3** 88
Masahiro Moritoki, Takeshi Kadowaki, Toshiro Niki, Daisuke Nakano,
Genichiro Soma, Hirohito Mori, Hideki Kobara, Tsutomu Masaki,
Masakazu Kohno and Mitsuomi Hirashima

Chapter 13   **Multiple Sites of the Cleavage of 21- and 25-Mer Encephalytogenic
Oligopeptides Corresponding to Human Myelin Basic Protein (MBP) by
Specific Anti-MBP Antibodies from Patients with Systemic Lupus Erythematosus** 98
Anna M. Timofeeva, Pavel S. Dmitrenok, Ludmila P. Konenkova,
Valentina N. Buneva and Georgy A. Nevinsky

Chapter 14   **Mesangial Cell-Binding Activity of Serum Immunoglobulin G in Patients with
Lupus Nephritis** 111
Desmond Y. H. Yap, Susan Yung, Qing Zhang, Colin Tang and Tak Mao Chan

Chapter 15   **Phagocytosis is the Main CR3-Mediated Function Affected by the
Lupus-Associated Variant of CD11b in Human Myeloid Cells** 119
Liliane Fossati-Jimack, Guang Sheng Ling, Andrea Cortini, Marta Szajna,
Talat H. Malik, Jacqueline U. McDonald, Matthew C. Pickering, H. Terence Cook,
Philip R. Taylor and Marina Botto

Chapter 16   **Flare, Persistently Active Disease and Serologically Active Clinically Quiescent
Disease in Systemic Lupus Erythematosus** 130
Fabrizio Conti, Fulvia Ceccarelli, Carlo Perricone, Francesca Miranda,
Simona Truglia, Laura Massaro, Viviana Antonella Pacucci, Virginia Conti,
Izabella Bartosiewicz, Francesca Romana Spinelli, Cristiano Alessandri and
Guido Valesini

Chapter 17   **Mannose-Binding Lectin Blunts Macrophage Polarization and Ameliorates
Lupus Nephritis** 136
Yanxing Cai, Weijuan Zhang and Sidong Xiong

Chapter 18   **Safety of Hormonal Replacement Therapy and Oral Contraceptives in Systemic
Lupus Erythematosus** 147
Adriana Rojas-Villarraga, July-Vianneth Torres-Gonzalez and
Ángela-María Ruiz-Sternberg

Chapter 19   **Increased Risk of Chronic Obstructive Pulmonary Disease in Patients with Systemic Lupus Erythematosus**..158
Te-Chun Shen, Cheng-Li Lin, Chia-Hung Chen, Chih-Yen Tu, Te-Chun Hsia,
Chuen-Ming Shih, Wu-Huei Hsu and Yen-Jung Chang

Chapter 20   **Clinical and Serological Features of Patients Referred through a Rheumatology Triage System because of Positive Antinuclear Antibodies**.......................................164
Christie Fitch-Rogalsky, Whitney Steber, Michael Mahler, Terri Lupton,
Liam Martin, Susan G. Barr, Dianne P. Mosher, James Wick and Marvin J. Fritzler

Chapter 21   **TRIpartite Motif 21 (TRIM21) Differentially Regulates the Stability of Interferon Regulatory Factor 5 (IRF5) Isoforms**..172
Elisa Lazzari, Justyna Korczeniewska, Joan Ní Gabhann, Siobhán Smith,
Betsy J. Barnes and Caroline A. Jefferies

Chapter 22   **Rapid Resolution Liquid Chromatography Coupled with Quadrupole Time-of-Flight Mass Spectrometry-Based Metabolomics Approach to Study the Effects of Jieduquyuziyin Prescription on Systemic Lupus Erythematosus**...................182
Xinghong Ding, Jinbo Hu, Chengping Wen, Zhishan Ding, Li Yao and
Yongsheng Fan

Chapter 23   **Meta-Analysis of Associations of IL1 Receptor Antagonist and Estrogen Receptor Gene Polymorphisms with Systemic Lupus Erythematosus Susceptibility**.........................193
Li Cai, Jin-wei Zhang, Xing-xin Xue, Zhi-gang Wang, Jia-jia Wang, Shai-di Tang,
Shao-wen Tang, Jie Wang, Yun Zhang and Xian Xia

Chapter 24   **Dysregulated Cytokine Production by Dendritic Cells Modulates B Cell Responses in the NZM2410 Mouse Model of Lupus**...203
Allison Sang, Ying-Yi Zheng, Yiming Yin, Igor Dozmorov, Hao Li, Hui-Chen Hsu,
John D. Mountz and Laurence Morel

Chapter 25   **Lupus-Prone Mice Fail to Raise Antigen-Specific T Cell Responses to Intracellular Infection**..215
Linda A. Lieberman and George C. Tsokos

Permissions

List of Contributors

Index

Preface

Systemic lupus erythematosus is a chronic inflammatory disease, in which the immune system attacks healthy tissues of the body. It is one of several diseases that mimics other illnesses. Its diagnosis can thus be elusive. Some of the initial and chronic signs associated with this condition are malaise, fever, joint pains, fatigue, rashes and muscle pains. Around 70% of people with lupus have skin symptoms. Multiple genes have an influence in the development of lupus. It may also be triggered by drug reactions but is largely reversible. The severity of the disease in an individual needs to be assessed correctly to successfully treat lupus. The treatment involves the use of non-steroidal anti-inflammatory drugs and anti-malarial drugs. Certain forms of lupus nephritis require cytotoxic drugs such as mycophenolate and cyclophosphamide. This book aims to shed light on some of the unexplored aspects of systemic lupus erythematosus and the recent researches in this condition. The various studies that are constantly contributing towards advancing the diagnosis and management of lupus are examined in detail. Those in search of information to further their knowledge will be greatly assisted by this book.

Various studies have approached the subject by analyzing it with a single perspective, but the present book provides diverse methodologies and techniques to address this field. This book contains theories and applications needed for understanding the subject from different perspectives. The aim is to keep the readers informed about the progresses in the field; therefore, the contributions were carefully examined to compile novel researches by specialists from across the globe.

Indeed, the job of the editor is the most crucial and challenging in compiling all chapters into a single book. In the end, I would extend my sincere thanks to the chapter authors for their profound work. I am also thankful for the support provided by my family and colleagues during the compilation of this book.

Editor

Anti-CD22/CD20 Bispecific Antibody with Enhanced Trogocytosis for Treatment of Lupus

Edmund A. Rossi[1,2], **Chien-Hsing Chang**[1,2], **David M. Goldenberg**[1,2,3]*

1 Immunomedics, Inc., Morris Plains, New Jersey, United States of America, 2 IBC Pharmaceuticals, Inc., Morris Plains, New Jersey, United States of America, 3 Center for Molecular Medicine and Immunology, Morris Plains, New Jersey, United States of America

Abstract

The humanized anti-CD22 antibody, epratuzumab, has demonstrated therapeutic activity in clinical trials of lymphoma, leukemia and autoimmune diseases, treating currently over 1500 cases of non-Hodgkin lymphoma, acute lymphoblastic leukemias, Waldenström's macroglobulinemia, Sjögren's syndrome, and systemic lupus erythematosus. Because epratuzumab reduces on average only 35% of circulating B cells in patients, and has minimal antibody-dependent cellular cytotoxicity and negligible complement-dependent cytotoxicity when evaluated *in vitro*, its therapeutic activity may not result completely from B-cell depletion. We reported recently that epratuzumab mediates Fc/FcR-dependent membrane transfer from B cells to effector cells via trogocytosis, resulting in a substantial reduction of multiple BCR modulators, including CD22, CD19, CD21, and CD79b, as well as key cell adhesion molecules, including CD44, CD62L, and β7 integrin, on the surface of B cells in peripheral blood mononuclear cells obtained from normal donors or SLE patients. Rituximab has clinical activity in lupus, but failed to achieve primary endpoints in a Phase III trial. This is the first study of trogocytosis mediated by bispecific antibodies targeting neighboring cell-surface proteins, CD22, CD20, and CD19, as demonstrated by flow cytometry and immunofluorescence microscopy. We show that, compared to epratuzumab, a bispecific hexavalent antibody comprising epratuzumab and veltuzumab (humanized anti-CD20 mAb) exhibits enhanced trogocytosis resulting in major reductions in B-cell surface levels of CD19, CD20, CD21, CD22, CD79b, CD44, CD62L and β7-integrin, and with considerably less immunocompromising B-cell depletion that would result with anti-CD20 mAbs such as veltuzumab or rituximab, given either alone or in combination with epratuzumab. A CD22/CD19 bispecific hexavalent antibody, which exhibited enhanced trogocytosis of some antigens and minimal B-cell depletion, may also be therapeutically useful. The bispecific antibody is a candidate for improved treatment of lupus and other autoimmune diseases, offering advantages over administration of the two parental antibodies in combination.

Editor: Michael P. Bachmann, Carl-Gustav Carus Technical University-Dresden, Germany

Funding: The authors have no support or funding to report.

Competing Interests: The authors have the following interests. All of the authors have full-time employment and or stock/options with Immunomedics, Inc. and it's wholly owned subsidiary, IBC Pharmaceuticals, Inc. David Goldenberg is on the Board of Directors for both Immunomedics, Inc. and IBC Pharmaceuticals, Inc. Reagents used in this study were gifted by Immunomedics, Inc.

* E-mail: dmg.gscancer@att.net

Introduction

Although the previous view of B cells in autoimmunity was as precursors of deleterious autoantibody-producing plasma cells, they have more recently been ascribed other roles in the pathogenesis of autoimmune diseases, including systemic lupus erythematosus (SLE or lupus), such as cytokine production, presentation of autoantigens, promotion of breakdown of T-cell tolerance, and possibly activation of populations of T cells with low affinity toward autoantigens [1–3]. Due to the central role of B cells in the pathogenesis of autoimmunity, targeted anti-B-cell immunotherapies should offer therapeutic opportunities in the treatment of SLE. Of note, belimumab, which was approved recently for the treatment of SLE, is a mAb that inhibits activation of B cells by blocking B-cell activating factor [4].

CD22, a B-lymphocyte-restricted member of the immunoglobulin superfamily that regulates B-cell activation and interaction with T cells [5–17], is yet another attractive target. The humanized mAb, epratuzumab (hLL2 or IMMU-103) [18,19],

has demonstrated therapeutic activity in clinical trials of lymphoma and autoimmune disease, having treated over 1500 cases of non-Hodgkin lymphoma (NHL) [1,20–25], acute lymphoblastic leukemias [26], Sjögren's syndrome [27], and SLE [28–31]. Although epratuzumab has indicated clinical activity [1,20–31], its mechanism of action (MOA) remains obscure. Because epratuzumab has modest antibody–dependent cellular cytotoxicity (ADCC) and negligible complement-dependent cytotoxicity (CDC) *in vitro* [5,6], we postulated that, unlike CD20-targeting mAbs, such as rituximab, its therapeutic action may not result from its moderate depletion of circulating B cells.

Recently, we identified trogocytosis as a previously unknown, and potentially important, MOA of epratuzumab, which may be pertinent to its therapeutic effects in B-cell-regulated autoimmune disease [32]. Trogocytosis [33], also referred to as shaving [34], is a mechanism of intercellular communication [35–38] where two different types of cells initially form an immunological synapse due to the interaction of receptors and ligands on acceptor and donor cells, respectively [39–41], after which the ligands and portions of the associated donor cell membrane are taken up and subsequently internalized by the acceptor cell. Importantly, trogocytosis may regulate immune responsiveness to disease-associated antigens and can either stimulate or suppress the immune response [39]. In studies with an *ex-vivo* model, we demonstrated that epratuzumab mediated a significant reduction of the B-cell surface levels of key B-cell antigen receptor (BCR) signal-modulating proteins, including CD22, CD19, CD21 and CD79b, and also important cell-adhesion molecules, such as CD44, CD62L and β7-integrin, that are involved in B-cell homeostasis, activation, recirculation, migration, and homing. The reduction of the surface proteins on B cells occurred via trogocytosis to FcγR-bearing effector cells, including monocytes, granulocytes and NK cells [32]. Importantly, we verified that these key proteins were reduced significantly on B cells of SLE patients receiving epratuzumab therapy, compared to treatment-naïve patients. We proposed that epratuzumab-mediated loss of BCR modulators and cell-adhesion molecules incapacitates B cells, rendering them unresponsive to activation by T-cell-dependent antigens, leading to therapeutic control in B-cell-mediated autoimmune disease [32].

The primary MOA of anti-CD20 mAbs in NHL and autoimmune disease is B-cell depletion. Whereas elimination of healthy B cells is likely unavoidable for effective therapy of NHL, it may be detrimental in the therapy of autoimmune diseases due to the increased susceptibility to serious, possibly life-threatening, infections. Although rituximab was approved in 2006 for rheumatoid arthritis [42], it failed to achieve the primary endpoint in the LUNAR trial of SLE [43], despite encouraging prior results. Moreover, an analysis of efficacy and safety data from BELONG, a phase III trial of ocrelizumab (humanized anti-CD20), found that the treatment did not significantly improve renal response rates compared with treatment controls, and was associated with a higher rate of serious infections [44]. In both trials, the anti-CD20 mAbs achieved numerically, but not statistically, better responses than the control group, which received standard lupus therapies including steroids, in part because many patients were unable to complete the designed regimen due to serious infections resulting from B-cell depletion. In fact, BELONG was terminated early because of this.

Since both CD20 and CD22 targets have shown activity with their respective antibodies given to patients with autoimmune disease, we postulated that a bispecific antibody (bsAb) targeting both antigens could have superior properties to either parental mAb alone or even a combination of both. Herein, we describe for the first time enhanced trogocytosis mediated by bispecific antibodies targeting neighboring cell-surface proteins. We have developed an anti-CD22/CD20 bispecific hexavalent antibody (bsHexAb), 22*-(20)-(20), that combines the advantages of both anti-CD20 and anti-CD22 therapies, with enhanced trogocytosis and reduced B-cell depletion, compared to the parental anti-CD22 and anti-CD20 mAbs, respectively. This bsAb, which was shown previously to have favorable pharmacokinetics and *in vivo* stability [45], could be highly effective in the therapy of autoimmune diseases, including SLE.

Methods

Antibodies, Cell Lines and Reagents

Epratuzumab (humanized anti-CD22 IgG1κ), veltuzumab (humanized anti-CD20 IgG1κ) [46], labetuzumab (humanized anti-CEACAM5 IgG1κ) [47], and hA19 (humanized anti-CD19 IgG1κ) were provided by Immunomedics, Inc. Rituximab was obtained from a commercial source. The Fc fragment was removed from rituximab and 22*-(20)-(20) by digestion with

pepsin at pH 4.0 (Figure 1). Daudi and Raji human Burkitt lymphoma cell lines were from ATCC (Manassas, VA). All cell lines, PBMCs and isolated blood cells were maintained in RPMI 1640 media (Life Technologies, Inc., Gaithersburg, MD), supplemented with 10% heat inactivated fetal bovine serum (Hyclone, Logan, UT).

Construction of bsHexAbs

The construction of 22*-(20)-(20) using the Dock-and-Lock (DNL^{TM}) method, and its biochemical characterization, have been described previously [45]. The 22*-(19)-(19) was assembled using the same method. Independent stable transfectant SpESFX-10 myeloma cell lines [48] produced C_k-AD2-IgG-epratuzumab (Figure 1A) and dimeric C_H3-DDD2-Fab modules of veltuzumab and hA19 (Figure 1B), which were isolated from culture broths by affinity chromatography using MAb-Select and Ni-Sepharose (GE Healthcare) resins. C_k-AD2-IgG-epratuzumab was combined with 2.1 mole equivalents (10% excess) of C_H3-DDD2-Fab-veltuzumab or C_H3-DDD2-Fab-hA19 to generate 22*-(20)-(20) or 22*-(19)-(19), respectively (Figure 1C). DNL conjugations were accomplished by overnight room temperature incubation of the mixtures with 1 mM reduced glutathione, followed by the addition of 2 mM oxidized glutathione. Homogeneous preparations of the bsHexAbs were purified from the reaction mixture with MAb-Select affinity chromatography (Figure 1E and F).

Ethical Approval

Because blood fractions from anonymous donors were purchased from a commercial source, and no animals were used, this study is not governed by the Declaration of Helsinki, and, consent and approval from an ethical committee were not required.

Preparation of Blood Cell Fractions

Heparinized whole blood (buffy coat) from anonymous healthy donors was purchased from The Blood Center of New Jersey (East Orange, NJ). PBMCs were isolated by density gradient centrifugation on UNI-SEP tubes (Novamed Ltd., Jerusalem, Israel). Depletion of NK cells and isolation of monocytes from PBMCs was accomplished using MACS separation technology (Miltenyi Biotec, Auburn, CA) with human anti-CD56 and anti-CD14 microbeads, respectively, according to the manufacturer's recommended protocol.

Ex vivo Experiments

For trogocytosis experiments, PBMCs (1.5×10^6 cells/mL) were treated in triplicate with 10 μg/mL mAbs or bsHexAbs overnight (16–18 h) at 37°C in non-tissue culture treated 48-well plates, before analysis by flow cytometry. For each antigen evaluated, incubation with the isotype control labetuzumab (anti-CEACAM5, irrelevant mAb) resulted in fluorescence staining that was indistinguishable from untreated cells. Surface antigen levels, shown as % of control, were obtained by dividing the mean fluorescent intensity (MFI) of the cells treated with a test agent by that of the cells treated under the same conditions with labetuzumab, and multiplying the quotient by 100.

For studying B-cell depletion, PBMCs were incubated for two days, before addition of anti-CD19-PE, anti-CD79b-APC, 7-AAD, and 30,000 CountBright Absolute Counting Beads (Life Technologies) to each tube. For each sample, 8,000 CountBright beads were counted as a normalized reference.

For CDC, cells were seeded in black 96-well plates (Nunc) at 5×10^4 cells in 50 μL/well and incubated with serial dilutions of test and control mAbs in the presence of human complement (1:20

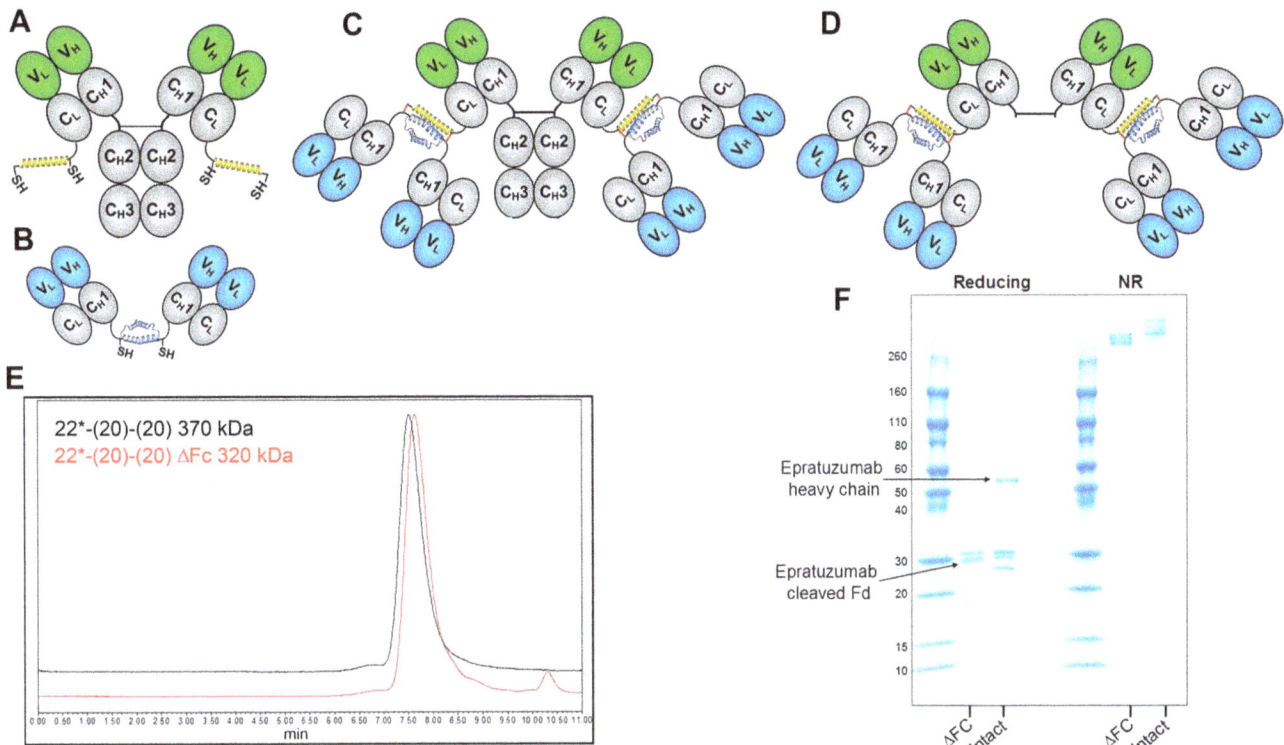

Figure 1. DNL modules and bsHexAb structures. (A) C_k-AD2-IgG-epratuzumab, an IgG-AD2 module with an AD2 fused to the carboxyl-terminal end of each kappa light chain. **(B)**. Dimeric C_H1-DDD2-Fab-veltuzumab, or C_H1-DDD2-Fab-hA9, Fab-DDD modules with DDD2 fused to the carboxyl-terminal end of the F_d chain **(C)**. Structure of 22*-(20)-(20) or 22*-(19)-(19), bsHexAbs comprising C_k-AD2-IgG-epratuzumab and two dimeric C_H1-DDD2-Fab-veltuzumab or C_H1-DDD2-Fab-hA19 modules, respectively. **(D)** Structure of 22*-(20)-(20) with the Fc removed. Variable (V, blue or green) and constant (C, grey) domains of IgG heavy (H) and light (L) chains are represented as ovals. The DDD2 (dimerization and docking domain) and AD2 (anchor domain) peptides are shown as blue and yellow helices, respectively, with the locations indicated for the reactive sulfhydryl groups (SH) and the "locking" disulfide bridges indicated as red lines. **(E)** SE-HPLC showing the homogeneity of 22*-(20)-(20) and the expected small shift in retention following removal of the Fc, which comprises 13% of the protein. **(F)** Reducing (left) and non-reducing (right) SDS-PAGE showing the elimination of the intact epratuzumab heavy chain (intact lane) and the appearance of the resulting cleaved epratuzumab Fd following removal of the Fc (ΔFc lane).

final dilution, Quidel Corp.) for 2 h at 37°C and 5% CO_2. Viable cells were then quantified using the Vybrant Cell Metabolic Assay Resazurin kit (Invitrogen). Controls included cells treated with 0.25% Triton X-100 (100% lysis) and cells treated with complement alone (background).

For ADCC, target cells were incubated with each test article in triplicate for 30 min at 37°C and 5% CO_2. Freshly isolated PBMCs were then added at a predetermined optimal effector to target ratio of 50:1. After a 4-h incubation, cell lysis was assessed by CytoTox-One (Promega).

Student's t-test was used to evaluate statistical significance ($P<$ .05).

Flow Cytometry

Cell mixtures were stained in a one-step procedure by incubating with mixed flourochrome-antibody cocktails in 1% BSA-PBS for 30 min at 4°C. Following staining, cells were washed twice with 1% BSA-PBS and samples were acquired on a FACSCalibur flow cytometer (Becton Dickinson, Franklin Lakes, NJ). For multi-color acquisition, compensation adjustments were performed using single color samples. The same instrument settings were maintained in acquiring all samples. Data were analyzed with Flowjo software (version 7.6.5, Treestar Inc., Ashland, OR). Lymphocytes were gated by forward and side scattering. B cells were identified from the lymphocyte gate using two B-cell specific markers (CD19, CD20, CD22 or CD79b),

depending on the specific antibody used for treatment, in order to avoid missing any cells where treatment reduced one marker to near background levels (Figure 2A).

Fluorochrome-antibody Conjugates Used with Flow Cytometry

The following fluorochrome-anti-human mAbs were used according to the manufacturer's recommendations. Anti-CD22 (FITC and APC, clone HIB22), anti-CD21 (FITC, clone LT21), anti-CD79b (APC and PE, clone CD3-1), and anti-CD19 (PE/Cy7, clone HIB19) were from Biolegend (San Diego, CA). Anti-CD19 (PE and FITC, clone LT19) and anti-CD20 (PE, clone LT20), were from Miltenyi Biotec. Anti-CD44 (FITC, clone L178), anti-β7 integrin (PE, clone FIB504), and anti-CD62L (FITC, clone DREG-56) were from BD Biosciences (San Jose, CA). Binding specificity was confirmed using isotype control mAbs. For exclusion of dead cells, 7-AAD (Life Technologies) was added prior to flow cytometry analysis. Preincubation of PBMCs or Daudi cells with epratuzumab or 22*-(20)-(20) at 4°C did not inhibit detection of CD22, CD19, CD21, or CD79b with anti-CD22 clone HIB22, anti-CD19 clone HIB19, anti-CD21 clone LT21, or anti-CD79b clone CD3-1, respectively. Preincubation with rituximab, veltuzumab, or 22*-(20)-(20) blocked detection of CD20 with anti-CD20 clone LT20. Preincubation with hA19 (humanized anti-CD19) or 22*-(19)-(19) blocked detection of CD19 with anti-CD19 clone LT19 (as well as 11 additional anti-CD19 mAbs).

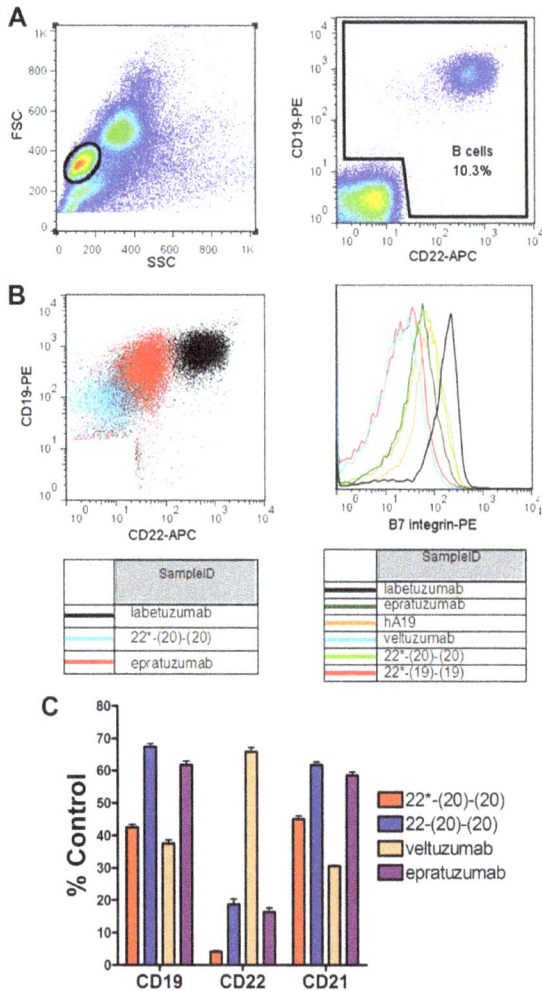

Figure 2. Analysis of trogocytosis by flow cytometry. PBMCs were incubated overnight with 10 μg/mL of various mAbs or bsHexAbs prior to measurement of surface antigens by flow cytometry. (**A**) Gating of lymphocytes by forward vs. side scattering (Left) and B cells from the lymphocyte gate using CD19 and CD22 staining (Right) following treatment with control mAb (labetuzumab). (**B**) Example dot-plots comparing CD19 and CD22 staining on B cells following treatment of PBMCs with 22*-(20)-(20), epratuzumab and labetuzumab (Left) and histograms showing β7 integrin staining following treatment with the indicated mAbs or bsHexAbs (Right). (**C**) Trogocytosis mediated by C_k and C_H3-based bsAbs. PBMCs were incubated overnight with 10 μg/mL 22*-(20)-(20), 22-(20)-(20), veltuzumab, epratuzumab or labetuzumab (control), prior to measurement of surface CD19, CD22 and CD21 by flow cytometry. Results are shown as the % MFI of the control treatment. Error bars, Std. Dev.

Fluorescence Microscopy

Monocytes were purified from freshly isolated PBMCs by positive selection and their plasma membranes were labeled with the PKH26-Red fluorescent cell labeling kit (Sigma, St. Louis, MO), following the manufacturer's recommended procedure. Daudi cell plasma membranes were labeled with the PKH67-Green fluorescent cell labeling kit (Sigma). Fluorescent-labeled monocytes and Daudi cells were mixed 2:1 (7.5×10^6/mL total cell density) and incubated at room temperature for 30 minutes in the presence of 10 μg/mL 22*-(20)-(20) or labetuzumab.

Results

Trogocytosis

The 22*-(20)-(20) bsHexAb (Figure 1C) exhibited the broadest and most extensive trogocytosis, reducing each of CD22, CD20, CD19, CD21, CD79b, CD44, CD62L, and β7-integrin more than epratuzumab, and to a similar extent as veltuzumab, except for CD22, which was reduced much more with the 22*-(20)-(20) (Table 1). The gating strategy (Figure 2A), example dot-plots (Figure 2B, left panel) and histograms (Figure 2B, right panel) demonstrating trogocytosis are shown in Figure 2. In general, 22*-(19)-(19) showed intermediate trogocytosis, with less antigen reduction than 22*-(20)-(20), but more than epratuzumab for select antigens, such as CD21 ($P = .0173$) and presumably CD19. We were unable to measure CD19 levels following treatment of PBMCs with hA19 or 22*-(19)-(19), because these antibodies block detection of the antigen (12 commercial CD19 mAbs tested). However, the considerable reduction of CD21 suggests a similar reduction of CD19. Similarly, CD20 detection was blocked with veltuzumab or 22*-(20)-(20), which each presumably remove most of the CD20 from B cells. The 22*-(20)-(20) mediated significantly ($P<.001$) more trogocytosis compared to 22-(20)-(20), which is a bsHexAb where the additional veltuzumab Fabs are fused at the end of the heavy chain, instead of at the end of the light chain (Figure 2C) [45,49].

The flow cytometry results demonstrating trogocytosis were further supported by fluorescence microscopy studies (Figure 3). Purified monocytes and Daudi (B-cell NHL) cells were membrane-labeled with red and green fluorochromes, respectively, and combined. Similar to what was observed previously with epratuzumab [32], addition of 22*-(20)-(20) to the cell mixture resulted in the rapid formation of immunological synapses and cell clustering between Daudi cells and monocytes, and subsequent trogocytosis of green Daudi membrane components to the red-stained monocytes (Figure 3A–C). Addition of the control mAb did not result in any evident trogocytosis, even where Daudi cells and monocytes were juxtaposed (Figure 3D).

B-cell Depletion

Treatment of PBMCs under the standard experimental conditions used for trogocytosis (10 μg/mL overnight) with either epratuzumab, hA19, or 22*-(19)-(19) caused minimal (<10%) B-cell depletion (not shown). The B-cell depletion caused by 22*-(20)-(20), specifically as compared to rituximab, was examined with PBMCs from multiple donors, which were treated at various concentrations for two days before counting viable B cells. The maximal level of B-cell depletion varied widely among donors, and for each donor, 22*-(20)-(20) (0–60% depletion) killed significantly ($P<.0001$) fewer B cells compared to rituximab (50–98% depletion) (Figure 4A). As shown using one of the more potent PBMCs (Donor 4), rituximab acted rapidly with considerable depletion after 24 h, whereas 22*-(20)-(20) did induce appreciable depletion at this time point; however, at higher concentrations of the bsHexAb (>1 nM), significant killing (40%) was evident after 2 days (Figure 4B). Both 22*-(20)-(20) and rituximab were considerably more effective at killing Daudi cells, which were spiked into PBMCs, compared to normal B cells (Figure 4C). It is unlikely that CDC is involved, because complement is expected to be removed during PBMC isolation. ADCC, mediated by Fc interactions with NK cells present in the PBMCs, is more likely involved in B-cell depletion. The effect of removal of NK cells (95%) from the PBMCs or deletion of the Fc from the antibodies (Figure 1) was examined using weak (Donor 1) and strong (Donor 2) B-cell-depleting PBMCs (Figure 4D). For rituximab, much less B-cell

Table 1. Percent reduction of B-cells antigens following overnight treatment of PBMCs.

Treatment	CD22	CD20	CD19	CD21	CD79b	CD62L	CD44	β7-Int
22*-(20)-(20)	96.2 (±1.3)[a]	n.d.	83.9 (±6.2)[c]	77.7 (±0.3)[c]	61.7 (±7.9)[a]	81.3 (±11.3)[d]	51.0 (±6.5)[d]	81.0 (±1.6)[d]
22*-(19)-(19)	93.7 (±1.6)[b]	25.3 (±5.4)[c]	n.d.	73.5 (±4.5)[c]	42.0 (±6.7)	64.5 (±7.0)	30.45 (±5.2)	57.7 (±3.5)
Epratuzumab	92.5 (±2.1)[b]	11.8 (±1.7)	56.1 (±6.0)	59.1 (±6.4)	39.4 (±4.5)	65.3 (±8.0)	31.3 (±3.9)	59.1 (±5.7)
Veltuzumab	58.5 (±6.2)	n.d.	92.9 (±2.3)[a]	84.8 (±0.5)[a]	45.0 (±10.3)	77.5 (±7.2)[e]	59.2 (±5.4)[e]	83.1 (±2.1)[e]
hA19	29.0 (±3.4)	17.3 (±8.2)	n.d.	68.0 (±3.1)[c]	32.8 (±7.6)	52.6 (±5.8)	31.9 (±4.6)	42.8 (±3.4)

Average % reduction from three experiments using PBMCs form independent donors. n.d., not measured due to blocked detection by the specific treatment. Significantly (P<0.05) more reduction than:
[a]all other agents;
[b]veltuzumab and hA19;
[c]epratuzumab;
[d]all but veltuzumab.
[e]Not significantly different from 22*-(20)-(20).

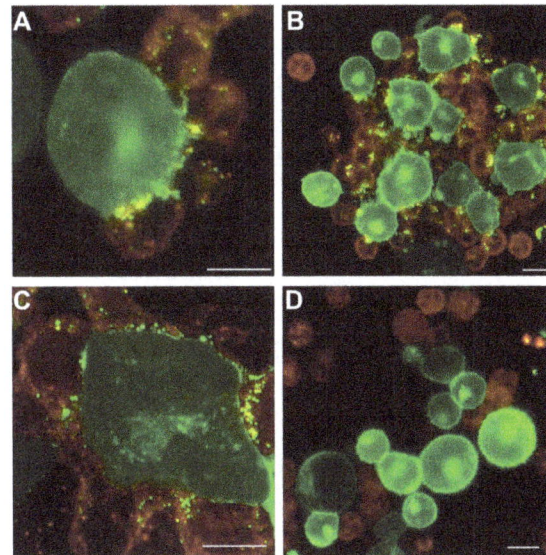

Figure 3. Fluorescence microscopy showing trogocytosis induced with 22*-(20)-(20). Purified monocytes labeled with PKH26-Red fluorescence were mixed 2:1 with Daudi cells labeled with PKH67-Green fluorescence, and treated with 22*-(20)-(20) (**A–C**) or labetuzumab (**D**) at 10 µg/mL. Fluorescent images were captured after 30 min at room temperature with an Olympus BX66 microscope (Shinjuko, Tokyo, Japan) equipped with a Mercury-100W laser (Chiu Technical Corp., Kings Park, NY), using an Olympus 40X/0.75 air objective lens and a Kodak DC290 Camera (Rochester, New York) set at 115X zoom. A WB filter was used to allow simultaneous fluorescence of both red and green fluorochromes. Images were captured and processed using Adobe Photoshop CS3 v.10 software with a Kodak Microscopy Documentation System 290 plug-in application. Bars: 10 µm.

depletion occurred when NK cells were removed from the PBMCs. It is possible that some ADCC still occurred with residual NK cells or neutrophils that were not eliminated during NK-cell removal and PBMC isolation, respectively. Removal of the Fc from rituximab had an even greater inhibitory effect on B-cell depletion, which was particularly evident with the strong Donor 2. For 22*-(20)-(20), removal of NK cells completely inhibited B-cell depletion with the strong donor. B cells were not depleted from the weak donor, even with intact PBMCs. Unexpectedly, deletion of the Fc from 22*-(20)-(20) did not affect B-cell depletion with the strong donor PBMCs, and markedly increased depletion with the weak donor PBMCs. These results suggest that there are two MOAs of 22*-(20)-(20) engaged in the *ex vivo* assay. ADCC is inhibited by depletion of NK cells. A putative signaling MOA is inhibited by trogocytosis. Removal of the Fc minimizes ADCC and also inhibits trogocytosis, whereas removal of NK cells only reduces ADCC, and not trogocytosis (Figure 4E), which is mostly mediated by monocytes.

Effector Functions

Veltuzumab and rituximab have potent ADCC, whereas hA19 and epratuzumab have moderate and low activity, respectively (Figure 5A). In repeated experiments using different target cell lines and PBMC donors, the bsHexAb 22*-(19)-(19) exhibited significantly lower ADCC than the humanized anti-CD19 mAb, hA19, and the activity was either similar or marginally higher than epratuzumab, depending on the experiment. The ADCC of 22*-(20)-(20) was compared to that of rituximab with titration experiments. Although the level of ADCC varied among donors,

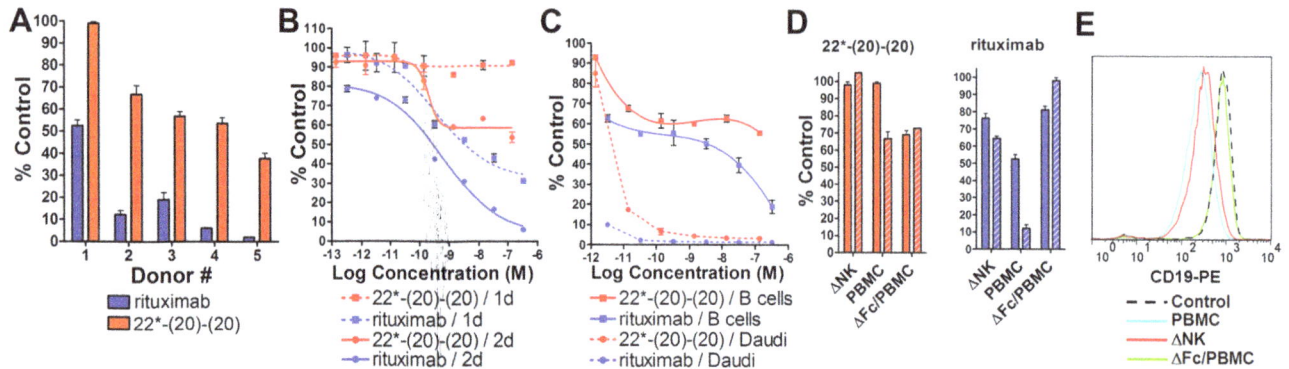

Figure 4. B-cell depletion. Freshly isolated PBMCs were incubated for two days with 22*-(20)-(20) (red) or rituximab (blue) prior to counting the viable B cells The relative viable B cell count is expressed as % Control, which was derived by dividing the specific B cell count by that measured following treatment with the control mAb (labetuzumab). Error bars, Std. Dev. (**A**) B-cell depletion with 140 nM rituximab or 22*-(20)-(20) in PBMCs from 6 unique donors. (**B**) B-cell depletion at 24 h and 48 h with antibody titrations using PBMCs from Donor 4. (**C**) Daudi Burkitt lymphoma cells were spiked in PBMCs from Donor 3 and treated with titrations of the antibodies. Daudi and normal B cells were separated by forward scattering and counted independently. (**D**) 140 nM of 22*-(20)-(20) (left, red) or rituximab (right, blue) were incubated with NK-depleted (ΔNK) or intact PBMCs, which were alternatively treated with Fc-deleted fragments (ΔFc/PBMC) of each antibody. Donor 1, solid bar; Donor 2, hatched bar. (**E**) Reduction of CD19 on B cells by trogocytosis. Control was PBMCs treated with labetuzumab (black dashed trace). Fc-deleted 22*-(20)-(20) was incubated with PBMCs (green trace). Intact 22*-(20)-(20) was incubated with PBMCs (blue trace) or NK cell-depleted PBMCs (red trace). Histograms show the fluorescence intensity for anti-CD19-PE.

rituximab consistently mediated more killing of Daudi cells, with approximately 2-fold greater maximal lysis compared to 22*-(20)-(20) (Figure 5B). Neither epratuzumab, hA19, nor 22*-(19)-(19) mediated CDC in vitro (Figure 5C). The CDC of 22*-(20)-(20) was more than 25-fold less potent than veltuzumab (Figure 5D).

Discussion

B-cell directed mAbs offer promising therapeutic options for SLE as well as other autoimmune diseases. Epratuzumab has shown clinical efficacy with minimal side-effects in SLE [1,28–31], and is in two worldwide Phase III EMBODY™ registration trials (NCT01262365). Rituximab, and possibly other anti-CD20 mAbs, are associated with increased risks of serious infections, due to near wholesale depletion of B cells. The "Black Box Warnings" for rituximab include the reactivation of hepatitis B virus and potentially fatal Progressive Multifocal Leukoencephalopathy (PML), which typically manifests only in individuals with severely compromised immune systems. Clinically, epratuzumab depletes only about 35–45% of circulating B cells and does not

increase the risk of infection [28–31]. Nonetheless, epratuzumab is effective in SLE and other diseases by mechanisms that remain unclear. Recently, we identified trogocytosis, whereby multiple key proteins, including BCR modulators and adhesion molecules, are stripped from the surface of B cells, as a potentially important MOA of epratuzumab in B-cell regulated autoimmune diseases [32]. We observed that the anti-CD20 mAbs, rituximab and veltuzumab, mediated an even stronger trogocytosis of each antigen (besides CD22). However, the potential of enhanced trogocytosis with anti-CD20 mAbs is diminished, because ultimately the B cells are all killed. Herein, we have identified a novel bsHexAb, 22*-(20)-(20), that mediates a broad and potent trogocytosis of multiple B-cell surface proteins with only moderate B-cell depletion.

An earlier version of an anti-CD22 x anti-CD20 bsHexAb, 22-(20)-(20), which has four Fabs of veltuzumab fused to the Fc of epratuzumab, demonstrated potent killing of lymphoma cell lines in vitro [49]. Subsequently, we reported that bsHexAbs of the "Ck" format, with the additional Fabs fused to the end of the light chain, has superior in vivo properties, including pharmacokinetics, neo-

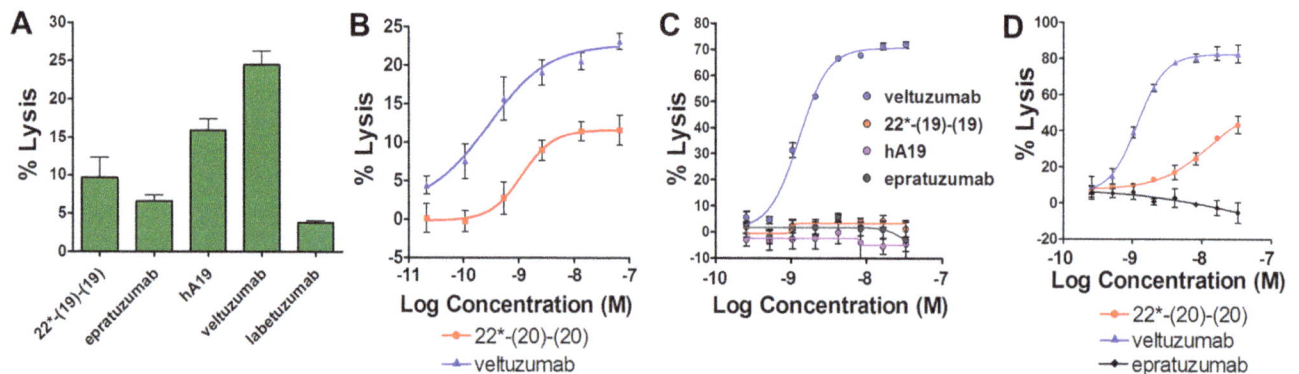

Figure 5. Effector functions. (**A+B**) ADCC. PBMCs were incubated with Daudi cells (50:1) for 4 h in the presence of the indicated agents at 33 nM (**A**) or with titration (**B**). Similar results were observed with Raji cells and a different PBMC donor. (**C+D**) CDC using Daudi as target cells. Error bars, Std. Dev.

natal FcR binding, and stability, compared to the original format, where Fabs are fused to the end of the heavy chain [45]. Here, we show that the Ck-based 22*-(20)-(20) mediates more trogocytosis compared to the Fc-based 22-(20)-(20). This is likely due to a stronger binding affinity for FcγRs (CD16 and CD64), as was found for FcRn binding.

Trogocytosis with 22*-(20)-(20) reduced the surface levels of CD19, CD21, CD79b, CD44, CD62L, and β7-integrin to similarly low levels as veltuzumab, which were considerably lower than with epratuzumab. Although we were unable to measure the level of CD20 after treatment, it is reasonable to assume that it is reduced to minimal levels, because it is one of the antigens specifically targeted by 22*-(20)-(20) and veltuzumab. Not surprisingly, CD22 is reduced to minimal levels by 22*-(20)-(20), but not with veltuzumab. Trogocytosis, the proposed MOA of epratuzumab, is enhanced with 22*-(20)-(20) by the addition of CD20-binding Fabs to epratuzumab. It is likely that targeting CD20 results in more trogocytosis compared to CD22 targeting, because the former is expressed at a higher level. Another important aspect is that following antibody ligation, CD22, but not CD20, is rapidly internalized [5,6], which is expected to compete with trogocytosis. Previously, we reported that the Fc-based bsHexAb, 22-(20)-(20), does not internalize rapidly [49], and it is likely that this is also the case for 22*-(20)-(20). The broad and potent trogocytosis mediated by 22*-(20)-(20) may modulate immune B cells more effectively than epratuzumab.

The key advantage of trogocytosis with 22*-(20)-(20) over rituximab or veltuzumab is that the bsHexAb kills less B cells. The extent of B-cell depletion varied considerably using PBMCs from different donors. "Weak" PBMCs had almost no B-cell depletion with 22*-(20)-(20) (50% with rituximab), whereas with "strong" PBMCs, up to 60% of the B cells were depleted with the bsHexAb and nearly 100% were killed with rituximab. Presumably, ADCC is the chief MOA involved in B-cell depletion in the *ex vivo* assay. We have found that *in-vitro* ADCC is highly variable among donors, which likely is responsible for the variability in B-cell depletion. We have observed a correlation between ADCC potency and B-cell depletion with a small number of PBMC specimens that were tested for both activities; however, a systematic study was not performed. Closer inspection of the dose-response curves suggests a biphasic shape, indicating that more than one MOA might be involved in the B-cell killing in the *ex vivo* assays (Fig. 4B and C). Removal of NK cells from the PBMCs, which is expected to eliminate ADCC, completely inhibited B-cell depletion with 22*-(20)-(20). Conversely, removal of the Fc, which eliminates trogocytosis as well as ADCC, resulted in enhanced B-cell depletion. This suggests that the second MOA is a result of the direct action on B cells, and is inhibited by trogocytosis. Previously, we described *in-vitro* cytotoxicity with the Fc-based 22-(20)-(20) on NHL cell lines resulting from signaling mechanisms involving Lyn, Syk, PLCγ2, AKT and NF-κB

pathways leading to apoptosis via signaling transduction mechanisms [49,50]. The Fc-based bsHexAb also caused some *ex-vivo* depletion of B cells [49] even though it has weak ADCC [45], suggesting that normal B-cell death resulted from signaling. The current results indicate that 22*-(20)-(20) also can induce apoptosis of normal B cells. However, stripping the antigens from the cell surface by trogocytosis diminishes the effects of signaling. This does not appear to be the case with rituximab, because removal of its Fc eliminates B-cell depletion. Although CDC is eliminated from the *ex vivo* system, it is likely to play a role *in vivo*. That 22*-(20)-(20) has considerably lower CDC than rituximab could widen the difference in B-cell depletion resulting from immunotherapy with these antibodies.

In this study, we compared two bsHexAbs, each comprising epratuzumab fused at the end of its light chains with four additional Fab fragments to either CD20 or CD19. In general, 22*-(20)-(20) induced more trogocytosis than 22*-(19)-(19), which reduced many of the proteins to a similar extent as epratuzumab. However, CD21, and presumably CD19, were reduced more with 22*-(19)-(19), compared to epratuzumab. Although we believe that 22*-(20)-(20) is a more promising candidate therapeutic for SLE, 22*-(19)-(19), having enhanced trogocytosis of some antigens and minimal B-cell depletion, may also be therapeutically useful.

Conclusion

The potentially ideal effects that might result from immunotherapy with 22*-(20)-(20), specifically, the extensive reduction via trogocytosis of many key B-cell surface proteins, including CD20, CD22, CD19 and CD21, with only moderate B-cell depletion, cannot be accomplished with a mixture of the two parent mAbs. While a mixture of veltuzumab (or rituximab) and epratuzumab may result in a similarly broad trogocytosis as the bsHexAb, inclusion of the anti-CD20 mAb will cause massive depletion of circulating B cells, rendering SLE patients susceptible to serious infections. Further, infusion of two mAbs, instead of a single agent, would be less convenient for both physicians and patients. Thus, 22*-(20)-(20) may offer an improved next-generation antibody for the therapy of SLE and possibly other autoimmune diseases, without the risk associated with rituximab or other potent anti-CD20 mAbs.

Acknowledgments

The authors thank Rosana Michel, John Kopinski and Diane Rossi for excellent technical assistance.

Author Contributions

Conceived and designed the experiments: EAR C-HC DMG. Performed the experiments: EAR. Analyzed the data: EAR C-HC DMG. Wrote the paper: EAR C-HC DMG.

References

1. Goldenberg DM (2006) Epratuzumab in the therapy of oncological and immunological diseases. Expert Rev Anticancer Ther 6: 1341–1353.
2. Looney RJ (2010) B cell-targeted therapies for systemic lupus erythematosus: an update on clinical trial data. Drugs 70: 529–540.
3. Mok MY (2010) The immunological basis of B-cell therapy in systemic lupus erythematosus. Int J Rheum. Dis 13: 3–11.
4. Navarra SV, Guzman RM, Gallacher AE, Hall S, Levy RA, et al. (2011) Efficacy and safety of belimumab in patients with active systemic lupus erythematosus: a randomised, placebo-controlled, phase 3 trial. Lancet 377: 721–731.
5. Carnahan J, Wang P, Kendall R, Chen C, Hu S, et al. (2003) Epratuzumab, a humanized monoclonal antibody targeting CD22: characterization of in vitro properties. Clin Cancer Res 9: 3982S–3990S.
6. Carnahan J, Stein R, Qu Z, Hess K, Cesano A, et al. (2007) Epratuzumab, a CD22-targeting recombinant humanized antibody with a different mode of action from rituximab. Mol Immunol 44: 1331–1341.
7. Haas KM, Sen S, Sanford IG, Miller AS, Poe JC, et al. (2006) CD22 ligand binding regulates normal and malignant B lymphocyte survival in vivo. J Immunol 177: 3063–3073.
8. John B, Herrin BR, Raman C, Wang YN, Bobbitt KR, et al. (2003) The B cell coreceptor CD22 associates with AP50, a clathrin-coated pit adapter protein, via tyrosine-dependent interaction. J Immunol 170: 3534–3543.
9. Kelm S, Gerlach J, Brossmer R, Danzer CP, Nitschke L (2002) The ligand-binding domain of CD22 is needed for inhibition of the B cell receptor signal, as demonstrated by a novel human CD22-specific inhibitor compound. J Exp Med 195: 1207–1213.

10. Lajaunias F, Nitschke L, Moll T, Martinez-Soria E, Semac I, et al. (2002) Differentially regulated expression and function of CD22 in activated B-1 and B-2 lymphocytes. J Immunol 168: 6078–6083.

11. Mills DM, Stolpa JC, Cambier JC (2004) Cognate B cell signaling via MHC class II: differential regulation of B cell antigen receptor and MHC class II/Ig-alpha beta signaling by CD22. J Immunol 172: 195–201.

12. Nitschke L (2009) CD22 and Siglec-G: B-cell inhibitory receptors with distinct functions. Immunol Rev 230: 128–143.

13. Onodera T, Poe JC, Tedder TF, Tsubata T (2008) CD22 regulates time course of both B cell division and antibody response. J Immunol 180: 907–913.

14. Richards S, Watanabe C, Santos L, Craxton A, Clark EA (2008) Regulation of B-cell entry into the cell cycle. Immunol Rev 224: 183–200.

15. Samardzic T, Gerlach J, Muller K, Marinkovic D, Hess J, et al. (2002) CD22 regulates early B cell development in BOB.1/OBF.1-deficient mice. Eur J Immunol 32: 2481–2489.

16. Szczepanik M, kahira-Azuma M, Bryniarski K, Tsuji RF, Kawikova I, et al. (2003) B-1 B cells mediate required early T cell recruitment to elicit protein-induced delayed-type hypersensitivity. J Immunol 171: 6225–6235.

17. Walker JA, Smith KG (2008) CD22: an inhibitory enigma. Immunology 123: 314–325.

18. Leung SO, Shevitz J, Pellegrini MC, Dion AS, Shih LB, et al. (1994) Chimerization of LL2, a rapidly internalizing antibody specific for B cell lymphoma. Hybridoma 13: 469–476.

19. Losman MJ, Hansen HJ, Dworak H, Krishnan IS, Qu Z, et al. (1997) Generation of a high-producing clone of a humanized anti-B-cell lymphoma monoclonal antibody (hLL2). Cancer 80: 2660–2666.

20. Goldenberg DM, Stein R, Leonard JP, Steinfeld SD, Dorner T, et al. (2006) B cell therapy with the anti-CD22 monoclonal antibody epratuzumab: comment on the editorial by St. Clair and Tedder. Arthritis Rheum. 54: 2344–2345.

21. Leonard JP, Coleman M, Ketas JC, Chadburn A, Ely S, et al. (2003) Phase I/II trial of epratuzumab (humanized anti-CD22 antibody) in indolent non-Hodgkin's lymphoma. J Clin Oncol 21: 3051–3059.

22. Leonard JP, Coleman M, Ketas JC, Chadburn A, Furman R, et al. (2004) Epratuzumab, a humanized anti-CD22 antibody, in aggressive non-Hodgkin's lymphoma: phase I/II clinical trial results. Clin Cancer Res 10: 5327–5334.

23. Leonard JP, Coleman M, Ketas J, Ashe M, Fiore JM, et al. (2005) Combination antibody therapy with epratuzumab and rituximab in relapsed or refractory non-Hodgkin's lymphoma. J Clin Oncol 23: 5044–5051.

24. Leonard JP, Goldenberg DM (2007) Preclinical and clinical evaluation of epratuzumab (anti-CD22 IgG) in B-cell malignancies. Oncogene 26: 3704–3713.

25. Leonard JP, Schuster SJ, Emmanouilides C, Couture F, Teoh N, et al. (2008) Durable complete responses from therapy with combined epratuzumab and rituximab: final results from an international multicenter, phase 2 study in recurrent, indolent, non-Hodgkin lymphoma. Cancer 113: 2714–2723.

26. Raetz EA, Cairo MS, Borowitz MJ, Blaney SM, Krailo MD, et al. (2008) Chemoimmunotherapy reinduction with epratuzumab in children with acute lymphoblastic leukemia in marrow relapse: a Children's Oncology Group Pilot Study. J Clin Oncol 26: 3756–3762.

27. Steinfeld SD, Tant L, Burmester GR, Teoh NK, Wegener WA, et al. (2006) Epratuzumab (humanised anti-CD22 antibody) in primary Sjogren's syndrome: an open-label phase I/II study. Arthritis Res Ther 8: R129.

28. Dorner T, Kaufmann J, Wegener WA, Teoh N, Goldenberg DM, et al. (2006) Initial clinical trial of epratuzumab (humanized anti-CD22 antibody) for immunotherapy of systemic lupus erythematosus. Arthritis Res Ther 8: R74.

29. Wallace DJ, Gordon C, Strand V, Hobbs K, Petri M, et al. (2013) Efficacy and safety of epratuzumab in patients with moderate/severe flaring systemic lupus erythematosus: results from two randomized, double-blind, placebo-controlled, multicentre studies (ALLEVIATE) and follow-up. Rheumatology. (Oxford) 52: 1313–1322.

30. Wallace DJ, Kalunian K, Petri MA, Strand V, Houssiau FA, et al. (2013) Efficacy and safety of epratuzumab in patients with moderate/severe active

systemic lupus erythematosus: results from EMBLEM, a phase IIb, randomised, double-blind, placebo-controlled, multicentre study. Ann Rheum Dis.

31. Wallace D, Kalunian K, Petri M, Strand V, Kilgallen B, et al. (2010) Epratuzumab demonstrates clinically meaningful improvements in patients with moderate to severe systemic lupus erythematosus (SLE): Results from EMBLEM^{TM}, a phase IIb study. Ann Rheum Dis (suppl 3): 558.

32. Rossi EA, Goldenberg DM, Michel R, Rossi DL, Wallace DJ, et al. (2013) Trogocytosis of multiple B-cell surface markers by CD22 targeting with epratuzumab. Blood 122: 3020–3029.

33. Joly E, Hudrisier D (2003) What is trogocytosis and what is its purpose? Nat Immunol 4: 815.

34. Beum PV, Kennedy AD, Williams ME, Lindorfer MA, Taylor RP (2006) The shaving reaction: rituximab/CD20 complexes are removed from mantle cell lymphoma and chronic lymphocytic leukemia cells by THP-1 monocytes. J Immunol 176: 2600–2609.

35. Ahmed KA, Xiang J (2011) Mechanisms of cellular communication through intercellular protein transfer. J Cell Mol Med 15: 1458–1473.

36. Davis DM (2007) Intercellular transfer of cell-surface proteins is common and can affect many stages of an immune response. Nat Rev Immunol 7: 238–243.

37. Rechavi O, Goldstein I, Kloog Y (2009) Intercellular exchange of proteins: the immune cell habit of sharing. FEBS Lett 583: 1792–1799.

38. Sprent J (2005) Swapping molecules during cell-cell interactions. Sci STKE. 2005: e8.

39. Ahmed KA, Munegowda MA, Xie Y, Xiang J (2008) Intercellular trogocytosis plays an important role in modulation of immune responses. Cell Mol Immunol 5: 261–269.

40. Caumartin J, Lemaoult J, Carosella ED (2006) Intercellular exchanges of membrane patches (trogocytosis) highlight the next level of immune plasticity. Transpl. Immunol 17: 20–22.

41. Lemaoult J, Caumartin J, Daouya M, Favier B, Le RS, et al. (2007) Immune regulation by pretenders: cell-to-cell transfers of HLA-G make effector T cells act as regulatory cells. Blood 109: 2040–2048.

42. Cohen SB, Emery P, Greenwald MW, Dougados M, Furie RA, et al. (2006) Rituximab for rheumatoid arthritis refractory to anti-tumor necrosis factor therapy: Results of a multicenter, randomized, double-blind, placebo-controlled, phase III trial evaluating primary efficacy and safety at twenty-four weeks. Arthritis Rheum 54: 2793–2806.

43. Gunnarsson I, Jonsdottir T (2013) Rituximab treatment in lupus nephritis-where do we stand? Lupus 22: 381–389.

44. Mysler EF, Spindler AJ, Guzman R, Bijl M, Jayne D, et al. (2013) Efficacy and safety of ocrelizumab in active proliferative lupus nephritis: results from the randomized, double-blind phase III BELONG study. Arthritis Rheum.

45. Rossi EA, Chang CH, Cardillo TM, Goldenberg DM (2013) Optimization of multivalent bispecific antibodies and immunocytokines with improved in vivo properties. Bioconjug. Chem 24: 63–71.

46. Goldenberg DM, Morschhauser F, Wegener WA (2010) Veltuzumab (humanized anti-CD20 monoclonal antibody): characterization, current clinical results, and future prospects. Leuk Lymphoma 51: 747–755.

47. Sharkey RM, Juweid M, Shevitz J, Behr T, Dunn R, et al. (1995) Evaluation of a complementarity-determining region-grafted (humanized) anti-carcinoembryonic antigen monoclonal antibody in preclinical and clinical studies. Cancer Res 55: 5935s–5945s.

48. Rossi DL, Rossi EA, Goldenberg DM, Chang CH (2011) A new mammalian host cell with enhanced survival enables completely serum-free development of high-level protein production cell lines. Biotechnol. Prog. 27: 766–775.

49. Rossi EA, Goldenberg DM, Cardillo TM, Stein R, Chang CH (2009) Hexavalent bispecific antibodies represent a new class of anticancer therapeutics: 1. Properties of anti-CD20/CD22 antibodies in lymphoma. Blood 113: 6161–6171.

50. Gupta P, Goldenberg DM, Rossi EA, Chang CH (2010) Multiple signaling pathways induced by hexavalent, monospecific, anti-CD20 and hexavalent, bispecific, anti-CD20/CD22 humanized antibodies correlate with enhanced toxicity to B-cell lymphomas and leukemias. Blood 116: 3258–3267.

Interleukin-17 Expression Positively Correlates with Disease Severity of Lupus Nephritis by Increasing Anti-Double-Stranded DNA Antibody Production in a Lupus Model Induced by Activated Lymphocyte Derived DNA

Zhenke Wen[1], Lin Xu[1], Wei Xu[2], Zhinan Yin[2], Xiaoming Gao[2], Sidong Xiong[1,2]*

1 Institute for Immunobiology, Shanghai Medical College of Fudan University, Shanghai, China, 2 Jiangsu Key Laboratory of Infection and Immunity, Institutes of Biology and Medical Sciences, Soochow University, Suzhou, Jiangsu Province, China

Abstract

Lupus nephritis is one of the most serious manifestations and one of the strongest predictors of a poor outcome in systemic lupus erythematosus (SLE). Recent evidence implicated a potential role of interlukin-17 (IL-17) in the pathogenesis of lupus nephritis. However, the correlation between IL-17 expression level and the severity of lupus nephritis still remains incompletely understood. In this study, we found that serum IL-17 expression level was associated with the severity of lupus nephritis, which was evaluated by histopathology of kidney sections and urine protein. Of note, we showed that enforced expression of IL-17 using adenovirus construct that expresses IL-17 could enhance the severity of lupus nephritis, while blockade of IL-17 using neutralizing antibody resulted in decreased severity of lupus nephritis. Consistently, we observed an impaired induction of lupus nephritis in IL-17-deficient mice. Further, we revealed that IL-17 expression level was associated with immune complex deposition and complement activation in kidney. Of interest, we found that IL-17 was crucial for increasing anti-double-stranded DNA (dsDNA) antibody production in SLE. Our results suggested that IL-17 expression level positively correlated with the severity of lupus nephritis, at least in part, because of its contribution to anti-dsDNA antibody production. These findings provided a novel mechanism for how IL-17 expression level correlated with disease pathogenesis and suggested that management of IL-17 expression level was a potential and promising approach for treatment of lupus nephritis.

Editor: Gayle E. Woloschak, Northwestern University Feinberg School of Medicine, United States of America

Funding: This work was supported by grants from the National Natural Science Foundation of China (30890141, 81273300), Major State Basic Research Development Program of China (2013CB530501), Program for Changjiang Scholars and Innovative Research Team in University (IRT1075), A Project Funded by the Priority Academic Program Development of Jiangsu Higher Education Institutions (PAPD), Shanghai STC grant (10JC1401400), and Mingdao Program for Medical Graduate Student in Fudan University (MDJH2012002). The funders had no role in study design, data collection and analysis, decision to publish, or preparation of the manuscript.

Competing Interests: The authors have declared that no competing interests exist.

* E-mail: sdxiongfd@126.com

Introduction

Systemic lupus erythematosus (SLE) is an autoantibody-mediated chronic autoimmune disease characterized by the deposition of immune complexes that contribute to severe organ damage. Lupus nephritis, which occurs most often within five years of lupus onset, is one of the most serious manifestations and one of the strongest predictors of a poor outcome [1]. In lupus nephritis, the pattern of glomerular injury is primarily related to the formation of the immune deposits in situ, which induces the inflammatory response by activation of adhesion molecules on endothelium and results in the recruitment of pro-inflammatory cells [2–5]. However, the exact mechanisms that lead to lupus nephritis are still unclear [2,6]. Thus, identification of crucial effectors which are correlated with disease severity of lupus nephritis would be of great prognostic value, and be helpful for providing targets in treatment of lupus nephritis.

Interleukin-17 (IL-17) is a pleiotropic cytokine that participates in tissue inflammation by inducing expression of proinflammatory cytokines, chemokines and matrix metalloproteases [7]. Recently, accumulating evidence has implicated a potential role of IL-17 in lupus [8–10]. An increase of IL-17 production from splenocytes and infiltration of IL-17-associated T cells in kidneys of SNF1 mice were reported [11]. Elevated numbers of IL-17-producing T cells were also infiltrated in the kidneys of patients with lupus nephritis [2,12]. Of note, laser microdissection-based cytokine analyses showed that elevated expression of IL-17 was correlated with clinical parameters in patients with lupus nephritis [13]. These data implicated a potential role of IL-17 in the pathogenesis of lupus nephritis. However, the correlation between IL-17 expression level and the severity of lupus nephritis still remains incompletely understood.

In our previous study, we demonstrated that compared with unactivated lymphocyte derived DNA (termed as UnALD-DNA), concanavalin A activated lymphocyte derived DNA (termed as ALD-DNA) was capable of inducing an autoimmune disease that closely resembled human SLE manifested by high levels of anti-dsDNA antibodies, glomerulonephritis and proteinuria in SLE-non-susceptible mice, which provided a lupus model to elucidate the SLE pathogenesis [14–19]. Here we characterized the association between IL-17 expression level and disease severity of lupus nephritis using the ALD-DNA induced lupus model. Up-regulation of IL-17 was performed using adenovirus construct that expresses IL-17, while in vivo blockade of IL-17 was achieved using neutralizing antibody. We found that management of IL-17 expression effectively modulated the severity of lupus nephritis. Consistently, we revealed that IL-17-deficient (IL-17$^{-/-}$) mice were resistant to development of lupus nephritis. Further, we demonstrated that IL-17 expression level was associated with immune complex deposition and complement activation in kidney. Of interest, we showed that IL-17 was crucial for elevating the generation of anti-dsDNA antibody in lupus. These findings could throw new light on the versatility of IL-17 in SLE pathogenesis, and be helpful for developing therapeutic strategy for treatment of lupus nephritis.

Materials and Methods

Ethics Statements

This study was carried out in strict accordance with the recommendations in the Guide for the Care and Use of Laboratory Animals of Shanghai Medical College of Fudan University, and was approved by the Committee on the Ethics of Animal Experiments of Fudan University (Permit Number: FDU20110306). All surgery was performed under sodium pentobarbital anesthesia, and all efforts were made to minimize suffering.

Mice

Female BALB/c mice between 6 and 8 weeks of age were purchased from the Center of Experimental Animals of Fudan University. The B6 IL-17$^{-/-}$ mice were kindly gifted by Prof. Zhinan Yin and all mice were housed in a pathogen-free mouse colony at our institution.

ALD-DNA Extraction and Purification

ALD-DNA extraction and purification was performed according to our previously described method [16–19].

Generation of ALD-DNA Induced Lupus Model

Generation of ALD-DNA induced lupus model was achieved according to our previously described method [16–19]. Briefly, groups of mice (n = 8) were subcutaneously injected under the dorsal skin with 0.2 ml of an emulsion containing ALD-DNA (50 μg/mouse) in PBS plus equal volume of complete Freund's adjuvant (CFA, Sigma-Aldrich) at week 0, followed by two booster immunizations of ALD-DNA (50 μg/mouse) emulsified with incomplete Freund's adjuvant (IFA, Sigma-Aldrich) at weeks 2 and 4. Mice receiving an equal volume of PBS plus CFA or IFA, or UnALD-DNA (50 μg/mouse) plus CFA or IFA were used as controls.

Anti-dsDNA Antibody Detection

Serological anti-dsDNA antibody was detected using mouse anti-dsDNA antibody ELISA Kit (Alpha Diagnostic International) as previously described [18,20].

Urine Protein Measurement

Urine protein was measured with the BCA Protein Assay Kit (Thermo Fisher Scientific) according to the manufacturer's instructions as previously described [18].

Study of kidney Sections

The immunofluorescence study of kidney sections was performed using polyclonal anti-mouse IgG-FITC (Sigma) or polyclonal anti-mouse complement C3-FITC (MP Biomedical) as previously described [17,21]. The intensity of fluorescence was evaluated with the ImageJ software (National Institute of Health) as previously described [17,22]. The histological signs of lupus nephritis were studied by two pathologists unaware of the immunized animals as described elsewhere [23]. In brief, the extent of the pathological lesions was graded on a semiquantitative scale ranging from 0 to 4 as follows: 0 = normal; 1, a small increase of cells in the glomerular mesanguim; 2, a larger number of cells in the mesangium; 3, glomerular lobular formation and thickened basement membrane; 4 glomerular crescent formation, sclerosis, tubular atrophy and casts. The score for each animal was calculated by dividing the total score for the number of glomeruli observed.

Treatment with Exogenous IL-17

Adenovirus construct that expresses murine IL-17 (Ad-mIL-17, 10^9 plaque-forming units per mouse) or the control vector that expresses β-galactosidase (Ad-Ctrl) was used as previously described [24,25].

Neutralization of IL-17 in vivo

In vivo blockade of IL-17 was achieved using the neutralizing antibody to IL-17 as previously described [26]. Briefly, groups of mice were injected intraperitoneal with 100 μg/mouse of either anti-IL-17 antibody (R&D Systems) or an isotype control antibody (R&D Systems) 24 h before ALD-DNA immunization and then were given at 3 day intervals for 10 weeks.

Statistical Analysis

Quantitative data were expressed as the mean ± SD. Unpaired t test and Pearson correlation were used for statistical analyses. A value of P<0.05 was considered statistically significant. All statistical analyses were performed by using SPSS statistical software version 16 (SPSS Inc.).

Results

Serological Expression Level of IL-17 was Associated with the Severity of Lupus Nephritis

To explore the association of IL-17 expression level and severity of lupus nephritis, we detected the serological level of IL-17 in ALD-DNA induced lupus mice. We found that the serological level of IL-17 was significantly elevated (Figure 1A, p<0.05). Then we analyzed the correlation between serological level of IL-17 and the pathology score of kidney in mice immunized with ALD-DNA for eight weeks. As shown in Figure 1B, we revealed that the IL-17 expression level was closely correlated with the pathology score of kidney (p<0.05). Consistently, we observed that serum IL-17 level was also associated with the level of urine protein in ALD-DNA induced lupus mice (Figure 1C, p<0.05). These data suggested the IL-17 expression level was correlated with disease severity of lupus nephritis.

A

B

C

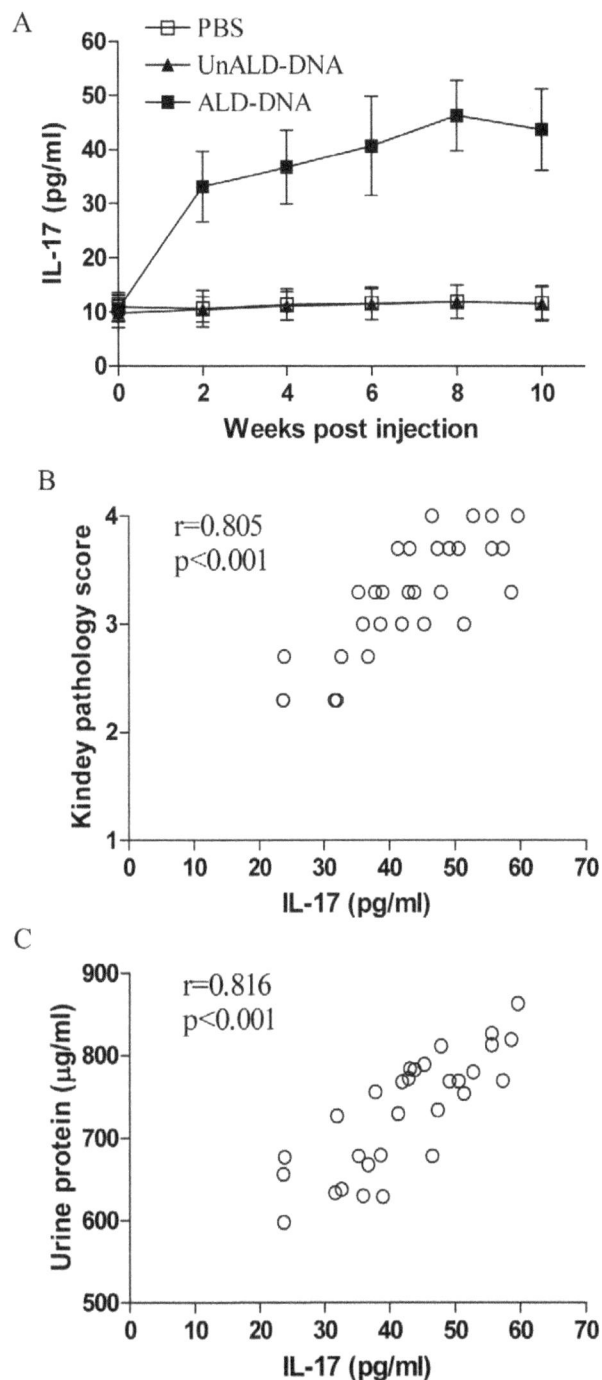

Figure 1. IL-17 expression level was associated with the severity of lupus nephritis. Groups of BALB/c mice were immunized with 50 μg of ALD-DNA as described in methods. (A) The serological level of IL-17 was determined at the indicated time. Data represented the means (±SD) for eight mice in each group. Shown was the represented data from one of four independent experiments. (B and C) The correlation between serological IL-17 expression level and the kidney pathology score, as well as the level of urine protein, was analyzed in thirty two mice eight weeks post ALD-DNA injection. Each dot represented the average value for triplicate in each mouse.

Up-regulation of IL-17 Expression Enhanced the Severity of Lupus Nephritis

To further evaluate the correlation between IL-17 expression level and severity of lupus nephritis, we detected whether up-regulation of IL-17 expression could modify the severity of lupus nephritis. Thus, groups of mice were injected with the adenovirus construct that expresses murine IL-17 (Ad-mIL-17) or with the control adenovirus vector (Ad-Ctrl) respectively, followed by immunization with ALD-DNA. We revealed that the kidney pathology score was significantly higher in mice treated with Ad-mIL-17 than that in control mice (Figure 2A and B, $p<0.05$). The kidney pathology score in mice treated with Ad-mIL-17 after ALD-DNA injection for six weeks was even higher than that in control mice after ALD-DNA injection for eight weeks (Figure 2A and B, $p<0.05$). Consistently, we found that the urine protein level in mice treated with Ad-mIL-17 was also significantly elevated compared with that in control mice (Figure 2C, $p<0.05$). These data demonstrated that up-regulation of IL-17 expression could enhance the severity of lupus nephritis. In addition, we observed that treatment with Ad-mIL-17 alone without ALD-DNA injection resulted in no significant induction of lupus nephritis (Figure 2A, B, C, $p>0.05$), suggesting that IL-17 was not the startup element for induction of lupus nephritis.

Blockade of IL-17 Ameliorated the Severity of Lupus Nephritis

To further detect whether blockade of IL-17 could ameliorate the severity of lupus nephritis, groups of mice were injected with neutralizing antibody to IL-17 and then immunized with ALD-DNA. Eight weeks later, we found that in vivo neutralization of IL-17 significantly abrogated the induction of nephritis (Figure 3A and B, $p<0.05$). Besides, we revealed that blockade of IL-17 resulted in decreased level of urine protein in ALD-DNA immunized mice (Figure 3C, $p<0.05$). These data demonstrated that blockade of IL-17 resulted in amelioration of lupus nephritis.

IL-17$^{-/-}$ Mice were Resistant to Induction of Lupus Nephritis

To further verify the correlation between IL-17 expression level and the severity of lupus nephritis, groups of IL-17$^{-/-}$ mice and wild type (WT) mice were immunized with ALD-DNA. Eight weeks later, we analyzed the pathology of kidney in ALD-DNA immunized IL-17$^{-/-}$ and WT mice. As shown in Figure 4A and B, ALD-DNA immunization effectively induced lupus nephritis in the WT mice. In contrast, we found that ALD-DNA failed to induce nephritis effectively in IL-17$^{-/-}$ mice (Figure 4A and B, $p<0.05$). Further, we observed that ALD-DNA induced high levels of urine protein in the WT mice but not in IL-17$^{-/-}$ mice (Figure 4C, $p<0.05$). To determine whether the immunization dose of ALD-DNA accounted for the impaired induction of lupus nephritis, groups of IL-17$^{-/-}$ mice were immunized with an increasing dose of ALD-DNA. Results showed that the increased dose of ALD-DNA still could not induce the apparent lupus nephritis in IL-17$^{-/-}$ mice (Figure 4D and E, $p>0.05$). These results demonstrated that IL-17$^{-/-}$ mice were resistant to induction of lupus nephritis.

IL-17 Expression Modified Immune Complex Deposition and Complement Activation in Kidney

In lupus nephritis, the pattern of glomerular injury is primarily related to the formation of the immune complex deposits in situ [2–5]. Therefore, to characterize the mechanisms account for the close correlation between IL-17 expression level and severity of

A

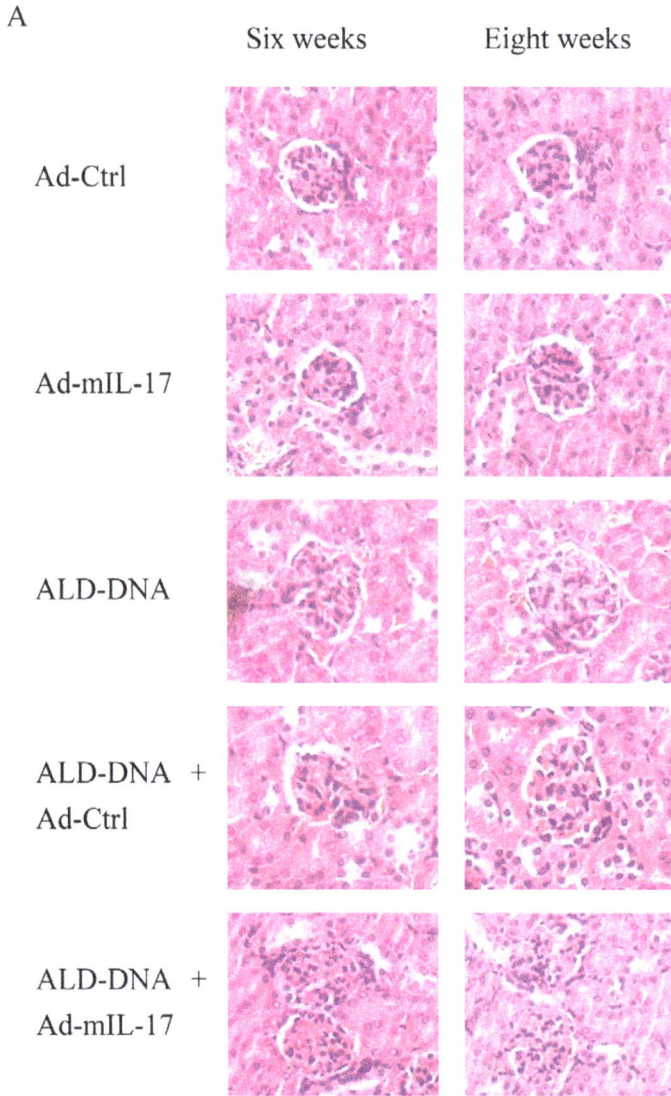

B

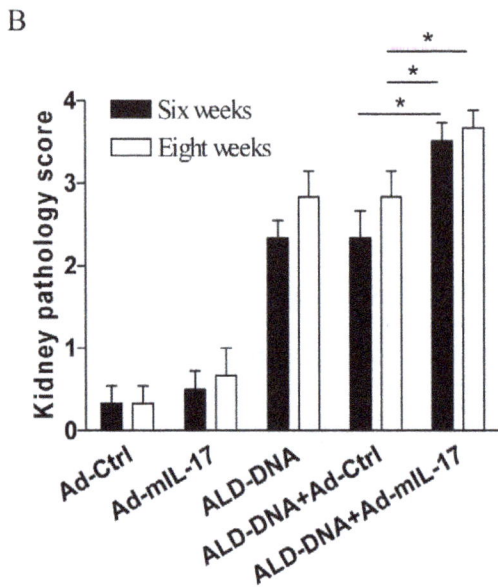

C

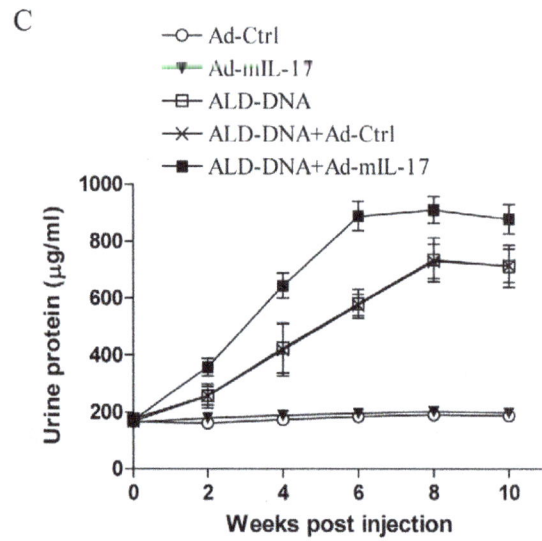

Figure 2. Treatment with Ad-mIL-17 enhanced the severity of lupus nephritis. Groups of BALB/c mice were treated with Ad-mIL-17 or Ad-Ctrl respectively, and then immunized with or without 50 µg of ALD-DNA. The kidney pathology (A and B) and the level of urine protein (C) were analyzed at the indicate time. Data represented the means (±SD) for eight mice in each group. *P<0.05.

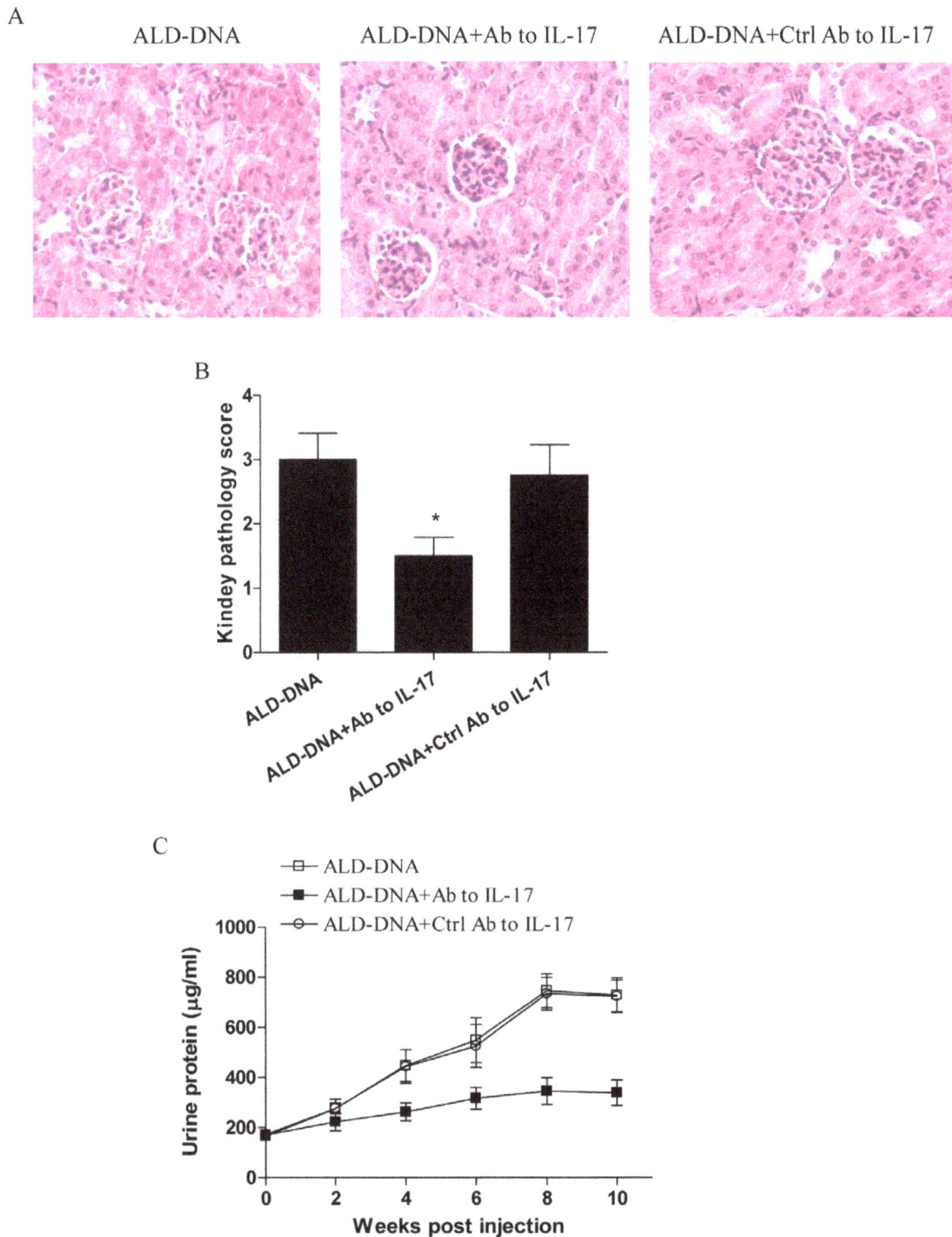

Figure 3. Blockade of IL-17 alleviated the severity of lupus nephritis. Groups of BALB/c mice were injected with neutralizing antibody to IL-17 or the control antibody, and then immunized with 50 µg of ALD-DNA. (A and B) The kidney histopathology and pathology score were analyzed eight weeks post ALD-DNA injection. (C) The level of urine protein was analyzed at the indicated time. Data represented the means (±SD) for eight mice in each group. *P<0.05.

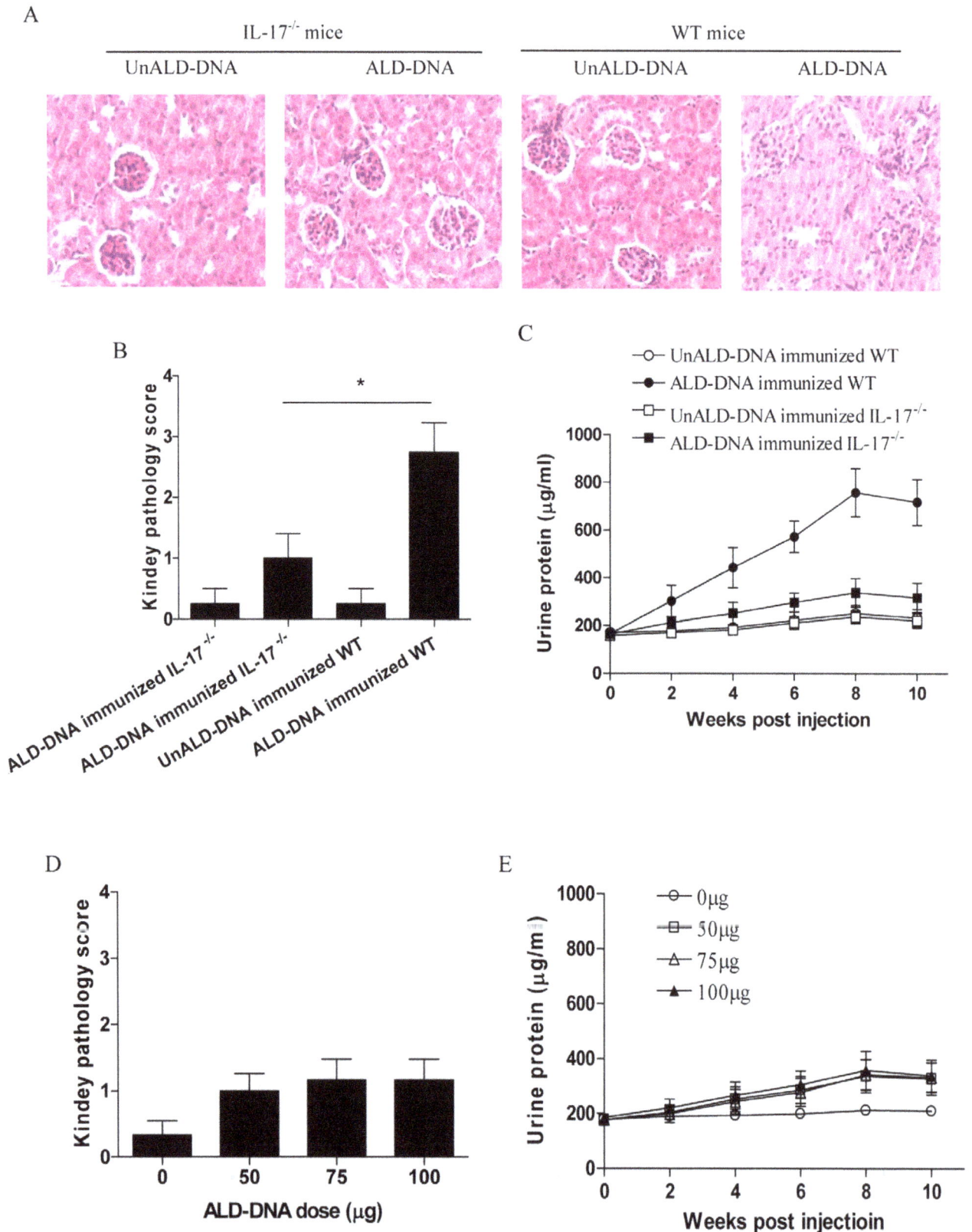

Figure 4. Impaired induction of lupus nephritis in IL-17$^{-/-}$ mice. (A-C) Groups of B6 WT mice or B6 IL-17$^{-/-}$ mice were immunized with 50 μg of the indicated DNA. The kidney histopathology and pathology score were analyzed eight weeks post ALD-DNA injection. The level of urine protein was determined at the indicated time. (D and E) Groups of B6 IL-17$^{-/-}$ mice were immunized with the indicated dose of ALD-DNA. The kidney pathology score was analyzed eight weeks post ALD-DNA injection. The level of urine protein was determined at the indicated time. Data represented the means (±SD) for eight mice in each group. *P<0.05.

lupus nephritis, kidney sections of ALD-DNA immunized mice were assayed for immune complex deposition and complement activation. As shown in Figure 5A and B, we showed that kidney sections from ALD-DNA immunized mice treated with Ad-mIL-17 exhibited elevated glomerular staining with anti-mouse IgG and anti-mouse complement C3 antibodies compared with the control group (p<0.05). Further, blockade of IL-17 significantly alleviated the glomerular staining with anti-mouse IgG and anti-mouse complement C3 antibodies in ALD-DNA immunized mice (Figure 5C and D, p<0.05). Consistently, we observed an impaired glomerular staining with anti-mouse IgG and anti-mouse complement C3 antibodies in IL-17$^{-/-}$ mice (Figure 5E and F, p<0.05). In addition, we found no significant staining with anti-mouse IgG and anti-mouse complement C3 antibodies in mice treated with Ad-mIL-17 alone without ALD-DNA injection (data not shown). These results suggested that management of IL-17 expression level could modify the immune complex deposition and complement activation in kidney, which might account for its positive correlation with the severity of lupus nephritis.

IL-17 was Crucial for Increasing Anti-dsDNA Antibody Production

It is well acknowledged that anti-dsDNA antibody, which is closely correlated with the clinical syndrome and hence of diagnostic and even prognostic value, is an important pathogenic autoantibody involved in immune complex deposition that resulted in development of lupus nephritis [27–29]. Thus, to elucidate why management of IL-17 expression level could modify the immune complex deposition and complement activation in kidney, we explored the potential role of IL-17 in anti-dsDNA antibody production. As shown in Figure 6A, we found that the serum IL-17 expression level was closely correlated with the serological level of anti-dsDNA antibody in ALD-DNA induced lupus mice (p<0.05). Of important, we revealed that treatment with exogenous IL-17 increased anti-dsDNA antibody production, while in vivo blockade of IL-17 decreased anti-dsDNA antibody production (Figure 6B and C, p<0.05). Furthermore, we observed that ALD-DNA could not induce anti-dsDNA antibody effectively in IL-17$^{-/-}$ mice (Figure 6D, p<0.05). When groups of IL-17$^{-/-}$ mice were immunized with an increased dose of ALD-DNA, we found that increased dose of ALD-DNA still failed to induce a high level of anti-dsDNA antibody in IL-17$^{-/-}$ mice (Figure 6E). These findings strongly demonstrated that IL-17 was crucial for increasing anti-dsDNA antibody production in lupus.

Discussion

IL-17 is believed to be important for host defense against various pathogens, while its inappropriate/excessive production is considered to be involved in the development of inflammatory autoimmune diseases [30,31]. In present study, we evaluated the association between IL-17 expression level and disease severity of lupus nephritis using ALD-DNA induced lupus model. We showed that IL-17 expression level was elevated and associated with the severity of lupus nephritis in ALD-DNA induced lupus mice. Of note, we found that treatment with exogenous IL-17 could enhance the severity of lupus nephritis, while blockade of IL-17 decreased the severity of lupus nephritis. In consistent, we found that IL-17$^{-/-}$ mice were resistant to development of lupus nephritis. Combing our findings demonstrated that IL-17 expression level was closely and positively correlated with the severity of lupus nephritis, implicating a potential and promising approach of IL-17-based therapy against lupus nephritis. However, the

mechanisms involved in the elevated expression of IL-17 in ALD-DNA induced lupus mice still needed successive studies.

Previous study showed that IL-17 could promote secretion of chemokines and other immune mediators from fibroblasts and epithelial cells, and thus may promote the recruitment of inflammatory cells to target organs including kidney [8]. In present study, we demonstrated the association of IL-17 expression level with immune complex deposition and complement activation in kidney. We showed that up-regulation of IL-17 enhanced the immune complex deposition and complement activation in kidney, while blockade of IL-17 alleviated the immune complex deposition and complement activation in kidney. We further confirmed this phenomenon and observed a weak intensity of immune complex deposition and complement activation in kidney of IL-17$^{-/-}$ mice. These findings could account for the close correlation of IL-17 expression level with the severity of lupus nephritis, and suggested that IL-17 was indeed a promising target for treatment of lupus nephritis. Consistently, recent study showed that down-regulation of IL-17 production by T cells was correlated with the amelioration of murine lupus after treatment with either low-dose peptide tolerance therapy or nasal anti-CD3 antibody [32,33]. However, it should be noted that a murine lupus model can not fully reproduce the complexity of clinical SLE in human patients. Further studies to reproduce our current findings in more clinically relevant models in primates and in clinical SLE patients were still needed. Of interest, two therapeutic human monoclonal antibodies against IL-17 (mAb AIN457 and LY2439821) have been developed and the clinical trials for uveitis, Crohn's disease, psoriasis and rheumatoid arthritis are underway [34–36]. Thus, our present findings indicated that this therapeutic approach might be useful for patients with lupus nephritis.

Recent evidence suggested that IL-17 was an effective and important player in antibody response [25,37–39]. IL-17 was responsible for the priming of collagen-specific T cells and IgG2a production, and thus the collagen-induced arthritis (CIA) was markedly suppressed in IL-17$^{-/-}$ mice [40]. The antigen-specific Ig production was also significantly decreased in IL-17$^{-/-}$ mice during allergic diseases such as methylated BSA-induced delayed-type hypersensitivity and ovalbumin (OVA)-induced airway inflammation [41]. In this study, we extended previous study by exploring the potential role of IL-17 in anti-dsDNA antibody production. We found that administration with exogenous IL-17 increased anti-dsDNA antibody production, while blockade of IL-17 decreased anti-dsDNA antibody production. Consistently, we observed an impaired generation of anti-dsDNA antibody in IL-17$^{-/-}$ mice. Thus, here we reported for the first time that IL-17 was vital for generation of anti-dsDNA antibody in SLE. In addition, we also found that other autoantibodies including anti-Sm and anti-rRNP antibody also decreased substantially in IL-17$^{-/-}$ mice compared with that in WT mice (data not shown), indicating a general effect of IL-17 on autoantibody production in SLE. Our results might partly explain the association of IL-17 expression level with the immune complex deposition and complement activation in kidney, and thus correlated with the severity of lupus nephritis. Besides, our data was also in line with previous study which showed that IL-17 could promote autoantibody production from peripheral blood mononuclear cells in patients with lupus nephritis [42]. In addition, recent study showed that IL-17 acted in synergy with B cell-activating factor to influence B cell survival, proliferation and differentiation into immunoglobulin-secreting cells [43], which might partly explain the crucial role of IL-17 in anti-dsDNA antibody production.

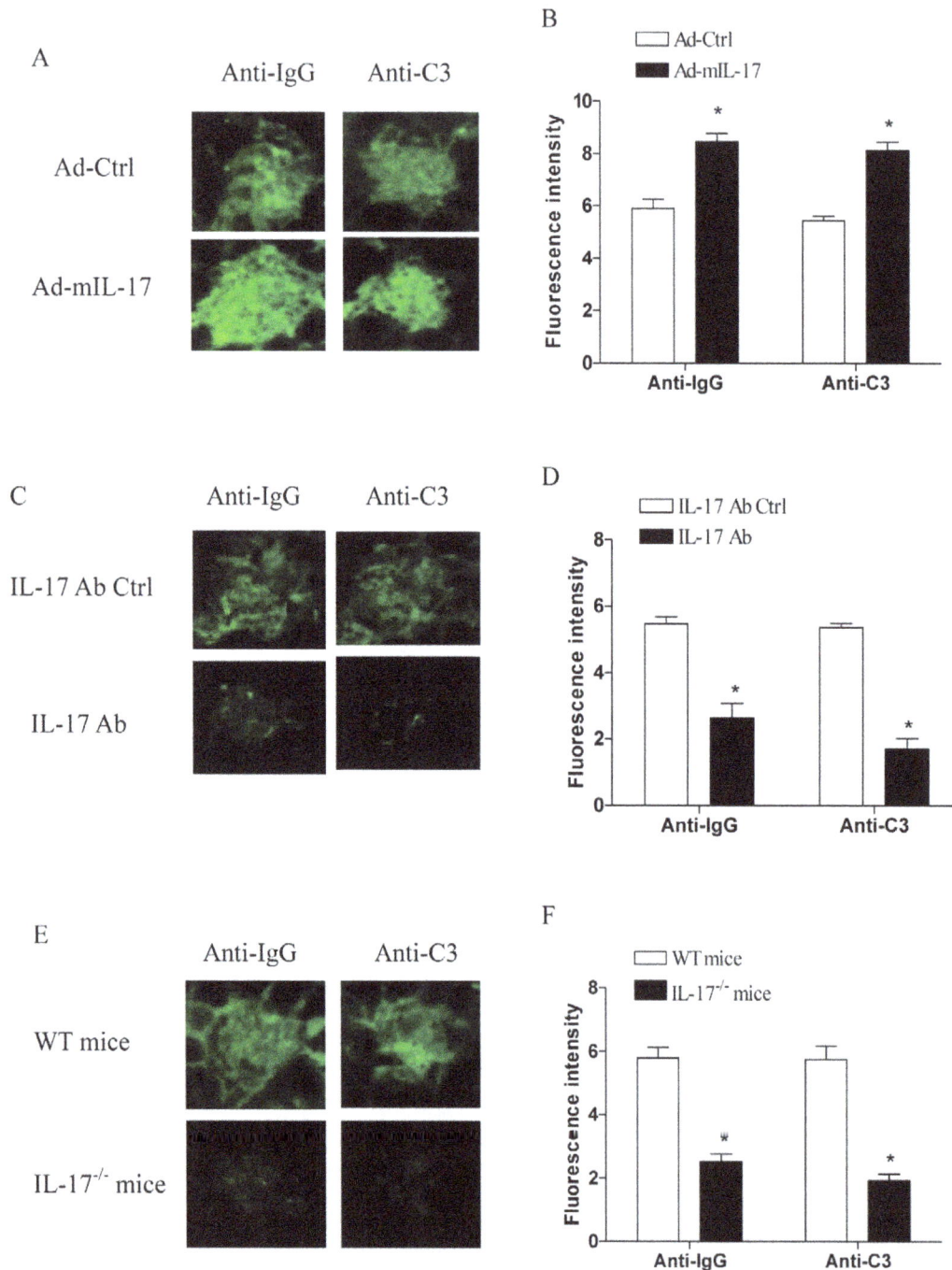

Figure 5. IL-17 was associated with immune complex deposition and complement activation in kidney. (A and B) Groups of BALB/c mice were treated with Ad-mIL-17 or Ad-Ctrl, and then immunized with 50 μg of ALD-DNA. Eight weeks later, the glomerular fluorescence was determined using anti-mouse IgG-FITC antibody or anti-mouse complement C3-FITC antibody. (C and D) Groups of BALB/c mice were injected with neutralizing antibody to IL-17 or the control antibody, and then immunized with 50 μg of ALD-DNA. Eight weeks later, the glomerular fluorescence was determined using anti-mouse IgG-FITC antibody or anti-mouse complement C3-FITC antibody. (E and F) Groups of IL-17$^{-/-}$ mice or WT mice were immunized with 50 μg of ALD-DNA. Eight weeks later, the glomerular fluorescence was determined using anti-mouse IgG-FITC antibody or anti-mouse complement C3-FITC antibody. The fluorescence image shown was the representative result. The data of fluorescence intensity represented means (±SD) for eight mice in each group. *$P < 0.05$.

However, the precise mechanisms for how IL-17 acted in generation of anti-dsDNA antibody still remain to be elucidated.

To conclude, here we demonstrated that IL-17 expression level was positively correlated with the severity of lupus nephritis. We did not focus on the proinflammatory effect of IL-17 in development of lupus nephritis. Instead, we reported the crucial role of IL-17 in anti-dsDNA antibody production, which might partly account for why IL-17 expression level was associated with the immune complex deposition in kidney and thus correlated with disease severity of lupus nephritis. Our findings provided a

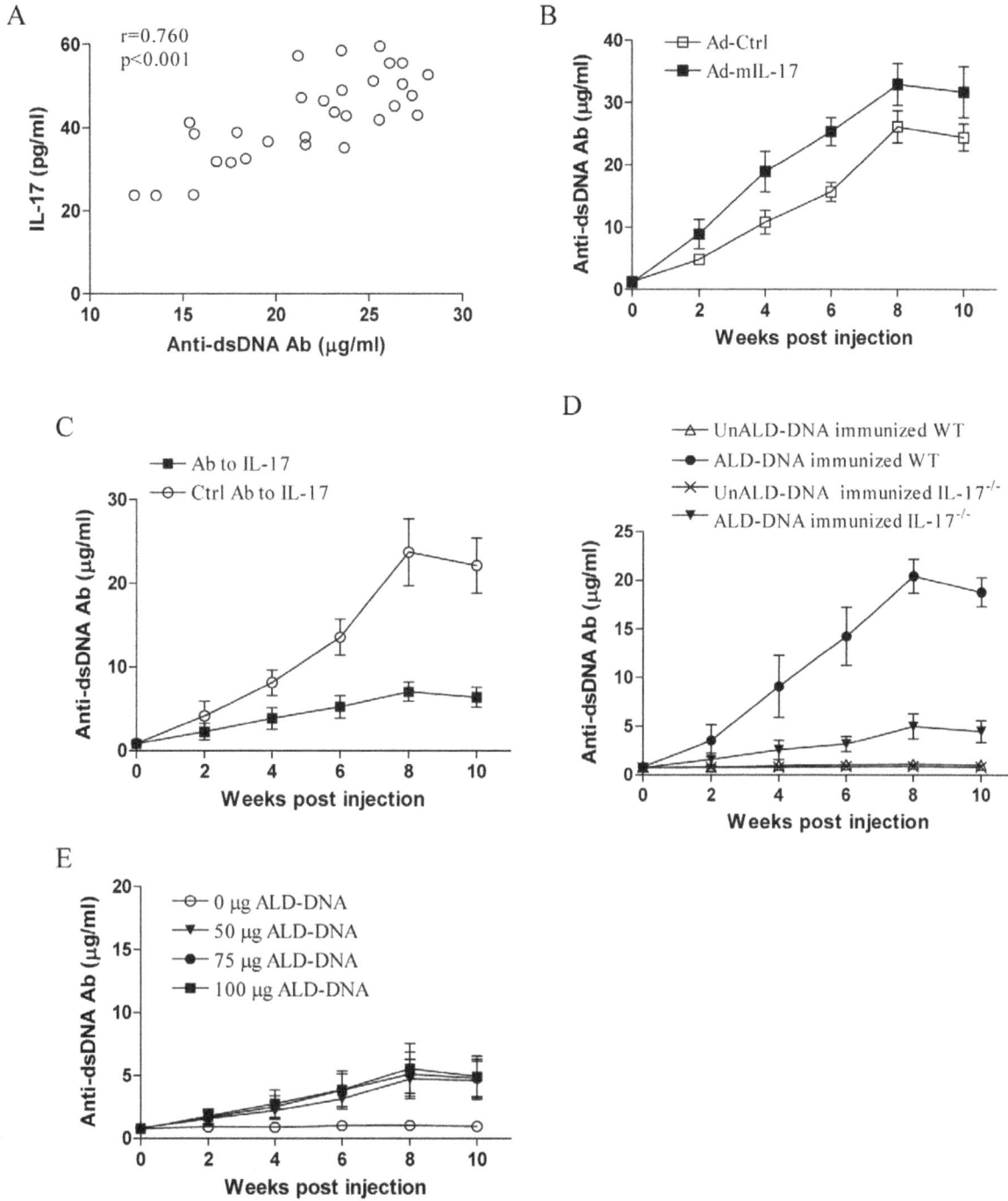

Figure 6. IL-17 increased anti-dsDNA antibody production. (A) Groups of BALB/c mice were immunized with 50 μg of ALD-DNA, and the correlation between serological level of IL-17 and anti-dsDNA antibody was analyzed in thirty two mice eight weeks post ALD-DNA injection. Each dot represented the average value for triplicate in each mouse. (B) Groups of BALB/c mice were treated with Ad-mIL-17 or Ad-Ctrl respectively, and then immunized with 50 μg of ALD-DNA. (C) Groups of BALB/c mice were injected with neutralizing antibody to IL-17 or the control antibody, and then immunized with 50 μg of ALD-DNA. (D) Groups of B6 WT mice or IL-17$^{-/-}$ mice were immunized with 50 μg of the indicated DNA. (E) Groups of IL-17$^{-/-}$ mice were immunized with the indicated dose of ALD-DNA. Data represented the means (±SD) for eight mice in each group. *P<0.05.

novel explanation through which IL-17 functioned in disease pathogenesis, and suggested that management of IL-17 expression level was a promising strategy for treatment of lupus nephritis.

Acknowledgments

We thank Ph.D Chun Wang for technical assistance and Ph.D Jun Gui for valuable discussions.

Author Contributions

Conceived and designed the experiments: SX. Performed the experiments: ZW LX. Analyzed the data: ZW SX. Contributed reagents/materials/analysis tools: WX ZY XG. Wrote the paper: ZW SX.

References

1. Alba P, Bento L, Cuadrado MJ, Karim Y, Tungekar MF, et al. (2003) Anti-dsDNA, anti-Sm antibodies, and the lupus anticoagulant: significant factors associated with lupus nephritis. Ann Rheum Dis 62: 556–560.
2. Apostolidis SA, Crispín JC, Tsokos GC (2011) IL-17-producing T cells in lupus nephritis. Lupus 20: 120–124.
3. Adalid-Peralta L, Mathian A, Tran T, Delbos L, Durand-Gasselin I, et al. (2008) Leukocytes and the kidney contribute to interstitial inflammation in lupus nephritis. Kidney Int 73: 172–180.
4. Cohen RA, Bayliss G, Crispin JC, Kane-Wanger GF, Van Beek CA, et al. (2008) T cells and in situ cryoglobulin deposition in the pathogenesis of lupus nephritis. Clin Immunol 128: 1–7.
5. Miyake K, Akahoshi M, Nakashima H (2011) Th subset balance in lupus nephritis. J Biomed Biotechnol 2011: 980286.
6. Xing Q, Wang B, Su H, Cui J, Li J (2012) Elevated Th17 cells are accompanied by FoxP3+ Treg cells decrease in patients with lupus nephritis. Rheumatol Int 32: 949–958.
7. Chen DY, Chen YM, Wen MC, Hsieh TY, Hung WT, et al. (2012) The potential role of Th17 cells and Th17-related cytokines in the pathogenesis of lupus nephritis. Lupus 21: 1385–1396.
8. Garrett-Sinha LA, John S, Gaffen SL (2008) IL-17 and the Th17 lineage in systemic lupus erythematosus. Curr Opin Rheumatol 20: 519–525.
9. Hemdan NY, Birkenmeier G, Wichmann G, Abu El-Saad AM, Krieger T, et al. (2010) Interleukin-17-producing T helper cells in autoimmunity. Autoimmun Rev 9: 785–792.
10. Chen XQ, Yu YC, Deng HH, Sun JZ, Dai Z, et al. (2010) Plasma IL-17A is increased in new-onset SLE patients and associated with disease activity. J Clin Immunol 30: 221–225.
11. Kang HK, Ecklund D, Liu M, Datta SK (2009) Apigenin, a non-mutagenic dietary flavonoid, suppresses lupus by inhibiting autoantigen presentation for expansion of autoreactive Th1 and Th17 cells. Arthritis Res Ther 11: R59.
12. Crispín JC, Oukka M, Bayliss G, Cohen RA, Van Beek CA, et al. (2008) Expanded double negative T cells in patients with systemic lupus erythematosus produce IL-17 and infiltrate the kidneys. J Immunol 181: 8761–8766.
13. Wang Y, Ito S, Chino Y, Goto D, Matsumoto I, et al. (2010) Laser microdissection-based analysis of cytokine balance in the kidneys of patients with lupus nephritis. Clin Exp Immunol 159: 1–10.
14. Qiao B, Wu J, Chu YW, Wang Y, Wang DP, et al. (2005) Induction of systemic lupus erythematosus-like syndrome in syngeneic mice by immunization with activated lymphocyte-derived DNA. Rheumatology (Oxford) 44: 1108–1114.
15. Wen ZK, Xu W, Xu L, Cao QH, Wang Y, et al. (2007) DNA hypomethylation is crucial for apoptotic DNA to induce systemic lupus erythematosus-like autoimmune disease in SLE-non-susceptible mice. Rheumatology (Oxford) 46: 1796–1803.
16. Zhang W, Xu W, Xiong S (2010) Blockade of Notch1 signaling alleviates murine lupus via blunting macrophage activation and M2b polarization. J Immunol 184: 6465–6478.
17. Zhang W, Wu J, Qiao B, Xu W, Xiong S (2011) Amelioration of lupus nephritis by serum amyloid p component gene therapy with distinct mechanisms varied from different stage of the disease. PLoS One 6: e22659.
18. Zhang W, Xu W, Xiong S (2011) Macrophage Differentiation and Polarization via Phosphatidylinositol 3-Kinase/Akt-ERK Signaling Pathway Conferred by Serum Amyloid P Component. J Immunol 187: 1764–1777.
19. Wen Z, Xu L, Xu W, Xiong S (2012) Production of anti-double-stranded DNA antibodies in activated lymphocyte derived DNA induced lupus model was dependent on CD4+ T cells. Lupus 21: 508–516.
20. Hutcheson J, Scatizzi JC, Siddiqui AM, Haines GK 3rd, Wu T, et al. (2008) Combined deficiency of proapoptotic regulators Bim and Fas results in the early onset of systemic autoimmunity. Immunity 28: 206–217.
21. Wang D, John SA, Clements JL, Percy DH, Barton KP, et al. (2005) Ets-1 deficiency leads to altered B cell differentiation, hyperresponsiveness to TLR9 and autoimmune disease. Int Immunol 17: 1179–1191.
22. Leng L, Chen L, Fan J, Greven D, Arjona A, et al. (2011) A small-molecule macrophage migration inhibitory factor antagonist protects against glomerulonephritis in lupus-prone NZB/NZW F1 and MRL/lpr mice. J Immunol 186: 527–538.

23. Nicoletti F, Di Marco R, Zaccone P, Xiang M, Magro G, et al. (2000) Dichotomic effects of IFN-gamma on the development of systemic lupus erythematosus-like syndrome in MRL-lpr/lpr mice. Eur J Immunol 30: 438–447.
24. Schwarzenberger P, La Russa V, Miller A, Ye P, Huang W, et al. (1998) IL-17 stimulates granulopoiesis in mice: use of an alternate, novel gene therapy-derived method for in vivo evaluation of cytokines. J Immunol 161: 6383–6389.
25. Hsu HC, Yang P, Wang J, Wu Q, Myers R, et al. (2008) Interleukin 17-producing T helper cells and interleukin 17 orchestrate autoreactive germinal center development in autoimmune BXD2 mice. Nat Immunol 9: 166–175.
26. Higgins SC, Jarnicki AG, Lavelle EC, Mills KH (2006) TLR4 mediates vaccine-induced protective cellular immunity to Bordetella pertussis: role of IL-17-producing T cells. J Immunol 177: 7980–7989.
27. Swaak AJ, Groenwold J, Aarden LA, Statius van Eps LW, Feltkamp EW (1982) Prognostic value of anti-dsDNA in SLE. Ann Rheum Dis 41: 388–395.
28. von Mühlen CA, Tan EM (1995) Autoantibodies in the diagnosis of systemic rheumatic diseases. Semin Arthritis Rheum 24: 323–358.
29. Rahman A, Isenberg DA (2008) Systemic lupus erythematosus. N Engl J Med 358: 929–939.
30. Gaffen SL (2011) Recent advances in the IL-17 cytokine family. Curr Opin Immunol 23: 613–619.
31. Korn T, Bettelli E, Oukka M, Kuchroo VK (2009) IL-17 and Th17 Cells. Annu Rev Immunol 27: 485–517.
32. Kang HK, Liu M, Datta SK (2007) Low-dose peptide tolerance therapy of lupus generates plasmacytoid dendritic cells that cause expansion of autoantigen-specific regulatory T cells and contraction of inflammatory CD4+IL-17-producing cells. J Immunol 178: 7849–7858.
33. Wu HY, Quintana FJ, Weiner HL (2008) Nasal anti-CD3 antibody ameliorates lupus by inducing an IL-10-secreting CD4+ CD25- LAP+ regulatory T cell and is associated with down-regulation of IL-17+ CD4+ ICOS+ CXCR5+ follicular helper T cells. J Immunol 181: 6038–6050.
34. Miossec P, Korn T, Kuchroo VK (2009) Interleukin-17 and type 17 helper T cells. N Engl J Med 361: 888–898.
35. Hueber W, Patel DD, Dryja T, Wright AM, Koroleva I, et al. (2010) Effects of AIN457, a fully human antibody to interleukin-17A, on psoriasis, rheumatoid arthritis, and uveitis. Sci Transl Med 2: 52ra72.
36. Genovese MC, Van den Bosch F, Roberson SA, Bojin S, Biagini IM, et al. (2010) LY2439821, a humanized anti-interleukin-17 monoclonal antibody, in the treatment of patients with rheumatoid arthritis: A phase I randomized, double-blind, placebo-controlled, proof-of-concept study. Arthritis Rheum 62: 929–939.
37. Mitsdoerffer M, Lee Y, Jäger A, Kim HJ, Korn T, et al. (2010) Proinflammatory T helper type 17 cells are effective B-cell helpers. Proc Natl Acad Sci U S A 107: 14292–14297.
38. Barbosa RR, Silva SP, Silva SL, Melo AC, Pedro E, et al. (2011) Primary B-cell deficiencies reveal a link between human IL-17-producing CD4 T-cell homeostasis and B-cell differentiation. PLoS One 6: e22848.
39. Mountz JD, Wang JH, Xie S, Hsu HC (2011) Cytokine regulation of B-cell migratory behavior favors formation of germinal centers in autoimmune disease. Discov Med 11: 76–85.
40. Nakae S, Nambu A, Sudo K, Iwakura Y (2003) Suppression of immune induction of collagen-induced arthritis in IL-17-deficient mice. J Immunol 171: 6173–6177.
41. Nakae S, Komiyama Y, Nambu A, Sudo K, Iwase M, et al. (2002) Antigen-specific T cell sensitization is impaired in IL-17-deficient mice, causing suppression of allergic cellular and humoral responses. Immunity 17: 375–387.
42. Dong G, Ye R, Shi W, Liu S, Wang T, et al. (2003) IL-17 induces autoantibody overproduction and peripheral blood mononuclear cell overexpression of IL-6 in lupus nephritis patients. Chin Med J (Engl) 116: 543–548.
43. Doreau A, Belot A, Bastid J, Riche B, Trescol-Biemont MC, et al. (2009) Interleukin 17 acts in synergy with B cell-activating factor to influence B cell biology and the pathophysiology of systemic lupus erythematosus. Nat Immunol 10: 778–785.

Gene–Gene and Gene-Sex Epistatic Interactions of *MiR146a, IRF5, IKZF1, ETS1* and *IL21* in Systemic Lupus Erythematosus

Rui-Xue Leng[1,2], Wei Wang[1,2], Han Cen[1,2], Mo Zhou[1,2], Chen-Chen Feng[1,2], Yan Zhu[1,2], Xiao-Ke Yang[1,2], Mei Yang[1,2], Yu Zhai[1,2], Bao-Zhu Li[1,2], Xiao-Song Wang[1,2], Rui Li[1,2], Gui-Mei Chen[1,2], Hong Chen[1,2], Hai-Feng Pan[1,2], Dong-Qing Ye[1,2]*

1 Department of Epidemiology and Biostatistics, School of Public Health, Anhui Medical University, Hefei, Anhui, People's Republic of China, 2 Anhui Provincial Laboratory of Population Health & Major Disease Screening and Diagnosis, Anhui Medical University, Hefei, Anhui, People's Republic of China

Abstract

Several confirmed genetic susceptibility loci involved in the interferon signaling and Th17/B cell response for SLE in Chinese Han populations have been described. Available data also indicate that sex-specific genetic differences contribute to SLE susceptibility. The aim of this study was to test for gene–gene/gene-sex epistasis (interactions) in these known lupus susceptibility loci. Six single-nucleotide polymorphisms (SNPs) in *MiR146a, IRF5, IKZF1, ETS1* and *IL21* were genotyped by Sequenom MassArray system. A total of 1,825 subjects (858 SLE patients and 967 controls) were included in the final analysis. Epistasis was tested by additive model, multiplicative model and multifactor dimensionality reduction (MDR) method. Additive interaction analysis revealed interactions between *IRF5* and *IKZF1* (OR 2.26, 95% CI 1.48–3.44 [P = 1.21 × 10^4]). A similar tendency was also observed between *IL21* and *ETS1* by parametric methods. In addition, multiple high dimensional gene-gene or gene-sex interactions (three-and four-way) were identified by MDR analysis. Our study identified novel gene–gene/gene-sex interactions in lupus. Furthermore, these findings highlight sex, interferon pathway, and Th17/B cells as important contributors to the pathogenesis of SLE.

Editor: Massimo Pietropaolo, University of Michigan Medical School, United States of America

Funding: This work was supported by grants from the National Natural Science Foundation of China (81102192, 30830089) and the Anhui Provincial Natural Science Foundation (11040606M183). The funders had no role in study design, data collection and analysis, decision to publish, or preparation of the manuscript.

Competing Interests: The authors have declared that no competing interests exist.

* E-mail: ydq@ahmu.edu.cn

Introduction

Systemic lupus erythematosus (SLE) is a prototypic, systemic, autoimmune disease, characterized by a diverse array of autoantibody production, complement activation and immune-complex deposition, which causes tissue and organ damage. The aetiology of SLE is incompletely understood, but genetic factors play an important role in the susceptibility to the disease.

Recent candidate gene and genome-wide association studies (GWAS) led to the discovery and validation of multiple susceptibility loci for SLE. The loci previously confirmed for SLE in Chinese include genes involved in the interferon signaling (eg. *IRF5, IRF7, Mir146a, IKZF1*) and Th17/B cell regulation (eg. *ETS1*) [1–3]. The reported effect of IL21 on B-cell differentiation into plasma cells and its effect on Th17-cell responses make *IL21* an attractive candidate gene for SLE [4]. Previous studies established and confirmed the genetic association between *IL21* and lupus in European descent [4–5]. In a recent case-control study (605 patients, 666 controls), Ding *et al* showed that polymorphisms of *IL21* gene have a marginal association with SLE susceptibility in the Chinese populations [6]. Most above pathway genes are known to play a key role in the pathogenesis of the disease. Since the heritability of SLE cannot be completely explained by the susceptibility loci already discovered. Herein, we

sought to examine gene–gene interactions (epistasis) in some of the previously established susceptibility loci for SLE in Chinese populations.

Current data also indicate that sex-specific genetic differences contribute to SLE susceptibility. For example, the frequency of the risk alleles in the *HLA, IRF5* and osteopontin (*SPP1*) locus was significantly higher in men than in women with SLE [7,8]. Interestingly, polymorphism in the *KIAA1542* locus was shown to be associated with lupus in women but not in men [7]. Therefore, we also investigated gene–sex interactions in above genes.

Results

Replication of Genetic Association with SLE in Chinese

After the quality control measures were applied, a total of 1,825 subjects (858 SLE patients and 967 controls) were included in the analysis. Table S1 shows demographic characteristics for study participants. The result of allelic association for single SNP is showed in Table 1. All SNPs in controls were under the Hardy-Weinberg equilibrium (HWE) (Table 1). In current study, 3 genes (*ETS1, IKZF1* and *IRF5*) previously reported in GWAS of Chinese Han populations were replicated. The SNP rs907715 in *IL21* showed association (P = 0.01) with SLE in Chinese. Association analysis using the genotype data (adjust for sex and age) generated

Table 1. Genotype characteristics of each single nucleotide polymorphism.

Gene	SNP	Function	Allele[a]	Case (MAF)	Control (MAF)	OR (95% CI)	P-value	HWE[b]
IL21	rs907715	Intron	A/G	0.420	0.463	0.84 (0.74–0.96)	0.01	0.37
IL21	rs2221903	Intron	G/A	0.115	0.098	1.19 (0.96–1.47)	0.11	0.18
IRF5	rs4728142	Flanking 5′ UTR	A/G	0.164	0.119	1.45 (1.20–1.75)	9.79×10^{-5}	0.92
IKZF1	rs4917014	Flanking 5′ UTR	G/T	0.267	0.331	0.74 (0.64–0.85)	2.56×10^{-5}	0.39
ETS1	rs6590330	Flanking 3′ UTR	A/G	0.407	0.345	1.30 (1.14–1.49)	1.15×10^{-4}	0.26
MiR146a	rs57095329	Promoter	G/A	0.214	0.200	1.09 (0.93–1.28)	0.29	0.62

MAF, minor allele frequency; 95% CI, 95% confidence intervals; HWE, Hardy-Weinberg Equilibrium.
[a]nor allele/major allele;
[b]P-value for HWE.

a more significant result (P = 0.004). In the current study, the power to detect a 1.3-fold increased risk, assuming an alpha value of 0.05, was 0.997 for rs907715. However, significant association with SLE was not observed in the selected SNP for *MiR146a*.

Additive Gene-gene Interactions Analysis by Direct Counting and Chi-square Test using a 2×2 Factorial Design

Because the numbers for some genotypes were small, and in most cases dominant models showed the better fit for association, we considered the dominant model in a further interaction analysis stage. In the current study, differences in risk genotype counts between patients and controls were high, which was particularly significant when risk genotypes were combined (Table S2). A significant additive interaction was observed between *IRF5* GA+AA and *IKZF1* GT+TT (OR 2.26, 95% CI 1.48–3.44 [P = 1.21×10^{4}]); the risk genotype combination contributed the most to the overall interaction, with the remaining combinations within being nonsignificant. The attributable proportion due to interaction (AP) was 0.41, and the relative excess risk due to interaction (RERI) was 0.93. A similar tendency was also observed between *IL21* rs907715 AG+GG and *IRF5* GA+AA (OR 2.03, 95% CI 1.49–2.78 [8.13×10^{6}] AP 0.14, RERI 0.29); *IL21* rs907715 AG+GG and *ETS1* GA+AA (OR 1.79, 95% CI 1.22–2.63 [P = 2.58×10^{3}] AP 0.34, RERI 0.60); *IKZF1* GT+TT and *ETS1* GA+AA (OR 2.10, 95% CI 1.23–3.57 [P = 5.25×10^{3}] AP 0.29, RERI 0.61).

Multiplicative Interaction Effect Analysis by Logistic Regression

We tested whether the log likelihood of the logistic model was significantly improved by adding an additional pairwise interaction term for the combined 2 SNPs. The result of genetic interactions for pairwise SNP is showed in Table 2. A marginal effect of gene-gene interaction was detected between *ETS1* and *IL21* rs2221903 in codominant model (β = 0.26, P = 0.02). Dominant model also showed a consistent tendency toward a gene–gene interaction between *ETS1* and *IL21* rs907715 (β = 0.58, P = 0.03). We have not observed any genetic interactions for other SNP combinations by the codominant, dominant and recessive models (P>0.05).

The result of pairwise gene-sex epistasis by logistic regression models is showed in Table S3. A marginal effect was detected between sex and *IL21* rs907715 in dominant model (β = 0.70, P = 0.03). We have not observed any multiplicative interactions for other gene-sex combinations by the codominant, dominant and

Table 2. Interaction analysis of gene-gene involved in systemic lupus erythematosus, by logistic regression*.

Gene	*IL21* (rs907715)	*IL21* (rs2221903)	*IRF5*	*IKZF1*	*ETS1*
IL21 (rs907715)					
IL21 (rs2221903)	0.84/0.24				
IRF5	0.62/0.73	0.49/0.74			
IKZF1	0.27/0.09	0.09/0.72	0.34/0.38		
ETS1	0.25/**0.03**	**0.02**/0.17	0.49/0.83	0.92/0.50	
Mir146a	0.45/0.37	0.51/0.65	0.86/0.72	0.37/0.27	0.15/0.30

*The data are presented as P values (codominant/dominant) for departure from a multiplicative interaction model, obtained by log-likelihood ratio tests between the models, with and without an interaction term. An interaction term was considered significant if P<0.05. The regression models were adjusted for the potential confounders, including age and sex.

recessive models (P>0.05). In order to corroborate the gene-sex interaction, we then compared risk allele frequencies between men and women with SLE (mean age was 35.75 years for male patients and 35.84 for female). There were no significant deviations in male-female frequencies (Table S4).

Gene-gene and Gene-sex Interaction by MDR

Next, we used MDR analysis to identify potential high dimensional gene-gene interactions. The two- to four-way gene-gene interaction models are listed in Table 3. The SNP in the *ETS1* gene had the highest testing-balanced accuracy among the 6 SNPs. The model of *IL21* rs907715 and *ETS1* showed the highest testing-balanced accuracy in two-way level (Figure S1a). The pairwise interaction was then validated based on 1000 permutations (p<0.03). A three-way interaction found between *IL21* rs907715, *IKZF1* and *ETS1* showed the highest testing-balanced accuracy and cross validation consistency in original data. Since our dataset is unbalanced, with 858 cases and 967 controls. An over- and under-sampling approach was applied to evaluate the high dimensional interaction. Based on the highest testing-balanced accuracy and cross validation consistency, a four-locus model (*IL21* rs907715, *IRF5*, *IKZF1*, *ETS1*) was chosen as the final model (Table S5).

Table 3. Summary of MDR gene-gene interaction results.

Model	Training Bal. Acc. (%)	Testing Bal. Acc. (%)	Cross-validation Consistency
ETS1	55.07	54.24	9/10
IL21(rs907715), ETS1	56.47	53.69	7/10
IL21(rs907715), IKZF1,ETS1	58.43	55.84	9/10
IL21(rs907715), IRF5, IKZF1,ETS1	60.19	55.72	9/10

Regarding high dimensional gene-sex interaction, a three-way interaction found between *IRF5*, *ETS1* and sex showed the highest testing-balanced accuracy and cross validation consistency in original data (Table 4, also see Figure S1b). The finding was further validated by over- and under-sampling approach (Table S6). In order to elucidate potential three-way gene-sex interactions in SLE, the top five three-way interaction models were listed (Table S7). The rank was determined by the training-balanced accuracy of MDR.

Discussion

Polymorphisms in *IRF5*, *IKZF1* and *ETS1* genes have been identified by recent GWAS in Chinese Han populations [1]. A functional variant (rs57095329) in *MiR146a* promoter also was found in 7,182 Asians by candidate gene approach [3]. The lupus-susceptibility gene *IL21* rs907715, identified in European descent [4–5], was replicated in current study. All these finding highlight that interferon signaling and Th17/B cell responses play an important role in the pathogenesis of SLE. Since previous studies have shown that polymorphisms in IFN pathway genes were especially associated with male SLE [7–10]. We then compared risk allele frequencies between men and women with SLE. The results showed that there was no significant difference in the patient group between men and women. It is noteworthy that the frequency of risk allele in the *IRF5* locus was significantly higher in men than in women with SLE in European descent [7]. In contrast, our data have not found a sex-specific genetic effect in *IRF5* rs4728142 (OR male-female = 1.06, P = 0.80), which previously were shown to be most significantly associated with SLE in Chinese [1].

It is well know that the best methodology for detecting interaction remains controversial. Combining several analytical methods may be optimal for detecting epistasis [11,12]. To test for gene–gene/sex interactions, we performed a 2-step analysis using a parametric approach, followed by a nonparametric analysis. Since available data indicate that gene-gene interactions may occur between different pathophysiological pathways [12,13], we examined gene-gene interactions for each SNP pair of the 5 genes.

The data showed that there were multiple tendencies toward interactions in above genes.

Ikaros family zinc finger 1, encoded by *IKZF1*, is lymphoid-restricted zinc finger transcription factors. Recently data has suggested that IKZF1 has an important role in the induction of Type I interferon [14]. In current study, we showed evidence for gene–gene interaction between the 2 independent lupus-associated SNPs within the *IRF5* and *IKZF1* (AP = 0.41, RERI = 0.93). This interaction emphasizes the role of the interferon pathway in the pathogenesis of lupus. Moreover, Fang *et al* recently identified the IRF-5-Ikaros axis as a critical modulator of the B-cell immuno-globulin (Ig) G2a/c class switching. They reported that IRF5 can control expression of IKZF1. Mechanism analysis further showed that IRF8 activates the IKZF1 promoter, and IRF-5 inhibits the transcriptional activity of IRF-8 [15].

The gene-gene interaction between the *IL21* and *ETS1* was identified in both additive and multiplicative model. This finding is very interesting, because it highlights a critical role for Th17 and B cells in lupus. IL21 play an essential role for the promotion of B-cell and Th17 activation and differentiation [4]. Available data has shown that patients with SLE have increased plasma IL21 levels and proportion of IL21[+] T-cells [16,17]. In contrast, ETS1 is a negative regulator for both pathogenic B cell and Th17 cell responses [18]. ETS1 is critical in maintaining B cell identity and its deficiency can drive terminal differentiation of B cells into Ig-secreting plasma cells [19,20]. Furthermore, ETS1-deficient Th cells differentiated more efficiently to Th17 cells than wild-type cells [21]. It is of note that the marginal effect (multiplicative interaction between *IL21* and *ETS1*) needs further replication on independent cohorts of SLE patients in order to be confident in the robustness of the results.

Except for the above interactions (*IRF5* and *IKZF1*, *IL21* and *ETS1*), we also identified additive interaction tendency between *IL21* rs907715 and *IRF5*; *IKZF1* and *ETS1*. Intriguingly, each of the four loci (*IL21*, *IRF5*, *IKZF1* and *ETS1*) can be mapped into B cell signaling pathways [4,14,15,18–20]. In addition, previous study reported that ETS1 levels can strongly affect *MiR146a* promoter activity in vitro. The authors also observed additive effects of the risk alleles of *MiR146a* rs57095329 and *ETS1* rs1128334 [3]. Therefore, we further investigated whether there is

Table 4. Summary of MDR gene-sex interaction results.

Model	Training Bal. Acc. (%)	Testing Bal. Acc. (%)	Cross-validation Consistency
Sex	60.54	60.54	10/10
Sex, IKZF1	61.25	58.32	5/10
Sex,IRF5, ETS1	62.62	61.89	9/10
Sex, IKZF1, ETS1, IL21(rs907715)	63.51	59.07	5/10

an interaction between the risk variants of the two genes, rs6590330 in *ETS1* and rs57095329 in *MiR146a*. No significant epistatic effect was detected between the two variants in any additive and multiplicative models.

To strengthen the reliability of the interactions observed in current study, we conducted functional analysis by method of bioinformatics. We assessed relational biological network (pathway analysis, see Figure S2) constructed using Pathway Studio Explore Affymetrix Edition Version 1.1. However, the protein-protein interact and transcription factors targets prediction analysis did not find any directly associations (data not shown). For further explain for biological significance of interactions, we provided information of location for these SNPs (Table 1). Moreover, we also searched expression quantitative trait locus (eQTL) information from public database. The date showed that rs4728142 is an eQTL for *IRF5* in Asians (CHB, Han Chinese in Beijing/JPT, Japanese in Tokyo). In addition, the genotype of rs57095329 is directly related to expression of *MiR146a* expression [3]. However, the eQTL information of SNPs in *IL21*, *ETS1* and *IKZF1* is not available from public database. It is noteworthy that rs1128334 (located at the 3'-UTR region of *ETS1*) have an effect on the expression level of *ETS1*. Intriguingly, the SNP have high linkage disequilibrium (LD) with *ETS1* rs6590330 ($r^2 = 0.97$) [22]. Nevertheless, further studies are required to comprehensively explore whether these SNPs is functional.

For two-way gene-sex interaction, we only detected a significant epistatic effect between sex and *IL21* rs907715 by logistic regression. However, we did not observe deviations in male-female frequencies that could corroborate their gene-sex interactions. An interaction between sex and *IRF5* locus, which was previously identified in patients with SLE of European descent [4], was not replicated in current study. It is of note that several limitations should be considered when interpreting the results of gene-sex interactions: First of all, the sample size of male patients with SLE is relatively small and is therefore of limited power, which may weaken the conclusion of this study. Secondly, it is unclear whether male SLE has the same disease severity or clinical features as female SLE. This question may be important because a more severe phenotype in lupus patients is often associated with higher total genetic risk [7].

MDR is a model-free method that can identify high dimensional gene-gene or gene-environment interactions [23,24]. We applied the non-parametrical approach and found many three-and four-way gene-gene and gene-sex epistasis on SLE. These findings may account for some of the "missing heritability" in GWAS or candidate gene–based case–control studies for complex diseases. Furthermore, the data emphasize sex-specific genetic effects contribute to SLE susceptibility. It should be noted that the end goal of the MDR analysis is hypothesis generation. Therefore, the approach may be preferred to reduce the risk of false negatives [25].The nonparametric analysis of this study reflects a joint effect consisting of the main genetic effect and the interaction effect.

In current study, we observed that the combined effect of 2 risk factors would differ from the sum of the effects of the individual factors. Moreover, we provided possible evidence that in patients with lupus, the presence of one risk allele can influence the presence or absence of other risk alleles, across different loci (marginal association for multiplicative interaction). In addition, gender may also have an important influence for genetic risk of SLE. Taken together, our study identified novel gene–gene/gene-sex epistatic effect in lupus. Furthermore, these findings highlight sex, the interferon pathway, and Th17/B cells as important contributors to the pathogenesis of SLE.

Materials and Methods

Ethics Statement
The study was approved by the medical ethics committee of Anhui Medical University and complied with the principles outlined in the Helsinki Declaration. All participants gave written informed consent.

Patients and Controls
Patients with SLE were recruited from the First Affiliated Hospital of Anhui Medical University and Anhui Provincial Hospital. The diagnosis of SLE was based on the presence of the combination of at least four criteria of 1997 American College of Rheumatology (ACR) revised criteria for the classification of SLE [26,27]. The healthy control subjects were matched to the patients geographically and ethnically.

SNPs Selection and Genotyping
SNP rs4728142 for *IRF5*, rs4917014 for *IKZF1* and rs6590330 for *ETS1*, which previously were shown to be most significantly associated with SLE in GWAS of Chinese Han populations [1], were selected for current case–control study. A novel Asian gene variant (rs57095329) in the promoter region of *MiR146a* was also selected [3]. Since previous study showed that polymorphisms of *IL21* gene have a marginal association with SLE susceptibility in the Chinese populations, we selected SNPs rs907715 and rs2221903 for *IL-21* genotyping [6]. *IRF7* rs1131665 is also a risk factor for the development of SLE in multiple populations including Chinese. However, the SNP was excluded in view of low allele frequency (MAF<5%) [2]. A total of 6 SNPs were included for further analysis (Table 1).

The genotyping was conducted using the Sequenom Massarray system (Sequenom, Inc., San Diego, CA, USA) according to the manufacturer's instructions to determine the genotypes. Only those individuals with 100% genotype success for all markers were included for final analysis.

Statistical Analysis
The genotype frequencies of the SNPs were tested for Hardy-Weinberg equilibrium in control subjects. Disease associations were analyzed by chi-square tests or by logistic regression analysis. Statistical power was estimated using Power and Sample Size Estimation Software (http://biostat.mc.vanderbilt.edu/wiki/Main/PowerSampleSize).

To test for additive gene-gene interactions, direct counting and chi-square tests were performed using a 2×2 factorial design to calculate the AP and RERI. Fisher's exact test was used when necessary. If there is no biologic interaction, RERI and AP are equal to 0 [11].

The multiplicative interactions of two-way gene-gene and gene-sex were estimated using multiple logistic regression models. For each individual, key variables were defined as a binary variable indicating case–control status, with SNP variables ranging from 0 to 2 indicating the number of risk alleles in an individual subject (Codominant model). Additionally, dominant and recessive models for gene were also tested [28]. For each SNP pair, a logistic regression model was built to predict case–control status (dependent variable) based on the indicator variables (sex and age) and the 2 SNP variables (independent variable), for a total of 4 variables and an intercept [11]. For two-way gene-sex interaction analysis, age was used as indicator variable. We tested whether the log likelihood of the model was significantly improved by adding an additional pairwise interaction term [11]. SPSS11.0 software was applied for the logistic regression analysis. Two-tailed P values less than 0.05 were considered significant.

Multifactor dimensionality reduction software (MDR; http://sourceforge.net/projects/mdr/) is a model-free and non-parametrical approach method [23]. Since previous studies have shown MDR to be a useful method for identifying high dimensional gene-gene or gene-environment interactions [24]. We then applied MDR analysis to detect three-and four-way gene-gene/sex epistasis on SLE. For those interaction models that showed higher testing-balanced accuracy, we further used permutation tests to validate the MDR interaction results [25]. Since our dataset is unbalanced, with 858 cases and 967 controls. An over- and under-sampling approach was applied to evaluate non-parametrical interaction effect [25]. A brief description of the MDR approach and of the meaning of its output has been shown in others papers [13,23,25].

Supporting Information

Figure S1 The optimal models as determined by MDR for *IL21* rs907715 and *ETS1* (a), Sex/*IRF5*/*ETS1* (b). (For SNP: 0 = no risk alleles, 1 = 1 risk allele, 2 = 2 risk alleles; For Sex: 1 = male, 2 = female). The numbers within each small square represent number of cases (left) and controls (right). For each square, dark-shading indicates high risk of disease, whereas light shading represents low risk of disease.

Figure S2 Relational gene network constructed using Pathway Studio Explore Affymetrix Edition Version 1.1 (a); Pathway Studio Explore Affymetrix Edition Version 1.1 was used to find linkages between 4 genes and diseases/cell biological processes (b).

Table S1 Characteristics of the patients and healthy controls studied.

Table S2 Additive interaction analysis of genes involved in SLE in genotype combinations by chi-square test using 2×2 factorial design.

Table S3 Interaction analysis of gene-sex involved in systemic lupus erythematosus, by logistic regression.

Table S4 Sex–gene disparities between men and women with systemic lupus erythematosus.

Table S5 Analysis of over- and under-sample data for gene-gene interaction.

Table S6 Analysis of over- and under-sampled data for gene-sex interaction.

Table S7 Three-way gene-sex interactions of MDR analysis.

Acknowledgments

We wish to thank Xiang-Pei Li, Jin-Hui Tao (Anhui Provincial Hospital) and Jian-Hua Xu (the First Affiliated Hospital of Anhui Medical University) for assistance in sample preparation and data collection.

Author Contributions

Conceived and designed the experiments: RXL WW. Performed the experiments: RXL WW HC MZ CCF. Analyzed the data: RXL WW. Contributed reagents/materials/analysis tools: RXL WW HC MZ CCF YZ XKY MY YZ BZL XSW RL GMC HC. Wrote the paper: RXL. Critical revising of manuscript: DQY HFP WW HC.

References

1. Han JW, Zheng HF, Cui Y, Sun LD, Ye DQ, et al. (2009) Genome-wide association study in a Chinese Han population identifies nine new susceptibility loci for systemic lupus erythematosus. Nat Genet 41: 1234–1237.
2. Fu Q, Zhao J, Qian X, Wong JL, Kaufman KM, et al. (2011) Association of a functional IRF7 variant with systemic lupus erythematosus. Arthritis Rheum 63: 749–754.
3. Luo X, Yang W, Ye DQ, Cui H, Zhang Y, et al. (2011) A functional variant in microRNA-146a promoter modulates its expression and confers disease risk for systemic lupus erythematosus. PLoS Genet 7: e1002128.
4. Sawalha AH, Kaufman KM, Kelly JA, Adler AJ, Aberle T, et al. (2008) Genetic association of interleukin-21 polymorphisms with systemic lupus erythematosus. Ann Rheum Dis 67: 458–461.
5. Hughes T, Kim-Howard X, Kelly JA, Kaufman KM, Langefeld CD, et al. (2011) Fine-mapping and transethnic genotyping establish IL2/IL21 genetic association with lupus and localize this genetic effect to IL21. Arthritis Rheum 63: 1689–1697.
6. Ding L, Wang S, Chen GM, Leng RX, Pan HF, et al. (2012) A Single Nucleotide Polymorphism of IL-21 Gene is associated with systemic lupus erythematosus in a Chinese population. Inflammation Doi: 10.1007/s10753-012-9497-7.
7. Hughes T, Adler A, Merrill JT, Kelly JA, Kaufman KM, et al. (2012) Analysis of autosomal genes reveals gene-sex interactions and higher total genetic risk in men with systemic lupus erythematosus. Ann Rheum Dis 71: 694–699.
8. Han S, Guthridge JM, Harley IT, Sestak AL, Kim-Howard X, et al. (2008) Osteopontin and systemic lupus erythematosus association: a probable gene-gender interaction. PLoS One 3: e0001757.
9. Shen N, Fu Q, Deng Y, Qian X, Zhao J, et al. (2010) Sex-specific association of X-linked Toll-like receptor 7 (TLR7) with male systemic lupus erythematosus. Proc Natl Acad Sci U S A 107: 15838–15843.
10. Kariuki SN, Crow MK, Niewold TB (2008) The PTPN22 C1858T polymorphism is associated with skewing of cytokine profiles toward high interferon-alpha activity and low tumor necrosis factor alpha levels in patients with lupus. Arthritis Rheum 58: 2818–2823.
11. Zhou XJ, Lu XL, Nath SK, Lv JC, Zhu SN, et al. (2012) Gene-gene interaction of BLK, TNFSF4, TRAF1, TNFAIP3, and REL in systemic lupus erythematosus. Arthritis Rheum 64: 222–231.
12. Hughes T, Adler A, Kelly JA, Kaufman KM, Williams AH, et al. (2012) Evidence for gene-gene epistatic interactions among susceptibility loci for systemic lupus erythematosus. Arthritis Rheum 64: 485–492.
13. Su MW, Tung KY, Liang PH, Tsai CH, Kuo NW, et al. (2012) Gene-gene and gene-environmental interactions of childhood asthma: a multifactor dimension reduction approach. PLoS One 7: e30694.
14. Hu SJ, Wen LL, Hu X, Yin XY, Cui Y, et al. (2012) IKZF1: a critical role in the pathogenesis of systemic lupus erythematosus? Mod Rheumatol Doi: 10.1007/s10165-012-0706-x.
15. Fang CM, Roy S, Nielsen E, Paul M, Maul R, et al. (2012) Unique contribution of IRF-5-Ikaros axis to the B-cell IgG2a response. Genes Immun 13: 421–430.
16. Dolff S, Abdulahad WH, Westra J, Doornbos-van der Meer B, Limburg PC, et al. (2011) Increase in IL-21 producing T-cells in patients with systemic lupus erythematosus. Arthritis Res Ther 13: R157.
17. Ettinger R, Kuchen S, Lipsky PE (2008) Interleukin 21 as a target of intervention in autoimmune disease. Ann Rheum Dis 67 Suppl 3: iii83–6.
18. Leng RX, Pan HF, Chen GM, Feng CC, Fan YG, et al. (2011) The dual nature of Ets-1: focus on the pathogenesis of systemic lupus erythematosus. Autoimmun Rev 10: 439–443.
19. Eyquem S, Chemin K, Fasseu M, Chopin M, Sigaux F, et al. (2004) The development of early and mature B cells is impaired in mice deficient for the Ets-1 transcription factor. Eur J Immunol 34: 3187–3196.
20. Wang D, John SA, Clements JL, Percy DH, Barton KP, et al. (2005) Ets-1 deficiency leads to altered B cell differentiation, hyperresponsiveness to TLR9 and autoimmune disease. Int Immunol 17: 1179–1191.
21. Moisan J, Grenningloh R, Bettelli E, Oukka M, Ho IC (2007) Ets-1 is a negative regulator of Th17 differentiation. J Exp Med 204: 2825–2835.
22. Yang W, Shen N, Ye DQ, Liu Q, Zhang Y, et al. (2010) Genome-wide association study in Asian populations identifies variants in ETS1 and WDFY4 associated with systemic lupus erythematosus. PLoS Genet 6: e1000841.

23. Hahn LW, Ritchie MD, Moore JH (2003) Multifactor dimensionality reduction software for detecting gene-gene and gene-environment interactions. Bioinformatics 19: 376–382.
24. Ritchie MD, Hahn LW, Moore JH (2003) Power of multifactor dimensionality reduction for detecting gene-gene interactions in the presence of genotyping error, missing data, phenocopy, and genetic heterogeneity. Genet Epidemiol 24: 150–157.
25. Motsinger AA, Ritchie MD (2006) Multifactor dimensionality reduction: an analysis strategy for modelling and detecting gene-gene interactions in human genetics and pharmacogenomics studies. Hum Genomics 2: 318–328.
26. Tan EM, Cohen AS, Fries JF, Masi AT, McShane DJ, et al. (1982) The 1982 revised criteria for the classification of systemic lupus erythematosus. Arthritis Rheum 25: 1271–1277.
27. Hochberg MC (1997) Updating the American College of Rheumatology revised criteria for the classification of systemic lupus erythematosus. Arthritis Rheum 40: 1725.
28. Kawasaki A, Ito S, Furukawa H, Hayashi T, Goto D, et al. (2010) Association of TNFAIP3 interacting protein 1, TNIP1 with systemic lupus erythematosus in a Japanese population: a case-control association study. Arthritis Res Ther 12: R174.

Platelet Activation and Anti-Phospholipid Antibodies Collaborate in the Activation of the Complement System on Platelets in Systemic Lupus Erythematosus

Christian Lood[1]*, **Helena Tydén**[1], **Birgitta Gullstrand**[2], **Gunnar Sturfelt**[1], **Andreas Jönsen**[1], **Lennart Truedsson**[2], **Anders A. Bengtsson**[1]

1 Department of Clinical Sciences Lund, Section of Rheumatology, Lund University and Skåne University Hospital, Lund, Sweden, **2** Department of Laboratory Medicine Lund, Section of Microbiology, Immunology and Glycobiology, Lund University, Lund, Sweden

Abstract

Anti-phospholipid (aPL) antibodies are important contributors to development of thrombosis in patients with the autoimmune rheumatic disease systemic lupus erythematosus (SLE). The underlying mechanism of aPL antibody-mediated thrombosis is not fully understood but existing data suggest that platelets and the complement system are key components. Complement activation on platelets is seen in SLE patients, especially in patients with aPL antibodies, and has been related to venous thrombosis and stroke. The aim of this study was to investigate if aPL antibodies could support classical pathway activation on platelets in vitro as well as in SLE patients. Furthermore, we investigated if complement deposition on platelets was associated with vascular events, either arterial or venous, when the data had been adjusted for traditional cardiovascular risk factors. Finally, we analyzed if platelet complement deposition, both C1q and C4d, was specific for SLE. We found that aPL antibodies supported C4d deposition on platelets in vitro as well as in SLE patients (p = 0.001 and p<0.05, respectively). Complement deposition on platelets was increased in SLE patients when compared with healthy individuals (p<0.0001). However, high levels of C4d deposition and a pronounced C1q deposition were also seen in patients with rheumatoid arthritis and systemic sclerosis. In SLE, C4d deposition on platelets was associated with platelet activation, complement consumption, disease activity and venous (OR = 5.3, p = 0.02), but not arterial, thrombosis, observations which were independent of traditional cardiovascular risk factors. In conclusion, several mechanisms operate in SLE to amplify platelet complement deposition, of which aPL antibodies and platelet activation were identified as important contributors in this investigation. Complement deposition on platelets was identified as a marker of venous, but not arterial thrombosis, in SLE patients independently of traditional risk factors and aPL antibodies. Further studies are needed to elucidate the role of complement deposition on platelets in development of venous thrombosis.

Editor: Gualtiero I. Colombo, Centro Cardiologico Monzino IRCCS, Italy

Funding: This work was supported by grants from the Medical Faculty at Lund University; The Crafoord Foundation; Swedish Combine Projects; Greta and Johan Kock's Foundation; King Gustaf V's 80th Birthday Foundation; Lund University Hospital; the Swedish Rheumatism Association; Swedish Society of Medicine; and the Foundation of the National Board of Health and Welfare and Österlund's Foundation. The funders had no role in study design, data collection and analysis, decision to publish, or preparation of the manuscript.

Competing Interests: The authors have declared that no competing interests exist.

* E-mail: Christian.Lood@med.lu.se

Introduction

Systemic lupus erythematosus (SLE) is an autoimmune rheumatic disease characterized by systemic inflammation affecting several organ systems including joints, kidney, skin and central nervous system [1]. SLE patients have a highly increased cardiovascular morbidity and mortality which can only be partly explained by traditional risk factors [2,3,4,5]. Anti-phospholipid (aPL) antibodies are a group of phospholipid-binding autoantibodies with overlapping, but partly different specificities. There are three main aPL tests used in clinical practice; anti-cardiolipin (aCL) antibodies, anti-beta 2 glycoprotein I (aB2GPI) antibodies and lupus anticoagulans (LA). Positivity in one or more of those assays is associated with development of venous thrombosis and stroke [6,7,8,9]. The underlying mechanism of aPL antibody-mediated thrombosis is not fully understood. It is known that aPL antibodies are able to bind to platelets and amplify platelet activation and aggregation through the p38 MAPK signaling pathway [10,11,12,13,14,15]. Furthermore, investigations in complement deficiency, both in mice and human, suggest that classical pathway activation of the complement system is essential in development of aPL antibody-mediated thrombosis [16,17,18,19,20,21]. Thus, even though the exact underlying mechanism for aPL antibody-mediated development of thrombosis is still not known, existing data suggest that two of the components behind the pro-thrombotic effects are platelets and the complement system.

Data from our group and from others have previously demonstrated that SLE patients have increased complement activation on platelets, especially patients with aPL antibodies [22,23,24]. It is known that some aPL antibodies have complement-fixing activity and allow complement activation through the classical pathway [25]. However, whether aPL antibodies support complement activation specifically on platelets is not known. In addition, complement activation on platelets may be caused by platelet activation and subsequent exposure of C1q binding epitopes on the activated platelet cell surface [23,26]. Currently, it is unclear which of these mechanisms, autoantibody-mediated complement activation or direct binding of C1q due to platelet activation, is operating in SLE to increase platelet complement deposition.

Complement deposition on platelets has been seen in cases of individuals with stroke, but is otherwise thought to be specific for SLE [22,27], although studies have not been extensive in other chronic inflammatory diseases. In SLE, increased C4d deposition on platelets is associated with vascular events [23,24,28]. However, there are discrepancies in the literature as to whether it is venous or arterial vascular events which are associated with complement deposition on platelets. In addition it is also important to note that none of the previous investigations adjusted data for traditional cardiovascular risk factors.

The aim of this study was to investigate if aPL antibodies could support classical pathway activation on platelets in vitro as well as in SLE patients. Furthermore, in data which had been adjusted to account for traditional cardiovascular risk factors and aPL antibodies, we investigated with which kind of vascular events, arterial or venous, complement deposition on platelets was associated. Finally, we analyzed if deposition of complement factors C1q and C4d on platelets was specific for SLE or also found in disease controls and healthy individuals. In brief we found that aPL antibodies supported activation of the classical pathway of the complement system on platelets by two separate mechanisms; amplification of platelet activation, and by providing complement-fixing antibodies on the platelet surface. Platelet activation was analyzed by flow cytometry measuring platelet P-selectin and CD69 expression. CD69 is constitutively expressed on platelets, but is increased upon activation and is important for platelet aggregation [29,30]. In SLE patients, deposition on platelets of both complement factor C1q and C4d, was associated with venous, but not arterial, thrombosis when the data was adjusted to account for traditional cardiovascular risk factors and aPL antibodies. These results suggest a possible link between aPL antibodies and development of venous thrombosis through mechanisms involving complement activation on platelets. Finally, complement deposition on platelets was not specific for SLE but high levels of both C1q and C4d on platelets were also found in other disease groups, in particular in patients with rheumatoid arthritis.

Materials and Methods

Patients

Patients with SLE (n = 148), rheumatoid arthritis (n = 20) and systemic sclerosis (n = 20) were recruited to participate in studies related to cardiovascular disease at the Department of Rheumatology, Skåne University Hospital, Lund, Sweden. Healthy volunteers (n = 79) were age- and sex-matched as a group to the SLE patients. Patients who had a recent myocardial infarction (within the previous year) but with no diagnosis of chronic inflammatory diseases (n = 39) were recruited at the Department of Cardiology, Skåne University Hospital, Lund, Sweden. The myocardial infarction patients were treated with Warfarin (n = 3), acetylsalicylic acid (n = 34) and the P2Y$_{12}$ receptor inhibitor Clopidogrel (n = 9). Furthermore, all patients with myocardial infarction used different anti-hypertension treatments, including beta blockers (n = 28). An overview of the clinical characteristics of the patients is presented in Tables 1, 2, and 3. Disease activity was assessed using SLEDAI-2K [31]. All but two

individuals fulfilled at least four American College of Rheumatology (ACR) 1982 criteria for SLE [32]. These two patients fulfilled three ACR criteria, had a clinical SLE diagnosis with at least two organ manifestations characteristic of SLE, autoimmune phenomena, and no other diagnosis that could better explain the symptoms. The following treatments were used in the SLE cohort at the time of blood sampling: glucocorticoids (n = 98, median dose = 5 mg, range 1–30 mg), hydroxychloroquine (n = 105), azathioprine (n = 32), mycophenolatmofetil (n = 20), methotrexate (n = 13), intravenous immunoglobulins (n = 2), non-steroidal anti-inflammatory drugs (n = 12), acetylsalicylic acid (n = 44) and Warfarin (n = 23). Previous episodes of myocardial infarction, claudicatio intermittens, cerebrovascular incidents (CVI), angina pectoris, deep venous thrombosis or pulmonary embolisms were defined by the Systemic Lupus International Collaborative Clinics/ACR Damage Index (SLICC/ACR-DI) [33]. Traditional cardiovascular risk factors; age, gender, smoking, diabetes, hypertension (systolic blood pressure equal or higher than 140 at the time of blood sampling or hypertensive treatment due to high blood pressure), body mass index (BMI) and LDL levels, were assessed at the visit to the clinic (Table 3). Complement proteins and autoantibodies were measured by routine standard analyses at the Department of Clinical Immunology and Transfusion Medicine, LabMedicin Skåne, Lund, Sweden.

Ethics statement

The study was approved by the regional ethics board (LU-06014520) and an informed written consent was obtained from all participants.

Complement deposition on platelets in SLE patients

Blood, collected in sodium-citrate tubes (BD Biosciences Pharmingen, Franklin Lakes, NJ, USA), was centrifuged at 280×g for 10 minutes to obtain platelet-rich plasma (PRP). Platelet purity was routinely analyzed by CD42a expression and was found to be more than 98% (mean: 98.8% (range 98.1–99.4%). Ethylenediaminetetraacetic acid (EDTA) was added to PRP to a final concentration of 10 mM to avoid complement activation during the isolation process, and then the platelets were centrifuged at 1125×g for 10 minutes. The platelets were resuspended in 10 mM N-2-hydroxyethylpiperazine-N′-2-ethane-sulfonic acid (HEPES) buffer pH 7.4, containing 145 mM NaCl and 5 mM KCl (HEPES buffer) and incubated with fluorescein isocyanate (FITC)-conjugated anti-C1q antibodies (Dako, Glostrup, Denmark) or antibodies against C4d (Quidel, San Diego, CA, USA) for 30 minutes at room temperature. For detection of C4d, the platelets were washed once in HEPES buffer and then incubated with FITC-conjugated rabbit anti-mouse IgG antibodies (Dako) for an additional 30 minutes at 4°C. The platelets were analyzed by flow cytometry on an Accuri C6 (BD).

In vitro complement deposition on activated platelets

PRP, 5 µl, was incubated with 5 µM ADP (Chrono-log, Havertown, PA, USA), for 30 minutes at room temperature in phosphate buffered saline pH 7.4 (PBS). The activation was terminated by incubation with 2% paraformaldehyde for 10 minutes. Activated and fixed platelets were isolated by centrifugation at 1125×g for 10 minutes. Purified platelets were resuspended in veronal buffered saline with 0.15 mM Ca^{2+} and 0.5 mM Mg^{2+} (VBS CaMg) containing 10% normal human serum and human IgG (Immuno AG, Vienna, Austria) or anti-cardiolipin IgG antibodies, at a final concentration of 20 µg/ml, (Antibodies-online.com, Atlanta, GA, USA) and incubated for 60 minutes at 37°C to allow complement activation. The platelets were washed

Table 1. Distribution of American College of Rheumatology (ACR) 1982 classification criteria for the 148 SLE patients.

ACR criteria, median (range)	5 (3–10)
Malar rash %	52
Discoid rash %	20
Photosensitivity %	56
Oral ulcers %	24
Arthritis %	78
Serositis %	39
Renal disease %	33
Neurological disorder %	6
Hematological manifestations %	55
Leukopenia %	37
Lymphopenia %	24
Thrombocytopenia %	14
Immunology %	69
Anti-dsDNA antibodies %	59
ANA %	98

once in PBS and incubated with an anti-C4d antibody (Quidel) for 30 minutes followed by a FITC-conjugated rabbit anti mouse IgG antibody (Dako) for an additional 30 minutes at 4°C. The platelets were analyzed by flow cytometry on an Accuri C6 (BD).

Platelet activation assay

PRP, 5 µl, was incubated with a suboptimal concentration of ADP (0.2 µM, established by titration curve (Figure 1B and Figure S1)), anti-cardiolipin IgG antibodies at a final concentration of 20 µg/ml, human IgG and PE-conjugated antibodies against P-selectin (BD) for 30 minutes at room temperature. The platelets were analyzed by flow cytometry on an Accuri C6 (BD). For detection of CD69, PRP was incubated with monoclonal

antibodies against CD69 (Santa Cruz Biotechnology, Santa Cruz, CA, USA), in PBS for 40 min at room temperature. The platelets were washed once in PBS and then incubated with FITC-conjugated rabbit anti-mouse Ig antibodies (Dako) for an additional 30 min at 4°C. The platelets were analyzed by flow cytometry on an Accuri C6 (BD).

Statistics

Spearman's correlation test was used to analyze correlations between C1q and C4d deposition on platelets. For paired analyses, Friedman test was followed by Wilcoxon matched-pairs signed rank test. For group analyses, Kruskal-Wallis test was followed by Mann-Whitney U test. Bonferroni correction was used as a post

Table 2. Clinical characteristics of the SLE patients.

Disease duration, median (range), years	11 (0–46)
SLEDAI score, median (range)	1.5 (0–18)
Serum C3 (g/L), median (range)	1.02 (0.36–2.46)
Serum C4 (g/L), median (range)	0.15 (0.03–0.58)
Serum C1q (%), median (range)	102 (8–200)
Serum C3dg (mg/L), median (range)	0 (0–25.10)
aCL at visit %	5
aCL titer (GPLU/mL)[a], median (range)	60 (42–158)
aCL ever %	28
aB2GP1 at visit %	7
aB2GP1 titer (U/mL)[a], median (range)	28 (16–100)
aB2GP1 ever %	11
Lupus anticoagulans visit %	11
Lupus anticoagulans ever %	11
SLICC/ACR-DI, median (range)	0 (0–8)

[a]Calculation only done for patients with detectable levels of autoantibodies. Abbreviations: SLEDAI; SLE disease activity index, aCL; anti-cardiolipin antibody, aB2GP1; anti-beta 2 glycoprotein 1 antibody.

Table 3. Distribution of traditional cardiovascular risk factors in the different cohorts included in the study.

Patient group	Healthy volunteers	SLE	RA	SSc	MI
Number	79	148	20	20	39
Female %	85	87	75	80	15
Age (median, range)	47 (18–81)	48 (20–82)	56 (28–67)	67 (19–82)	69 (61–77)
LDL concentration (mM), mean and SD	3.16±0.87	3.06±0.95	3.28±0.87	2.91±1.10	2.41±1.08
Smoking %	9	21	30	20	0
Diabetes %	1	3	5	5	15
Hypertension[a] %	18	43	30	35	69
Body mass index	23.5±3.1	25.5±4.9	26.5±4.2	22.5±3.0	25.7±2.9

[a]Hypertension was defined as systolic blood pressure equal or higher than 140 at time point of blood sampling or hypertensive treatment due to high blood pressure. Abbreviations: LDL; low-density lipoproteins.

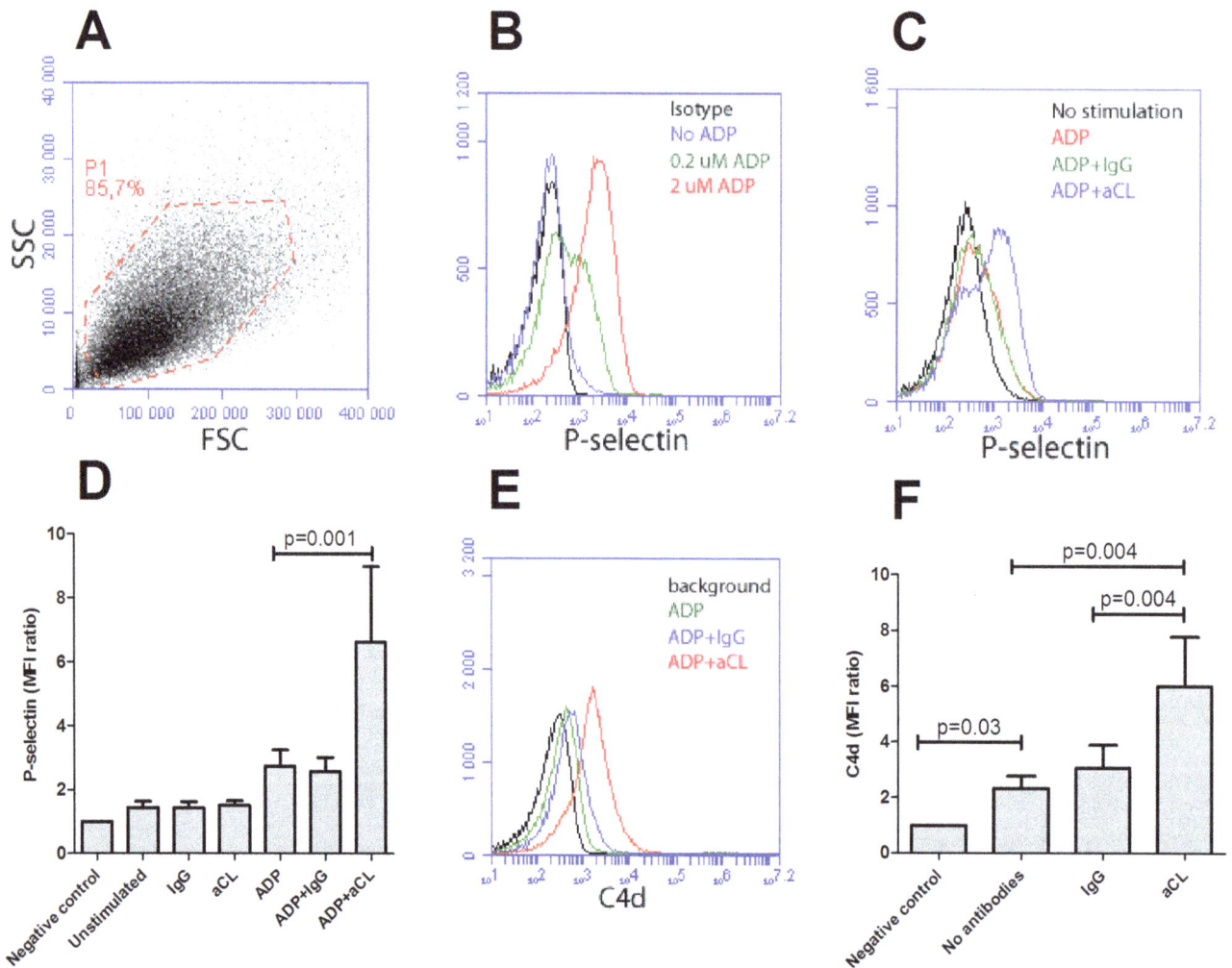

Figure 1. Anti-phospholipid (aPL) antibody-mediated platelet activation and complement deposition. A) Isolated platelets from healthy individuals were gated by flow cytometry (P1) and had consistently purity above 98%. B) Platelet activation after ADP stimulation was detected as P-selectin expression. The lower concentration (0.2 μM) was used for sub-optimal activation. C) Representative figure of P-selectin expression in sub-optimal activated platelets with or without addition of anti-cardiolipin antibodies (aCL). D) A summary of the data presented in Figure 1C. The results are the mean and standard deviation of six or more independent experiments. E–F) Activated and fixed platelets were incubated with or without aCL antibodies in presence of normal human serum. Complement deposition was analyzed with flow cytometry and illustrated as E) a representative histogram and F) a summary of the mean and standard deviation of six or more independent experiments.

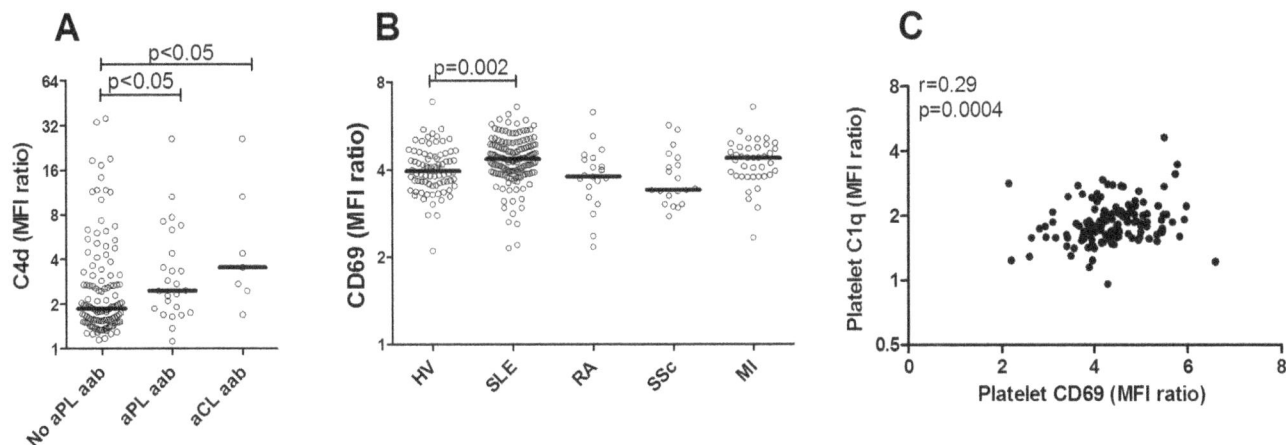

Figure 2. Complement deposition on platelets in SLE patients is associated with aCL antibodies and platelet activation. A) Platelet expression of C4d was analyzed in 148 SLE patients and grouped into patients with or without anti-phospholipid (aPL) or anti-cardiolipin (aCL) antibodies at the time of blood sampling. The line represents the median value in each group. B) Platelet expression of CD69 was measured by flow cytometry in healthy volunteers (HV), patients with systemic lupus erythematosus (SLE), rheumatoid arthritis (RA), systemic sclerosis (SSc) and myocardial infarction (MI). The line represents the median value in each group. C) Correlation analysis between C1q deposition on platelets and platelet activation marker CD69 in the 148 SLE patients.

hoc test for all analyses. Platelet deposition of C1q and C4d did not assume Gaussian distribution why the variables were normalized through logarithms and associations determined by logarithmic regression analysis. The odds ratio (OR) describes the OR for the investigated variable if it increases by one standard deviation. The cut-off for high C1q and C4d deposition on platelets was determined by the 95 percentile of the healthy individuals. A p-value <0.05 was considered statistically significant.

Results

Anti-cardiolipin antibodies mediate platelet activation and complement deposition in vitro

Studies have shown that aPL antibodies can interact with platelets and amplify platelet activation [10,11,12,13,14,15]. However, it is not known whether or not aPL antibodies contribute to complement activation on platelets. In this study, isolated platelets were first incubated with anti-cardiolipin (aCL) antibodies, or human IgG, and P-selectin expression measured by flow cytometry as a marker of platelet activation. Using sub-optimally ADP-activated platelets, this study found that aCL antibodies, but not purified human IgG, were able to amplify platelet activation (p = 0.001, Figures 1C and 1D). However, this effect was not seen in non-activated platelets, indicating that low grade platelet activation was necessary to allow aCL antibody interactions with the platelets (Figure 1D). Thus, the data presented herein validated the methodology used and supports the observation that aCL antibodies were able to amplify platelet activation, which is in agreement with previous investigations [10,11,12,13,14,15].

In addition, the ability of aCL antibodies to support complement activation on platelets was tested. Purified platelets were activated with ADP and subsequently fixed with paraformaldehyde to end the activation process. The fixation of the platelets also prevented extensive complement-mediated lysis of the activated platelets during the course of the experiment. Once activated and fixed, serum from a healthy individual supplemented with either human IgG or aCL antibodies was added. Addition of aCL antibodies, but not human IgG, markedly increased the C4d

deposition on activated fixed platelets (p = 0.004, Figures 1E and 1F). Even in the absence of additional antibodies, using human serum from a healthy individual, the classical pathway of the complement system was activated and C4d was readily measured on the surface of activated platelets (p = 0.03, Figure 1F). Thus, in vitro, activated platelets supported classical pathway activation and subsequent deposition of C4d and this process was amplified in the presence of aCL antibodies.

Anti-phospholipid antibody-mediated complement deposition in SLE patients

The presence of aPL antibodies has previously been statistically associated with complement deposition on platelets in SLE patients [22,23,24], but to date it has not been established whether aPL antibodies truly support complement activation on platelets in SLE patients. At the time-point of blood sampling, 25/148 SLE patients (17%) had anti-cardiolipin or anti-B2GP1 antibodies of IgG type, or presence of lupus anticoagulant (LA). Presence of any of these factors was associated with increased C4d deposition on platelets (p<0.05, Figure 2A). When analyzed separately, anti-cardiolipin antibodies were associated with increased C4d deposition on platelets (p<0.05 Figure 2A). Using a cut-off for high levels of C4d deposition on platelets, presence of anti-cardiolipin antibodies at the time point of blood sampling was highly associated with increased C4d deposition on platelets (OR = 7.1 (1.1–44.3), p = 0.04).

However, patients without any detectable levels of aPL antibodies also had high levels of C4d on platelets. Thus, aPL antibodies did not explain all complement deposition on platelets, but clearly other factors also contributed. As described in Figure 1F, as well as previously [23,26], platelet activation, even in the absence of autoantibodies, supported complement activation. SLE patients are known to have increased platelet activation and accordingly, increased platelet expression of CD69 (p = 0.002, Figure 2B) was demonstrated in this study, which correlated to complement deposition on platelets (r = 0.29, p = 0.0004, Figure 2C). Thus, our results suggest that both platelet activation and aPL antibodies can act synergistically to support complement deposition and activation on platelets in SLE patients.

Complement deposition on platelets is associated with venous, but not arterial, thrombosis in SLE patients

In SLE patients, increased C4d deposition on platelets has been suggested to be associated with vascular events [23,24,28]. However, there are discrepancies in these investigations as to which vascular events, venous or arterial, complement deposition on platelets is associated.

In this study we observed no associations between C1q and C4d deposition on platelets and arterial vascular disease including myocardial infarction (OR = 1.2 (0.4–3.9), p = 0.81 and OR = 2.4 (0.7–8.1), p = 0.16, respectively) and cerebrovascular insult (OR = 0.8 (0.4–1.5), p = 0.44 and OR = 0.4 (0.1–1.2), p = 0.09, respectively, Table 4) in SLE patients using a logistic regression model adjusting for traditional cardiovascular risk factors. Not even when combining all arterial vascular diseases (claudicatio intermittens, angina pectoris, myocardial infarction and cerebrovascular insult) could an association with C1q or C4d deposition on platelets be found (OR = 0.8 (0.5–1.4), p = 0.50 and OR = 0.7 (0.4–1.3), p = 0.23, respectively, Table 4). Thus, in this study's SLE cohort, complement deposition on platelets was not associated with arterial vascular events. However, both C1q and C4d deposition on platelets were clearly associated with deep venous thrombosis (OR = 2.3 (1.2–4.2), p = 0.008, and OR = 2.0 (1.2–3.4), p = 0.01, respectively), independent of traditional cardiovascular risk factors: age, gender, smoking, hypertension, hyperglycemia, diabetes and obesity. Combining all venous manifestations the association with C1q and C4d levels on platelets remained statistically significant (p = 0.04 and p = 0.03, respectively, Table 4). For both arterial and venous thrombosis, adjusting for presence of aPL antibodies in the logistic regression model did not affect the results significantly (Table 4).

Whereas our statistical model uses a continuous variable, other investigators have used a cut-off to describe complement deposition on platelets as a dichotomized variable [22,28]. Using the cut-off as described in the material and methods section C4d deposition on platelets still remained highly associated with venous thrombosis (OR = 5.3 (1.3–22.1), p = 0.02) after adjusting for traditional risk factors and aPL antibodies. However, using the same cut-off, C4d deposition on platelets was associated with a decreased frequency of arterial thrombosis (OR = 0.2 (0.1–0.8), p = 0.03) as well as stroke (OR = 0.2 (0.0–1.0), p<0.05), adjusted for traditional cardiovascular risk factors and presence of aPL antibodies. Thus, in SLE patients, increased complement deposition on platelets was clearly associated with venous, and not arterial, thrombosis independently of traditional cardiovascular risk factors and aPL antibodies.

Complement deposition on platelets is not specific for SLE patients

C4d deposition on platelets has been suggested to be highly specific for SLE [22]. However, whether C1q deposition on platelets is specific for SLE had not been investigated previously. Complement deposition of both C1q and C4 on platelets were markedly increased in SLE patients as compared to healthy volunteers (p<0.0001 for both analyses, Figure 3). Patients with rheumatoid arthritis had increased C1q deposition (p = 0.002, Figure 3B) as well as increased C4d deposition (p<0.0001, Figure 3D) whereas patients with systemic sclerosis only were found to have increased C4d deposition (p<0.05, Figure 3D) on platelets as compared to healthy volunteers. Notably, some of the apparently healthy individuals had increased C4d deposition on their platelets. Using the cut-off value for high and low complement deposition on platelets 12% of the SLE patients,

Table 4. Associations between complement deposition on platelets and cardiovascular disease and venous thromboembolism.

Manifestation		N	OR (95% CI)	p-value	OR (95% CI)[a]	p-value[a]	OR (95%CI)[d]	p-value[d]
Arterial[b]	C1q	25	1.0 (0.7–1.5)	0.98	0.8 (0.5–1.4)	0.50	0.8 (0.5–1.4)	0.40
	C4d		0.8 (0.5–1.3)	0.28	0.7 (0.4–1.3)	0.23	0.6 (0.3–1.2)	0.18
CVI	C1q	14	0.9 (0.5–1.6)	0.75	0.8 (0.4–1.5)	0.44	0.7 (0.4–1.3)	0.23
	C4d		0.5 (0.2–1.2)	0.12	0.4 (0.1–1.2)	0.09	0.3 (0.1–1.0)	<0.05
MI	C1q	8	1.0 (0.5–2.1)	0.92	1.2 (0.4–3.9)	0.81	2.0 (0.4–11.6)	0.42
	C4d		1.3 (0.7–2.4)	0.44	2.4 (0.7–8.1)	0.16	2.9 (0.8–11.5)	0.12
DVT	C1q	12	2.2 (1.3–3.8)	0.005	2.3 (1.2–4.2)	0.008	2.2 (1.2–4.2)	0.01
	C4d		1.7 (1.0–2.7)	0.04	2.0 (1.2–3.4)	0.01	2.0 (1.1–3.3)	0.01
Venous[c]	C1q	17	1.7 (1.0–2.7)	0.03	1.7 (1.0–2.9)	0.04	1.7 (1.0–2.9)	0.04
	C4d		1.4 (0.9–2.2)	0.11	1.7 (1.1–2.8)	0.03	1.7 (1.1–2.8)	0.03

[a] Adjusted for traditional risk factors; age, gender, smoking, hypertension, hyperglycemia and diabetes.
[b] Arterial disease includes cerebrovascular insult (CVI), myocardial infarction (MI), angina pectoris and claudicatio intermittens.
[c] Venous thrombosis includes deep venous thrombosis (DVT) and pulmonary embolism.
[d] Further adjusted for presence of aPL antibodies at time-point of blood sampling.

35% of the rheumatoid arthritis patients, 10% of the systemic sclerosis patients, 12% of the myocardial infarction patients and 5% of the healthy individuals were regarded as having high levels of C1q on platelets (Figure 3B). For the C4d deposition on platelets, 35% of the SLE patients, 20% of the rheumatoid arthritis patients, 5% of the systemic sclerosis patients, 8% of the myocardial infarction patients and 4% of the healthy individuals were regarded as having high levels (Figure 3D). There was a correlation between C1q and C4d deposition on platelets (r = 0.41, p<0.0001, Figure 3E). Only 67% of the SLE patients positive for C1q deposition were also positive for C4d deposition on platelets suggesting that complement activation does not always proceed after C1q binding. Furthermore, of the SLE patients negative for C1q deposition, 31% had increased deposition of C4d on platelets, indicating that small amounts of C1q might be enough to activate C4.

Complement deposition on platelets is associated with disease activity

To investigate the clinical relevance of our findings we first assessed if complement deposition on platelets was associated with disease activity. C4d deposition on platelets, but not C1q deposition, was positively correlated to SLEDAI (r = 0.27,

p = 0.001). Furthermore, patients with active disease (SLEDAI ≥ 5) had highly increased C4d deposition on their platelets (p = 0.008) compared to SLE patients with no or low disease activity. Patients treated with Prednisone had a higher C4d deposition on platelets (p = 0.006), most likely due to increased disease activity seen in this group (p = 0.01). None of the other immunosuppressive treatments affected C1q or C4d deposition on platelets in a statistically significant manner. Even though not correlated to disease activity in general, C1q deposition on platelets was increased in SLE patients with ongoing arthritis (p = 0.01). For C4d deposition, no associations were found with any specific clinical disease manifestation. Instead C4d deposition correlated with the presence in serum of anti-dsDNA antibodies (p = 0.03) and low levels of either C3 or C4 (p<0.0001). The deposition of C4d on platelets was inversely correlated with serum levels of both C3 and C4 (r = −0.38, p<0.0001 for both analyses, Figures 4A and 4B) as well as positively correlated with the complement split product C3dg (r = 0.44, p<0.0001, Figure 4C). Finally, even when using a modified SLEDAI excluding any score for anti-dsDNA antibodies or low complement levels, C4d deposition on platelets remained statistically significantly correlated to disease activity, even though the association was weak (r = 0.17, p = 0.04).

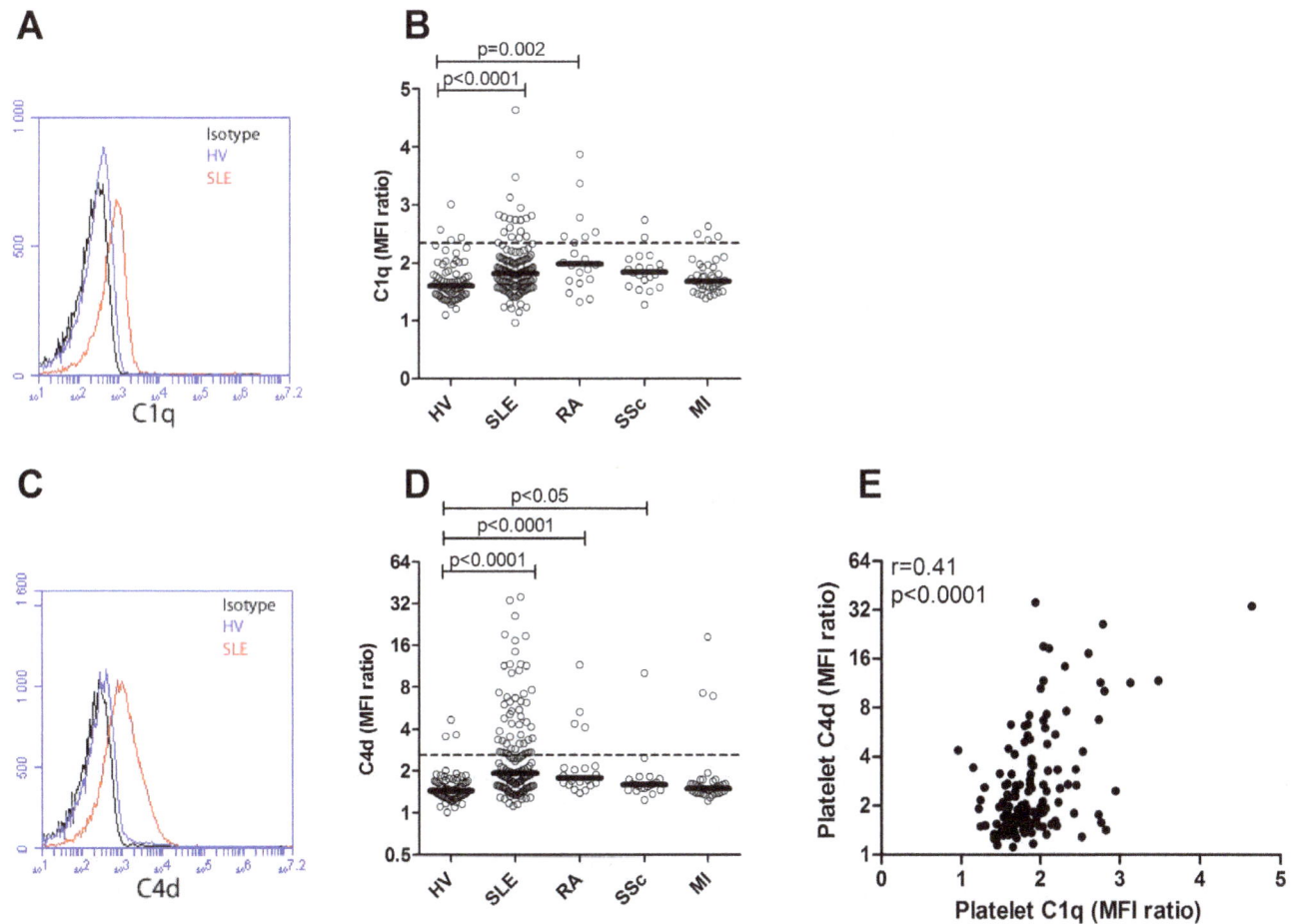

Figure 3. Increased complement deposition on platelets in SLE patients. A) Deposition of C1q and C) C4d was analyzed by flow cytometry and illustrated as representative flow cytometry histograms. Deposition of B) C1q and D) C4d on platelets from healthy volunteers (HV), patients with systemic lupus erythematosus (SLE), rheumatoid arthritis (RA), systemic sclerosis (SSc) and myocardial infarction (MI). The dotted lines represent the 95th percentile of the healthy volunteers and depict the cut-off level for positivity in each analysis. E) Correlation analysis between C1q and C4d deposition on platelets in the SLE patients.

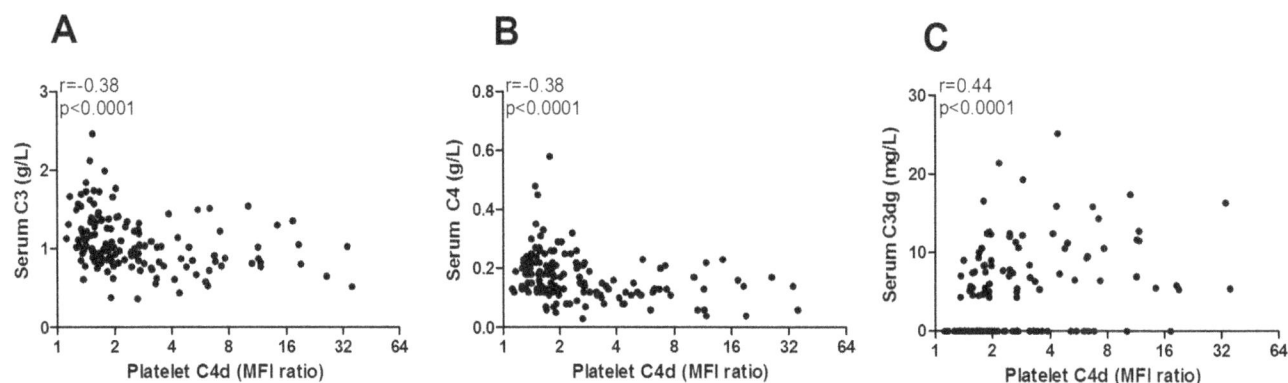

Figure 4. Platelet C4d deposition is associated with complement consumption and activation. C4d deposition on platelets from SLE patients was correlated to A) serum level of C3, B) serum level of C4, and C) the complement activation split fragment C3dg.

Discussion

Anti-phospholipid antibodies are well-known important pro-thrombotic factors contributing to development of venous thrombosis and stroke in SLE patients [9,34,35]. The molecular mechanism of how aPL antibodies mediate development of thrombosis is not fully understood but may involve activation of both platelets and the classical pathway of the complement system [16,17,23]. In human C2 deficiency (C2D), anti-cardiolipin antibodies are frequently seen but virtually never lead to development of venous thrombosis [17]. Furthermore, in mouse, C3, C5a and C6 are all necessary for development of aPL antibody-mediated thrombosis [16,18,19,20,21]. In this investigation we have studied the role of aPL antibodies in mediating complement activation on the surface of platelets and if this could be a possible mechanism linking aPL antibodies, complement activation, platelet activation and vascular events in SLE patients. Furthermore, we present a detailed examination of associations between complement deposition on platelets and other clinical variables.

Increased complement activation has been seen on platelets in SLE patients, especially in patients with aPL antibodies [22,23,24]. However, it was not known if aPL antibodies could support complement activation on platelets. Data presented herein demonstrates that aPL antibodies indeed allow complement activation on platelets by two separate mechanisms, both of which could be operating in SLE patients. Firstly, aPL antibodies contribute to platelet activation-mediated complement deposition. It is well-established that aPL antibodies amplify platelet activation [10,11,12,13,14,15], which was verified in this investigation. Activated platelets expose several molecules including phosphatidylserine and chondroitinsulfate which support binding of C1q and subsequent complement activation [26]. Supporting the hypothesis of platelet activation being sufficient to allow complement activation we observed that sera from healthy individuals supported complement activation on the surface of activated platelets (Figure 1F) also confirming observations in one of our previous studies [23].

Secondly, we hypothesized that the complement-fixing ability of some anti-PL antibodies [25] may allow C1q binding with subsequent activation of the classical pathway on platelets. To test the validity of this model, normal human serum, supplemented with purified aPL antibodies, was added to activated fixed platelets. Using this experimental approach it was found that aPL antibodies also mediated complement activation on platelets independently of their ability to also support platelet activation.

Those results are strongly supported by the current as well as previous investigations demonstrating associations between aPL antibodies and complement deposition on platelets [22,23,24]. Thus, we suggest that aPL antibodies, through both platelet activation and binding of complement-fixing antibodies, support complement activation on platelets.

However, aPL antibodies are not indispensable in activating the complement system on platelets, and several mechanisms may operate to mediate complement activation on platelets. This was highlighted by the significant number of SLE patients having no detectable aPL antibodies but still having high levels of both C1q and C4d on platelets. One explanation for this may be presence of other anti-platelet antibodies, including anti-GPIIb/IIIa [36,37,38], but more likely, complement deposition on platelets can be explained by increased platelet activation. In this study we could demonstrate that SLE patients had increased platelet activation and the platelet activation correlated with complement deposition on the platelet surface. The cause for the initial platelet activation in SLE is not known but may include immune complexes, shear stress, type I IFNs or endothelial damage with exposure of extracellular matrix proteins and collagen [39,40,41]. Furthermore, oxidized LDL (oxLDL), which is increased in SLE patients [42], may also participate in the initial platelet activation [43]. Thus, based on our results, we suggest that complement deposition is increased in SLE patients due to ongoing platelet activation and this process, both platelet activation and complement activation on platelets, is amplified in the presence of aPL antibodies.

Earlier studies have established that anti-PL antibodies are associated with development of venous thrombosis and stroke in SLE patients [9], and previous studies have demonstrated an association between increased complement deposition on platelets and vascular events [23,24,28]. However, there are some discrepancies in the literature with regard to which type of vascular event, venous or arterial, complement deposition on platelets is associated with. Furthermore, none of the previous studies have taken into account the role of traditional cardiovascular risk factors in their statistical analyses. In the current investigation we found that complement deposition on platelets was associated with venous, but not arterial, thrombosis, which is in line with our previous study [23]. However, in this study, data demonstrated that the association to venous thrombosis was independent of traditional cardiovascular risk factors and aPL antibodies. Previous studies have suggested that aPL antibodies found in patients with venous thrombosis have increased complement-fixing ability compared to aPL antibodies found in patients with arterial thrombosis [25] and this may be one reason for the increased complement deposition on platelets in patients with aPL antibodies and venous thrombosis.

C4d deposition on platelets has been suggested to be highly specific for SLE [22] but it was not known if C1q deposition on platelets could be seen in inflammatory diseases other than SLE. In contrast to a previous investigation [22] increased C4d and C1q deposition could be readily observed on platelets in patients with rheumatoid arthritis, increased C4d deposition on platelets was found in patients with systemic sclerosis, as well as high levels of complement deposition found on platelets in some apparently healthy individuals. Thus, complement activation on platelets is not specific for SLE but associated with platelet activation in general. However, different patterns of C1q and C4d deposition were found in SLE patients and patients with rheumatoid arthritis. Patients with rheumatoid arthritis had a high frequency of elevated C1q levels on platelets but a relatively low frequency of C4d, whereas SLE patients had the opposite with high frequency of elevated C4d levels compared to a relatively low frequency of C1q. This suggests that different mechanisms of complement activation and regulation might be operating in the two diseases. Interestingly, SLE patients with ongoing arthritis had increased C1q deposition on platelets compared to SLE patients with no arthritis. Even though the pathogenesis of arthritis is different between rheumatoid arthritis and lupus, platelet activation has been demonstrated in the joints of patients with rheumatoid arthritis, but the contribution of complement activation on platelets to this is not known [44]. Further studies are needed to elucidate how complement activation on platelets is regulated in different conditions and contributes to disease manifestations.

In conclusion, we suggest that aPL antibodies are able to amplify C4d deposition on platelets through two separate mechanisms; amplification of platelet activation, and providing complement-fixing antibodies on platelets. Complement deposition on platelets is associated with venous, but not arterial, thrombosis in SLE patients, independent of traditional cardiovascular risk factors and aPL antibodies. Further studies are needed to elucidate the underlying mechanisms linking complement activation on platelets to cardiovascular disease.

Supporting Information

Figure S1   Dose-response curve for ADP. ADP, at different concentrations, was incubated with platelets for 15 minutes at room temperature and platelet activation analyzed by P-selectin expression by flow cytometry. Concentrations ranging between 0.2-0.4 µM ADP were found to induce sub-optimal platelet activation.

Author Contributions

Conceived and designed the experiments: CL HT BG GS AJ LT AAB. Performed the experiments: CL HT BG. Analyzed the data: CL HT BG GS AJ LT AAB. Contributed reagents/materials/analysis tools: HT GS AJ AAB. Wrote the paper: CL AAB. Critically revised the manuscript: HT BG GS AJ LT.

References

1. Crispin JC, Liossis SN, Kis-Toth K, Lieberman LA, Kyttaris VC, et al. (2010) Pathogenesis of human systemic lupus erythematosus: recent advances. Trends Mol Med 16: 47–57.

2. Esdaile JM, Abrahamowicz M, Grodzicky T, Li Y, Panaritis C, et al. (2001) Traditional Framingham risk factors fail to fully account for accelerated atherosclerosis in systemic lupus erythematosus. Arthritis Rheum 44: 2331–2337.

3. Manzi S, Meilahn EN, Rairie JE, Conte CG, Medsger TA Jr, et al. (1997) Age-specific incidence rates of myocardial infarction and angina in women with systemic lupus erythematosus: comparison with the Framingham Study. Am J Epidemiol 145: 408–415.

4. Jonsson H, Nived O, Sturfelt G (1989) Outcome in systemic lupus erythematosus: a prospective study of patients from a defined population. Medicine (Baltimore) 68: 141–150.

5. Rubin LA, Urowitz MB, Gladman DD (1985) Mortality in systemic lupus erythematosus: the bimodal pattern revisited. Q J Med 55: 87–98.

6. Al-Homood IA (2012) Thrombosis in systemic lupus erythematosus: a review article. ISRN Rheumatol 2012: 428269.

7. Koskenmies S, Vaarala O, Widen E, Kere J, Palosuo T, et al. (2004) The association of antibodies to cardiolipin, beta 2-glycoprotein I, prothrombin, and oxidized low-density lipoprotein with thrombosis in 292 patients with familial and sporadic systemic lupus erythematosus. Scand J Rheumatol 33: 246–252.

8. Sallai KK, Nagy E, Bodo I, Mohl A, Gergely P (2007) Thrombosis risk in systemic lupus erythematosus: the role of thrombophilic risk factors. Scand J Rheumatol 36: 198–205.

9. Vikerfors A, Johansson AB, Gustafsson JT, Jonsen A, Leonard D, et al. (2013) Clinical manifestations and anti-phospholipid antibodies in 712 patients with systemic lupus erythematosus: evaluation of two diagnostic assays. Rheumatology (Oxford) 52: 501–509.

10. Betts NA, Ahuja KD, Adams MJ (2013) Anti-beta2GP1 antibodies have variable effects on platelet aggregation. Pathology 45: 155–161.

11. Nojima J, Kuratsune H, Suehisa E, Kitani T, Iwatani Y, et al. (2004) Strong correlation between the prevalence of cerebral infarction and the presence of anti-cardiolipin/beta2-glycoprotein I and anti-phosphatidylserine/prothrombin antibodies—Co-existence of these antibodies enhances ADP-induced platelet activation in vitro. Thromb Haemost 91: 967–976.

12. Wiener HM, Vardinon N, Yust I (1991) Platelet antibody binding and spontaneous aggregation in 21 lupus anticoagulant patients. Vox Sang 61: 111–121.

13. Lin YL, Wang CT (1992) Activation of human platelets by the rabbit anticardiolipin antibodies. Blood 80: 3135–3143.

14. Wang L, Su CY, Chou KY, Wang CT (2002) Enhancement of human platelet activation by the combination of low concentrations of collagen and rabbit anticardiolipin antibodies. Br J Haematol 118: 1152–1162.

15. Vega-Ostertag M, Harris EN, Pierangeli SS (2004) Intracellular events in platelet activation induced by antiphospholipid antibodies in the presence of low doses of thrombin. Arthritis Rheum 50: 2911–2919.

16. Pierangeli SS, Vega-Ostertag M, Liu X, Girardi G (2005) Complement activation: a novel pathogenic mechanism in the antiphospholipid syndrome. Ann N Y Acad Sci 1051: 413–420.

17. Jönsson G, Sjöholm AG, Truedsson L, Bengtsson AA, Braconier JH, et al. (2007) Rheumatological manifestations, organ damage and autoimmunity in hereditary C2 deficiency. Rheumatology (Oxford) 46: 1133–1139.

18. Girardi G, Berman J, Redecha P, Spruce L, Thurman JM, et al. (2003) Complement C5a receptors and neutrophils mediate fetal injury in the antiphospholipid syndrome. J Clin Invest 112: 1644–1654.

19. Salmon JE, de Groot PG (2008) Pathogenic role of antiphospholipid antibodies. Lupus 17: 405–411.

20. Carrera-Marin A, Romay-Penabad Z, Papalardo E, Reyes-Maldonado E, Garcia-Latorre E, et al. (2012) C6 knock-out mice are protected from thrombophilia mediated by antiphospholipid antibodies. Lupus 21: 1497–1505.

21. Holers VM, Girardi G, Mo L, Guthridge JM, Molina H, et al. (2002) Complement C3 activation is required for antiphospholipid antibody-induced fetal loss. J Exp Med 195: 211–220.

22. Navratil JS, Manzi S, Kao AH, Krishnaswami S, Liu CC, et al. (2006) Platelet C4d is highly specific for systemic lupus erythematosus. Arthritis Rheum 54: 670–674.

23. Lood C, Eriksson S, Gullstrand B, Jonsen A, Sturfelt G, et al. (2012) Increased C1q, C4 and C3 deposition on platelets in patients with systemic lupus erythematosus - a possible link to venous thrombosis? Lupus 21: 1423–1432.

24. Peerschke E, Yin W, Alpert D, Roubey R, Salmon J, et al. (2009) Serum complement activation on heterologous platelets is associated with arterial thrombosis in patients with systemic lupus erythematosus and antiphospholipid antibodies. Lupus 18: 530–538.

25. Shinzato MM, Bueno C, Trindade Viana VS, Borba EF, Goncalves CR, et al. (2005) Complement-fixing activity of anticardiolipin antibodies in patients with and without thrombosis. Lupus 14: 953–958.

26. Hamad OA, Ekdahl KN, Nilsson PH, Andersson J, Magotti P, et al. (2008) Complement activation triggered by chondroitin sulfate released by thrombin receptor-activated platelets. J Thromb Haemost 6: 1413–1421.

27. Mehta N, Uchino K, Fakhran S, Sattar MA, Branstetter BFt, et al. (2008) Platelet C4d is associated with acute ischemic stroke and stroke severity. Stroke 39: 3236–3241.

28. Kao AH, McBurney CA, Sattar A, Lertratanakul A, Wilson NL, et al. (2013) Relation of Platelet C4d with All-Cause Mortality and Ischemic Stroke in Patients with Systemic Lupus Erythematosus. Transl Stroke Res.

29. Testi R, Pulcinelli F, Frati L, Gazzaniga PP, Santoni A (1990) CD69 is expressed on platelets and mediates platelet activation and aggregation. J Exp Med 172: 701–707.

30. Testi R, Pulcinelli FM, Cifone MG, Botti D, Del Grosso E, et al. (1992) Preferential involvement of a phospholipase A2-dependent pathway in CD69-mediated platelet activation. J Immunol 148: 2867–2871.

31. Gladman DD, Ibanez D, Urowitz MB (2002) Systemic lupus erythematosus disease activity index 2000. J Rheumatol 29: 288–291.

32. Tan EM, Cohen AS, Fries JF, Masi AT, McShane DJ, et al. (1982) The 1982 revised criteria for the classification of systemic lupus erythematosus. Arthritis Rheum 25: 1271–1277.

33. Gladman D, Ginzler E, Goldsmith C, Fortin P, Liang M, et al. (1996) The development and initial validation of the Systemic Lupus International Collaborating Clinics/American College of Rheumatology damage index for systemic lupus erythematosus. Arthritis Rheum 39: 363–369.

34. Hughes G (2007) Hughes Syndrome: the antiphospholipid syndrome—a clinical overview. Clin Rev Allergy Immunol 32: 3–12.

35. Hughes GR, Khamashta MA (1994) The antiphospholipid syndrome. J R Coll Physicians Lond 28: 301–304.

36. Tsubakio T, Tani P, Curd JG, McMillan R (1986) Complement activation in vitro by antiplatelet antibodies in chronic immune thrombocytopenic purpura. Br J Haematol 63: 293–300.

37. Ziakas PD, Routsias JG, Giannouli S, Tasidou A, Tzioufas AG, et al. (2006) Suspects in the tale of lupus-associated thrombocytopenia. Clin Exp Immunol 145: 71–80.

38. Anderson GP, van de Winkel JG, Anderson CL (1991) Anti-GPIIb/IIIa (CD41) monoclonal antibody-induced platelet activation requires Fc receptor-dependent cell-cell interaction. Br J Haematol 79: 75–83.

39. Lood C, Amisten S, Gullstrand B, Jönsen A, Allhorn M, et al. (2010) Platelet transcriptional profile and protein expression in patients with systemic lupus erythematosus: up-regulation of the type I interferon system is strongly associated with vascular disease. Blood 116: 1951–1957.

40. Larsson A, Egberg N, Lindahl TL (1994) Platelet Activation and Binding of Complement Components to Platelets Induced by Immune-Complexes. Platelets 5: 149–155.

41. Shanmugavelayudam SK, Rubenstein DA, Yin W (2011) Effects of physiologically relevant dynamic shear stress on platelet complement activation. Platelets.

42. Svenungsson E, Jensen-Urstad K, Heimburger M, Silveira A, Hamsten A, et al. (2001) Risk factors for cardiovascular disease in systemic lupus erythematosus. Circulation 104: 1887–1893.

43. Wraith KS, Magwenzi S, Aburima A, Wen Y, Leake D, et al. (2013) Oxidized low-density lipoproteins induce rapid platelet activation and shape change through tyrosine kinase and Rho kinase-signaling pathways. Blood 122: 580–589.

44. Boilard E, Nigrovic PA, Larabee K, Watts GF, Coblyn JS, et al. (2010) Platelets amplify inflammation in arthritis via collagen-dependent microparticle production. Science 327: 580–583.

Lipid Anti-Lipid Antibody Responses Correlate with Disease Activity in Systemic Lupus Erythematosus

Vojislav Jovanović[1], Nurhuda Abdul Aziz[1], Yan Ting Lim[1], Amanda Ng Ai Poh[1], Sherlynn Jin Hui Chan[1], Eliza Ho Xin Pei[1], Fei Chuin Lew[1], Guanghou Shui[4], Andrew M. Jenner[5], Li Bowen[4], Eoin F. McKinney[2,3], Paul A. Lyons[2,3], Michael D. Kemeny[1], Kenneth G. C. Smith[2,3], Markus R. Wenk[4], Paul A. MacAry[1]*

1 Immunology Programme and Department of Microbiology, National University of Singapore, Singapore, 2 Cambridge Institute for Medical Research, Cambridge, United Kingdom, 3 Department of Medicine, University of Cambridge, School of Clinical Medicine, Addenbrooke's Hospital, Cambridge, United Kingdom, 4 Department of Biochemistry, National University of Singapore, Singapore, 5 School of Biological Sciences, Illawara Health and Medical Research Institute, University of Wollongong, Australia

Abstract

Systemic Lupus Erythematosus (SLE) is a chronic autoimmune disorder characterized by broad clinical manifestations including cardiovascular and renal complications with periodic disease flares and significant morbidity and mortality. One of the main contributing factors to the pathology of SLE is the accumulation and impaired clearance of immune complexes of which the principle components are host auto-antigens and antibodies. The contribution of host lipids to the formation of these autoimmune complexes remains poorly defined. The aim of the present study was to identify and analyze candidate lipid autoantigens and their corresponding anti–lipid antibody responses in a well-defined SLE patient cohort using a combination of immunological and biophysical techniques. Disease monitoring in the SLE cohort was undertaken with serial British Isles Lupus Assessment Group (BILAG) scoring. Correlations between specific lipid/anti-lipid responses were investigated as disease activity developed from active flares to quiescent during a follow up period. We report a significant negative correlation between anti-lipid antibodies for 24S-hydroxycholesterol, cardiolipin and phosphatidylserine with SLE disease activity. Taken together, these data suggest that lipid autoantigens represent a new family of biomarkers that can be employed to monitor disease activity plus the efficacy of therapeutic intervention in SLE.

Editor: Leah J. Siskind, MUSC SC College of Pharmacy, United States of America

Funding: This work was supported by a grant from the Singapore National Research Foundation NRF370062-HUJ-NUS, "Generation of monoclonal antibodies as tools for targeting inflammatory diseases" (to P.A.M. and D.M.K); a grant from the Singapore National Medical Research Council NMRC/1164/2008, "A comparative transcriptional analysis of Systemic Lupus Erythematosus in UK (Caucasian) and Singapore (Chinese) Patients" (to P.A.M. and D.M.K); National Medical Research Council, "STOP-Dengue TCR", NMRC-182-003-220-275, and NCIS C-000-999-002-001 and the National Research Foundation NRF-182-000-218-281 and NRF2-182-005-172-281 (to P.A.M). K.G.C.S was supported by the Wellcome Trust and NIHR Cambridge Biomedical Research Centre. M.R.W. was supported by Singapore National Research Foundation under CRPAward No. 2007-04 and the Biomedical Research Council of Singapore (R-183-000-211-305).

Competing Interests: The authors have declared that no competing interests exist.

* E-mail: micpam@nus.edu.sg

Introduction

Systemic Lupus Erythematosus (SLE) is a chronic inflammatory autoimmune disease found predominantly in women. Complex interactions amongst immune, genetic, environmental and hormonal factors have been implicated in SLE susceptibility and pathogenesis [1]. Numerous mouse and human studies have implicated dysfunctional cellular and immune components including autoimmune T and B lymphocytes [2,3,4]; elevated levels of pro- inflammatory cytokines [5]; formation of antinuclear antibodies [6]; accumulation and impaired clearance of post-apoptotic cell remnants [7,8] or failure of FcγR-mediated clearance of immune complexes [9] in the pathology of Systemic Lupus Erythematosus.

The role of lipids and anti-lipid responses in Systemic Lupus Erythematosus and other autoimmune diseases remains poorly defined in comparison to proteins and genetic factors based on the technical challenges inherent in their analysis. A summary of studies linking oxysterols, phospholipids and prostaglandin derivatives with autoimmune, degenerative and age-related diseases including SLE is provided in Table 1. Thus there is a requirement for a broader and more detailed analysis of the role of lipids in these diseases.

Oxysterols represent the family of host lipids most strongly implicated in autoimmune conditions (Table 1). These are oxygenated derivatives of cholesterol that are intermediates in the cholesterol excretion pathway [10]. Cholesterol oxidation is either through attack by reactive oxygen species (ROS) that oxygenate the sterol ring at the C7-position or by enzymatic hydroxylation of cholesterol side-chains that generate 24S-, 25- and 27-hydroxycholesterol respectively [11]. 24S-hydroxycholesterol is specifically generated in the central nervous system [12–13] and plasma levels of this lipid have been implicated in diseases linked to CNS inflammation including Alzheimer's and Vascular dementia [14].

Elevated plasma levels of 24S-hydroxycholesterol was reported in Multiple Sclerosis (MS) patients with positive cranial MRI scans indicating an acute inflammatory episode of demyelination [15]. Oxidized phosphatidylcholine and their corresponding autoantibodies have also been implicated in MS [16]. Other lipid markers including F(2)-isoprostanes, 7-β-hydroxycholesterol, 7-ketocholesterol and 27-hydroxycholesterol have been linked to Parkinson's

Table 1. A summary of reported lipids and anti-lipid antibodies involved in autoimmune, degenerative and age-related diseases.

Pathologies	Organ involved	Associated oxidized lipid/anti-lipid Ab	Origin of oxidized lipid	Method of detection	Reference
Alzheimer disease, vascular demented patients	CNS	24S-hydroxycholesterol	Plasma	ID-MS	[14]
Alzheimer disease	CNS	24S-hydroxycholesterol	Plasma, cerebrospinal fluid	ID-MS	[49]
Multiple sclerosis	CNS	24S-hydroxycholesterol	Plasma, cerebrospinal fluid	ID-MS	[15]
Alzheimer disease	CNS	27-hydroxycholesterol	Brain tissue	GC-MS	[50]
Hereditary spastic paresis	CNS	27-hydroxycholesterol, 25-hydroxycholesterol	Plasma, cerebrospinal fluid	ID-MS	[51]
Atherosclerosis	Cardiovascular	27-hydroxycholesterol, 25-hydroxycholesterol, 7β- hydroxycholesterol	Plasma	HP-LC	[52]
Parkinson disease	CNS	F(2)-isoprostanes, hydroxyeicosatetraenoic acid products, 7β- hydroxycholesterol, 27-hydroxycholesterol, 7-ketocholesterol, neuroprostanes(F(4)NPs)	Plasma	GC-MS	[17]
Multiple sclerosis	CNS	7-ketocholesterol	Serum, CSF	ID-MS	[53]
Multiple sclerosis	CNS	Oxidized phosphatidylcholine (OxPC) Anti-OxPC (T15 Idiotype) antibodies	Brain extracts, CSF	Western blotting,	[16]
SLE	Different organ systems	Anti-cardiolipin Ab	Serum	ELISA	[54]
Immunoglobulin A deficiency	Different organ systems	Anti-cardiolipin Ab	Serum	ELISA	[55]
Antiphospholipid syndrome	Different organ systems	Anti-cardiolipin Ab	Serum	ELISA	[56]
Systemic Lupus Erythematosus	Different organ systems	15-F2t-IsoP	Serum	ELISA	[57]
Systemic Lupus Erythematosus	Different organ systems	15-F2t-IsoP	Plasma	GC-MS	[58]
Systemic Lupus Erythematosus; Antiphospholipid syndrome	Cardiovascular system	Anti-phosphatidylserine Ab, Anti-cardiolipin Ab	Plasma	ELISA	[59]
Alzheimer disease	CNS	24S-hydroxycholesterol	Plasma	LC-MS	[60]

disease [17]. 7-ketocholesterol may also be involved in the pathophysiology of atherosclerosis where it is suspected of inducing apoptosis in the cells of the vascular wall including monocytes/macrophages [18]. This lipid is also known to be related to oxidized-LDL-mediated cytotoxicity [19]. 7-β hydroxycholesterol is proposed to promote human NK cell death and may also be involved in atherosclerosis [20]. This study focuses on the role of oxidized lipids and anti-lipid responses in Systemic Lupus Erythematosus (SLE).

Materials and Methods

Patients

The patient cohort employed was composed of individuals referred to Addenbrooke's Hospital, Cambridge, UK between 2004 and 2008. All patients provided written informed consent and ethical approval was obtained from the Cambridge Local Research Ethics Committee (Ref: 04/023). Blood was collected at two time points: the moment of disease [21] - flare; and during the follow-up period. Follow-up was defined as the period between 3-months and 12-months post therapy. Disease monitoring was undertaken with serial BILAG scoring [22]. All patients were enrolled with active disease with an average BILAG score of 16.01 prior to treatment. Patients on treatment entered clinical remission and the average BILAG score in the follow up period was reduced

to 2.4+/−2.1. For all patients, a full haematological, biochemical and immunological profiling was done [21]. BILAG scores for 3 time-points and clinical data for patients with flare are included (Supplementary table). Thirteen paired SLE patients' samples were used to analyze changes in lipid and anti-lipid IgG levels between the flare and follow-up period (between 3–12 months post-therapy). Twenty patients with flare (including 13 previously mentioned patients) were used for the correlation analysis.

Blood Processing

Blood was collected in EDTA tubes and peripheral blood mononuclear cells (PBMC) separated on Ficoll-Paque PLUS gradient (GE Healthcare, Sweden). Plasma was stored at −80°C prior to use.

Lipid Standards and Chemicals

Phosphatidylcholine, oxidized phosphatidylcholine, cardiolipin, phosphatidylserine, were obtained from Avanti Polar Lipids (Alabaster, AL, USA). 7-ketocholesterol, 7 alpha-hydroxycholesterol, 7 beta-hydroxycholesterol, and cholesterol which were purchased from Sigma (St. Louis, MO, USA), 24S-hydroxycholesterol was obtained from Steraloids (Newport, RI, USA). 7-α-hydroxycholesterol-d7, 7-β-hydroxycholesterol-d7, 26 (27)-OH cholesterol-d5, 24S-hydroxycholesterol-d6, 7-ketocholesterol-d7, lathosterol, and lathosterol-d4 were purchased from CDN Isotopes (Quebec, Canada). Arachidonic acid, arachidonic acid-d_8, 8-Iso-PGF$_2$a (8-iso-prostaglandin F$_{2a}$ or 15-F$_{2t}$-IsoP or iPF$_{2a}$-III), 8-iso-PGF$_{2a}$-d_4, 8-F$_{2t}$-IsoP-d$_4$ (iPF$_{2a}$-IV or 5S,9a,11a,-trihydroxy-1a,1b,1g-trihomo-18,19,20-trinor-8b-prosta-2Z,6E-dien-1-oic acid) and 5-F$_{2t}$-IsoP (iPF$_{2a}$-VI-d_4 or 5S,9a,11a,-trihydroxy-(8b)-prosta-6E,14Z-dien-1-oic acid) were purchased from Cayman Chemical (Ann Arbor, MI USA). All solvents used were HPLC grade.

Enzyme-linked Immunosorbent Assay (ELISA) and Lipid Quantification

Maxi-sorp plates (NUNC, Denmark) were coated with 5 ug/ml of lipids in EtOH evaporated for 2 hrs at RT. Plates were blocked with 0.8% collagen in PBS (Sigma-Aldrich, USA). Anti-lipid IgG responses were detected using goat-anti human IgG antibody conjugated with horseradish peroxidase (HRP) (Thermo Scientific Pierce, USA). TMB substrate (BD OptEIA^{TM}, BD Biosciences) was employed for 15 mins and colour development assayed at 450 nm using a Perkin-Elmer Victor^{3}V plate reader.

Lipid Extraction and Gas Chromatography-mass Spectrometry (GC- MS)

Lipids were extracted using a modified Folch method and hydrolysed in methanolic KOH [23]. COPs and F$_2$-Isoprostanes were then purified into 2 separate fractions by solid phase extraction on mixed mode anion exchange columns, dried under a stream of nitrogen, derivatised and injected onto an Agilent 5973/6890 GC-MS system as described previously [24]. Briefly, cholesterol oxidative products (COPs) were derivatised to generate their trimethyl silyl ether derivatives and analysed in the EI (electron ionization) mode. F$_2$-isoprostanes were derivatised to form their pentafluorobenzyl (PFB) ester, trimethyl silyl ether derivatives and analysed in the NCI (negative chemical ionization) mode. Quantification was achieved by relating peak area of samples with respective deuterated internal standards according to the previously published method [25]. 8-Iso-PGF$_2$a and 5-F$_{2t}$-IsoP F$_2$-isoprostane isomers co-eluted and were measured together as a single peak.

Lipid Extraction and Liquid Chromatography – Mass Spectrometry (LC – MS)

Phospholipids were extracted according to a modified protocol of Bligh and Dyer, 1959 [26]. Synthetic lipids obtained from Avanti Polar Lipids (Alabaster, AL, USA) were spiked as internal standards. The extracted lipids were measured using ABI 3200QT (Applied Biosystems, Foster City, CA) interfaced to a HPLC system using multiple reaction-monitoring mode [27]. Phospholipids were separated on a Phenomenex Luna 3 μ C18 column (150 mm×2 mm)(Phenomenex, Torrance, CA, USA). Signal intensities obtained for each lipid class were normalized to the appropriate internal standard.

Statistical Analysis

Differential levels of lipids or anti-lipid IgGs between time points were assessed in Prism (GraphPad Software) using the Wilcoxon nonparametric matched pairs test with a p<0.05 value considered significant in all cases. A correlation between different clinical parameters and anti-lipid IgG levels was examined using a Spearman nonparametric correlation and Linear regression tests.

Results

Total IgG Levels in SLE Patients Remain Unchanged during Therapy

A reduction in BILAG score was employed as the principal indicator for treatment success in our SLE patient cohort. We observed a decrease in this score as patients progressed from flare through follow-up period (Fig. 1a). Absolute levels of IgG in the patients' plasma remain unchanged at these time points (Fig. 1b).

In Table S1, we present BILAG scores for 8 systems: General (Gen), Mucocutaneous (Muc), Neurological (Cns), Musculoskeletal (Msk), Cardiovascular and Respiratory (Car), Vasculitis (Vas), Renal (Ren) and Haematological (Hae). As documented in this table, BILAG scores in SLE patients at 3-months and 12-months indicate that these patients have quiescent disease and can thus be combined as our follow-up cohort.

SLE Patients with Active Disease Exhibit Increased Levels of Lipid and Anti-lipid Responses

Gas chromatography-mass spectrometry (GC-MS) analyses indicate significantly higher levels of oxidized cholesterols in patients during flare versus follow-up. Specifically, 7-β-hydroxycholesterol, 7-ketocholesterol (Fig. 2bi, 2ci) were significantly increased. At the same time, 24S-hydroxycholesterol and 7-α-hydroxycholesterol levels remained unchanged (Fig. 2ai, 2di). Only five of the patients had a form of therapy aimed at reducing cholesterol levels-a combination of fenofibrate, pravastatin or simvastatin (Table S2). In four out of five patients, administration of lipid-lowering drugs started from the moment of flare and lasted over next 12 months. Administration of statins will reduce cholesterol levels. However, we have not addressed to what extent statins will affect levels of oxidized cholesterols over time in these patients. Anti-7-α-hydroxycholesterol IgG responses against oxysterols were significantly higher in patients with flare in comparison with the results obtained during the follow-up period (Fig. 2aii). The same trend was seen in anti-7-β-hydroxycholesterol and anti-7-ketocholesterol IgGs though these differences were not significant (Fig. 2bii and 2cii). Anti-24S-hydroxycholesterol IgG levels did not change over time (Fig. 2dii).

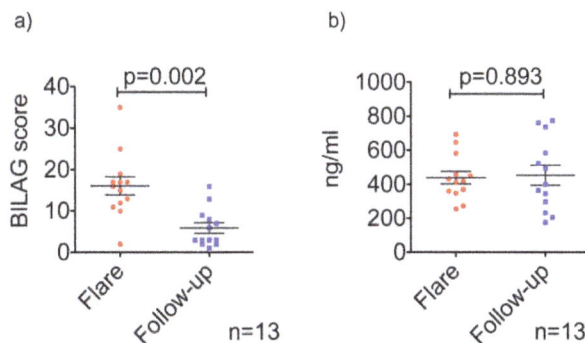

Figure 1. SLE disease activity score measured with the BILAG index reduces significantly over the time while total IgG levels remain the same. The British Isles Lupus Assessment Group (BILAG) index score during disease flare and the follow-up period. Figure 1a. A significant improvement is detectable over the time. Figure 1b. A level of total IgGs in patients' blood is similar during disease flares and in the follow-up period. p<0.05 value considered significant in Wilcoxon test.

38

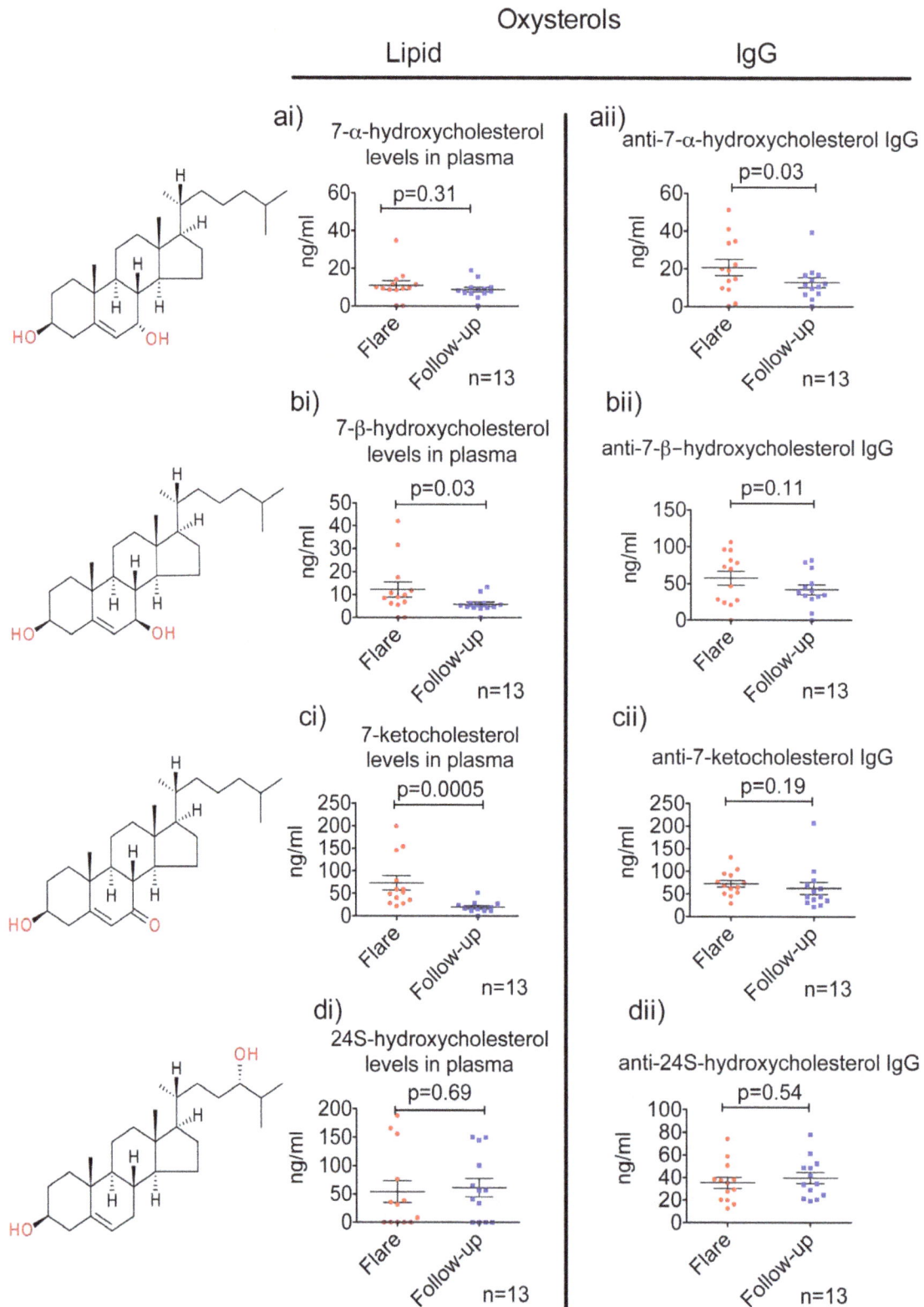

Figure 2. Levels of oxysterol and anti-oxysterol IgG in SLE patients' plasma. Analysis by GC-MS and ELISA show higher levels of oxidized cholesterols or anti-cholesterol IgGs in patients during flare versus follow-up period. Figure 2ai and 2 aii. 7-α-hydroxycholesterol levels and anti-7-α-hydroxycholesterol IgG levels in plasma. Figure 2bi and 2bii. 7-β-hydroxycholesterol levels and anti-7-β-hydroxycholesterol IgG levels in plasma. Figure 2ci and 2cii. 7-ketocholesterol levels and anti-7-ketocholesterol IgG levels in plasma. Figure 2di and 2dii. 24S-hydroxycholesterol levels and anti-24S-hydroxycholesterol IgG levels in plasma. $p < 0.05$ value was considered as significant in Wilcoxon test.

Levels of Oxidatively Modified Unsaturated Fatty Acids and Anti-lipid Antibodies Change during Therapy

Mass-spectroscopy analyses of phosphatidylserine during the flare and follow-up period suggest a reduction in this lipid over time (Fig. 3ai). Also, anti-phosphatidylserine IgG levels tend to increase during the follow-up period (Fig. 3aii).

Normalized values for isoprostanes (normalized against arachidonic acid (AA)) significantly decrease from the moment of flare (Fig. 3bi and 3ci). We employed 15-F2t-IsoP as the antigen in this assay where we measured anti-isoprostane IgG response (Fig. 3bii). Anti-15-F2t-IsoP IgG exhibited a trend of higher levels in flare compared to follow-up.

Anti-lipid IgG Levels for Other Lipids also Change during Therapy

Lathosterol is a precursor of cholesterol and we detected significantly higher anti-lathosterol IgG responses in patients with flare (Fig. 4ai). Phospholipids and anti-phospholipid antibodies are often seen in autoimmune disorders and are associated with cerebrovascular disease or moderate-to-severe cognitive dysfunction. In our study we detected significantly higher levels of anti-cardiolipin (Fig. 4aii) and anti-oxidized phopsphatidylcholine in flare (Fig. 4bii). Anti-phopsphatidylcholine IgG in patients with flare was also increased (Fig. 4bi).

Levels of Anti-lipid Antibodies Negatively Correlate with BILAG Scores

We analyzed our lipid anti-lipid data for correlations with a score of disease activity in SLE. For those analyses we included an additional 7 SLE patients for which we had BILAG scores during the flare. In total we analyzed 20 patients. Spearman correlation and linear regression tests showed that anti-24S hydroxycholesterol IgG, anti-cardiolipin IgG and anti-phosphatidylserine IgG, negatively correlate with BILAG score – the disease activity index (Fig. 5ai, 5aii, 5bi respectively). A similar, although not significant trend was seen in anti-7-α hydroxycholesterol IgGs (Fig. 5bii). A higher level of these anti-lipid antibodies was observed in patients with lower BILAG scores suggesting that these may be markers for improved prognosis.

Discussion

In SLE, the heterogeneity of disease presentations in patient populations combined with a poor understanding of the underlying pathological mechanisms result in challenges for successful disease management. The American College of Rheumatology classification utilizes 11 criteria for diagnosis of lupus, of which a patient must meet four [28]. Several computerised indices for measuring clinical disease activity in Systemic Lupus Erythematosus are employed in clinical practice- BILAG, SLEDAI, LUMINA [29–32]. Despite advances in treatment protocols there remains a dearth of good diagnostic and prognostic biomarkers to facilitate improvements in disease characterization and management [33–35]. Moreover, the immune modulating treatment used for SLE remains a significant problem with many patients developing treatment-associated complications [36]. Thus, the identification of biomarkers that correlate with a good response to therapy will have an impact on treatment-associated side-effects where less-aggressive approaches can be employed [33].

In our lipidomic and immunologic approaches we have identified a new corpus of biomarkers relevant to this disease. This study focused on a clinically well-defined SLE cohort that was monitored over a period of 12 months. Based on clinical score and

statistical tests, we grouped samples provided between 3 and 12 months post-therapy as our follow-up cohort. This approach enabled us to apply statistical tests for paired samples.

We were also interested in correlations between lipid/anti-lipid IgG levels and BILAG scores during disease flares. In this case we did not need paired samples and thus employed 20 samples in total.

We have identified new targets that correlate with disease score. Our approach employed gas chromatography-mass spectrometry (GC-MS) and liquid chromatography-mass spectrometry (LC-MS) to investigate the lipids of interest. The presence of anti-lipid autoantibodies was confirmed by an enzyme-linked immunosorbent assay where we focused on the immunoglobulin isotype G.

Our high-resolution analysis has identified a cohort of new anti-lipid autoantibodies. Whilst total IgG levels remain consistent during therapy, we detected differential levels of anti-lipid IgGs for four different lipid species: lathosterol; enzymatically produced oxysterols 7-α-hydroxycholesterol and oxidatively modified phospholipids – cardiolipin, and oxidized phosphatidylcholine.

The measurement of oxygenated cholesterol species remains technically challenging based on the proposed auto-oxidation that can occur during lipid derivation, processing or storage from biological samples. [37–39]. In our study plasma levels of oxysterols showed a general trend of decrease over time. Thus, if auto-oxidation occurs, it should happen at a similar level in all samples tested without a significant influence on absolute ratios. The main conclusion of this study concerns relationships between anti-lipid antibodies and BILAG score. Anti-lipid antibodies identified in lupus patients' plasma are part of an autoimmune response that targets lipid antigens. These develop as a result of pathogenic processes in the afflicted patients. Thus, antibodies from SLE patient's plasma should not target oxidized cholesterols that are result of in vitro auto-oxidation processes (e.g. during the ELISA plate coating with lipid-antigen). We found similar levels of anti-24S-hydroxycholesterol IgGs between flare and follow-up (Fig. 2dii). There was no significant difference in IgG levels against 27-hydroxycholesterol when analyzing the same time points (data not shown). Phosphatidylserine levels in plasma showed a trend of reduction over the time. Anti-cardiolipin antibodies are one of several anti-phospholipid antibodies that have been previously identified in SLE patients [40] where cardiolipin present on the surface of apoptotic cells acts as an immunologic trigger for the production of the autoantibodies [41].

Isoprostanes are generated by the free radical-mediated peroxidation of arachidonic acid (AA) [42]. 15-F2t-IsoP is a marker of free radical damage and lipid peroxidation in vivo that is formed by free radical catalysis of arachidonic acid [43]. Serum levels of 15-iso-PGF2alpha and 8-iso-PGF2alpha in SLE patients showed a significantly higher level at flare compared to the post-therapy period.

BILAG is currently accepted as the best disease activity score in SLE [22] and thus we analyzed which if any of our lipid/anti-lipid parameters correlate. We observed that anti-phosphatidylserine, anti-cardiolipin and anti-24S hydroxycholesterol IgG negatively correlate with the BILAG score. Anti-7-α-hydroxycholesterol IgGs also show trend of negative correlation with BILAG score. However, for this anti-lipid response we were not able to confirm a statistically significant correlation.

At the same time points we were not able to detect statistically significant correlations between BILAG scores and one traditional SLE biomarker - anti-DNA antibodies (data not shown). This can potentially be explained by the fact that anti-DNA antibodies are found in only 60% of SLE patients and those antibodies are particularly associated with lupus nephritis [44].

Unsaturated fatty acids

| Lipid | IgG |

ai)

Phosphatidylserine levels in plasma

p=0.057

aii)

anti-phosphatidylserine IgG

p=0.278

bi)

F2-isoprostanes $(15-F_{2t}\text{-IsoP} + 5-F_{2t}\text{-IsoP})$/AA levels in plasma

p=0.01

bii)

anti-15-F_{2t}-IsoP IgG

p=0.21

ci)

F2-isoprostanes $(8-F_{2t}\text{-IsoP})$/AA levels in plasma

p=0.0002

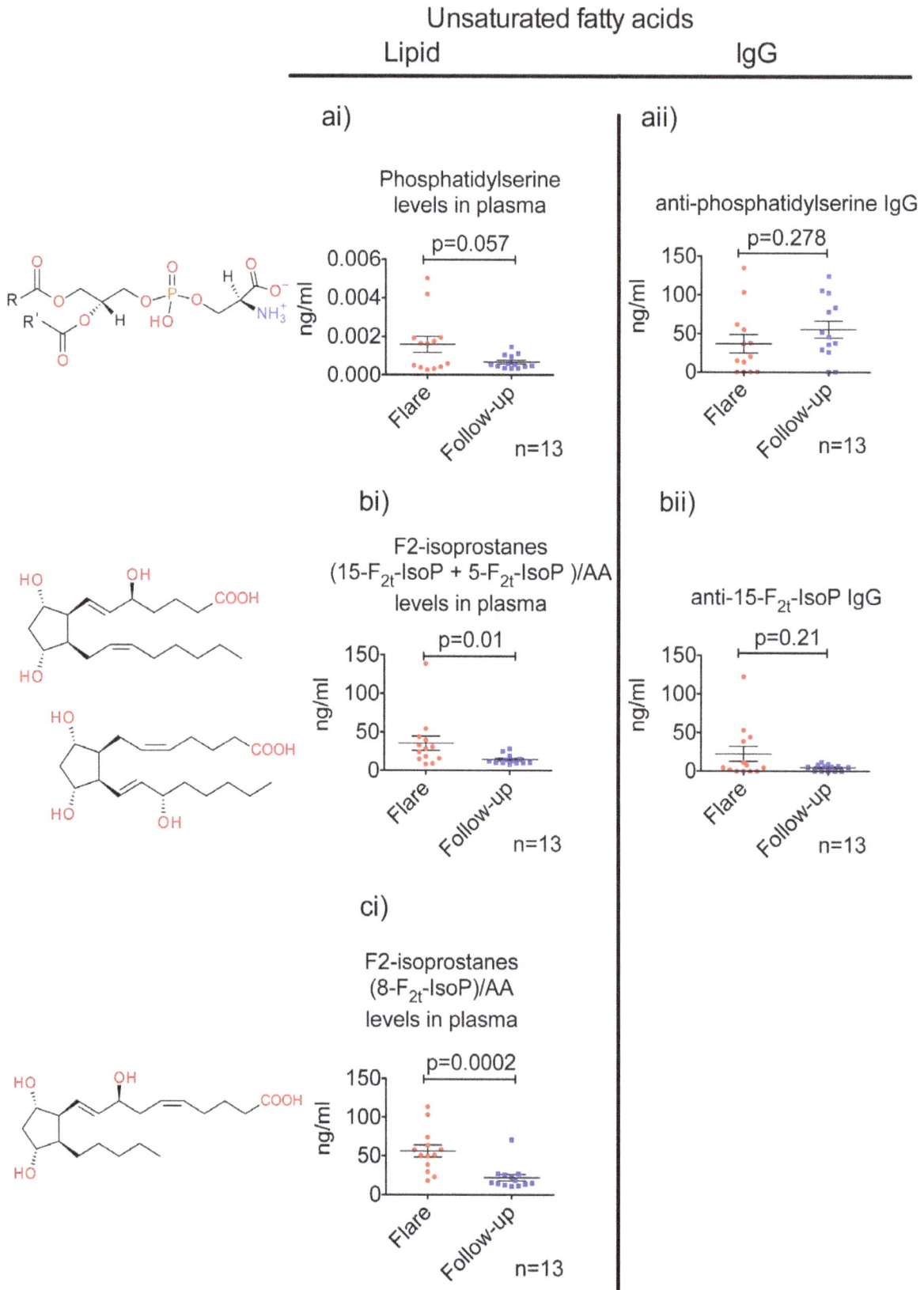

Figure 3. Levels of unsaturated fatty acids and anti-unsaturated fatty acids IgG in SLE patients' plasma. Figure 3ai and 3aii. Phosphatidylserine levels and anti-phosphatidylserine IgG levels in plasma. Figure 3bi and 3bii. Isoprostane (15-F_{2t}-IsoP +5-F_{2t}-IsoP) levels normalized against AA values and anti-15-F_{2t}-IsoP IgG levels in plasma. Figure 3ci. Isoprostane (8-F_{2t}-IsoP) levels normalized against AA values. $p<0.05$ value was considered as significant in Wilcoxon test.

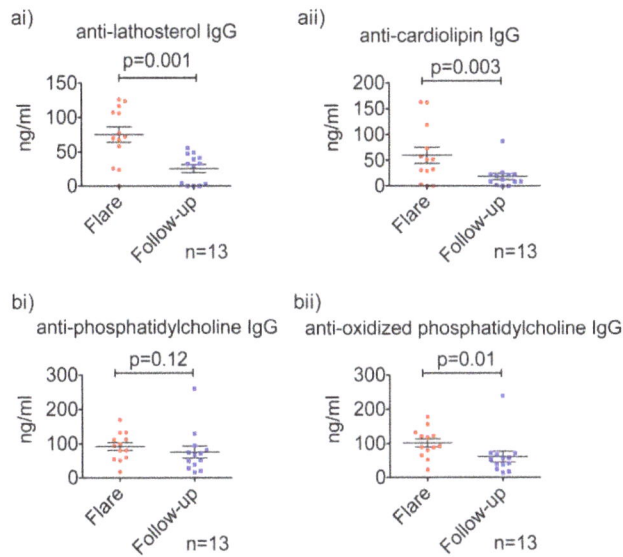

Figure 4. Anti-lipid responses against lathosterol, cardiolipin, phosphatidylcholine and oxidized-phosphatidylcholine. Figure 4ai anti-lathosterol IgG levels in plasma. Figure 4aii anti-cardiolipin IgG levels in plasma. Figure 4bi anti-phosphatidylcholine IgG levels in plasma. Figure 4bi anti-oxidized phosphatidylcholine IgG levels in plasma. $p < 0.05$ value considered significant in Wilcoxon test.

cells in the liver [45–46]; or reduced levels of lipids and their corresponding anti-lipid antibodies in plasma are a consequence of deposition of immune complexes in the tissues. Both of these mechanisms are currently under investigation in our laboratory.

It is an interesting observation that levels of anti-lipid IgGs for 24S-hydroxycholesterol and phosphatidylserine remained very similar over the time period of study. Since levels of these antibodies negatively correlate with BILAG score at the time of flare, one explanation could be that their presence during the post-flare period might have a protective role. For the actual levels of phosphatidylserine we saw a trend of reduction between flare and follow-up. This phenomenon suggests that either oxidation processes in unsaturated fatty acids were reduced or the development of phosphatidylserine immune complexes intensified over time.

IgM autoantibodies have been linked to apoptosis-associated antigen clearance [47–48]. IgM anti-phosphorylcholine was shown to be notably higher in patients with low SELENA-SLEDAI disease activity index [47]. Those patients encountered less cardiovascular and renal problems and high levels of IgM are attributed to the homeostatic and protective roles [47]. The panel of auto-antigens that appear during the apoptosis is large and further identification of protective IgG and IgM antibodies is required.

Clinical and laboratory markers currently used in SLE have moderate utility based on specificity and sensitivity. Based on our findings, we suggest that the measurement of anti-lipid IgGs for 24S-hydroxycholesterol, cardiolipin and phosphatidylserine may be used as a sensitive and non-invasive method of surveillance during treatment. These therefore represent improved biomarkers for the evaluation and development of better therapeutic strategies aimed at reducing treatment associated morbidity and mortality, a significant problem in SLE.

The negative correlations observed can be explained by two possible mechanisms: the presence of anti-lipid IgG during flare may be beneficial and aid immune complex clearance through IgG receptors expressed on phagocytic cells such as the Kuppfer

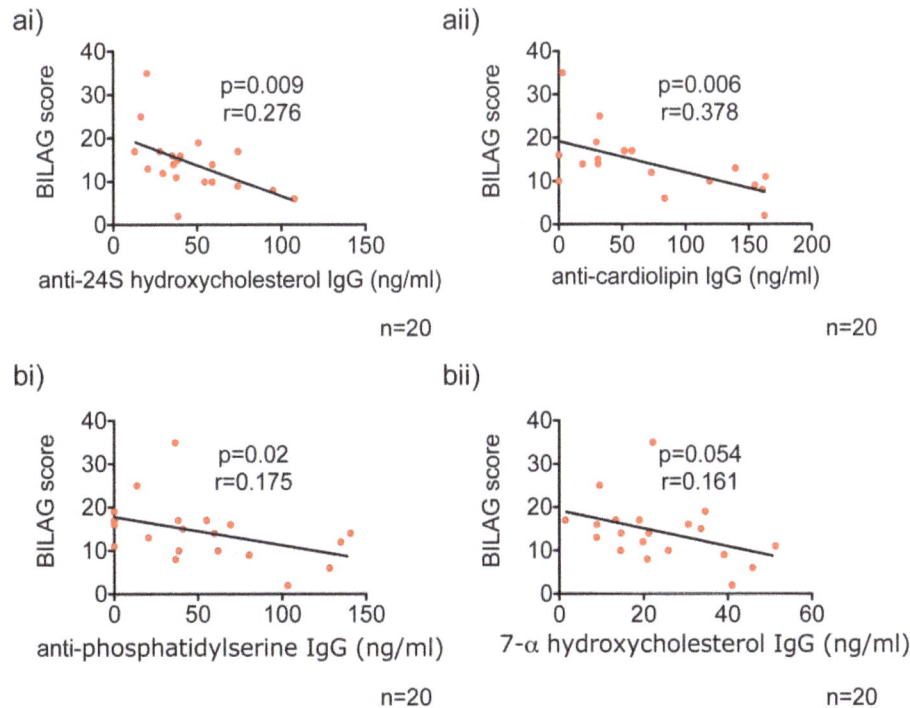

Figure 5. Biomarker candidates that correlate with BILAG scores. Figure 5ai, 5bi, 5ci. Anti-24S hydroxycholesterol IgG, anti-cardiolipin IgG and anti-phosphatidylserine IgG levels negatively correlate with BILAG scores. Figure 5bii. Anti-7-α-hydroxycholesterol IgG levels also show trend of negative correlation with BILAG scores. $p < 0.05$ value was considered as significant in Spearman correlation and Linear regression tests.

Supporting Information

Table S1 BILAG scores summary for three different time-points. BILAG scores (A-E) for 8 headings: General (Gen), Mucocutaneous (Muc), Neurological (Cns), Musculoskeletal (Msk), Cardiovascular and Respiratory (Car), Vasculitis (Vas), Renal (Ren) and Haematological (Hae). Time point of flare is represented with 13 patients' samples (patients C4, C5, C8, C10, C13, C15, C16, C17, C18, C19, C20, C22 and C24). Follow-up group consists of patients' samples from time-point of 3 months (patients C4, C5, C13, C15, C16, C17, C18 and C24) and time-point of 12 months post treatment (patients C8, C10, C19, C20 and C22).

Table S2 Statin administration in SLE patients. Five SLE patients out of thirteen received cholesterol-lowering therapy.

Acknowledgments

We thank the SLE patients and blood donors from Addenbrooke's Hospital, Cambridge, UK.

Author Contributions

Conceived and designed the experiments: VJ NAZ YTL ANAP SJHC EHXP FCL GS AMJ LB EFM PAL MDK KGCS MRW PAM. Performed the experiments: VJ NAZ YTL ANAP SJHC EHXP FCL GS AMJ. Analyzed the data: VJ NAZ YTL ANAP EHXP FCL AMJ LB EFM PAL MDK KGCS MRW PAM. Contributed reagents/materials/analysis tools: VJ NAZ YTL ANAP GS AMJ LB EFM PAL MDK KGCS MRW PAM. Wrote the paper: VJ NAZ YTL ANAP SJHC EHXP FCL GS AMJ LB EFM PAL MDK KGCS MRW PAM.

References

1. Mok CC, Lau CS (2003) Pathogenesis of systemic lupus erythematosus. J Clin Pathol 56: 481–490.
2. Tenbrock K, Juang YT, Kyttaris VC, Tsokos GC (2007) Altered signal transduction in SLE T cells. Rheumatology (Oxford) 46: 1525–1530.
3. Jenks SA, Sanz I (2009) Altered B cell receptor signaling in human systemic lupus erythematosus. Autoimmun Rev 8: 209–213.
4. Pascual V, Banchereau J, Palucka AK (2003) The central role of dendritic cells and interferon-alpha in SLE. Curr Opin Rheumatol 15: 548–556.
5. Kirou KA, Salmon JE, Crow MK (2006) Soluble mediators as therapeutic targets in systemic lupus erythematosus: cytokines, immunoglobulin receptors, and the complement system. Rheum Dis Clin North Am 32: 103–119, ix.
6. Munoz LE, Gaipl US, Herrmann M (2008) Predictive value of anti-dsDNA autoantibodies: importance of the assay. Autoimmun Rev 7: 594–597.
7. Munoz LE, Lauber K, Schiller M, Manfredi AA, Herrmann M (2010) The role of defective clearance of apoptotic cells in systemic autoimmunity. Nat Rev Rheumatol 6: 280–289.
8. Gaipl US, Kuhn A, Sheriff A, Munoz LE, Franz S, et al. (2006) Clearance of apoptotic cells in human SLE. Curr Dir Autoimmun 9: 173–187.
9. Niederer HA, Willcocks LC, Rayner TF, Yang W, Lau YL, et al. (2010) Copy number, linkage disequilibrium and disease association in the FCGR locus. Hum Mol Genet 19: 3282–3294.
10. Bjorkhem I, Meaney S, Diczfalusy U (2002) Oxysterols in human circulation: which role do they have? Curr Opin Lipidol 13: 247–253.
11. Brown AJ, Jessup W (2009) Oxysterols: Sources, cellular storage and metabolism, and new insights into their roles in cholesterol homeostasis. Mol Aspects Med 30: 111–122.
12. Lutjohann D, Breuer O, Ahlborg G, Nennesmo I, Siden A, et al. (1996) Cholesterol homeostasis in human brain: evidence for an age-dependent flux of 24S-hydroxycholesterol from the brain into the circulation. Proc Natl Acad Sci U S A 93: 9799–9804.
13. Bjorkhem I, Lutjohann D, Diczfalusy U, Stahle L, Ahlborg G, et al. (1998) Cholesterol homeostasis in human brain: turnover of 24S-hydroxycholesterol and evidence for a cerebral origin of most of this oxysterol in the circulation. J Lipid Res 39: 1594–1600.
14. Lutjohann D, Papassotiropoulos A, Bjorkhem I, Locatelli S, Bagli M, et al. (2000) Plasma 24S-hydroxycholesterol (cerebrosterol) is increased in Alzheimer and vascular demented patients. J Lipid Res 41: 195–198.
15. Leoni V, Masterman T, Diczfalusy U, De Luca G, Hillert J, et al. (2002) Changes in human plasma levels of the brain specific oxysterol 24S-hydroxycholesterol during progression of multiple sclerosis. Neurosci Lett 331: 163–166.
16. Qin J, Goswami R, Balabanov R, Dawson G (2007) Oxidized phosphatidylcholine is a marker for neuroinflammation in multiple sclerosis brain. J Neurosci Res 85: 977–984.
17. Seet RC, Lee CY, Lim EC, Tan JJ, Quek AM, et al. (2010) Oxidative damage in Parkinson disease: Measurement using accurate biomarkers. Free Radic Biol Med 48: 560–566.
18. Berthier A, Lemaire-Ewing S, Prunet C, Montange T, Vejux A, et al. (2005) 7-Ketocholesterol-induced apoptosis. Involvement of several pro-apoptotic but also anti-apoptotic calcium-dependent transduction pathways. FEBS J 272: 3093–3104.
19. Kritharides L, Kus M, Brown AJ, Jessup W, Dean RT (1996) Hydroxypropyl-beta-cyclodextrin-mediated efflux of 7-ketocholesterol from macrophage foam cells. J Biol Chem 271: 27450–27455.
20. Li W, Johnson H, Yuan XM, Jonasson L (2009) 7beta-hydroxycholesterol induces natural killer cell death via oxidative lysosomal destabilization. Free Radic Res 43: 1072–1079.
21. McKinney EF, Lyons PA, Carr EJ, Hollis JL, Jayne DR, et al. (2010) A CD8+ T cell transcription signature predicts prognosis in autoimmune disease. Nat Med 16: 586–591, 581p following 591.
22. Isenberg DA, Rahman A, Allen E, Farewell V, Akil M, et al. (2005) BILAG 2004. Development and initial validation of an updated version of the British Isles Lupus Assessment Group's disease activity index for patients with systemic lupus erythematosus. Rheumatology (Oxford) 44: 902–906.
23. Folch J, Lees M, Sloane Stanley GH (1957) A simple method for the isolation and purification of total lipides from animal tissues. J Biol Chem 226: 497–509.
24. Kim JH, Jittiwat J, Ong WY, Farooqui AA, Jenner AM (2010) Changes in cholesterol biosynthetic and transport pathways after excitotoxicity. J Neurochem 112: 34–41.
25. Cheng D, Jenner AM, Shui G, Cheong WF, Mitchell TW, et al. (2011) Lipid pathway alterations in Parkinson's disease primary visual cortex. PLoS One 6: e17299.
26. Bligh EG, Dyer WJ (1959) A rapid method of total lipid extraction and purification. Can J Biochem Physiol 37: 911–917.
27. Shui G, Stebbins JW, Lam BD, Cheong WF, Lam SM, et al. (2011) Comparative plasma lipidome between human and cynomolgus monkey: are plasma polar lipids good biomarkers for diabetic monkeys? PLoS One 6: e19731.
28. Tan EM, Cohen AS, Fries JF, Masi AT, McShane DJ, et al. (1982) The 1982 revised criteria for the classification of systemic lupus erythematosus. Arthritis Rheum 25: 1271–1277.
29. Hay EM, Bacon PA, Gordon C, Isenberg DA, Maddison P, et al. (1993) The BILAG index: a reliable and valid instrument for measuring clinical disease activity in systemic lupus erythematosus. Q J Med 86: 447–458.
30. Isenberg DA, Gordon C (2000) From BILAG to BLIPS–disease activity assessment in lupus past, present and future. Lupus 9: 651–654.
31. Bombardier C, Gladman DD, Urowitz MB, Caron D, Chang CH (1992) Derivation of the SLEDAI. A disease activity index for lupus patients. The Committee on Prognosis Studies in SLE. Arthritis Rheum 35: 630–640.
32. Alarcon GS, Roseman J, Bartolucci AA, Friedman AW, Moulds JM, et al. (1998) Systemic lupus erythematosus in three ethnic groups: II. Features predictive of disease activity early in its course. LUMINA Study Group. Lupus in minority populations, nature versus nurture. Arthritis Rheum 41: 1173–1180.
33. Smith MF Jr, Hiepe F, Dorner T, Burmester G (2009) Biomarkers as tools for improved diagnostic and therapeutic monitoring in systemic lupus erythematosis. Arthritis Res Ther 11: 255.
34. Francis L, Perl A (2009) Pharmacotherapy of systemic lupus erythematosus. Expert Opin Pharmacother 10: 1481–1494.
35. Liu CC, Manzi S, Ahearn JM (2005) Biomarkers for systemic lupus erythematosus: a review and perspective. Curr Opin Rheumatol 17: 543–549.
36. Smith RM, Clatworthy MR, Jayne DR (2010) Biological therapy for lupus nephritis-tribulations and trials. Nat Rev Rheumatol 6: 547–552.
37. Bjorkhem I, Lovgren-Sandblom A, Piehl F, Khademi M, Pettersson H, et al. (2011) High levels of 15-oxygenated steroids in circulation of patients with multiple sclerosis: fact or fiction? J Lipid Res 52: 170–174.
38. Griffiths WJ, Wang Y (2010) Are 15-oxygenated sterols present in the human circulation? J Lipid Res 52: 4–5.
39. Bjorkhem I, Diczfalusy U, Olsson T, Russell DW, McDonald JG, et al. (2011) Detecting oxysterols in the human circulation. Nat Immunol 12: 577; author reply 577–578.
40. Descloux E, Durieu I, Cochat P, Vital Durand D, Ninet J, et al. (2008) Paediatric systemic lupus erythematosus: prognostic impact of antiphospholipid antibodies. Rheumatology (Oxford) 47: 183–187.
41. Sorice M, Circella A, Misasi R, Pittoni V, Garofalo T, et al. (2000) Cardiolipin on the surface of apoptotic cells as a possible trigger for antiphospholipids antibodies. Clin Exp Immunol 122: 277–284.

42. Morrow JD, Hill KE, Burk RF, Nammour TM, Badr KF, et al. (1990) A series of prostaglandin F2-like compounds are produced in vivo in humans by a non-cyclooxygenase, free radical-catalyzed mechanism. Proc Natl Acad Sci U S A 87: 9383–9387.

43. Basu S (2008) F2-isoprostanes in human health and diseases: from molecular mechanisms to clinical implications. Antioxid Redox Signal 10: 1405–1434.

44. Smith PP, Gordon C (2010) Systemic lupus erythematosus: clinical presentations. Autoimmun Rev 10: 43–45.

45. Bilzer M, Roggel F, Gerbes AL (2006) Role of Kupffer cells in host defense and liver disease. Liver Int 26: 1175–1186.

46. Kosugi I, Muro H, Shirasawa H, Ito I (1992) Endocytosis of soluble IgG immune complex and its transport to lysosomes in hepatic sinusoidal endothelial cells. J Hepatol 16: 106–114.

47. Gronwall C, Akhter E, Oh C, Burlingame RW, Petri M, et al. (2012) IgM autoantibodies to distinct apoptosis-associated antigens correlate with protection from cardiovascular events and renal disease in patients with SLE. Clin Immunol 142: 390–398.

48. Mehrani T, Petri M (2011) IgM anti-beta2 glycoprotein I is protective against lupus nephritis and renal damage in systemic lupus erythematosus. J Rheumatol 38: 450–453.

49. Leoni V, Masterman T, Mousavi FS, Wretlind B, Wahlund LO, et al. (2004) Diagnostic use of cerebral and extracerebral oxysterols. Clin Chem Lab Med 42: 186–191.

50. Shafaati M, Marutle A, Pettersson H, Lovgren-Sandblom A, Olin M, et al. (2011) Marked accumulation of 27-hydroxycholesterol in the brain of Alzheimer patients with the Swedish APP 670/671 mutation. J Lipid Res.

51. Schule R, Siddique T, Deng HX, Yang Y, Donkervoort S, et al. (2010) Marked accumulation of 27-hydroxycholesterol in SPG5 patients with hereditary spastic paresis. J Lipid Res 51: 819–823.

52. Yasunobu Y, Hayashi K, Shingu T, Yamagata T, Kajiyama G, et al. (2001) Coronary atherosclerosis and oxidative stress as reflected by autoantibodies against oxidized low-density lipoprotein and oxysterols. Atherosclerosis 155: 445–453.

53. Leoni V, Lutjohann D, Masterman T (2005) Levels of 7-oxocholesterol in cerebrospinal fluid are more than one thousand times lower than reported in multiple sclerosis. J Lipid Res 46: 191–195.

54. Navarra SV, Ishimori ML, Uy EA, Hamijoyo L, Sama J, et al. (2010) Studies of Filipino patients with systemic lupus erythematosus (SLE): Autoantibody profile of first degree relatives. Lupus.

55. Fusaro AE, Fahl K, Cardoso EC, de Brito CA, Jacob CM, et al. (2010) Profile of autoantibodies against phosphorylcholine and cross-reactivity to oxidation-specific neoantigens in selective IgA deficiency with or without autoimmune diseases. J Clin Immunol 30: 872–880.

56. Ortona E, Capozzi A, Colasanti T, Conti F, Alessandri C, et al. (2010) Vimentin/cardiolipin complex as a new antigenic target of the antiphospholipid syndrome. Blood 116: 2960–2967.

57. Abou-Raya A, el-Hallous D, Fayed H (2004) 8-Isoprostaglandin F2 alpha: a potential index of lipid peroxidation in systemic lupus erythematosus. Clin Invest Med 27: 306–311.

58. Ames PR, Alves J, Murat I, Isenberg DA, Nourooz-Zadeh J (1999) Oxidative stress in systemic lupus erythematosus and allied conditions with vascular involvement. Rheumatology (Oxford) 38: 529–534.

59. Szodoray P, Tarr T, Tumpek J, Kappelmayer J, Lakos G, et al. (2009) Identification of rare anti-phospholipid/protein co-factor autoantibodies in patients with systemic lupus erythematosus. Autoimmunity 42: 497–506.

60. Zuliani G, Donnorso MP, Bosi C, Passaro A, Dalla Nora E, et al. (2011) Plasma 24S-hydroxycholesterol levels in elderly subjects with late onset Alzheimer's disease or vascular dementia: a case-control study. BMC Neurol 11: 121.

Association of Increased Frequencies of *HLA-DPB1*05:01* with the Presence of Anti-Ro/SS-A and Anti-La/SS-B Antibodies in Japanese Rheumatoid Arthritis and Systemic Lupus Erythematosus Patients

Hiroshi Furukawa[1]*, Shomi Oka[1], Kota Shimada[2], Shoji Sugii[2], Atsushi Hashimoto[3], Akiko Komiya[1], Naoshi Fukui[1], Tatsuo Nagai[4], Shunsei Hirohata[4], Keigo Setoguchi[5], Akira Okamoto[6], Noriyuki Chiba[7], Eiichi Suematsu[8], Taiichiro Miyashita[9], Kiyoshi Migita[9], Akiko Suda[10], Shouhei Nagaoka[10], Naoyuki Tsuchiya[11], Shigeto Tohma[1]

1 Clinical Research Center for Allergy and Rheumatology, Sagamihara Hospital, National Hospital Organization, Sagamihara, Japan, 2 Department of Rheumatology, Tokyo Metropolitan Tama Medical Center, Fuchu, Japan, 3 Department of Rheumatology, Sagamihara Hospital, National Hospital Organization, Sagamihara, Japan, 4 Department of Rheumatology and Infectious Disease, Kitasato University School of Medicine, Sagamihara, Japan, 5 Allergy and Immunological Diseases, Tokyo Metropolitan Cancer and Infectious Diseases Center Komagome Hospital, Tokyo, Japan, 6 Department of Rheumatology, Himeji Medical Center, National Hospital Organization, Himeji, Japan, 7 Department of Rheumatology, Morioka Hospital, National Hospital Organization, Morioka, Japan, 8 Department of Internal Medicine and Rheumatology, Clinical Research Institute, National Hospital Organization, Kyushu Medical Center, Fukuoka, Japan, 9 Nagasaki Medical Center, National Hospital Organization, Omura, Japan, 10 Department of Rheumatology, Yokohama Minami Kyosai Hospital, Yokohama, Japan, 11 Molecular and Genetic Epidemiology Laboratory, Faculty of Medicine, University of Tsukuba, Tsukuba, Japan

Abstract

Introduction: Autoantibodies to ribonucleoprotein are associated with a variety of autoimmune diseases, including rheumatoid arthritis (RA). Many studies on associations between human leukocyte antigen (HLA) alleles and RA have been reported, but few have been validated in RA subpopulations with anti-La/SS-B or anti-Ro/SS-A antibodies. Here, we investigated associations of *HLA class II* alleles with the presence of anti-Ro/SS-A or anti-La/SS-B antibodies in RA.

Methods: An association study was conducted for *HLA-DRB1, DQB1,* and *DPB1* in Japanese RA and systemic lupus erythematosus (SLE) patients that were positive or negative for anti-Ro/SS-A and/or anti-La/SS-B antibodies.

Results: An increased prevalence of certain class II alleles was associated with the presence of anti-Ro/SS-A antibodies as follows: *DRB1*08:03* ($Pc = 3.79 \times 10^{-5}$, odds ratio [OR] 3.06, 95% confidence interval [CI] 1.98–4.73), *DQB1*06:01* ($Pc = 0.0106$, OR 1.70, 95%CI 1.26–2.31), and *DPB1*05:01* ($Pc = 0.0040$, OR 1.55, 95%CI 1.23–1.96). On the other hand, *DRB1*15:01* ($Pc = 0.0470$, OR 3.14, 95%CI 1.63–6.05), *DQB1*06:02* ($Pc = 0.0252$, OR 3.14, 95%CI 1.63–6.05), and *DPB1*05:01* ($Pc = 0.0069$, OR 2.27, 95% CI 1.44–3.57) were associated with anti-La/SS-B antibodies. The *DPB1*05:01* allele was associated with anti-Ro/SS-A ($Pc = 0.0408$, OR 1.69, 95% CI 1.19–2.41) and anti-La/SS-B antibodies ($Pc = 2.48 \times 10^{-5}$, OR 3.31, 95%CI 2.02–5.43) in SLE patients.

Conclusion: HLA-DPB1*05:01 was the only allele associated with the presence of both anti-Ro/SS-A and anti-La/SS-B antibodies in Japanese RA and SLE patients.

Editor: Silke Appel, University of Bergen, Norway

Funding: This work was supported by Grants-in-Aid for Scientific Research (B, C) (22390199, 22591090) and for Young Scientists (24791018) from the Japan Society for the Promotion of Science, Health and Labour Science Research, Grants from the Ministry of Health, Labour, and Welfare of Japan, Grants-in-Aid for Clinical Research from National Hospital Organization, Research Grants from Daiwa Securities Health Foundation, Research Grants from Japan Research Foundation for Clinical Pharmacology, Research Grants from The Nakatomi Foundation, Research Grants from the Takeda Science Foundation, and research grants from pharmaceutical companies: Abbott Japan Co., Ltd., Astellas Pharma Inc., Chugai Pharmaceutical Co., Ltd., Eisai Co., Ltd., Mitsubishi Tanabe Pharma Corporation, Merck Sharp and Dohme Inc., Pfizer Japan Inc., Takeda Pharmaceutical Company Limited and Teijin Pharma Limited. The funders had no role in study design, data collection and analysis, decision to publish, or preparing the manuscript.

Competing Interests: HF has the following conflicts. The following funders are supported in whole or in part by the indicated pharmaceutical companies. The Japan Research Foundation for Clinical Pharmacology is run by Daiichi Sankyo, the Takeda Science Foundation is supported by an endowment from Takeda Pharmaceutical Company and the Nakatomi Foundation was established by Hisamitsu Pharmaceutical Co., Inc. The Daiwa Securities Health Foundation was established by Daiwa Securities Group Inc. ST was supported by research grants from nine pharmaceutical companies: Abbott Japan Co., Ltd., Astellas Pharma Inc., Chugai Pharmaceutical Co., Ltd., Eisai Co., Ltd., Mitsubishi Tanabe Pharma Corporation, Merck Sharp and Dohme Inc., Pfizer Japan Inc., Takeda Pharmaceutical Company Limited, and Teijin Pharma Limited. NT is supported by the Takeda Science Foundation, which is supported by an endowment from the Takeda Pharmaceutical Company. The other authors declare no financial or commercial conflicts of interest.

* E-mail: h-furukawa@sagamihara-hosp.gr.jp

Table 1. Characteristics of RA and SLE patients.

	Ro(+)La(−)RA	Ro(+)La(+)RA	Ro(−)La(−)RA	P [Ro(+)La(−) vs. Ro(−)La(−)]	P [Ro(+)La(+) vs. Ro(−)La(−)]
Number	181	40	704		
Mean age, years (SD)	59.8 (13.1)	59.6 (12.2)	63.9 (11.8)	0.0002*	0.0390*
Male, n (%)	15 (8.3)	0 (0.0)	143 (20.5)	0.0001	0.0003
Disease duration, years (SD)	14.3 (10.3)	17.7 (13.5)	14.3 (10.9)	0.9940*	0.1017*
Steinbrocker stage III and IV, n (%)	75 (51.0)	18 (62.1)	311 (57.4)	0.1897	0.7019
Association of secondary SS, n (%)	34 (18.8)	12 (30.0)	26 (3.7)	1.41×10^{-10}	1.07×10^{-7}
Rheumatoid factor positive, n (%)	146 (89.0)	30 (88.2)	545 (87.6)	0.6878	1.0000
ACPA positive, n (%)	135 (87.1)	30 (96.8)	506 (91.8)	0.0832	0.4999

	Ro(+)La(−)SLE	Ro(+)La(+)SLE	Ro(−)La(−)SLE	P [Ro(+)La(−) vs. Ro(−)La(−)]	P [Ro(+)La(+) vs. Ro(−)La(−)]
Number	129	45	137		
Mean age, years (SD)	49.1 (15.3)	46.0 (15.5)	50.0 (14.7)	0.7118*	0.1676*
Male, n (%)	11 (8.5)	2 (4.4)	15 (10.9)	0.5417	0.2483
Disease duration, years (SD)	13.3 (12.1)	7.2 (5.8)	15.6 (12.1)	0.1656*	0.0001*
Association of secondary SS, n (%)	6 (4.7)	3 (6.7)	1 (0.7)	0.0598	0.0473
Anti-dsDNA antibody positive, n (%)	104 (80.6)	31 (68.9)	104 (75.9)	0.3948	0.2720

SS: Sjögren's syndrome, RA: rheumatoid arthritis, SLE: systemic lupus erythematosus, ACPA: anti-citrullinated peptide antibody, dsDNA: double-stranded-DNA, Ro(+)La(−): anti-Ro/SS-A-positive but anti-La/SS-B-negative, Ro(+)La(+): anti-Ro/SS-A- and anti-La/SS-B-positive, Ro(−)La(−): anti-Ro/SS-A- and anti-La/SS-B-negative. Association was tested by Fisher's exact test using 2×2 contingency tables or Student's t-test. *Student's t-test was employed.

Introduction

Rheumatoid arthritis (RA) is a chronic systemic inflammatory disease susceptibility to which is associated with genetic and environmental factors [1,2,3]. Altered frequencies of human leukocyte antigen (HLA) alleles are known to be associated with RA in most ethnic groups studied. Some *HLA-DR* alleles are reported to be positively associated with RA susceptibility [4]. A conserved amino acid sequence at position 70–74 (QKRAA, RRRAA, or QRRAA) in the HLA-DRβ chain is shared between the RA-associated *HLA-DR* alleles; this was therefore designated the shared epitope (SE) [4].

The presence of autoantibodies to ribonucleoprotein is associated with a variety of autoimmune diseases, including Sjögren's Syndrome (SS), systemic lupus erythematosus (SLE), and RA. Anti-La/SS-B antibodies share many features with anti-Ro/SS-A antibodies, and almost all anti-La/SS-B antibody-positive RA patients also have anti-Ro/SS-A antibodies, whereas about one fifth of anti-Ro/SS-A antibody-positive RA patients also have anti-La/SS-B antibodies. HLA-DR2 (*DRB1*15* and **16*) and DR3 are strongly associated with anti- Ro/SS-A or anti-La/SS-B antibodies in European primary SS populations [5,6,7,8]. On the other hand, *DRB1*08:03* was reported to be associated with anti-La/SS-B antibodies and **15:01* with anti-Ro/SS-A antibodies in primary SS, SLE, and asymptomatic individuals in the Japanese population [9]. However, few studies have focused on the association of anti-La/SS-B and anti-Ro/SS-A antibodies with HLA alleles in RA [10]. Here, we elucidate *HLA class II* associations with the presence of autoantibody in Japanese RA patients.

Materials and Methods

Patients and Controls

Nine hundred twenty five RA and 622 SLE patients were recruited at Sagamihara Hospital, Nagasaki Medical Center, Yokohama Minami Kyosai Hospital, Tama Medical Center, Kitasato University, Komagome Hospital, Himeji Medical Center, Morioka Hospital, and Kyushu Medical Center. All patients were native Japanese living in Japan. All patients with RA fulfilled the 1988 American College of Rheumatology Criteria for RA [11] and did not overlap any other collagen diseases. All patients with SLE fulfilled the American College of Rheumatology criteria for SLE [12]. The RA patients with SS also fulfilled the Japanese Ministry of Health Criteria for the diagnosis of SS [13]. This study was reviewed and approved by the research ethics committees of each participating institute, Sagamihara Hospital Research Ethics Committee, Nagasaki Medical Center Research Ethics Committee, Yokohama Minami Kyosai Hospital Research Ethics Committee, Tama Medical Center Research Ethics Committee, University of Tsukuba Research Ethics Committee, Kitasato University Ethics Committee, Komagome Hospital Ethics Committee, Himeji Medical Center Ethics Committee, Morioka Hospital Ethics Committee, and Kyushu Medical Center Ethics Committee. Written informed consent was obtained from all study participants. This study was conducted in accordance with the principles expressed in the Declaration of Helsinki. Anti-Ro/SS-A and anti-La/SS-B antibodies were detected using Mesacup-2 test (Medical & Biological Laboratories, Nagoya, Japan), or Ouchterlony double immunodiffusion method (TFB, Hachioji, Japan). RA patients who visited Sagamihara Hospital (n = 1538) were classified as anti-Ro/SS-A antibodies positive RA (n = 225, 14.6%) and anti-La/SS-B antibodies positive RA (n = 37, 2.4%).

Table 2. HLA allele frequencies in Ro(+)La(−) RA patients.

	Ro(+) La(−)	Ro(−) La(−)	P	OR	Pc	95%CI
DRB1*01:01	21 (5.8)	110 (7.8)	0.2162	0.73	NS	
DRB1*04:01	6 (1.7)	52 (3.7)	0.0667	0.44	NS	
DRB1*04:03	5 (1.4)	20 (1.4)	1.0000	0.97	NS	
DRB1*04:04	0 (0.0)	3 (0.2)	1.0000	0.55	NS	
DRB1*04:05	92 (25.4)	406 (28.8)	0.2132	0.84	NS	
DRB1*04:06	7 (1.9)	25 (1.8)	0.8256	1.09	NS	
DRB1*04:07	0 (0.0)	3 (0.2)	1.0000	0.55	NS	
DRB1*04:10	4 (1.1)	33 (2.3)	0.2136	0.47	NS	
DRB1*07:01	0 (0.0)	6 (0.4)	0.6086	0.30	NS	
DRB1*08:02	11 (3.0)	21 (1.5)	0.0727	2.07	NS	
DRB1*08:03	38 (10.5)	52 (3.7)	1.35×10^{-6}	3.06	3.79×10^{-5}	(1.98–4.73)
DRB1*08:23	1 (0.3)	0 (0.0)	0.2045	11.69		
DRB1*09:01	42 (11.6)	243 (17.3)	0.0082	0.63	0.2283	(0.44–0.89)
DRB1*10:01	3 (0.8)	12 (0.9)	1.0000	0.97	NS	
DRB1*11:01	3 (0.8)	17 (1.2)	0.7809	0.68	NS	
DRB1*12:01	14 (3.9)	39 (2.8)	0.2985	1.41	NS	
DRB1*12:02	7 (1.9)	20 (1.4)	0.4724	1.37	NS	
DRB1*13:01	1 (0.3)	3 (0.2)	1.0000	1.30	NS	
DRB1*13:02	7 (1.9)	60 (4.3)	0.0434	0.44	NS	(0.20–0.98)
DRB1*14:02	0 (0.0)	2 (0.1)	1.0000	0.78	NS	
DRB1*14:03	8 (2.2)	10 (0.7)	0.0180	3.16	0.5051	(1.24–8.06)
DRB1*14:05	3 (0.8)	14 (1.0)	1.0000	0.83	NS	
DRB1*14:06	9 (2.5)	15 (1.1)	0.0689	2.37	NS	
DRB1*14:07	0 (0.0)	1 (0.1)	1.0000	1.29	NS	
DRB1*14:54	13 (3.6)	34 (2.4)	0.2041	1.51	NS	
DRB1*15:01	28 (7.7)	75 (5.3)	0.1006	1.49	NS	
DRB1*15:02	36 (9.9)	124 (8.8)	0.5373	1.14	NS	
DRB1*16:02	2 (0.6)	8 (0.6)	1.0000	0.97	NS	
DQB1*02:01	0 (0.0)	6 (0.4)	0.6086	0.30	NS	
DQB1*03:01	39 (10.8)	133 (9.4)	0.4280	1.16	NS	
DQB1*03:02	22 (6.1)	73 (5.2)	0.5134	1.18	NS	
DQB1*03:03	46 (12.7)	229 (16.3)	0.1038	0.75	NS	
DQB1*03:06	0 (0.0)	3 (0.2)	1.0000	0.55	NS	
DQB1*04:01	96 (26.5)	432 (30.7)	0.1384	0.82	NS	
DQB1*04:02	7 (1.9)	35 (2.5)	0.6987	0.77	NS	
DQB1*05:01	25 (6.9)	125 (8.9)	0.2461	0.76	NS	
DQB1*05:02	14 (3.9)	27 (1.9)	0.0471	2.06	0.7071	(1.07–3.97)
DQB1*05:03	6 (1.7)	29 (2.1)	0.8322	0.80	NS	
DQB1*06:01	72 (19.9)	179 (12.7)	0.0007	1.70	0.0106	(1.26–2.31)
DQB1*06:02	27 (7.5)	75 (5.3)	0.1291	1.43	NS	
DQB1*06:03	1 (0.3)	3 (0.2)	1.0000	1.30	NS	
DQB1*06:04	6 (1.7)	57 (4.0)	0.0259	0.40	0.3884	(0.17–0.93)
DQB1*06:09	1 (0.3)	1 (0.1)	0.3673	3.90	NS	
DPB1*01:01	1 (0.3)	0 (0.0)	0.2045	11.69	NS	
DPB1*02:01	87 (24.0)	387 (27.5)	0.2061	0.83	NS	
DPB1*02:02	15 (4.1)	59 (4.2)	1.0000	0.99	NS	
DPB1*03:01	16 (4.4)	56 (4.0)	0.6573	1.12	NS	
DPB1*04:01	10 (2.8)	55 (3.9)	0.3498	0.70	NS	
DPB1*04:02	30 (8.3)	171 (12.1)	0.0409	0.65	0.6540	(0.44–0.98)

Table 2. Cont.

	Ro(+) La(−)	Ro(−) La(−)	P	OR	Pc	95%CI
DPB1*05:01	165 (45.6)	493 (35.0)	0.0002	1.55	0.0040	(1.23–1.96)
DPB1*06:01	0 (0.0)	9 (0.6)	0.2181	0.20	NS	
DPB1*09:01	24 (6.6)	112 (8.0)	0.4400	0.82	NS	
DPB1*13:01	4 (1.1)	16 (1.1)	1.0000	0.97	NS	
DPB1*14:01	5 (1.4)	25 (1.8)	0.8194	0.77	NS	
DPB1*17:01	0 (0.0)	5 (0.4)	0.5900	0.35	NS	
DPB1*19:01	2 (0.6)	5 (0.4)	0.6368	1.56	NS	
DPB1*38:01	0 (0.0)	3 (0.2)	1.0000	0.55	NS	
DPB1*41:01	1 (0.3)	7 (0.5)	1.0000	0.55	NS	
DPB1*47:01	0 (0.0)	3 (0.2)	1.0000	0.55	NS	

RA: rheumatoid arthritis, Ro(+)La(−)RA: anti-Ro/SS-A-positive but anti-La/SS-B-negative RA, Ro(−)La(−)RA: ani-Ro/SS-A- and anti-La/SS-B-negative RA. OR: odds ratio, CI: confidence interval, Pc: corrected P value, NS: not significant. Allele frequencies are shown in parenthesis (%). Associations were established by Fisher's exact test using 2×2 contingency tables.

Genotyping

Genotyping of *HLA-DRB1*, *DQB1*, and *DPB1* was performed by polymerase chain reaction using sequence-specific oligonucleotide probes, WAKFlow HLA typing kits (Wakunaga, Hiroshima, Japan), using a Bio-Plex 200 system (Bio-Rad, Hercules, CA). *HLA-DRB1* alleles encoding the SE are as follows: *01:01, *04:01, *04:04, *04:05, *04:10, *10:01, *14:02, and *14:06 [14]. One of each *DRB1* and *DQB1* locus could not be typed in the present study. These were revealed to be novel HLA alleles, *DRB1* 08:36:02 and DQB1*06:51*, by sequencing of the isolated alleles [15].

Statistical Analysis

Differences of RA characteristics, allele frequencies, or amino acid residue frequencies were analyzed by Student's t-test or Fisher's exact test using 2×2 contingency tables. Adjustment for multiple comparisons was performed using the Bonferroni method. Corrected P (Pc) values were calculated by multiplying the P value by the number of alleles or amino acid residues tested.

Results

Characteristics of Anti-Ro/SS-A and/or Anti-La/SS-B Antibody-positive RA and SLE Patients

Characteristics of anti-Ro/SS-A-positive but anti-La/SS-B-negative [Ro(+)La(−)] RA and anti-Ro/SS-A- and anti-La/SS-B-positive [Ro(+)La(+)] RA patients are given in Table 1. Mean age and percentage of males in the Ro(+)La(−)RA and Ro(+)La(+)RA groups were lower than in the anti-Ro/SS-A- and anti-La/SS-B-negative [Ro(−)La(−)] patients. Percentage of secondary SS in the Ro(+)La(−)RA and Ro(+)La(+)RA was higher than in the Ro(−)La(−)RA. There were no significant differences in terms of disease duration, rheumatoid factor or anti-citrullinated peptide antibody positivity, or Steinbrocker stage.

Characteristics of Ro(+)La(−) and Ro(+)La(+) SLE patients are also given in Table 1. Disease duration in the Ro(+)La(+) groups was shorter than in the Ro(−)La(−). Percentage of secondary SS in the Ro(+)La(+)SLE was higher than in the Ro(−)La(−)SLE. There were no significant differences in terms of mean age,

Table 3. HLA allele frequencies in Ro(+)La(+) RA patients.

	Ro(+) La(+)	Ro(−) La(−)	P	OR	Pc	95%CI
DRB1*01:01	3 (3.8)	110 (7.8)	0.2739	0.46	NS	
DRB1*03:01	1 (1.3)	0 (0.0)	0.0538	53.15	NS	
DRB1*04:01	0 (0.0)	52 (3.7)	0.1097	0.16	NS	
DRB1*04:03	0 (0.0)	20 (1.4)	0.6214	0.42	NS	
DRB1*04:04	0 (0.0)	3 (0.2)	1.0000	2.49	NS	
DRB1*04:05	15 (18.8)	406 (28.8)	0.0555	0.57	NS	
DRB1*04:06	1 (1.3)	25 (1.8)	1.0000	0.70	NS	
DRB1*04:07	0 (0.0)	3 (0.2)	1.0000	2.49	NS	
DRB1*04:10	5 (6.3)	33 (2.3)	0.0492	2.78	NS	(1.05–7.32)
DRB1*07:01	1 (1.3)	6 (0.4)	0.3213	2.96	NS	
DRB1*08:02	4 (5.0)	21 (1.5)	0.0414	3.48	NS	(1.16–10.38)
DRB1*08:03	5 (6.3)	52 (3.7)	0.2280	1.74	NS	
DRB1*09:01	6 (7.5)	243 (17.3)	0.0205	0.39	0.5728	(0.17–0.90)
DRB1*10:01	0 (0.0)	12 (0.9)	1.0000	0.69	NS	
DRB1*11:01	1 (1.3)	17 (1.2)	1.0000	1.04	NS	
DRB1*12:01	4 (5.0)	39 (2.8)	0.2865	1.85	NS	
DRB1*12:02	3 (3.8)	20 (1.4)	0.1223	2.70	NS	
DRB1*13:01	0 (0.0)	3 (0.2)	1.0000	2.49	NS	
DRB1*13:02	4 (5.0)	60 (4.3)	0.7735	1.18	NS	
DRB1*14:02	0 (0.0)	2 (0.1)	1.0000	3.49	NS	
DRB1*14:03	1 (1.3)	10 (0.7)	0.4566	1.77	NS	
DRB1*14:05	2 (2.5)	14 (1.0)	0.2111	2.55	NS	
DRB1*14:06	3 (3.8)	15 (1.1)	0.0681	3.62	NS	
DRB1*14:07	0 (0.0)	1 (0.1)	1.0000	5.83	NS	
DRB1*14:54	2 (2.5)	34 (2.4)	1.0000	1.04	NS	
DRB1*15:01	12 (15.0)	75 (5.3)	0.0017	3.14	0.0470	(1.63–6.05)
DRB1*15:02	7 (8.8)	124 (8.8)	1.0000	0.99	NS	
DRB1*16:02	0 (0.0)	8 (0.6)	1.0000	1.02	NS	
DQB1*02:01	2 (2.5)	6 (0.4)	0.0647	5.99	0.9710	
DQB1*03:01	12 (15.0)	133 (9.4)	0.1183	1.69	NS	
DQB1*03:02	4 (5.0)	73 (5.2)	1.0000	0.96	NS	
DQB1*03:03	6 (7.5)	229 (16.3)	0.0392	0.42	0.5886	(0.18–0.97)
DQB1*03:06	0 (0.0)	3 (0.2)	1.0000	2.49	NS	
DQB1*04:01	15 (18.8)	432 (30.7)	0.0238	0.52	0.3573	(0.29–0.92)
DQB1*04:02	6 (7.5)	35 (2.5)	0.0198	3.18	0.2974	(1.30–7.80)
DQB1*05:01	3 (3.8)	125 (8.9)	0.1484	0.40	NS	
DQB1*05:02	1 (1.3)	27 (1.9)	1.0000	0.65	NS	
DQB1*05:03	3 (3.8)	29 (2.1)	0.2450	1.85	NS	
DQB1*06:01	12 (15.0)	179 (12.7)	0.4962	1.21	NS	
DQB1*06:02	12 (15.0)	75 (5.3)	0.0017	3.14	0.0252	(1.63–6.05)
DQB1*06:03	0 (0.0)	3 (0.2)	1.0000	2.49	NS	
DQB1*06:04	4 (5.0)	57 (4.0)	0.5656	1.25	NS	
DQB1*06:09	0 (0.0)	1 (0.1)	1.0000	5.83	NS	
DPB1*02:01	11 (13.8)	387 (27.5)	0.0061	0.42	0.0913	(0.22–0.80)
DPB1*02:02	1 (1.3)	59 (4.2)	0.3713	0.29	NS	
DPB1*03:01	5 (6.3)	56 (4.0)	0.3746	1.61	NS	
DPB1*04:01	2 (2.5)	55 (3.9)	0.7656	0.63	NS	
DPB1*04:02	4 (5.0)	171 (12.1)	0.0506	0.38	0.7591	
DPB1*05:01	44 (55.0)	493 (35.0)	0.0005	2.27	0.0069	(1.44–3.57)

Table 3. Cont.

	Ro(+) La(+)	Ro(−) La(−)	P	OR	Pc	95%CI
DPB1*06:01	0 (0.0)	9 (0.6)	1.0000	0.92	NS	
DPB1*09:01	6 (7.5)	112 (8.0)	1.0000	0.94	NS	
DPB1*13:01	2 (2.5)	16 (1.1)	0.2517	2.23	NS	
DPB1*14:01	4 (5.0)	25 (1.8)	0.0660	2.91	0.9907	
DPB1*17:01	0 (0.0)	5 (0.4)	1.0000	1.58	NS	
DPB1*19:01	0 (0.0)	5 (0.4)	1.0000	1.58	NS	
DPB1*38:01	0 (0.0)	3 (0.2)	1.0000	2.49	NS	
DPB1*41:01	0 (0.0)	7 (0.5)	1.0000	1.16	NS	
DPB1*47:01	1 (1.3)	3 (0.2)	0.1985	5.93	NS	

RA: rheumatoid arthritis, Ro(+)La(+)RA: anti-Ro/SS-A- and anti-La/SS-B-positive RA, Ro(−)La(−)RA: anti-Ro/SS-A- and anti-La/SS-B-negative RA. OR: odds ratio, CI: confidence interval, Pc: corrected P value, NS: not significant. Allele frequencies are shown in parenthesis (%). Associations were established by Fisher's exact test using 2×2 contingency tables.

percentage of males or anti-double-stranded-DNA antibody positivity.

Association of HLA Class II Allele Frequencies with the Presence of Anti-Ro/SS-A Antibodies

We tested whether *HLA class II* was associated with the presence of anti-Ro/SS-A antibodies, comparing the Ro(+)La(−)RA and Ro(−)La(−)RA groups. A significant positive association was found for *DRB1*08:03* and anti-Ro/SS-A antibodies ($Pc = 3.79 \times 10^{-5}$, odds ratio [OR] 3.06, 95% confidence interval [CI] 1.98–4.73, Table 2). The *DQB1*06:01* allele was also associated with the presence of anti-Ro/SS-A antibodies ($Pc = 0.0106$, OR 1.70, 95% CI 1.26–2.31, Table 2). Further, the *HLA-DPB1*05:01* allele was associated with anti-Ro/SS-A antibodies ($Pc = 0.0040$, OR 1.55, 95% CI 1.23–1.96). Frequencies of DR4 and SE alleles were lower in Ro(+)La(−)RA than in Ro(−)La(−)RA ($P = 0.0146$, OR 0.73, 95% CI 0.57–0.94 and $P = 0.0089$, OR 0.73, 95% CI 0.57–0.92, respectively). Frequencies of DR2 alleles (*DRB1*15* and *16*) in Ro(+)La(−)RA and Ro(−)La(−)RA were not significantly different ($P = 0.1028$, OR 1.29). Thus, there were positive associations between certain alleles of *HLA-DRB1, DQB1,* and *DPB1* and the presence of anti-Ro/SS-A antibodies in RA patients.

Association of HLA Class II Allele Frequencies with the Presence of Anti-La/SS-B Antibodies

We then compared Ro(+)La(+)RA and Ro(−)La(−)RA *HLA class II* allele frequencies to seek associations with anti-La/SS-B antibodies. A significant positive association was found for *DRB1*15:01* and anti-La/SS-B antibodies ($Pc = 0.0470$, OR 3.14, 95%CI 1.63–6.05, Table 3). The *DQB1*06:02* allele was also associated with the presence of anti-La/SS-B antibodies ($Pc = 0.0252$, OR 3.14, 95% CI 1.63–6.05, Table 3). Further, the *HLA-DPB1*05:01* allele was also associated with anti-La/SS-B antibodies ($Pc = 0.0069$, OR 2.27, 95%CI 1.44–3.57, Table 3). Frequencies of SE and DR4 alleles were lower in Ro(+)La(+)RA than Ro(−)La(−)RA ($P = 0.0367$, OR 0.59, 95%CI 0.36–0.95, $P = 0.0324$, OR 0.57, 95%CI 0.34–0.95, respectively). Frequencies of DR2 alleles in Ro(+)La(+)RA were higher than Ro(−)La(−)RA patients ($P = 0.0364$, OR 1.81, 95%CI 1.06–3.09). Thus, there was

Table 4. HLA class II allele frequencies in RA cases with or without specific class II alleles.

	allele positivity		Ro(+)La(−)	Ro(−)La(−)	P	OR	Pc	95%CI
DRB1*08:03	(−)	DQB1*06:01	32 (10.9)	124 (9.5)	0.4481	1.16	NS	
	(−)	DPB1*05:01	143 (48.6)	456 (34.9)	1.41×10^{-5}	1.77	0.0002	(1.37–2.28)
	(+)	DQB1*06:01	40 (58.8)	55 (53.9)	0.6364	1.22	NS	
	(+)	DPB1*05:01	22 (32.4)	37 (36.3)	0.6254	0.84	NS	
DQB1*06:01	(−)	DRB1*08:03	0 (0.0)	2 (0.2)	1.0000	0.91	NS	
	(−)	DPB1*05:01	119 (50.4)	421 (39.1)	0.0016	1.59	0.0264	(1.20–2.11)
	(+)	DRB1*08:03	38 (30.2)	50 (15.2)	0.0005	2.42	0.0141	(1.49–3.93)
	(+)	DPB1*05:01	46 (36.5)	72 (21.8)	0.0018	2.06	0.0294	(1.32–3.22)
DPB1*05:01	(−)	DRB1*08:03	14 (17.5)	22 (3.7)	1.41×10^{-5}	5.59	0.0004	(2.73–11.45)
	(−)	DQB1*06:01	23 (28.8)	111 (18.4)	0.0357	1.78	0.5356	(1.05–3.02)
	(+)	DRB1*08:03	24 (8.5)	30 (3.7)	0.0023	2.41	0.0654	(1.38–4.19)
	(+)	DQB1*06:01	49 (17.4)	68 (8.4)	0.0001	2.28	0.0011	(1.54–3.39)

	allele positivity		Ro(+)La(+)	Ro(−)La(−)	P	OR	Pc	95%CI
DRB1*15:01	(−)	DQB1*06:02	0 (0.0)	0 (0.0)				
	(−)	DPB1*05:01	32 (53.3)	430 (34.0)	0.0033	2.22	0.0490	(1.32–3.74)
	(+)	DQB1*06:02	12 (60.0)	75 (52.8)	0.6356	1.34	NS	
	(+)	DPB1*05:01	12 (60.0)	63 (44.4)	0.2337	1.88	NS	
DQB1*06:02	(−)	DRB1*15:01	0 (0.0)	2 (0.2)	1.0000	4.19	NS	
	(−)	DPB1*05:01	32 (53.3)	431 (33.9)	0.0033	2.22	0.0488	(1.32–3.74)
	(+)	DRB1*15:01	12 (60.0)	73 (52.9)	0.6353	1.34	NS	
	(+)	DPB1*05:01	12 (60.0)	62 (44.9)	0.2368	1.84	NS	
DPB1*05:01	(−)	DRB1*15:01	2 (20.0)	26 (4.3)	0.0724	5.54	NS	
	(−)	DQB1*06:02	2 (20.0)	27 (4.5)	0.0771	5.32	NS	
	(+)	DRB1*15:01	10 (14.3)	49 (6.1)	0.0205	2.57	0.5739	(1.24–5.34)
	(+)	DQB1*06:02	10 (14.3)	48 (6.0)	0.0195	2.63	0.2918	(1.27–5.46)

RA: rheumatoid arthritis, Ro(+)La(−)RA: anti-Ro/SS-A-positive but anti-La/SS-B-negative RA, Ro(−)La(−)RA: anti-Ro/SS-A- and anti-La/SS-B-negative RA, Ro(+)La(+)RA: anti-Ro/SS-A- and anti-La/SS-B-positive RA, OR: odds ratio, CI: confidence interval, Pc: corrected P value, NS: not significant. Allele frequencies are shown in parenthesis (%). Associations were established by Fisher's exact test using 2×2 contingency tables.

Table 5. HLA class II allele frequency in the RA cases without SE alleles.

	Ro(+)La(−)	Ro(−)La(−)	P	OR	Pc	95%CI
DRB1*0803	29 (21.0)	29 (7.4)	4.60×10^{-5}	3.33	0.0008	(1.91–5.82)
DQB1*0601	47 (34.1)	79 (20.2)	0.0016	2.05	0.0191	(1.33–3.15)
DPB1*0501	60 (43.5)	131 (33.4)	0.0392	1.53	0.5887	(1.03–2.28)

	Ro(+)La(+)	Ro(−)La(−)	P	OR	Pc	95%CI
DRB1*1501	7 (20.6)	36 (9.2)	0.0660	2.56	NS	
DQB1*0602	7 (20.6)	36 (9.2)	0.0660	2.56	0.7915	
DPB1*0501	15 (44.1)	131 (33.4)	0.2579	1.57	NS	

SE: shared epitope, OR: odds ratio, CI: confidence interval, Pc: corrected P value, NS: not significant. Allele frequencies are shown in parenthesis (%). Associations were established by Fisher's exact test using 2×2 contingency tables.

an association of *HLA class II alleles* with anti-La/SS-B antibodies in RA patients.

Independent Associations of DRB1 and DPB1 with the Presence of Anti-Ro/SS-A Antibodies

A two-locus analysis was performed to identify the primary role of *DRB1*08:03*, *DQB1*06:01*, or *DPB1*05:01* for the production of anti-Ro/SS-A antibodies in RA patients. The OR for *DRB1*08:03* in patients lacking *DQB1*06:01* was 0.91 (not significant), while the OR for *DQB1*06:01* in patients without *DRB1*08:03* was 1.16 (not significant, Table 4). These differences did not reach statistical significance because of the strong linkage disequilibrium (LD) between *DRB1*08:03* and *DQB1*06:01* which results in a low frequency of *DRB1*08:03* in patients without *DQB1*06:01*. On the other hand, the OR for *DRB1*08:03* in patients lacking *DPB1*05:01* was 5.59 ($Pc = 0.0004$), while it was 1.77 for *DPB1*05:01* in patients without *DRB1*08:03*($Pc = 0.0002$, Table 4). This suggests independent effects of *DRB1*08:03* and *DPB1*05:01* on the production of anti-Ro/SS-A antibodies in RA.

The two-locus analysis was also performed to identify the primary role of *DRB1*15:01*, *DQB1*06:02*, or *DPB1*05:01* for the production of anti-La/SS-B antibodies in RA patients. OR for *DPB1*05:01* was 2.22 in patients without *DRB1*15:01*

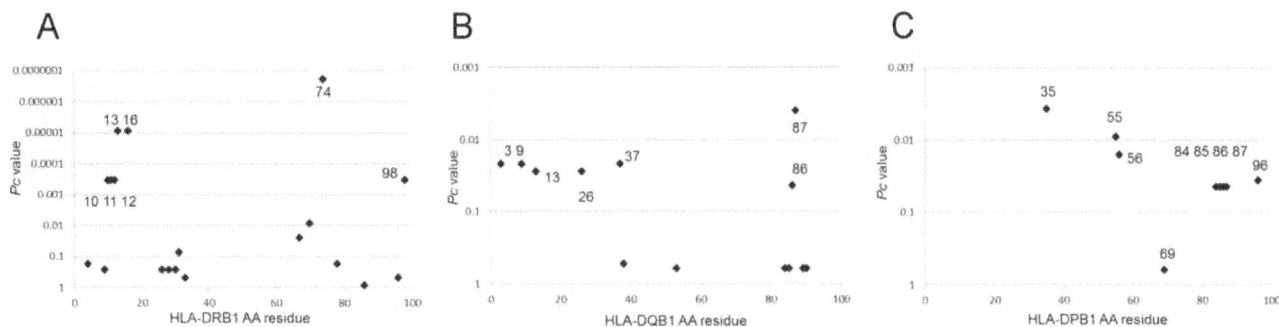

Figure 1. Associations of amino acid residues in DRβ (A), DQβ (B), and DPβ chains (C) with the presence of anti-Ro/SS-A antibodies.
Corrected P (Pc) values were calculated by multiplying the P value by the number of amino acid residues tested. Associations were established by Fisher's exact test using 2×2 contingency tables.

(Pc = 0.0490, Table 4) and was 2.22 in patients without DQB1*06:02 (Pc = 0.0490, Table 4). This might suggests independent effects of DPB1*05:01 and DRB1*15:01 or DQB1*06:02 on the production of anti-La/SS-B antibodies in RA.

Effects of SE on the Association of HLA Class II Alleles

We examined whether the positive association of DRB1*08:03, DQB1*06:01, and DPB1*05:01 alleles is secondary to the decrease of SE in the Ro(+)La(−)RA patients. When the patients with SE were excluded from the analysis, the DRB1*08:03 and DQB1*06:01 allele frequencies were significantly higher in Ro(+)La(−)RA than Ro(−)La(−)RA (Pc = 0.0008, OR 3.33, 95%CI 1.91–5.82, and Pc = 0.0191, OR 2.05, 95%CI 1.33–3.15, respectively, Table 5). On the other hand, DPB1*05:01 frequency was still higher in Ro(+)La(−)RA than Ro(−)La(−)RA, although the effect was not statistically significant (Pc = 0.5887, OR 1.53, 95%CI 1.03–2.28, Table 5).

We also examined whether the positive association of DRB1*15:01, DQB1*06:02, and DPB1*05:01 alleles is secondary to the decrease of SE in the Ro(+)La(+)RA patients. When the patients with SE were excluded from the analysis, these allele frequencies were still higher in the Ro(+)La(+)RA than Ro(−)La(−)RA, although the effect was not statistically significant (Table 5).

Effects of Secondary SS on the Association of HLA Class II Alleles

The associations of anti-Ro/SS-A and anti-La/SS-B antibodies with secondary SS were described in Table 1, and the association

of secondary SS with HLA class II alleles was investigated. No association was observed between DPB1*05:01 or anti-Ro/La antibody-associated HLA alleles and secondary SS. The associations of DRB1*08:03 (Pc = 0.0001, OR 3.13, 95%CI 1.97–4.96), DQB1*06:01 (Pc = 0.0173, OR 1.75, 95%CI 1.27–2.43), or DPB1*05:01 (Pc = 0.0064, OR 1.59, 95%CI 1.23–2.05) with anti-Ro/SS-A antibodies remain significant after excluding RA patients with secondary SS. However, the associations of DRB1*15:01 (Pc = 0.3450, OR 2.93, 95%CI 1.34–6.42), DQB1*06:02 (Pc = 0.1848, OR 2.93, 95%CI 1.34–6.42), or DPB1*05:01 (Pc = 0.0941, OR 2.16, 95%CI 1.26–3.70) with anti-La/SS-A antibodies did not reach statistical significance after excluding RA patients with secondary SS, because of reduced sample numbers after the exclusion.

Certain Amino Acid Residues in the DRβ, DQβ, and DPβ Chains are Associated with the Presence of Anti-Ro/SS-A Antibodies

Amino acid residues in HLA-DRβ, DQβ, and DPβ chains were analyzed for their potential associations with anti-Ro/SS-A antibodies. Amino acid positions 13, 16, and 74 in the DRβ chain showed strong associations with the presence of anti-Ro/SS-A antibodies (Figure 1A). The amino acid residue at position 74 associated with anti-Ro/SS-A is different from the SE at that position; these three amino acid residues (13, 16 and 74) are shared by DRB1*08:02, *08:03, and *08:23. The amino acid position 87 in the DQβ chain showed associations with anti-Ro/SS-A antibodies (Figure 1B). Finally, amino acid positions 35, 55, and 56 in the DPβ chain showed associations with anti-Ro/SS-A

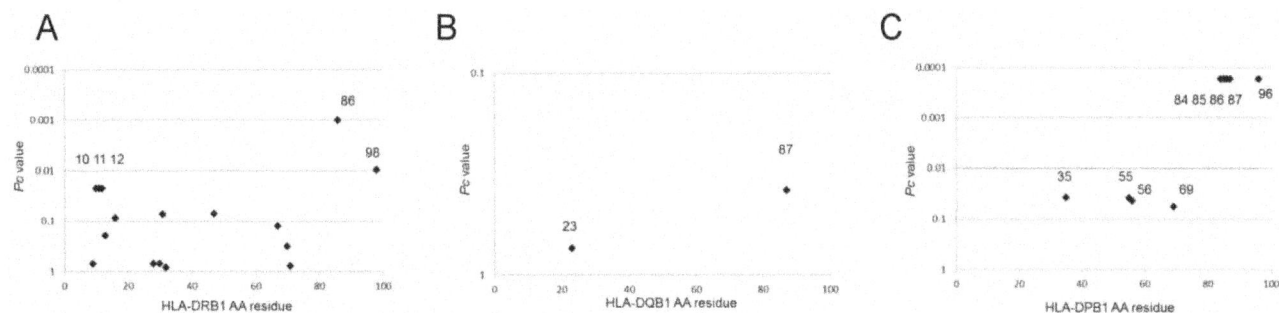

Figure 2. Associations of amino acid residues in DRβ (A), DQβ (B), and DPβ chains (C) with the presence of anti-La/SS-B antibodies.
Corrected P (Pc) values were calculated by multiplying the P value by the number of amino acid residues tested. Associations were established by Fisher's exact test using 2×2 contingency tables.

Table 6. *HLA-DPB1* allele frequency in the SLE patients.

	Ro(+)La(−)	Ro(+)La(+)	Ro(−)La(−)	Ro(+)La(−) vs. Ro(−)La(−)				Ro(+)La(+) vs. Ro(−)La(−)			
				P	OR	Pc	95%CI	P	OR	Pc	95%CI
DPB1*01:01	0 (0.0)	1 (1.1)	0 (0.0)					0.2473	9.20	NS	
DPB1*02:01	49 (19.0)	10 (11.1)	73 (26.6)	0.0393	0.65	0.4711	(0.43–0.97)	0.0022	0.34	0.0283	(0.17–0.70)
DPB1*02:02	11 (4.3)	3 (3.3)	19 (6.9)	0.1939	0.60	NS		0.3084	0.46	NS	
DPB1*03:01	13 (5.0)	3 (3.3)	10 (3.6)	0.5239	1.40	NS		1.0000	0.91	NS	
DPB1*04:01	6 (2.3)	0 (0.0)	9 (3.3)	0.6045	0.70	NS		0.1198	0.15	NS	
DPB1*04:02	27 (10.5)	7 (7.8)	25 (9.1)	0.6622	1.16	NS		0.8315	0.84	NS	
DPB1*05:01	118 (45.7)	56 (62.2)	91 (33.2)	0.0034	1.69	0.0408	(1.19–2.41)	1.91×10^{-6}	3.31	2.48×10^{-5}	(2.02–5.43)
DPB1*06:01	1 (0.4)	0 (0.0)	2 (0.7)	1.0000	0.53	NS		1.0000	0.60	NS	
DPB1*09:01	18 (7.0)	4 (4.4)	23 (8.4)	0.6264	0.82	NS		0.2544	0.51	NS	
DPB1*13:01	6 (2.3)	3 (3.3)	10 (3.6)	0.4509	0.63	NS		1.0000	0.91	NS	
DPB1*14:01	8 (3.1)	2 (2.2)	8 (2.9)	1.0000	1.06	NS		1.0000	0.76	NS	
DPB1*19:01	1 (0.4)	0 (0.0)	2 (0.7)	1.0000	0.53	NS		1.0000	0.60	NS	
DPB1*38:01	0 (0.0)	0 (0.0)	2 (0.7)	0.4995	0.21	NS		1.0000	0.60	NS	

SLE: systemic lupus erythematosus, Ro(+)La(−): anti-Ro/SS-A-positive but anti-La/SS-B-negative, Ro(+)La(+): anti-Ro/SS-A- and anti-La/SS-B-positive, Ro(−)La(−): anti-Ro/SS-A- and anti-La/SS-B-negative SLE patients. OR: odds ratio, CI: confidence interval, Pc: corrected P value, NS: not significant. Allele frequencies are shown in parenthesis (%). Associations were established by Fisher's exact test using 2×2 contingency tables.

antibodies (Figure 1C). These three residues are shared by *DPB1*05:01 and *38:01*. Thus, certain amino acid residues in the DRβ, DQβ, and DPβ chains are associated with the presence of anti-Ro/SS-A antibodies.

Certain Amino Acid Residues in the DRβ, DQβ, and DPβ Chains are Associated with the Presence of Anti-La/SS-B Antibodies

Amino acid residues in HLA-DRβ, DQβ, and DPβ chains were also analyzed for associations with anti-La/SS-B antibodies. Positions 86 in the DRβ chain showed strong associations with anti-La/SS-B antibodies (Figure 2A). No associations were observed for any residues in the DQβ chain (Figure 2B), whereas positions 84–87 and 96 in the DPβ chain showed associations with anti-La/SS-B antibodies (Figure 2C). Thus, association analysis suggested roles for certain defined amino acid residues in DRβ and DPβ.

Association of HLA-DPB1*05:01 with the Presence of Anti-Ro/SS-A and Anti-La/SS-B Antibodies in SLE Patients

We also tested whether *HLA-DPB1* was associated with the presence of anti-Ro/SS-A or anti-La/SS-B antibodies in SLE patients. The *DPB1*05:01* allele was associated with anti-Ro/SS-A (Pc = 0.0408, OR 1.69, 95% CI 1.19–2.41, Table 6) and anti-La/SS-B antibodies (Pc = 2.48×10⁻⁵, OR 3.31, 95%CI 2.02–5.43, Table 6). A significant negative association was found for *DPB1*02:01* and anti-La/SS-B antibodies (Pc = 0.0283, OR 0.34, 95%CI 0.17–0.70, Table 6). Thus, there was an association of *DPB1*05:01* allele with anti-Ro/SS-A and anti-La/SS-B antibodies in SLE patients.

Discussion

Several studies have shown that certain *HLA-DR* alleles are associated with the presence of anti-Ro/SS-A or anti-La/SS-B antibodies in patients with autoimmune diseases. However, few studies have focused on the association of HLA alleles with anti-

Ro/SS-A or anti-La/SS-B antibodies in RA. To the best of our knowledge, this is the first report of a positive association of *HLA-DPB1*05:01* with anti-Ro/SS-A and anti-La/SS-B antibodies in RA, although a tendency towards a higher frequency of this allele in Japanese patients with anti-Ro/SS-A or anti-La/SS-B antibodies has been reported before [9]. Recent studies have noted associations of *DPB1* alleles with several diseases [16,17,18,19,20], but here we report an association of *DPB1*05:01* with anti-Ro/SS-A and anti-La/SS-B antibodies in Japanese RA and SLE patients.

It was reported that RA patients with anti-Ro/SS-A antibodies had a more severe disease course, and that they were less frequently DR4-positive than patients without such antibodies [21,22]. In contrast, the presence of anti-Ro/SS-A antibodies in RA was reported to be positively associated with DR4 in some other studies [10,23]. Here, we found that frequencies of DR4 and the SE were lower in anti-Ro/SS-A-positive RA patients (Figure 2). Although the implications of this finding are not clear, it might suggest that the role of SE may not be as important in anti-Ro/SS-A-positive RA. Alternatively, the genetic background of anti-Ro/SS-A-positive and -negative RA may be different, and genetic factors other than SE may play a significant role in the former.

It was reported that anti-Ro/SS-A-positive patients were more frequently DR3- or DR2-positive in the context of other autoimmune diseases like primary SS and SLE in European populations [5]. An association of *DRB1*15:01* and anti-Ro/SS-A antibodies has been reported in the Japanese population [9]. Such an association of DR2 with the presence of anti-Ro/SS-A was not confirmed in our study on RA patients, but an association of DR2 with the presence of anti-La/SS-B was observed. Although *DRB1*08:03* was reported to be associated with anti-La/SS-B in Japanese [9], we observed here that it was associated with the presence of anti-Ro/SS-A antibodies in our RA patients. These could be explained by differences in the pathogenesis of RA and SLE.

Amino acid residues 13, 16 and 74 of the HLA-DRβ chain were found to be associated with the presence of anti-Ro/SS-A antibodies (Figure 1). Residues 13 and 74 form the HLA-DR peptide-binding groove [24]. Amino acid residues 84–87 and 96 in the DPβ chain were associated with anti-La/SS-B antibodies. Similarly, amino acid residues 85 and 86 form the peptide-binding grooves of HLA-DP molecules. These data suggest the involvement of peptide antigens bound to specific HLA molecules in controlling the production of anti-Ro/SS-A or anti-La/SS-B antibodies.

It has been determined that patients with anti-Ro/SS-A antibodies are more prone to develop adverse effects when treated with gold salts and other drugs [25,26,27]. Recent studies have shown that adverse drug reactions are associated with drug-specific *HLA class I* alleles, for example *A*31:01* and *B*15:02* with carbamazepine, and *A*31:01* with methotrexate [28,29,30]. Furthermore, *A*31:01* is in LD with *DRB1*08:03* and *15:01* (0.56% and 0.63% of haplotype frequency, respectively, see http://hla.or.jp/haplo/haplonavi.php?type = haplo&lang = en). Frequencies of these class II alleles were higher in anti-Ro/SS-A or anti-La/SS-B antibody- positive RA patients (Tables 2, 3). Large scale association studies for *HLA class I* and anti-Ro/SS-A or anti-La/SS-B antibodies should be performed. Because of the limited sample size of the present study, the observed significance

of the statistical association was modest. The association with *HLA-DP* needs to be confirmed in future independent studies. Because the allelic distribution of *HLA* in other ethnic populations is different from that in the Japanese, the role of *HLA-DP* in anti-Ro/SS-A or anti-La/SS-B antibody production in RA in other populations should be determined.

This is the first identification of an association of *HLA-DPB1*05:01* with positivity for anti-Ro/SS-A or anti-La/SS-B antibodies in RA. Our findings support the role of *HLA-DP*, as well as *DR*, in the pathogenesis of autoantibody production.

Acknowledgments

We thank Ms. Mayumi Yokoyama (Sagamihara Hospital) for secretarial assistance.

Author Contributions

Conceived and designed the experiments: HF NT ST. Performed the experiments: HF SO. Analyzed the data: HF. Contributed reagents/materials/analysis tools: HF K. Shimada SS AH AK NF TN SH K. Setoguchi AO NC ES TM KM AS SN ST. Wrote the paper: HF NT ST.

References

1. Perricone C, Ceccarelli F, Valesini G (2011) An overview on the genetic of rheumatoid arthritis: a never-ending story. Autoimmun Rev 10: 599–608. Epub 2011 Apr 2022.
2. Scott IC, Steer S, Lewis CM, Cope AP (2011) Precipitating and perpetuating factors of rheumatoid arthritis immunopathology: linking the triad of genetic predisposition, environmental risk factors and autoimmunity to disease pathogenesis. Best Pract Res Clin Rheumatol 25: 447–468.
3. Lewis SN, Nsoesie E, Weeks C, Qiao D, Zhang L (2011) Prediction of disease and phenotype associations from genome-wide association studies. PLoS ONE 6: e27175. Epub 22011 Nov 27174.
4. Reveille JD (1998) The genetic contribution to the pathogenesis of rheumatoid arthritis. Curr Opin Rheumatol 10: 187–200.
5. Hernandez-Molina G, Leal-Alegre G, Michel-Peregrina M (2010) The meaning of anti-Ro and anti-La antibodies in primary Sjogren's syndrome. Autoimmun Rev 10: 123–125.
6. Rischmueller M, Lester S, Chen Z, Champion G, Van Den Berg R, et al. (1998) HLA class II phenotype controls diversification of the autoantibody response in primary Sjogren's syndrome (pSS). Clin Exp Immunol 111: 365–371.
7. Gottenberg JE, Busson M, Loiseau P, Cohen-Solal J, Lepage V, et al. (2003) In primary Sjogren's syndrome, HLA class II is associated exclusively with autoantibody production and spreading of the autoimmune response. Arthritis Rheum 48: 2240–2245.
8. Tzioufas AG, Wassmuth R, Dafni UG, Guialis A, Haga HJ, et al. (2002) Clinical, immunological, and immunogenetic aspects of autoantibody production against Ro/SSA, La/SSB and their linear epitopes in primary Sjogren's syndrome (pSS): a European multicentre study. Ann Rheum Dis 61: 398–404.
9. Miyagawa S, Shinohara K, Nakajima M, Kidoguchi K, Fujita T, et al. (1998) Polymorphisms of HLA class II genes and autoimmune responses to Ro/SS-A-La/SS-B among Japanese subjects. Arthritis Rheum 41: 927–934.
10. Schneeberger E, Citera G, Heredia M, Maldonado Cocco J (2008) Clinical significance of anti-Ro antibodies in rheumatoid arthritis. Clin Rheumatol 27: 517–519.
11. Arnett FC, Edworthy SM, Bloch DA, McShane DJ, Fries JF, et al. (1988) The American Rheumatism Association 1987 revised criteria for the classification of rheumatoid arthritis. Arthritis Rheum 31: 315–324.
12. Hochberg M (1997) Updating the American College of Rheumatology revised criteria for the classification of systemic lupus erythematosus. Arthritis Rheum 40: 1725.
13. Tsuboi H, Matsumoto I, Wakamatsu E, Nakamura Y, Iizuka M, et al. (2010) New epitopes and function of anti-M3 muscarinic acetylcholine receptor antibodies in patients with Sjogren's syndrome. Clin Exp Immunol 162: 53–61.
14. Furukawa H, Oka S, Shimada K, Sugii S, Ohashi J, et al. (2012) Association of human leukocyte antigen with interstitial lung disease in rheumatoid arthritis: A protective role for shared epitope. PLoS ONE 7: e33133.
15. Oka S, Furukawa H, Kashiwase K, Tsuchiya N, Tohma S (2012) Identification of a novel HLA allele, HLA-DQB1*06:51, in a Japanese rheumatoid arthritis patient. Tissue Antigens 80: 386–387.
16. Kamatani Y, Wattanapokayakit S, Ochi H, Kawaguchi T, Takahashi A, et al. (2009) A genome-wide association study identifies variants in the HLA-DP locus associated with chronic hepatitis B in Asians. Nat Genet 41: 591–595.
17. Noguchi E, Sakamoto H, Hirota T, Ochiai K, Imoto Y, et al. (2011) Genome-wide association study identifies HLA-DP as a susceptibility gene for pediatric asthma in Asian populations. PLoS Genet 7: e1002170.
18. Kominami S, Tanabe N, Ota M, Naruse TK, Katsuyama Y, et al. (2009) HLA-DPB1 and NFKBIL1 may confer the susceptibility to chronic thromboembolic pulmonary hypertension in the absence of deep vein thrombosis. J Hum Genet 54: 108–114.
19. Raychaudhuri S, Sandor C, Stahl EA, Freudenberg J, Lee HS, et al. (2012) Five amino acids in three HLA proteins explain most of the association between MHC and seropositive rheumatoid arthritis. Nat Genet 44: 291–296.
20. Lyons PA, Rayner TF, Trivedi S, Holle JU, Watts RA, et al. (2012) Genetically distinct subsets within ANCA-Associated Vasculitis. N Engl J Med 367: 214–223.
21. Boire G, Menard HA (1988) Clinical significance of anti-Ro(SSA) antibody in rheumatoid arthritis. J Rheumatol 15: 391–394.
22. Boire G, Menard HA, Gendron M, Lussier A, Myhal D (1993) Rheumatoid arthritis: anti-Ro antibodies define a non-HLA-DR4 associated clinicoserological cluster. J Rheumatol 20: 1654–1660.
23. Tishler M, Moutsopoulos HM, Yaron M (1992) Genetic studies of anti-Ro (SSA) antibodies in families with rheumatoid arthritis. J Rheumatol 19: 234–236.
24. Jardetzky TS, Brown JH, Gorga JC, Stern LJ, Urban RG, et al. (1994) Three-dimensional structure of a human class II histocompatibility molecule complexed with superantigen. Nature 368: 711–718.
25. Tishler M, Golbrut B, Shoenfeld Y, Yaron M (1994) Anti-Ro(SSA) antibodies in patients with rheumatoid arthritis–a possible marker for gold induced side effects. J Rheumatol 21: 1040–1042.
26. Tishler M, Nyman J, Wahren M, Yaron M (1997) Anti-Ro (SSA) antibodies in rheumatoid arthritis patients with gold-induced side effects. Rheumatol Int 17: 133–135.
27. Kamada N, Kinoshita K, Togawa Y, Kobayashi T, Matsubara H, et al. (2006) Chronic pulmonary complications associated with toxic epidermal necrolysis: report of a severe case with anti-Ro/SS-A and a review of the published work. J Dermatol 33: 616–622.
28. Chung WH, Hung SI, Hong HS, Hsih MS, Yang LC, et al. (2004) Medical genetics: a marker for Stevens-Johnson syndrome. Nature 428: 486.
29. McCormack M, Alfirevic A, Bourgeois S, Farrell JJ, Kasperaviciute D, et al. (2011) HLA-A*3101 and carbamazepine-induced hypersensitivity reactions in Europeans. N Engl J Med 364: 1134–1143.
30. Furukawa H, Oka S, Shimada K, Rheumatoid Arthritis-Interstitial Lung Disease Study Consortium, Tsuchiya N, et al. (2012) HLA-A*31:01 and methotrexate-induced interstitial lung aisease in Japanese rheumatoid arthritis patients: A multi-drug hypersensitivity marker? Ann Rheum Dis in press.

The Tolerogenic Peptide, hCDR1, Down-Regulates the Expression of Interferon-α in Murine and Human Systemic Lupus Erythematosus

Zev Sthoeger[1,2]*, Heidy Zinger[1], Amir Sharabi[1], Ilan Asher[2], Edna Mozes[1]*

1 Department of Immunology, The Weizmann Institute of Science, Rehovot, Israel, **2** Department of Internal Medicine B and Clinical Immunology, Kaplan Medical Center, Rehovot, Israel

Abstract

Background: The tolerogenic peptide, hCDR1, ameliorated manifestations of systemic lupus erythematosus (SLE) via the immunomodulation of pro-inflammatory and immunosuppressive cytokines and the induction of regulatory T cells. Because type I interferon (IFN-α) has been implicated to play a role in SLE pathogenesis, we investigated the effects of hCDR1 on IFN-α in a murine model of SLE and in human lupus.

Methodology/Principal Findings: (NZBxNZW)F1 mice with established SLE were treated with hCDR1 (10 weekly injections). Splenocytes were obtained for gene expression studies by real-time RT-PCR. hCDR1 down-regulated significantly IFN-α gene expression (73% inhibition compared to vehicle treated mice, p = 0.002) in association with diminished clinical manifestations. Further, hCDR1 reduced, in vitro, IFN-α gene expression in peripheral blood mononuclear cells (PBMC) of 10 lupus patients (74% inhibition compared to medium, p = 0.002) but had no significant effects on the expression levels of IFN-α in PBMC of primary anti-phospholipid syndrome patients or of healthy controls. Lupus patients were treated for 24 weeks with hCDR1 (5) or placebo (4) by weekly subcutaneous injections. Blood samples collected, before and after treatment, were frozen until mRNA isolation. A significant reduction in IFN-α was determined in hCDR1 treated patients (64.4% inhibition compared to pretreatment expression levels, p = 0.015). No inhibition was observed in the placebo treated patients. In agreement, treatment with hCDR1 resulted in a significant decrease of disease activity. IFN-α appears to play a role in the mechanism of action of hCDR1 since recombinant IFN-α diminished the immunomodulating effects of hCDR1 on IL-1β, TGFβ and FoxP3 gene expression.

Conclusions/Significance: We reported previously that hCDR1 affected various cell types and immune pathways in correlation to disease amelioration. The present studies demonstrate that hCDR1 is also capable of down-regulating significantly (and specifically to lupus) IFN-α gene expression. Thus, hCDR1 has a potential role as a novel, disease specific treatment for lupus.

Editor: Ari Waisman, Johannes Gutenberg University of Mainz, Germany

Funding: The authors have no support or funding to report.

Competing Interests: The authors have declared that no competing interests exist.

* E-mail: sthoeger@gmail.com (ZS); edna.mozes@weizmann.ac.il (EM)

Introduction

Systemic lupus erythematosus (SLE) is an autoimmune disorder characterized by the production of autoantibodies and impaired function of B and T cells accompanied by systemic clinical manifestations [1]. Various cytokines [2,3], factors affecting B cell activation and survival [4], apoptosis [5,6] and dysfunction of regulatory T-cells [7,8] were shown to be involved in the pathogenesis of murine and human SLE. Our laboratory designed a peptide, designated hCDR1 [9], that is based on the sequence of the complementarity determining region 1 (CDR1) of a human anti-DNA monoclonal antibody that bears a major idiotype (Id), namely the 16/6 Id [10]. hCDR1 was shown to ameliorate the serological and clinical manifestations of experimental SLE in mice with either induced (BALB/c) or spontaneous (NZBxNZW)F1 lupus [11]. The beneficial effects of hCDR1 were associated with a reduced production and expression of inflam-

matory cytokines (e.g. IL-1β, IFN-γ, TNF-α,) [11,12] and up regulation of the immunosuppressive cytokine TGFβ [11,13]. hCDR1 was shown to inhibit T cell receptor signaling following its binding to class II major histocompatibility complex (MHC) [14]. The induction of CD4 and CD8 regulatory T cells play a key role in the mechanism of action of hCDR1 [15–17]. Further, hCDR1 was shown to diminish T cell apoptosis [18,19]. Treatment with hCDR1 affected the B cell compartment as well. Thus, it down regulated the rate of maturation, differentiation and survival of B cells by reducing the levels of B cell activating factor (BAFF, BLyS) [20] as well as of molecules of the CD74/MIF pathway on B cells [21]. In addition, hCDR1 was shown to induce dendritic cells with immature phenotype and suppressed function that down regulate autoreactive T cells [22].

We have further demonstrated similar immunomodulatory effects of hCDR1 on peripheral blood mononuclear cells (PBMC)

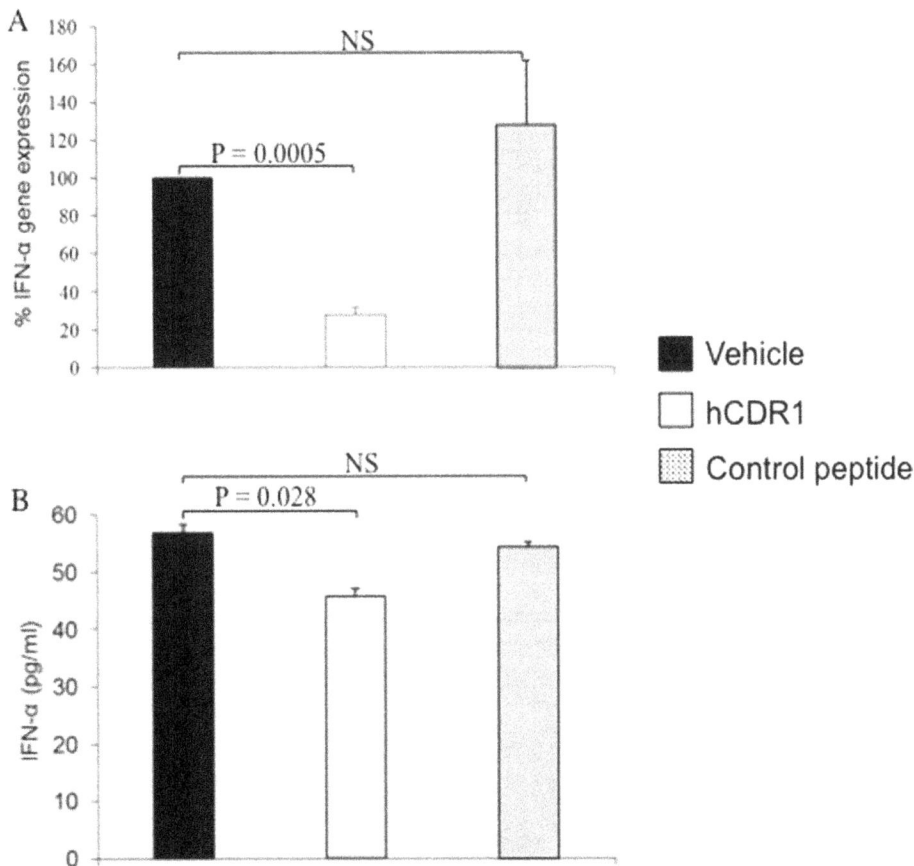

Figure 1. Treatment of SLE afflicted (NZBxNZW)F1 mice with hCDR1 results in the down regulation of IFN-α. (A) Mean percentage (±SE) results of 4 independent experiments in which the mRNA expression of IFN-α was determined in pools of spleen derived cells of SLE afflicted mice (10–12 mice per group) treated with vehicle, hCDR1, or the control, scrambled, peptide. The levels of gene expression were determined by real-time RT-PCR and calculated relatively to levels in cells from vehicle-treated mice (considered as 100%). (B) Mean concentrations (±SE) of IFN-α determined by ELISA in sera of the same groups of mice.

obtained from lupus patients. Thus, incubation of PBMC of lupus patients (but not of healthy volunteers) with hCDR1 resulted in a significant down regulation of gene expression of pro-inflammatory cytokines, apoptotic factors, and BLyS and up regulation of gene expression of immunosuppressive factors (Foxj1, Foxo3a, TGFβ, Foxp3) [23]. In addition, hCDR1 increased the number as well as the function of CD4+CD25+Foxp3+regulatory T-cells in PBMC of lupus patients [23]. Further, we reported the beneficial effects of in vivo treatment with hCDR1 in five lupus patients with mild to moderate disease [24]. In agreement with its clinical beneficial effects, hCDR1 was shown to immunomodulate in vivo the expression of genes that play a role in SLE thus restoring the global immune dysregulation in those patients [24].

Type I interferons, mainly interferon (IFN)-α, were suggested to play a major role in the pathogenesis of murine and human SLE [25]. Thus, elevated levels of IFN-α were demonstrated in sera of SLE afflicted mice as well as in sera of lupus patients [26,27], and IFN-α levels were reported to correlate with disease activity [28]. Similarly, high levels of IFN-α inducible gene expression ("IFN-signature") were shown in blood cells of lupus patients [29]. Moreover, type I IFN receptor deficiency was reported to reduce significantly lupus like disease in a mouse model [30] and IFN-α neutralizing antibodies were shown to prevent the clinical manifestations in a lupus flare murine model [31]. Hence, IFN-

α has been considered recently as a therapeutic target for the treatment of human SLE.

Since we have demonstrated that hCDR1 was capable of restoring the cytokine dysregulation observed in SLE and of down regulating the maturation and function of dendritic cells (that are activated by IFN-α and are a source for IFN-α production as well) we investigated, in the present studies, the effects of hCDR1 on IFN-α in a murine model of SLE and in human lupus.

Results

Treatment of SLE afflicted (NZBxNZW)F1 mice with hCDR1 down regulated gene expression of IFN-α

Eight month old (NZBxNZW)F1 female mice were treated with 10 subcutaneously weekly injections of hCDR1 (50 μg/mouse), control (scrambled) peptide (50 μg/mouse) or the vehicle alone (10–12 mice per group in 4 independent experiments). Mice were bled periodically for the determination of sera anti-dsDNA autoantibody and IFN-α levels and were tested for proteinuria levels. All mice were sacrificed at the end of treatment, their kidneys were evaluated for immune complex deposits and spleen derived lymphocytes were used for mRNA preparation.

Figure 1A shows the effect of treatment with hCDR1 on IFN-α gene expression. The results are of 4 independent experiments in which mRNA was prepared from pools of spleen derived

Table 1. Effects of treatment with hCDR1 on SLE manifestations in mice.

Treatment [a]	dsDNA Ab [b](OD)	p [c]	Proteinuria [d] (g/L)	p [c]	ICD [e]	p [c]
Vehicle	0.50±0.08	—	8.36±1.86	—	2.43±0.2	—
hCDR1	0.30±0.05	0.04	1.94±0.45	0.03	1.57±0.2	0.002
Control[f]	0.52±0.08	NS	8.94±1.86	NS	2.78±0.2	NS

[a]SLE-afflicted (NZB×NZW)F1 mice (10–12 mice per group in 4 independent experiments) were treated with weekly subcutaneous injections of the vehicle, hCDR1, or a control (scrambled peptide) for 10 weeks.
[b]Results are of sera from mice that were bled after the end of treatment. Dilution of sera 1:1250.
[c]Statistical evaluation was based on the Mann-Whitney U test to compare post –treatment effects between the vehicle –treated groups and the remaining treatment groups.
[d]Proteinuria was always measured at about the same time of day and all mice in an experimental cohort were tested together.
[e]Immune complex deposits (ICD) were assessed at sacrifice.
[f]$p = 0.04$, 0.02 and 0.0001 between the control peptide and hCDR1 treated mice for dsDNA specific antibodies, proteinuria and ICD, respectively.

lymphocytes of SLE-afflicted mice treated with vehicle, hCDR1 or control peptide. The gene expression of IFN-α was determined by real-time RT-PCR. The results are expressed as percentage gene expression relatively to that observed for vehicle treated mice, considered as 100%. As can be seen in the Figure, treatment with hCDR1 down-regulated significantly ($p = 0.0005$) the gene expression of IFN-α as compared to levels of the vehicle treated mice. No such effects were observed in splenocytes of mice treated with the control peptide. In spite of the limited sensitivity of the ELISA assay, the levels of IFN-α (56.83 ± 1.4 pg/ml) detected in sera of vehicle treated mice were similar to those reported for the sera of SLE patients [32]. As can been seen in Figure 1B, treatment with hCDR1 but not with the control peptide decreased significantly ($p = 0.028$) the sera levels of IFN-α. Thus, our studies demonstrated that hCDR1 treatment decreased IFN-α gene expression (Figure 1A) and its sera levels (Figure 1B).

In agreement, treatment with hCDR1 ameliorated disease manifestations in the experimental mice. As can be seen in Table 1, that summarizes the beneficial effects of hCDR1 treatment, a significant reduction was determined in the levels of dsDNA autoantibodies, in proteinuria levels as well as in glomerular immune complex deposits (ICD) as compared to mice that were treated with the vehicle alone. It is also seen in the Table that no such effects were observed in mice that were treated with the control peptide.

Immunohistology of kidney sections of representative mice of each group are shown in Figure 2. As can been seen in the Figure, intense ICD are demonstrated in the kidney sections of the vehicle and the control peptide treated mice but not in the hCDR1 treated group of mice.

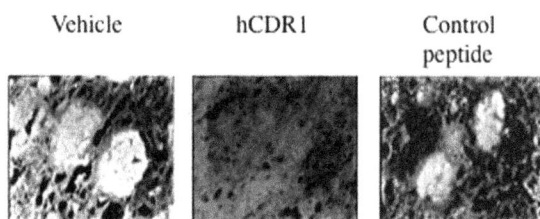

Figure 2. hCDR1 down regulates immune complex deposits in kidney sections. Immunohistology of kidney sections of representative mice of each experimental group (vehicle, hCDR1 and control peptide treated mice). Magnification X400.

Effects of hCDR1 on IFN-α gene expression of PBMC of lupus patients

We further studied the in vitro effects of hCDR1 on IFN-α in lupus patients. To this end, PBMC were obtained from 10 lupus patients (8 females, 2 males) aged 32–65 years that were diagnosed with SLE according to four or more ACR diagnostic criteria [33]. Their main current clinical manifestations were arthritis (60%), mucocutaneous (50%), renal (20%) and pleuritis/pericarditis (20%). Eight patients were treated with Plaquonil (400 mg/d) and five with corticosteroids (2.5–10 mg/d of Prednisone) at the time of the study. The patients' PBMC were cultured for 48 hours in the presence of hCDR1 (25 μg/ml) or medium alone. Thereafter, mRNA was isolated from the cells and IFN-α gene expression was determined by real-time RT-PCR. For control we cultured concomitantly PBMC that were obtained from 5 healthy volunteers and PBMC of 5 patients with primary anti-phospho-lipid syndrome (APS) that did not have lupus (either clinically or serologically). Figure 3 shows the results of these experiments. It can be seen that in vitro incubation of PBMC of lupus patients with hCDR1 diminished significantly ($p = 0.004$) the IFN-α gene expression as compared with PBMC of the same patients cultured with medium (considered as 100%). It should be noted that the baseline levels of IFN-α gene expression in PBMC of SLE patients were 3 folds higher than those determined for the healthy controls ($p = 0.028$). Figure 3 also shows that in vitro incubation of hCDR1 with PBMC of healthy donors or of patients with primary APS did not down regulate the levels of IFN-α gene expression in the treated cells. Thus, these results suggest that the hCDR1-induced reduction of IFN-α gene expression is specific to lupus patients.

We also tested the supernatants of the lupus PBMC cultured with hCDR1 (or medium alone) for the presence of IFN-α by ELISA but apparently the assay was not sensitive enough and IFN-α could not be detected in the cultures.

The effect of in vivo treatment of lupus patients with hCDR1 on IFN-α gene expression

We have further evaluated the effect of hCDR1 treatment on IFN-α gene expression in 9 lupus patients with mild to moderate disease. The patients were treated with weekly subcutaneous injections of either hCDR1 (5 patients) or vehicle alone (4 patients). The inclusion and exclusion criteria, patients' characterization and clinical outcome were described previously [24]. Blood samples were collected from the patients in PAXgene tubes prior and following 24 weeks of treatment for the preparation of mRNA. The in vivo effect of weekly administration of hCDR1 to

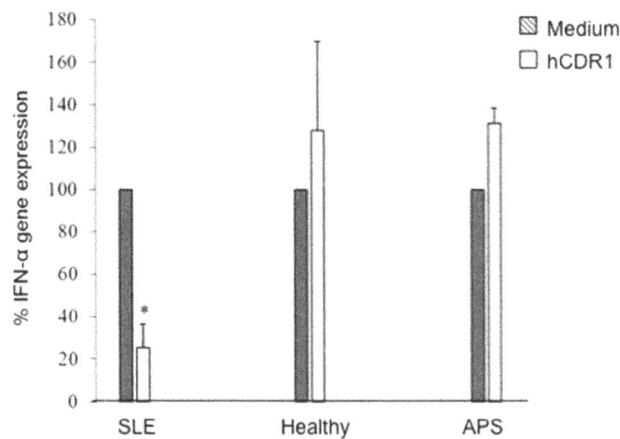

Figure 3. hCDR1 down regulates IFN-α gene expression in PBMC of SLE patients. PBMC of 10 SLE, 5 primary APS patients and 5 healthy controls were cultured (5×10^6 cells/well) for 48 hours in the presence of medium or hCDR1 (25 µg/ml). Gene expression was determined by real-time RT-PCR. Results are presented as the mean±SE percentage of gene expression compared with cultures with medium (considered as 100%). * $p = 0.004$.

the SLE patients on IFN-α gene expression was then determined. Table 2 shows the expression of the IFN-α gene for the individual patients and Figure 4 presents the mean percent of gene expression at week 24 compared to the level prior to hCDR1 or vehicle treatment, at week 0 (defined as 100%; dotted line). As can be seen in Table 2 and Figure 4, treatment for 24 weeks with hCDR1 diminished significantly ($p = 0.0005$) the gene expression of IFN-α in the 5 treated patients. No significant effects were observed in the 4 lupus patients that were treated with the vehicle alone (placebo group; Table 2, Figure 4).

Figure 4 also shows that the significant inhibition of IFN-α gene expression following treatment with hCDR1 was in agreement with the observed clinical effects. Thus, as shown in the Figure, lupus disease activity as determined by the BILAG score decreased significantly ($p = 0.03$) in the hCDR1 treated but not in the placebo treated group of patients. Not shown in the Figure are the

SLEDAI scores of the treated patients. In agreement, a significant decrease in the SLEDAI-2K score (45% reduction, $p = 0.02$) was observed in the hCDR1 treated patients but not in the placebo treated patients [24].

The role of IFN-α in the hCDR1-induced immunomodulation in SLE

We further studied the possible mechanistic role of IFN-α in the hCDR1-induced immunomodulation in SLE. To this end, PBMC obtained from 3 SLE patients were cultured in triplicates for 48 hours in the presence of medium alone, hCDR1 (25 µg/ml) or hCDR1 (25 µg/ml) with human recombinant IFN-α at concentrations of 100–10,000 U/ml. Thereafter, mRNA was isolated from the cells and IL-1β, TGFβ and FoxP3 gene expression was determined by real-time RT-PCR. Figure 5 shows the results of these experiments using human recombinant IFN-α at a concentration of 5,000 U/ml (shown to have the optimal effect). It can been seen that, as was previously shown [23], hCDR1 significantly down-regulated IL-1β and up-regulated TGFβ and FoxP3 gene expression in lupus PBMC ($p = 0.05$, 0.03 and 0.03 for IL-1β, TGFβ and FoxP3, respectively). The addition of IFN-α to the cultures abolished completely those effects ($p = 0.05$, 0.016 and 0.028 between cultures of PBMC with hCDR1 and those with hCDR1+recombinant IFN-α for IL-1β, TGFβ and FoxP3, respectively) suggesting that IFN-α plays a role in the immunomodulating effects of hCDR1 in SLE.

Discussion

The main finding of the present study is that the tolerogenic peptide hCDR1 is capable of suppressing IFN-α gene expression in a murine SLE model and in lupus patients. This suppressive effect was specific since it was not observed following treatment of (NZBxNZW) F1 lupus prone mice with the control scramble peptide, or in PBMC obtained from healthy volunteers or APS patients. Moreover, the down regulation of IFN-α gene expression correlates to the therapeutic beneficial effects of hCDR1 in murine and in human lupus.

In previous studies, we were able to demonstrate that the tolerogenic peptide, hCDR1, ameliorates manifestations of SLE in murine models [9] and in a small cohort of lupus patients [24].

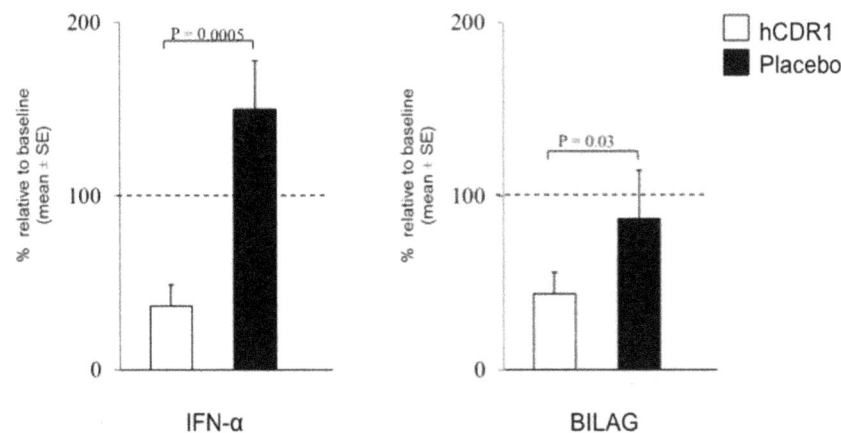

Figure 4. hCDR1 down regulates in vivo IFN-α gene expression in SLE patients. SLE patients were treated (subcutaneously, once a week) with either hCDR1 (0.5, 1, or 2.5 mg) or placebo. Gene expression in blood samples obtained from the patients was determined by real-time RT-PCR. Results are presented as mean percentage of gene expression (±SE) at week 24 compared to the levels at week 0 (defined as 100%; dotted line). Also shown in the Figure is the mean percent reduction in the BILAG score following 24 weeks of treatment with either hCDR1 or placebo as compared to the baseline score (week 0) considered as 100% (dotted line).

Table 2. The effect of in vivo treatment with hCDR1 on IFN-α gene expression in PBMC of SLE patients.

Patient No.	Treatment	Dose (mg)	IFN-α (% Expression relative to baseline)
70103	hCDR1	0.5	20
70106	hCDR1	0.5	20
70101	hCDR1	1.0	17
70403	hCDR1	1.0	44
70104	hCDR1	2.5	82
70404	Placebo	—	135
70405	Placebo	—	141
70102	Placebo	—	228
70107	Placebo	—	96

SLE patients with mild and moderate disease manifestations were treated (subcutaneously) with either hCDR1 or placebo. IFN-α gene expression in blood samples was determined by real-time RT-PCR. Results are presented as the percentage of gene expression at week 24 compared to that at week 0 (before the study was initiated), defined as100%.

Those beneficial effects resulted from the effects of hCDR1 on different immune cell types (including dendritic [22], T [9,17,34] and B cells [20,21,35]) and on cytokines [9,11]. Thus, hCDR1 down regulated (in vivo and in vitro, in murine SLE models and in human lupus) pro-inflammatory cytokines [11,23,24], apoptotic factors [18,19,23,24,36], B-cell stimulatory factors (BAFF/BLyS) [20,24] and up regulated immunosuppressive cytokines [9,11,23,24,37] with the induction of CD4+CD25+FoxP3+regulatory T-cells [15,23].

We demonstrate here a significant down regulation of IFN-α gene expression by hCDR1 in three different lupus related experimental systems. First, treatment of (NZBxNZW) F1 lupus prone mice with hCDR1, but not with the vehicle or the control (scrambled) peptide, resulted in significant down regulation of IFN-α gene expression (Figure 1A) and IFN-α sera levels (Figure 1B) which correlated to the serological and clinical beneficial effects of hCDR1 in this model (Table 1, Figure 2).

Second, hCDR1 significantly decreased, in vitro, IFN-α gene expression in PBMC of lupus patients but not in PBMC obtained from healthy volunteers or primary APS patients (Figure 3). Thus, as was previously shown for other cytokines and immunosuppressive factors [9,23], the effect of hCDR1 on IFN-α is specific to lupus. Third, treatment of five lupus patients with hCDR1 for twenty-four consecutive weeks resulted in significant inhibition of IFN-α gene expression (Table 2, Figure 4). Concomitantly, disease activity (defined by both, BILAG and SLEDAI) in the hCDR1 treated patients decreased significantly (Figure 4 and [24]). No such effects were observed in the four other lupus patients who were treated with the vehicle alone [Table 2, Figure 4]. Taken together, the present studies clearly demonstrated lupus-specific inhibitory effects of our tolerogenic peptide on IFN-α in SLE.

We have previously demonstrated the ability of the tolerogenic peptide, hCDR1, to ameliorate SLE manifestations by immunomodulating specifically a variety of cytokines, molecules and cell

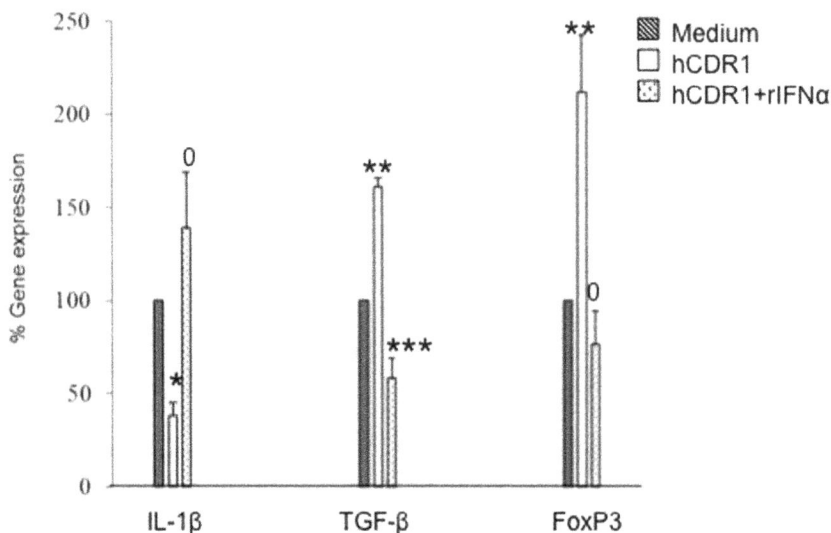

Figure 5. IFN-α diminishes hCDR1 immunomodulatory effects on PBMC of SLE patients. PBMC of 3 SLE patients were cultured (5×10^6 cells/well) for 48 hours in the presence of medium, hCDR1 (25 μg/ml) or hCDR1 (25 μg/ml) and human recombinant IFN-α (rIFN-α) at a concentration of 5,000 U/ml. Gene expression (for IL-1β, TGFβ and FoxP3) were determined by real-time RT-PCR. Results are presented as the mean±SEpercentage of gene expression compared with cultures of PBMC incubated with medium alone (considered as 100%). *p = 0.05, **p = 0.03, ***p = 0.015 and ⁰ = not significant.

types that are involved in the pathogenicity of lupus. In the present study we demonstrated down regulating effect of hCDR1 on one of the important cytokines that is involved in lupus etiology and pathogenesis, namely IFN-α. Recent reports showing that IFN-α has the potential to influence the development and progression of SLE suggest this cytokine as a therapeutic target. A number of mechanisms were suggested to account for the pathogenic effects of IFN-α. It has been reported that dendritic cells mature and become more prone to activate T cells in the presence of IFN-α [38]. Further, activity of regulatory T cells (Tregs) was shown to be suppressed by the in vitro treatment of dendritic cells with IFN-α [39] and the increased levels of IFN-α in lupus patients were reported to contribute, at least in part, to the diminished Tregs activity observed in patients with SLE [40]. Type 1 interferons were shown to directly improve B-cell survival in vitro [41] and to reduce the sensitivity of B cells to FasL-mediated apoptosis [42]. In addition, IFN-α may affect B cell survival, maturation and differentiation, indirectly by inducing dendritic cells and macrophages to produce BLyS [43]. Moreover, the present study suggests that IFN-α plays a mechanistic role in the immunomodulating effects of hCDR1 in SLE since the addition of recombinant IFN-α diminished the effects of hCDR1 on cytokine expression in PBMC of SLE patients (Figure 5). In agreement, the addition of anti-IFN-α-antibodies to PBMC of SLE patients (in the absence of hCDR1) down regulated IL-1β and up regulated TGFβ and FoxP3 gene expression, similarly to the immunomodulation of these genes by hCDR1 (Mozes et al., unpublished results) further supporting the role of IFN-α.

Thus, the diminished expression of IFN-α following treatment with hCDR1 demonstrated in our study may affect SLE manifestations via any or all the above suggested mechanisms. Indeed, we have previously reported that treatment with hCDR1 down regulated the maturation and activation of dendritic cells [22] resulting in the induction of functional Tregs and suppressed autoreactive T cell activity in SLE models and in lupus patients [9]. Furthermore, hCDR1 was shown to reduce BAFF/BLyS production and to up-regulate B cell apoptosis via the up regulation of pro-apoptotic molecules (e.g. Caspase 8) and the down regulation of anti-apoptotic molecules (Bcl-2, Bcl-xL) [20,24]. Nevertheless, it should be kept in mind that even though the effects of IFN-α can explain many SLE features, only a fraction of SLE patients displays elevated levels of IFN-α. Furthermore, other pathogenic cytokines that function together with IFN-α or independently, and cell marker molecules [2,44] were shown to be involved in lupus and therefore, reducing IFN-α probably affects only partially this complex, multifactorial disease. Thus, blocking a single cytokine might not be the full answer for controlling SLE. Indeed, we have previously shown that treatment with hCDR1 leads to a cascade of events that affect activated dendritic cells, T and B cells and their products as well as important pathways involved in the pathogenesis of lupus [9,45,46].

An important aim in the treatment of lupus, as well as any other diseases, is to suppress the SLE related autoimmune responses and, at the same time, to spare the normal function of the immune system. One of the challenges using therapeutic means that neutralize IFN-α is to inhibit the SLE-related over production of IFN-α and to leave intact the anti-viral activity of IFN-α. A similar problem arises when certain cell types (e.g., B cells) are depleted in order to suppress autoimmune responses. We have shown, in the present study that the inhibitory effect of hCDR1 on the expression of the IFN-α gene is specific to lupus and it does not affect healthy controls and patients with APS (Figure 3). In agreement, we have previously shown that hCDR1 inhibited in vitro murine and human T cell proliferation as well as IFN-γ and

IL-2 production only in cases of lupus associated responses [14,34,37,45] and did not affect responses to unrelated antigens. Similarly, we demonstrated that treatment of SLE–like disease in SCID mice, transplanted with PBMC of SLE patients, led to the suppressed production of the human anti-dsDNA autoantibodies as well as to the amelioration of SLE manifestations. Nevertheless, no significant effects could be observed on the levels of human anti-tetanus toxoid antibodies [47] in the treated mice. Moreover, only Tregs induced by hCDR1 ameliorated disease manifestations when transferred into SLE afflicted (NZBxNZW)F1 mice [15]. Tregs originating from a control peptide or the vehicle treated mice did not have a significant clinical effect on mice with established lupus [15]. The specific effect of hCDR1 was further confirmed by the fact that hCDR1 induced functional Tregs were not capable of inhibiting myasthenia gravis associated responses (Mozes E. et al. unpublished results).

Thus, the efficient and specific beneficial effects of hCDR1 at the different checkpoints and on the various factors involved in lupus, as exemplified in the present study by its effect on one of the central cytokine, IFN-α, suggest a potential role for this tolerogenic peptide in the treatment of lupus patients.

Materials and Methods

Mice

Female (NZBxNZW)F1 mice were purchased from The Jackson Laboratory (Bar harbor, ME, USA). Murine experiments were approved by the Animal Care and Use Committee of the Weizmann Institute of Science.

Synthetic peptides

A peptide, GYYWSWIRQPPGKGEEWIG, (hCDR1) [37] that is based on the complementarity determining region (CDR) 1 of the human anti-DNA monoclonal antibody, bearing a major idiotype (16/6 Id) [10] was synthesized by Polypeptide Laboratories (CA, USA). A peptide, SKGIPQYGGWEGWRYEI, containing the same amino acids as hCDR1 in a scrambled order was used as a control.

Treatment of (NZBxNZW)F1 mice

Eight-month old female mice (10–12 mice per group) with established lupus manifestations were treated in 4 independent experiments with 10 weekly subcutaneous injections of hCDR1 (50 μg/mouse), control peptide (50 μg/mouse) or vehicle alone (phosphate buffered saline).

Evaluation of murine lupus disease activity

Anti-dsDNA autoantibody levels were measured using λ phage dsDNA, as previously described [11]. Proteinuria was measured by a standard semi-quantitative test, using an Albustix kit (Bayer Diagnostic, Newbury, UK). Detection of glomerular immune complex deposits was performed as described earlier [11]. The intensity of immune complex deposits (immunohistology) was graded as follows: 0, no immune complex deposits; 1, low intensity; 2, moderate intensity; and 3, high intensity of immune complexes. The analysis was performed by two people blinded to whether the mice belonged to control or experimental groups.

Patients

Ten lupus patients (8 females and 2 males), 5 patients (all females) with primary APS and 5 (4 females and 1 male) age matched healthy controls participated in the in vitro experiments. We also present here data of 9 lupus patients (8 females and 1 male) from two Israeli Medical Centers. These patients participated in a large clinical trial with hCDR1 (Edratide) [24]. Included are all patients from the two Medical Centers who completed the study and from whom blood samples were taken at least twice (before treatment initiation and at week 24) for mRNA preparation. All lupus patients were diagnosed according to the American College of Rheumatology (ACR) diagnostic criteria [33]. All participants signed an informed consent form prior to the initiation of the studies. The studies were approved by the Ethic Committees of the Medical Centers and were conducted according to all good clinical practice (GCP) rules.

In vitro experiments

Peripheral blood mononuclear cells (PBMC) were isolated from heparinized venous blood using UNI-SEP maxi for density gradient separation (NOVAmed Ltd., Jerusalem, Israel). PBMC (5×10^6/ml) were cultured in triplicates in enriched RPMI-1640 medium containing 10% fetal calf serum [23] for 48 hours in the presence of hCDR1 (25 µg/ml) or medium alone as control. In some experiments, PBMC were also cultured with hCDR1 (25 µg/ml) and various concentrations (100–10,000 U/ml) of human recombinant IFN-α (Millipore, Temacula, Ca, USA). PBMC were then washed (x3 in RPMI-1640) and mRNA was extracted for gene expression as described below.

In vivo studies

The 9 lupus patients that participated in the clinical study had a mild to moderate disease with SLE-disease activity index 2000 (SLEDAI-2K) [48] of 6–12 (inclusive) and stable lupus-related medications [24]. hCDR1 dissolved in Captisol (Sulfobutyl ether cyclodextrin sodium, CyDex, Inc., KS, USA) was injected subcutaneously weekly for 24 consecutive weeks at doses of 0.5 mg (2 patients), 1 mg (2 patients) or 2.5 mg (1 patient). Four patients were treated with Captisol alone. Patients were evaluated clinically by the SLEDAI-2K and the British Islets Lupus Assessment Group (BILAG) [49] scores. Venous blood samples prior (week 0) and following treatment (week 24) were collected in PAXgene (PreanalytiX, Switzerland) tubes and frozen at -70°C until mRNA isolation.

Real-time RT-PCR

Total RNA was isolated from spleen derived murine lymphocytes, human PBMC or blood samples collected in PAXgene tubes. The RNA was reversed transcribed to prepare cDNA using Moloney murine leukemia virus reverse transcribtase (Promega, Madison, WI, USA). The resulting cDNA was subjected to real-time RT-PCR using Light Cycler ((Roche Mannheim, Germany) according to the manufacturer's instructions. Primer sequences (forward and reversed, respectively) were: mouse IFN-α1 (5′-CTGCAAGGCTGTCTGA-3′, 5′-GCACATTGGCAGAGGA-3′), mouse β-actin, (5′-GTGACGTTGACATCCG-3′, 5′-CAG-TAACAGTCCGCCT-3′), human IFNα1 (5′-TGTGATCTCCCTGAGACC-3′, 5′-AGATGGAGTCCG-CATT-3′), human IL-1β (5′-CAGAAAACATGCCCGT-3′, 5′-GCACTACCCTAAGGCAG-3′), human TGF-β (5′-GCAA-GACTATCGACATGG-3′, 5′-ACTTGTCATA-GATTTCGTTGTG-3′), human FoxP3 (5′-CCACAACATG-GACTACTT-3′, 5′-CGTTTCTTGCGGAACT-3′), and human GAPDH (5′-CTGCCAACGTGTCAGT-3′, 5′- GTTGAGGG-CAATGCCA-3′). The levels of β-actin (murine studies) and GAPDA (human studies) were used to normalize the gene expression levels of the other genes.

ELISA assays for IFN-α

IFN-α levels in murine sera and in human PBMC supernatants were determined by Platinum ELISA sets (eBioscience, San Diego, Ca.) according to the manufacturer's instructions.

Statistical analysis

Results are presented as Mean±standard error (SE). The nonparametric Mann-Whitney and unpaired Student's T tests were used for statistical analysis. p values of 0.05 or less were considered statistically significant.

Author Contributions

Conceived and designed the experiments: ZS EM. Performed the experiments: ZS HZ IA. Analyzed the data: ZS HZ EM. Contributed reagents/materials/analysis tools: ZS EM. Wrote the paper: ZS AS EM.

References

1. Tsokos GC (2011) Systemic lupus erythematosus. N Engl J Med 365: 2110–2121.
2. Horwitz DA, Jacob CO (1994) The cytokine network in the pathogenesis of systemic lupus erythematosus and possible therapeutic implications. Springer Semin Immunopathol 16: 181–200.
3. Segal R, Bermas BL, Dayan M, Kalush F, Shearer GM, et al. (1997) Kinetics of cytokine production in experimental systemic lupus erythematosus: involvement of T helper cell 1/T helper cell 2-type cytokines in disease. J Immunol 158: 3009–3016.
4. Cheema GS, Roschke V, Hilbert DM, Stohl W (2011) Elevated serum B lymphocyte stimulator levels in patients with systemic immune-based rheumatic diseases. Arthritis Rheum 44: 1313–1319.
5. Trébéden-Nègre H, Weill B, Fournier C, Batteux F (2003) B cell apoptosis accelerates the onset of murine lupus. Eur J Immunol 33: 1603–1612.
6. Emlen W, Niebur J, Kadera R (1994) Accelerated in vitro apoptosis of lymphocytes from patients with systemic lupus erythematosus. J Immunol 152: 3685–3692.
7. Valencia X, Yarboro C, Illei G, Lipsky PE (2007) Deficient CD4+CD25high T regulatory cell function in patients with active systemic lupus erythematosus. J Immunol 178: 2579–2588.
8. Paust S, Cantor H (2005) Regulatory T cells and autoimmune disease. Immunol Rev 204: 195–207.
9. Mozes E, Sharabi A (2010) A novel tolerogenic peptide, hCDR1, for the specific treatment of systemic lupus erythematosus. Autoimmun Rev 10: 22–26.
10. Waisman A, Shoenfeld Y, Blank M, Ruiz PJ, Mozes E (1995) The pathogenic human monoclonal anti-DNA that induces experimental systemic lupus erythematosus in mice is encoded by a VH4 gene segment. Int Immunol 7: 689–696.
11. Luger D, Dayan M, Zinger H, Liu JP, Mozes E (2004) A peptide based on the complementarity determining region 1 of a human monoclonal autoantibody

ameliorates spontaneous and induced lupus manifestations in correlation with cytokine immunomodulation. J Clin Immunol 24: 579–590.
12. Sharabi A, Haviv A, Zinger H, Dayan M, Mozes E (2006) Amelioration of murine lupus by a peptide, based on the complementarity determining region-1 of an autoantibody as compared to dexamethasone: different effects on cytokines and apoptosis. Clin Immunol 119: 146–155.
13. Sela U, Hershkoviz R, Cahalon L, Lider O, Mozes E (2005) Down-regulation of stromal cell-derived factor-1alpha-induced T cell chemotaxis by a peptide based on the complementarity-determining region 1 of an anti-DNA autoantibody via up-regulation of TGF-beta secretion. J Immunol 174: 302–309.
14. Sela U, Dayan M, Hershkoviz R, Cahalon L, Lider O, et al. (2006) The negative regulators Foxj1 and Foxo3a are up-regulated by a peptide that inhibits systemic lupus erythematosus-associated T cell responses. Eur J Immunol 36: 2971–2980.
15. Sharabi A, Zinger H, Zborowsky M, Stoeger ZM, Mozes E (2006) A peptide based on the complementarity-determining region 1 of an autoantibody ameliorates lupus by up-regulating CD4+CD25+cells and TGF-beta. Proc Natl Acad Sci U S A 103: 8810–8815.
16. Sharabi A, Mozes E (2008) The suppression of murine lupus by a tolerogenic peptide involves foxp3-expressing CD8 cells that are required for the optimal induction and function of foxp3-expressing CD4 cells. J Immunol 181: 3243–3251.
17. Arazi A, Sharabi A, Zinger H, Mozes E, Neumann AU (2009) In vivo dynamical interactions between CD4 Tregs, CD8 Tregs and CD4+CD25- cells in mice. PLoS One 4: e8447.
18. Rapoport MJ, Sharabi A, Aharoni D, Bloch O, Zinger H, et al. (2005) Amelioration of SLE-like manifestations in (NZBxNZW)F1 mice following treatment with a peptide based on the complementarity determining region 1 of an autoantibody is associated with a down-regulation of apoptosis and of the pro-apoptotic factor JNK kinase. Clin Immunol 117: 262–270.

19. Sharabi A, Luger D, Ben-David H, Dayan M, Zinger H, et al. (2007) The role of apoptosis in the ameliorating effects of a CDR1-based peptide on lupus manifestations in a mouse model. J Immunol 179: 4979–4987.
20. Parameswaran R, Ben David H, Sharabi A, Zinger H, Mozes E (2009) B-cell activating factor (BAFF) plays a role in the mechanism of action of a tolerogenic peptide that ameliorates lupus. Clin Immunol 131: 223–232.
21. Lapter S, Ben-David H, Sharabi A, Zinger H, Telerman A, et al. (2011) A role for the B-cell CD74/macrophage migration inhibitory factor pathway in the immunomodulation of systemic lupus erythematosus by a therapeutic tolerogenic peptide. Immunology 132: 87–95.
22. Sela U, Sharabi A, Dayan M, Hershkoviz R, Mozes E (2009) The role of dendritic cells in the mechanism of action of a peptide that ameliorates lupus in murine models. Immunology 128: e395–405.
23. Sthoeger ZM, Sharabi A, Dayan M, Zinger H, Asher I, et al. (2009) The tolerogenic peptide hCDR1 downregulates pathogenic cytokines and apoptosis and upregulates immunosuppressive molecules and regulatory T cells in peripheral blood mononuclear cells of lupus patients. Hum Immunol 70: 139–145.
24. Sthoeger ZM, Sharabi A, Molad Y, Asher I, Zinger H, et al. (2009) Treatment of lupus patients with a tolerogenic peptide, hCDR1 (Edratide): immunomodulation of gene expression. J Autoimmun 33: 77–82.
25. Lee PY, Reeves WH (2006) Type I interferon as a target of treatment in SLE. Endocr Metab Immune Disord Drug Targets 6: 323–330.
26. Crow MK, Kirou KA (2004) Interferon-alpha in systemic lupus erythematosus. Curr Opin Rheumatol 16: 541–547.
27. Ytterberg SR, Schnitzer TJ (1982) Serum interferon levels in patients with systemic lupus erythematosus. Arthritis Rheum 25: 401–406.
28. Kirou KA, Lee C, George S, Louca K, Peterson MG, et al. (2005) Activation of the interferon-alpha pathway identifies a subgroup of systemic lupus erythematosus patients with distinct serologic features and active disease. Arthritis Rheum 52: 1491–1503.
29. Baechler EC, Batliwalla FM, Karypis G, Gaffney PM, Ortmann WA, et al. (2003) Interferon-inducible gene expression signature in peripheral blood cells of patients with severe lupus. Proc Natl Acad Sci U S A 100: 2610–2615.
30. Santiago-Raber ML, Baccala R, Haraldsson KM, Choubey D, Stewart TA, et al. (2003) Type-I interferon receptor deficiency reduces lupus-like disease in NZB mice. J Exp Med 197: 777–788.
31. Zagury D, Le Buanec H, Mathian A, Larcier P, Burnett R, et al. (2009) IFNalpha kinoid vaccine-induced neutralizing antibodies prevent clinical manifestations in a lupus flare murine model. Proc Natl Acad Sci U S A 106: 5294–5299.
32. Shahin D, El-Refaey AM, El-Hawary AK, Salam AA, Machaly S, et al. (2011) Serum Interferon-alpha level in first degree relatives of systemic lupus erythematosus patients: correlation with autoantibodies titers. The Egyptian J Med Hum Genetics12:139–146.
33. Tan EM, Cohen AS, Fries JF, Masi AT, McShane DJ, et al. (1982) The 1982 revised criteria for the classification of systemic lupus erythematosus. Arthritis Rheum 25: 1271–1277.
34. Sela U, Mauermann N, Hershkoviz R, Zinger H, Dayan M, et al. (2005) The inhibition of autoreactive T cell functions by a peptide based on the CDR1 of an anti-DNA autoantibody is via TGF-beta-mediated suppression of LFA-1 and CD44 expression and function. J Immunol 175: 7255–7263.
35. Ben-David H, Sharabi A, Parameswaran R, Zinger H, Mozes E (2009) A tolerogenic peptide down-regulates mature B cells in bone marrow of lupus-afflicted mice by inhibition of interleukin-7, leading to apoptosis. Immunology 128: 245–252.
36. Sharabi A, Lapter S, Mozes E (2010) Bcl-xL is required for the development of functional regulatory CD4 cells in lupus-afflicted mice following treatment with a tolerogenic peptide. J Autoimmun 34: 87–95.
37. Sthoeger ZM, Dayan M, Tcherniack A, Green L, Toledo S, et al. (2003) Modulation of autoreactive responses of peripheral blood lymphocytes of patients with systemic lupus erythematosus by peptides based on human and murine anti-DNA autoantibodies. Clin Exp Immunol 131: 385–392.
38. Farkas A, Tonel G, Nestle FO (2008) Interferon-alpha and viral triggers promote functional maturation of human monocyte-derived dendritic cells. Br J Dermatol 158: 921–929.
39. Gigante M, Mandic M, Wesa AK, Cavalcanti E, Dambrosio M, et al. (2008) Interferon-alpha (IFN-alpha)-conditioned DC preferentially stimulate type-1 and limit Treg-type in vitro T-cell responses from RCC patients. J Immunother 31: 254–262.
40. Yan B, Ye S, Chen G, Kuang M, Shen N, et al. (2008) Dysfunctional CD4+,CD25+regulatory T cells in untreated active systemic lupus erythematosus secondary to interferon-alpha-producing antigen-presenting cells. Arthritis Rheum 58: 801–812.
41. Braun D, Caramalho I, Demengeot J (2002) IFN-alpha/beta enhances BCR-dependent B cell responses. Int Immunol 14: 411–419.
42. Badr G, Saad H, Waly H, Hassan K, Abdel-Tawab H, et al. (2010) Type I interferon (IFN-alpha/beta) rescues B-lymphocytes from apoptosis via PI3K-delta/Akt, Rho-A, NFkappaB and Bcl-2/Bcl(XL). Cell Immunol 263: 31–40.
43. Litinskiy MB, Nardelli B, Hilbert DM, He B, Schaffer A, et al. (2002) DCs induce CD40-independent immunoglobulin class switching through BLyS and APRIL. Nat Immunol 3: 822–829.
44. Mitani Y, Takaoka A, Kim SH, Kato Y, Yokochi T, et al. (2001) Cross talk of the interferon-alpha/beta signalling complex with gp130 for effective interleukin-6 signalling. Genes Cells 6: 631–640.
45. Sela U, Dayan M, Hershkoviz R, Lider O, Mozes E (2008) A peptide that ameliorates lupus up-regulates the diminished expression of early growth response factors 2 and 3. J Immunol 180: 1584–1591.
46. Sharabi A, Sthoeger ZM, Mahlab K, Lapter S, Zinger H, et al. (2009) A tolerogenic peptide that induces suppressor of cytokine signaling (SOCS)-1 restores the aberrant control of IFN-gamma signaling in lupus-affected (NZB×NZW)F1 mice. Clin Immunol 132: 61–68.
47. Mauermann N, Sthoeger Z, Zinger H, Mozes E (2004) Amelioration of lupus manifestations by a peptide based on the complementarity determining region 1 of an autoantibody in severe combined immunodeficient (SCID) mice engrafted with peripheral blood lymphocytes of systemic lupus erythematosus (SLE) patients. Clin Exp Immunol 137: 513–520.
48. Gladman DD, Ibañez D, Urowitz MB (2002) Systemic lupus erythematosus disease activity index 2000. J Rheumatol 29: 288–291.
49. Yee CS, Isenberg DA, Prabu A, Sokoll K, Teh LS, et al. (2008) BILAG-2004 index captures systemic lupus erythematosus disease activity better than SLEDAI-2000. Ann Rheum Dis 67: 873–876.

8

The Clinical Significance of Vitamin D in Systemic Lupus Erythematosus

Rajalingham Sakthiswary*, Azman Ali Raymond

Department of Medicine, Universiti Kebangsaan Malaysia Medical Centre, Cheras, Kuala Lumpur, Malaysia

Abstract

Background: Vitamin D deficiency is more prevalent among SLE patients than the general population. Over the past decade, many studies across the globe have been carried out to investigate the role of vitamin D in SLE from various clinical angles. Therefore, the aim of this systematic review is to summarise and evaluate the evidence from the published literature; focusing on the clinical significance of vitamin D in SLE.

Methods: The following databases were searched: MEDLINE, Scopus, Web of Knowledge and CINAHL, using the terms "lupus", "systemic lupus erythematosus", "SLE and "vitamin D". We included only adult human studies published in the English language between 2000 and 2012.The reference lists of included studies were thoroughly reviewed in search for other relevant studies.

Results: A total of 22 studies met the selection criteria. The majority of the studies were observational (95.5%) and cross sectional (90.9%). Out of the 15 studies which looked into the association between vitamin D and SLE disease activity, 10 studies (including the 3 largest studies in this series) revealed a statistically significant inverse relationship. For disease damage, on the other hand, 5 out of 6 studies failed to demonstrate any association with vitamin D levels. Cardiovascular risk factors such as insulin resistance, hypertension and hypercholesterolaemia were related to vitamin D deficiency, according to 3 of the studies.

Conclusion: There is convincing evidence to support the association between vitamin D levels and SLE disease activity. There is paucity of data in other clinical aspects to make firm conclusions.

Editor: Paul Proost, University of Leuven, Rega Institute, Belgium

Funding: The authors have no funding or support to report.

Competing Interests: The authors have declared that no competing interests exist.

* E-mail: sakthis5@hotmail.com

Introduction

The link between vitamin D and systemic lupus erythematosus (SLE) was first described in 1995 [1]. The discovery of vitamin D receptor expression by cells of the immune system has spurred more research on the immunomodulatory properties of vitamin D over the past decade. Both the innate and adaptive immune systems have a wide array of cells such as macrophages, dendritic cells, T cells, and B cells which express vitamin D receptors that may respond to the biologically active form of vitamin D (1,25-dihydroxyvitamin D) [2]. Several studies across the globe have reported that vitamin D deficiency is more prevalent among SLE patients than the general population [3]. A possible explanation for this is the sun avoidance by SLE patients, which is an established trigger of lupus flares.

To date, there are over a hundred studies on SLE and vitamin D. The investigators of these studies have tried to establish the prevalence of vitamin D deficiency and its significance in various clinical aspects such as disease activity, disease damage and laboratory parameters. A question which is yet to be answered is whether or not vitamin D deficiency truly alters the course and prognosis of SLE. The answer to this question has important clinical implications, as it may offer potential therapeutic possibilities with vitamin D supplementation. Therefore, the aim of this systematic review is to summarise and evaluate the evidence from published literature focusing on the clinical significance of vitamin D in SLE.

Methodology

Search Strategy

We used the terms "lupus", "systemic lupus erythematosus", "SLE", "vitamin D" and 'SLE and vitamin D" to search the following databases: MEDLINE, Scopus, Web of Knowledge and CINAHL. Furthermore, the references of all retrieved articles were reviewed for relevant citations.

Inclusion Criteria

All adult human cohort and case-control studies written in English, which investigated the role and effects of vitamin D in SLE published between the years 2000 and 2012 were included.

Exclusion Criteria

Studies in other languages apart from English, case reports, case series, animal studies letters to the editor and review articles were excluded. Regarding the justification for excluding paediatric studies; apart from the age factor, paediatric SLE runs a more aggressive clinical course than adult SLE with higher rates of organ involvement and the disease tends to be more severe at presentation [4,5]. Besides, studies on vitamin D receptor gene polymorphisms were not selected. Most of the aforementioned studies lacked emphasis on and were not powered to investigate the correlation between measured vitamin D levels (25[OH]D) and its clinical significance [6,7,8]. Stringent selection criteria were applied in order to achieve a high level of homogeneity in the studies included in this systematic review.

Screening of Articles for Eligibility

Retrieved articles were screened for eligibility based on titles and abstracts and were subsequently classified as 'include', 'possible' and 'exclude' categories. The 'include' and 'possible' categories comprised studies reporting (1) measured vitamin D levels and/or vitamin D supplementation, and (2) disease activity, disease damage, laboratory parameters and/or organ involvement in SLE. In the 'possible' category, there were uncertainties concerning the study design, sample population or objectives. For articles falling into the 'include' and 'possible' categories, where available, the full texts were obtained and assessed. Both authors participated in the selection of articles and only articles which were agreed upon by both were finally included in the review. Throughout the selection process, both authors reached consensus in every instance. Figure 1 summarises the algorithm followed in the selection of studies.

Data Extraction

The following data were extracted from the selected studies: study design; country; year; sample size; disease activity and damage scoring systems; organ involvement and findings. The relevant and particularly, significant statistical values were recorded (odds ratios [OR], p values, rho [r]).

Results

A total of 22 studies met the eligibility criteria. The vast majority of the studies were observational (95.5%) and cross-sectional (90.9%). Eight case-control studies and 14 cohort studies were included. The number of studies originating from each continent is as follows: 8 from America, 6 from Europe, 6 from Asia, 1 from Australia and 1 from Africa. Study sample sizes varied from 37 to 378 subjects. All studies used 25-hydroxyvitamin D to determine the vitamin D level. Table 1 highlights the findings of the selected studies.

Vitamin D and its Association with SLE Disease Activity and Damage

The disease activity was assessed in most studies with validated scoring systems such as SLEDAI (Systemic Lupus Erythematosus Disease Activity Index), BILAG (British Isles Lupus Activity Group), and ECLAM (European Consensus of Lupus Activity Measurement). In 6 of the studies, the disease damage was investigated with the Systemic Lupus International Collaborating Clinics Damage Index (SDI) [9,10,11,12,13,14]. Across the studies, the correlation between vitamin D levels and SLE disease activity has been rather inconsistent. Out of the 15 studies which looked into this aspect, two third of the studies (10/15) reported a significant inverse association between vitamin D and the measured disease activity [10,14,15,16,17,18,19,20,21,22]. There were no significant methodological variations between the 10 studies showing an inverse relationship between vitamin D and the

disease activity and the 5 studies that did not show such relationship. The outcome measurement used in all the 5 studies was SLEDAI [9,11,12,13,23]. Similarly, 90% (9/10) of the studies which demonstrated a significant inverse relationship used SLEDAI. Of note, 3 out of the 5 negative studies in this regard were Spanish [9,11,13], and 2 of them were by the same authors [9,11].The damage scores, on the other hand, in 5 out of 6 studies failed to demonstrate a significant association with vitamin D levels [9,11,12,13,14].

In clinical practice, anti double stranded (ds) DNA and complement levels are simple, yet useful tools to monitor SLE disease activity. High titres of antidsDNA and low complement levels are associated with lupus flares [24].The majority of studies showed a significant inverse relationship between vitamin D levels and the former [14,18,19] and a direct relationship with the latter [12,19]. Along this line, Ritterhouse et al. [25] found that that vitamin D deficiency was associated with significantly higher B cell activation and interferon alpha activity. Bogaczewicz et al. [26] had conflicting results in this regard with their finding of vitamin D deficiency being associated with lower concentrations of interleukin 23.

Vitamin D and VAS (Visual Analogue Score)

The VAS was used to evaluate the patients' global assessment [9,20,27] and level of fatigue [11,23,28]. The findings of these studies showed no consistent pattern with respect to the relationship between the VAS and vitamin D levels. Only half of the studies found significant inverse correlation between these parameters [11,20,27]. The remaining studies found no significant association.

Vitamin D and Cardiovascular Risk Factors

There were 4 studies which investigated the relationship between vitamin D deficiency and cardiovascular risk factors such as hypercholesterolaemia, insulin resistance/diabetes mellitus and hypertension [10,20,22,29]. Wu et al. [10] found a significant association with insulin resistance which was consistent with the results of the study by Reynolds et al. [22]. Mok et al. [20] demonstrated a higher total/high density lipoprotein (HDL) cholesterol ratio in vitamin D deficient subjects supporting the findings of Wu et al. [10] of higher low density lipoprotein (LDL) cholesterol with lower vitamin D levels. Reynolds et al. [22] and Ravenell et al. [29] had conflicting results on the correlation with carotid plaque. Ravenell et al. [29] discovered that vitamin D levels inversely correlated with age-adjusted total plaque area while Reynolds et al. [22] found the opposite. The latter, however demonstrated a significant increase in aortic stiffness with reducing levels of vitamin D.

Discussion

The results of this systematic review indicate that there is substantial evidence to convince us of the association between vitamin D levels and SLE disease activity. However, one may argue that a few of the studies refute this finding and cast doubts on the aforementioned link. It is noteworthy that the 3 largest studies with sample sizes of 378,290 and 181 subjects, revealed strong inverse correlations between vitamin D levels and SLEDAI scores with p values of 0.018,<0.001 and 0.001, respectively [10,14,16]. Mok et al. [14] concluded that vitamin D deficiency is a marker of SLE disease activity with comparable specificity to anti-C1q. The conflicting results of the few studies could be due to the diverse study populations, methodological variations and the power of several studies [11,13,23] was probably too low to

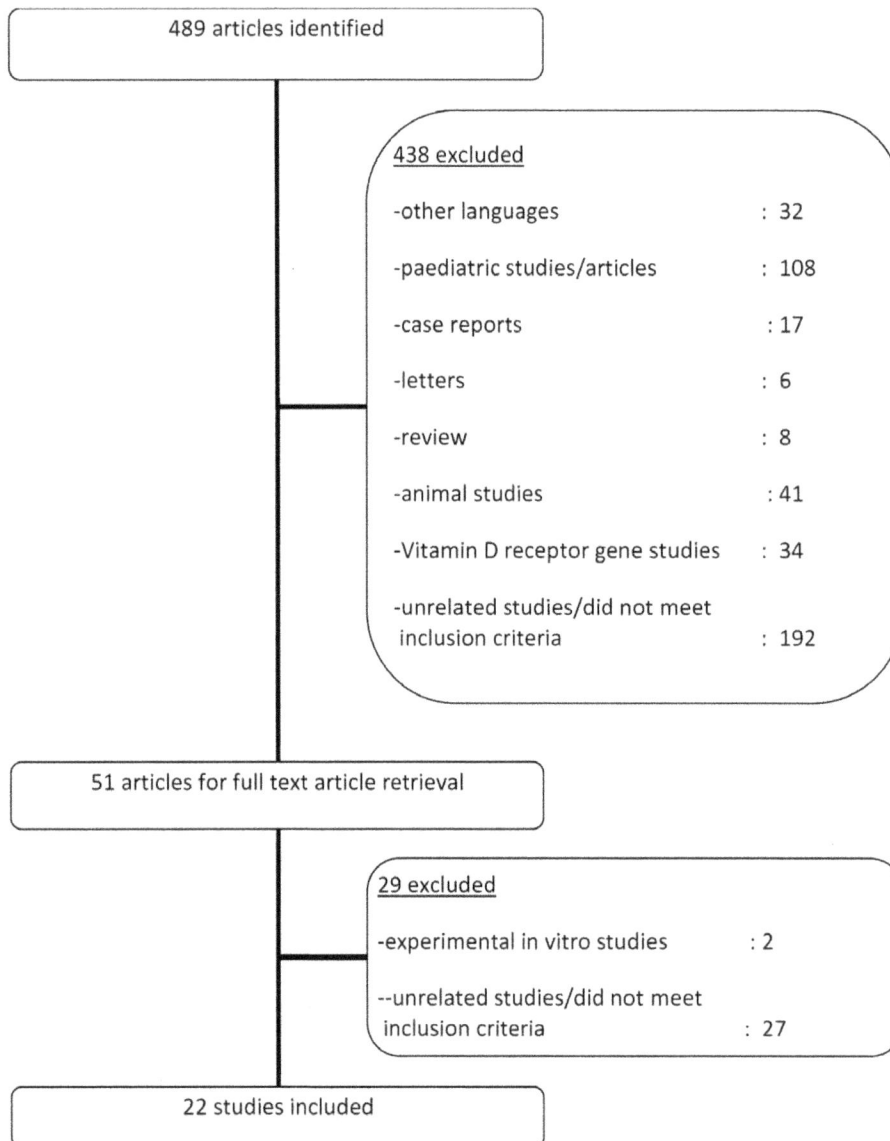

Figure 1. The algorithm for selection of studies in this systematic review.

achieve statistical significance. While the results of these observational studies are helpful for generating hypotheses concerning the effects of vitamin D on the clinical course of SLE, it is unwise to make causal inferences from these studies.

Lupus disease activity predicts the risk of subsequent organ damage [30]. Intriguingly, the majority of studies consistently demonstrated that vitamin D level is not associated with organ damage [9,11,12,13,14]. The authors are unable to provide any valid evidence-based explanation for this observation. This finding limits or perhaps, deters the use of vitamin D levels as a prognostication tool. Kamen et al. (4) and Bogaczewicz et al. (22) found an association between vitamin D levels and renal disease. Similarly, Reynolds et al. (24) and Ravenell et al. (25) pointed out a significant relationship with the cardiovascular system. These findings need to be tested rigorously by larger prospective studies to make firm conclusions. As these studies are too few in number, there is still profound lack of evidence to support the role of vitamin D in the management of the individual organ system.

Nevertheless, this is an area worthy of further research due to the biologic plausibility of a link between vitamin D deficiency and especially, cardiovascular and renal disease in SLE.

Our systematic review has limitations. We did not include articles in other languages which may have had valuable information or additional evidence related to this topic. It is reasonable to assume that some studies with negative or null results were simply not published; a well recognised publication bias. The cross sectional study design used in the majority of these studies does not give us a clear picture as to whether vitamin D deficiency confers a poorer outcome of SLE in the long term. Future research on vitamin D in SLE will hopefully address more practical concerns and provide answers to the following questions : the most appropriate phase of SLE to assess vitamin D (ie, at the time of diagnosis or while in remission); the cutoff value of 'normal' versus 'insufficient' vitamin D levels in lupus patients as compared to the general population; potential confounding factors such as medications, age, body size, geographic location, ethnicity,

Table 1. Summary of the selected studies.

Ref.	Year	Country	Study design	Study population	Findings/Conclusions	Statistical findings
[31]	2006	United States	Cross sectional Case-control	123 recently diagnosed SLE 240 controls	Lower vitamin D levels is associated with a. presence of renal disease b. photosensitivity.	OR 13.3, p<0.01 OR 12.9, p<0.01
[9]	2008	Spain	Cross sectional Cohort	92 SLE	No relation was seen between vitamin D and disease duration, SLEDAI, SLICC-ACR or VAS indexes.	
[27]	2008	United States	Cross sectional Cohort	37 female SLE	Vitamin D deficiency was associated with a. lower global assessment scores, However, levels of dsDNA were higher in the group with levels of vitamin D that were greater than 47.7 nmol/L	p< or =0.003 p=0.0069
[32]	2009	Canada	Cross sectional Cohort	124 SLE	Vitamin D levels showed no correlation with bone mineral density	p=0.26
[15]	2009	Brazil	Cross sectional Case-control	36 SLE 26 controls	Vitamin D level was associated with a. SLEDAI, b. osteocalcin c. bone-specific alkaline phosphatase.	r=−0.65, p<0.001) r=0.35 r=−0.17,
[10]	2009	United States	Cross sectional Cohort	181 female SLE	Lower vitamin D levels were significantly associated with higher a. diastolic blood pressure b. low-density lipoprotein cholesterol, c. lipoprotein(a) d.fibrinogen levels e. self-reported hypertension f. diabetes mellitus g. SLEDAI h. SLICC. With further adjustment for BMI, these associations were no longer significant.	p=0.034 p=0.013 p=0.024 p=0.000 p=0.016,OR 0.68 p=0.032, OR 0.49 p=0.001 p=0.003
[11]	2010	Spain	Prospective cohort, those with low baseline vitamin D levels were supplemented with oral vitamin D(3)	80 SLE	Inverse significant correlations between vitamin D levels and the VAS(fatigue) Changes in vitamin D levels correlated with changes in the VAS in patients with baseline vitamin D levels <30 ng/ml No significant correlations between the vitamin D levels and: a. SLEDAI b. SDI	p=0.001 p=0.017 p=0.87 p=0.63
[16]	2010	Israel	Cross sectional Cohort study	378 SLE (European and Israeli patients)	A significant negative correlation between the serum concentration of vitamin D and the SLEDAI-2K and ECLAM scales	r=−0.12, p=0.018.
[17]	2011	Egypt	Cross sectional Case-control	60 SLE 60 controls	Serum vitamin D levels were lower with a. increased SLEDAI score, b. frequency of photosensitivity	OR: 2.72, p=0.002 OR: 3.6, p<0.01
[18]	2011	Iran	Cross sectional Cohort study	40 SLE	Serum vitamin D concentration was inversely correlated with the BILAG index score. Vitamin D deficiency was associated with a. higher concentrations of liver enzymes, b. lower serum albumin and hemoglobin concentrations c. higher titers of antibodies to double-stranded DNA (ds-DNA).	r=−0.486, p=0.001 p<0.05 p<0.05 p<0.001
[25]	2011	United States	Cross sectional Case-control	32 SLE 32 controls	Vitamin D deficiency was associated with a. higher B cell activation b. higher serum IFNalpha activity	p=0.009 p=0.02
[12]	2011	Korea	Cross sectional Case-control	104 SLE 49 controls	The serum vitamin D levels, were positively correlated only with a. hemoglobin b. serum complement 3 but not with a. SLEDAI b. SLICC	beta=0.256, p=0.018 beta=0.365, p=0.002 beta=−0.04,p=0.742 beta =−0.052, p=0.62

Table 1. Cont.

Ref.	Year	Country	Study design	Study population	Findings/Conclusions	Statistical findings
[19]	2011	Hungary	Cross sectional Cohort	177 SLE	Reduced vitamin D levels were associated with : a. pericarditis b. neuropsychiatric diseases c. deep vein thrombosis d. higher SLEDAI score e. higher anti-double-stranded (ds)DNA autoantibody concentrations, f. higher anti-Smith antigen (anti-Sm) concentrations g. lower C4 levels h. higher immunoglobulin (Ig)G concentration	p = 0.013 p = 0.010 p = 0.014 p = 0.038 p = 0.021 p < 0.001 p = 0.027 p = 0.034
[28]	2012	Australia	Cross sectional Case-control	24 SLE 21 controls	Fatigue was not related to vitamin D status	
[13]	2012	Spain	Cross sectional Cohort study	73 SLE	No correlation between vitamin D deficiency and a. SLEDAI score b. SLICC/ACR score	p = 0.310 p = 0.820
[14]	2012	Hong Kong	Cross sectional Cohort study	290 SLE	Vitamin D correlated inversely and significantly with a. clinical SLE activity b. anti-C1q c. anti-dsDNA titers, d. but not with complement levels or damage scores.	r = −0.26; p < 0.001 r = −0.14; p = 0.020 r = −0.13; p = 0.020
[20]	2012	Hong Kong	Cross sectional Cohort	290 SLE	Levels of vitamin D correlated inversely with a. PGA, b. total SLEDAI scores vitamin D deficiency had significantly higher a. total/high-density lipoprotein(HDL) cholesterol ratio b. prevalence of antiphospholipid syndrome No association could be demonstrated between vitamin D level and atherosclerosis	beta −0.20; p = 0.003 beta −0.19; p = 0.003 p = 0.02 p = 0.007
[21]	2012	Malaysia	Prospective Cohort	38 premenopausal SLE	There was a significant negative correlation between SLEDAI scores and vitamin D levels.	p = 0.033
[26]	2012	Poland	Cross sectional Case-control	49 SLE. 49 controls	Vitamin D deficiency was associated with a. renal disease b. leucopenia c. lower serum concentrations of IL-23)	p = 0.006 p = 0.047 p = 0.037
[23]	2012	Brazil	Cross sectional Case control	78 SLE 64 controls	No statistically significant association was observed between vitamin D deficiency and the following: a. disease activity (SLEDAI >6) b. fatigue c. anti-DNA	p = 0.971 p = 0.808 p = 0.435
[22]	2012	United Kingdom	Cross sectional Cohort	75 SLE	Patients with vitamin D deficiency had higher a. BMI b. insulin resistance. c. SLEDAI-2K Aortic stiffness was inversely associated with serum vitamin D independently of BMI, CVD risk factors and serum insulin. There was no association between vitamin D and carotid plaque and intima media thickness.	p = 0.014 p = 0.023 p = 0.031 beta = −0.0217 p = 0.010
[29]	2012	United States	Cross sectional Cohort	51 SLE	vitamin D levels inversely correlated with age-adjusted total plaque area.	r = −0.33, p = 0.018

sun protective behaviours; and genetic variation in the metabolism of vitamin D.

Much emphasis has been placed on vitamin D in SLE in recent years. Apart from its significant association with disease activity, based on the evidence highlighted in this systematic review, it is premature and would be fallacious to make any definitive claims for or against the role of vitamin D in other clinical aspects.

Author Contributions

Conceived and designed the experiments: RS AAR. Performed the experiments: RS. Analyzed the data: AAR. Wrote the paper: RS AAR.

References

1. Muller K, Kriegbaum NJ, Baslund B, Sorensen OH, Thymann M, et al. (1995) Vitamin D3 metabolism in patients with rheumatic diseases: low serum levels of 25-hydroxyvitamin D3 in patients with systemic lupus erythematosus. Clinical rheumatology 14: 397–400.
2. Adorini L, Penna G (2008) Control of autoimmune diseases by the vitamin D endocrine system. Nat Clin Pract Rheumatol 4: 404–412.
3. Kamen DL, Aranow C (2008) The link between vitamin D deficiency and systemic lupus erythematosus. Curr Rheumatol Rep 10: 273–280.
4. Brunner HI, Gladman DD, Ibanez D, Urowitz MD, Silverman ED (2008) Difference in disease features between childhood-onset and adult-onset systemic lupus erythematosus. Arthritis and rheumatism 58: 556–562.
5. Pradhan V, Patwardhan M, Rajadhyaksha A, Ghosh K (2012) Clinical and Immunological Profile of Systemic Lupus Erythematosus. Indian pediatrics.
6. Abbasi M, Rezaieyazdi Z, Afshari JT, Hatef M, Sahebari M, et al. (2010) Lack of association of vitamin D receptor gene BsmI polymorphisms in patients with systemic lupus erythematosus. Rheumatology international 30: 1537–1539.
7. Huang CM, Wu MC, Wu JY, Tsai FJ (2002) No association of vitamin D receptor gene start codon fok 1 polymorphisms in Chinese patients with systemic lupus erythematosus. The Journal of rheumatology 29: 1211–1213.
8. Huang CM, Wu MC, Wu JY, Tsai FJ (2002) Association of vitamin D receptor gene BsmI polymorphisms in Chinese patients with systemic lupus erythematosus. Lupus 11: 31–34.
9. Ruiz-Irastorza G, Egurbide MV, Olivares N, Martinez-Berriotxoa A, Aguirre C (2008) Vitamin D deficiency in systemic lupus erythematosus: prevalence, predictors and clinical consequences. Rheumatology 47: 920–923.
10. Wu PW, Rhew EY, Dyer AR, Dunlop DD, Langman CB, et al. (2009) 25-hydroxyvitamin D and cardiovascular risk factors in women with systemic lupus erythematosus. Arthritis & Rheumatism: Arthritis Care & Research 61: 1387–1395.
11. Ruiz-Irastorza G, Gordo S, Olivares N, Egurbide MV, Aguirre C (2010) Changes in vitamin D levels in patients with systemic lupus erythematosus: Effects on fatigue, disease activity, and damage. Arthritis care & research 62: 1160–1165.
12. Kim HA, Sung JM, Jeon JY, Yoon JM, Suh CH (2011) Vitamin D may not be a good marker of disease activity in Korean patients with systemic lupus erythematosus. Rheumatology international 31: 1189–1194.
13. Munoz-Ortego J, Torrente-Segarra V, Prieto-Alhambra D, Salman-Monte T, Carbonell-Abello J (2012) Prevalence and predictors of vitamin D deficiency in non-supplemented women with systemic lupus erythematosus in the Mediterranean region: a cohort study. Scandinavian journal of rheumatology.
14. Mok CC, Birmingham DJ, Ho LY, Hebert LA, Song H, et al. (2012) Vitamin D deficiency as marker for disease activity and damage in systemic lupus erythematosus: a comparison with anti-dsDNA and anti-C1q. Lupus 21: 36–42.
15. Borba VZ, Vieira JG, Kasamatsu T, Radominski SC, Sato EI, et al. (2009) Vitamin D deficiency in patients with active systemic lupus erythematosus. Osteoporosis international : a journal established as result of cooperation between the European Foundation for Osteoporosis and the National Osteoporosis Foundation of the USA 20: 427–433.
16. Amital H, Szekanecz Z, Szucs G, Danko K, Nagy E, et al. (2010) Serum concentrations of 25-OH vitamin D in patients with systemic lupus erythematosus (SLE) are inversely related to disease activity: is it time to routinely supplement patients with SLE with vitamin D? Annals of the rheumatic diseases 69: 1155–1157.
17. Hamza RT, Awwad KS, Ali MK, Hamed AI (2011) Reduced serum concentrations of 25-hydroxy vitamin D in Egyptian patients with systemic lupus erythematosus: relation to disease activity. Medical science monitor : international medical journal of experimental and clinical research 17: CR711–718.
18. Bonakdar ZS, Jahanshahifar L, Jahanshahifar F, Gholamrezaei A (2011) Vitamin D deficiency and its association with disease activity in new cases of systemic lupus erythematosus. Lupus 20: 1155–1160.
19. Szodoray P, Tarr T, Bazso A, Poor G, Szegedi G, et al. (2011) The immunopathological role of vitamin D in patients with SLE: data from a single centre registry in Hungary. Scandinavian journal of rheumatology 40: 122–126.
20. Mok CC, Birmingham DJ, Leung HW, Hebert LA, Song H, et al. (2012) Vitamin D levels in Chinese patients with systemic lupus erythematosus: relationship with disease activity, vascular risk factors and atherosclerosis. Rheumatology 51: 644–652.
21. Yeap SS, Othman AZ, Zain AA, Chan SP (2012) Vitamin D levels: its relationship to bone mineral density response and disease activity in premenopausal Malaysian systemic lupus erythematosus patients on corticosteroids. International journal of rheumatic diseases 15: 17–24.
22. Reynolds JA, Haque S, Berry JL, Pemberton P, Teh LS, et al. (2012) 25-Hydroxyvitamin D deficiency is associated with increased aortic stiffness in patients with systemic lupus erythematosus. Rheumatology 51: 544–551.
23. Fragoso TS, Dantas AT, Marques CD, Rocha Junior LF, Melo JH, et al. (2012) 25-Hydroxyivitamin D3 levels in patients with systemic lupus erythematosus and its association with clinical parameters and laboratory tests. Revista brasileira de reumatologia 52: 60–65.
24. Giles BM, Boackle SA (2012) Linking complement and anti-dsDNA antibodies in the pathogenesis of systemic lupus erythematosus. Immunol Res.
25. Ritterhouse LL, Crowe SR, Niewold TB, Kamen DL, Macwana SR, et al. (2011) Vitamin D deficiency is associated with an increased autoimmune response in healthy individuals and in patients with systemic lupus erythematosus. Annals of the rheumatic diseases 70: 1569–1574.
26. Bogaczewicz J, Sysa-Jedrzejowska A, Arkuszewska C, Zabek J, Kontny E, et al. (2012) Vitamin D status in systemic lupus erythematosus patients and its association with selected clinical and laboratory parameters. Lupus 21: 477–484.
27. Thudi A, Yin S, Wandstrat AE, Li QZ, Olsen NJ (2008) Vitamin D levels and disease status in Texas patients with systemic lupus erythematosus. The American journal of the medical sciences 335: 99–104.
28. Stockton KA, Kandiah DA, Paratz JD, Bennell KL (2012) Fatigue, muscle strength and vitamin D status in women with systemic lupus erythematosus compared with healthy controls. Lupus 21: 271–278.
29. Ravenell RL, Kamen DL, Spence JD, Hollis BW, Fleury TJ, et al. (2012) Premature Atherosclerosis Is Associated With Hypovitaminosis D and Angiotensin-Converting Enzyme Inhibitor Non-use in Lupus Patients. The American journal of the medical sciences 344: 268–273.
30. Lopez R, Davidson JE, Beeby MD, Egger PJ, Isenberg DA (2012) Lupus disease activity and the risk of subsequent organ damage and mortality in a large lupus cohort. Rheumatology (Oxford) 51: 491–498.
31. Kamen DL, Cooper GS, Bouali H, Shaftman SR, Hollis BW, et al. (2006) Vitamin D deficiency in systemic lupus erythematosus. Autoimmunity reviews 5: 114–117.
32. Toloza SM, Cole DE, Gladman DD, Ibanez D, Urowitz MB (2010) Vitamin D insufficiency in a large female SLE cohort. Lupus 19: 13–19.

9

Evidence of New Risk Genetic Factor to Systemic Lupus Erythematosus: The *UBASH3A* Gene

Lina-Marcela Diaz-Gallo[1]*, **Elena Sánchez**[1], **Norberto Ortego-Centeno**[2], **Jose Mario Sabio**[3],
Francisco J. García-Hernández[4], **Enrique de Ramón**[5], **Miguel A. González-Gay**[6], **Torsten Witte**[7],
Hans-Joachim Anders[8], **María F. González-Escribano**[9], **Javier Martin**[1]

1 Cellular Biology and Immunology Department, Instituto de Parasitología y Biomedicina "López-Neyra", Consejo Superior de Investigaciones Científicas (IPBLN- Consejo Superior de Investigaciones Científicas), Granada, Spain, 2 Department of Internal Medicine, Hospital Clínico San Cecilio, Granada, Spain, 3 Department of Internal Medicine, Hospital Virgen de las Nieves, Granada, Spain, 4 Department of Internal Medicine, Hospital Virgen del Rocío, Sevilla, Spain, 5 Department of Internal Medicine, Hospital Carlos Haya, Málaga, Spain, 6 Department of Rheumatology, Instituto de Formación e Investigación Marqués de Valdecilla, Hospital Universitario Marqués de Valdecilla, Santander, Spain, 7 Department of Clinical Immunology and Rheumatology, Hannover Medical School, Hannover, Germany, 8 Medical department and policlinic IV, Klinikum der Universität, München, Munich, Germany, 9 Department of Immunology, Hospital Virgen del Rocío, Sevilla, Spain

Abstract

The ubiquitin associated and Src-homology 3 (SH3) domain containing A (*UBASH3a*) is a suppressor of T-cell receptor signaling, underscoring antigen presentation to T-cells as a critical shared mechanism of diseases pathogenesis. The aim of the present study was to determine whether the *UBASH3a* gene influence the susceptibility to systemic lupus erythematosus (SLE) in Caucasian populations. We evaluated five *UBASH3a* polymorphisms (rs2277798, rs2277800, rs9976767, rs13048049 and rs17114930), using TaqMan® allelic discrimination assays, in a discovery cohort that included 906 SLE patients and 1165 healthy controls from Spain. The SNPs that exhibit statistical significance difference were evaluated in a German replication cohort of 360 SLE patients and 379 healthy controls. The case-control analysis in the Spanish population showed a significant association between the rs9976767 and SLE (Pc = 9.9E-03 OR = 1.21 95%CI = 1.07–1.37) and a trend of association for the rs2277798 analysis (P = 0.09 OR = 0.9 95%CI = 0.79–1.02). The replication in a German cohort and the meta-analysis confirmed that the rs9976767 (Pc = 0.02; Pc = 2.4E-04, for German cohort and meta-analysis, respectively) and rs2277798 (Pc = 0.013; Pc = 4.7E-03, for German cohort and meta-analysis, respectively) *UBASH3a* variants are susceptibility factors for SLE. Finally, a conditional regression analysis suggested that the most likely genetic variation responsible for the association was the rs9976767 polymorphism. Our results suggest that *UBASH3a* gene plays a role in the susceptibility to SLE. Moreover, our study indicates that *UBASH3a* can be considered as a common genetic factor in autoimmune diseases.

Editor: Xiao-Ping Miao, MOE Key Laboratory of Environment and Health, School of Public Health, Tongji Medical College, Huazhong University of Science and Technology, China

Funding: This work was partially supported by RETICS Program, RD08/0075 (RIER) from Instituto de Salud Carlos III, within the VI PN de I+D+i 2008-2011 (FEDER) and grant KFO 250, TP 03, WI 1031/6-1 LMDG was supported by the "Ayudas Predoctorales de Formación en Investigación en Salud (PFIS - FI09/00544)" from the "Instituto de Salud Carlos III". The funders had no role in study design, data collection and analysis, decision to publish, or preparation of the manuscript.

Competing Interests: The authors have declared that no competing interests exist.

* E-mail: lina.diaz@ipb.csic.es

Introduction

The T cell ubiquitin ligand proteins (TULA) family is characterized by function as suppressors of T cell receptor signalling. One of the members of the TULA family proteins is the ubiquitin associated and Src-homology 3 (SH3) domain containing A (*UBASH3a*) which is expressed only in lymphoid cells and facilitates apoptosis induced in T cells by certain stimuli, such as growth factor withdrawal [1]. *UBASH3a* gene spans 40 kb, contains 15 exons and is located on human chromosome 21q22.3 [2]. The lack of TULA proteins resulted in hyper-reactivity of T cells [1]. Evidence for both B and T lymphocyte hyper-reactivity is typically observed in autoimmune disorders [2]. These disorders are characterized by an inappropriate, ultimately excessive, inflammatory response against self, resulting in tissue destruction. Although many individuals affected by autoimmune diseases demonstrate multiorgan involvement, the primary end-organ

target (e.g., autoimmune destruction of pancreatic islet cells in type 1 diabetes mellitus) typically drives the clinical presentation and disease definition. Recent studies have showed that single nucleotide polymorphisms (SNPs) of the *UBASH3a* gene are associated with some autoimmune diseases, like type 1 diabetes (T1D), celiac disease (CD), rheumatoid arthritis (RA) and vitiligo, suggesting that this gene could play an important role in the pathogenesis of autoimmune disorders [3–8].

Systemic lupus erythematosus (SLE) is a prototypic autoimmune diseases characterized by the production of autoantibodies, immune-complex deposition, and subsequent multiple organ damage. The complex aetiology of autoimmune diseases includes environmental, hormonal and genetic factors. Some of those factors remained to be defined [3,4]. Based on these insights, the aim of the present study was to evaluate the role of five *UBASH3a* polymorphism in SLE.

Table 1. Genotype and minor allele frequencies of *UBASH3a* SNPs located in Caucasian SLE patients and healthy controls from Spain, the discovery cohort.

SNP	1/2	Subgroup (N)	Genotype, N (%)			Alleles, N(%)		Allele test	
			1/1	1/2	2/2	1	2	P-value*	OR [CI 95%]****
rs2277798	G/A	Controls (n = 1165)	477 (40.94)	529 (45.41)	159 (13.65)	1483 (63.6)	847 (36.4)		
		SLE (n = 906)	402 (44.37)	394 (43.49)	110 (12.14)	1198 (66.1)	614 (33.9)	0.0993**	0.90 [0.79-1.02]
rs2277800	C/T	Controls (n = 1165)	1080 (92.70)	84 (7.21)	1 (0.09)	2244 (96.3)	86 (3.7)		
		SLE (n = 906)	832 (91.83)	73 (8.06)	1 (0.11)	1737 (95.9)	75 (4.1)	0.4592	1.13 [0.82–1.55]
rs9976767	A/G	Controls (n = 1165)	363 (31.16)	558 (47.90)	244 (20.94)	1284 (55.1)	1046 (44.9)		
		SLE (n = 906)	230 (25.39)	451 (49.78)	225 (24.83)	911 (503)	901 (49.7)	1.99E-03***	1.21 [1.07–1.37]
rs13048049	G/A	Controls (n = 1165)	1038 (89.10)	126 (10.82)	1 (0.09)	2202 (94.5)	128 (5.5)		
		SLE (n = 906)	808 (89.18)	96 (10.60)	2 (0.22)	1712 (94.5)	100 (5.5)	0.9719	1.01 [0.77–1.32]
rs17114930	C/G	Controls (n = 1165)	1066 (91.50)	95 (8.15)	4 (0.34)	2227 (95.6)	103 (4.4)		
		SLE (n = 906)	811 (89.51)	93 (10.26)	2 (0.22)	1715 (94.6)	97 (5.4)	0.1649	1.22 [0.92–1.63]

*All P-values have been calculated for the allelic model. ** Pc = 0.248 Benjamini & Hochberg (1995). ***Pc = 9.9E-03 Benjamini & Hochberg (1995) step-up FDR control. ****Odds ratio for the minor allele.

Materials and Methods

Ethics Statement

Written informed consent was obtained from all participants and the respectively ethics committee approved the study according to the principles expressed in the Declaration of Helsinki.

The case-control study included 906 SLE patients and 1165 healthy controls from a white Spanish population. The replication cohort from white Germans comprehends 360 SLE patients and 379 healthy controls. All the patients met the American College of Rheumatology criteria for classification of SLE [5]. Written informed consent was obtained from all participants and the respectively ethics committee approved the study. DNA was obtained from peripheral blood using standard methods. The samples were genotyped for the *UBASH3a* rs2277798, rs2277800, rs9976767, rs13048049 and rs17114930 polymorphisms via TaqMan® 5′allelic discrimination technology using a predesigned SNPs genotyping assays provided by Applied Biosystems (assay ID: C___1724055_10, C__15885522_20, C___1724067_10,

C___1724073_20 and C___25622591_10, respectively; Figure S1). At the moment of the design of the study the only confirmed case-control associated SNP with autoimmune diseases was the rs9976767 [6]. The other four SNPs were selected because they were not included in previous SLE genetic studies and they are non-synonymous changes located in different exons of the *UBASH3a* gene. Moreover, the minor allele frequency (MAF) of those SNPs was reported in Caucasian populations and they exhibited moderated LD with at least one SNP in the loci. Deviation from Hardy-Weinberg equilibrium (HWE) was tested by standard chi-square analysis. The differences in genotype distribution and allele frequency among cases and controls were calculated by contingency tables and when necessary by Fisher's exact test. Odds ratios (OR), and 95% confidence intervals (CI), were calculated according to Woolf's method. Combined data were analysed by Mantel-Haenszel tests under fixed effect model and the Breslow-Day (BD) test was used to estimate the OR heterogeneity amongst the two cohorts. An association was considered statistically significant if P<0.05. Benjamini & Hochberg (1995) step-up false discovery rate (FDR) control correction

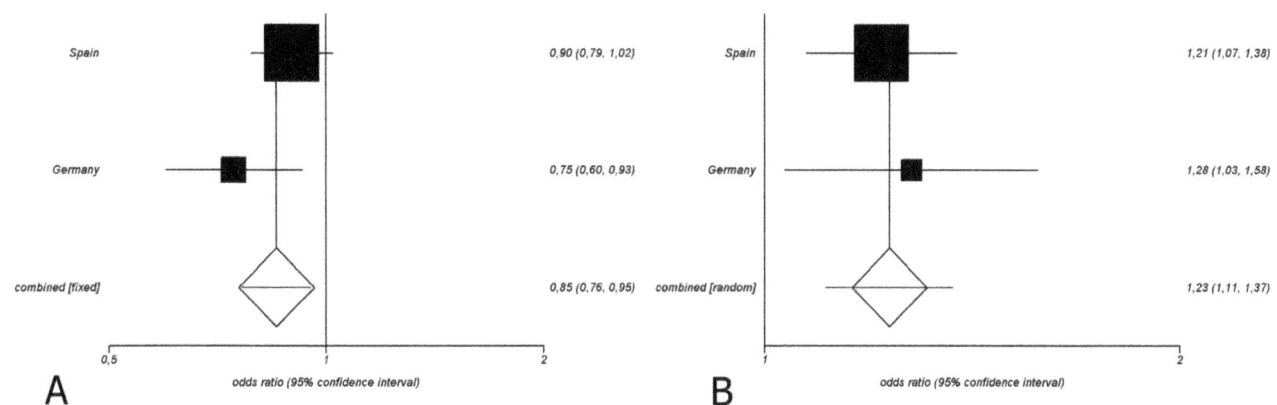

Figure 1. Graphical representation of the meta-analysis (A) Forest plot for the meta-analysis of the *UBASH3a* rs2277798 polymorphism in SLE in two Caucasian cohorts. (B) Forest plot for the meta-analysis of the *UBASH3a* rs9976767 polymorphism in SLE in two Caucasian cohorts.

Table 2. Genotype and minor allele frequencies of *UBASH3a* SNPs located in Caucasian SLE patients and healthy controls from Germany.

SNP	$\frac{1}{2}$	Subgroup (N)	Genotype, N (%)			Alleles, N(%)		Allele test		
			1/1	1/2	2/2	1	2	*P*-value*	P_{FR}**	OR [CI 95%]***
rs2277798	G/A	Controls (n = 379)	184 (48.55)	132 (34.83)	63 (16.62)	448 (59.1)	310 (40.9)			
		SLE(n = 360)	149 (41.39)	163 (45.28)	48 (13.33)	475 (66)	245 (34)	0.0064	0,0128	0.75 [0.60–0.92]
rs9976767	A/G	Controls (n = 379)	186 (49.08)	136 (35.88)	57 (15.04)	458 (60.4)	300 (39.4)			
		SSc (n = 360)	180 (50.00)	106 (29.44)	74 (20.56)	392 (54.4)	328 (45.6)	0.0201	0,0201	1.28 [1.04–1.57]

*All P-values have been calculated for the allelic model. ** Benjamini & Hochberg (1995) step-up FDR control. ***Odds ratio for the minor allele.

[7] for multiple testing was applied to the P-values in both the independent analysis and the combined meta-analysis (P_c). Linkage disequilibrium (LD) measurement (r^2) between the studied SNPs was estimated by expectation-maximization algorithm using HAPLOVIEW (version 4.2; Broad Institute of MIT and Harvard). Finally, the dependency of the association between each SNP and every studied genetic variant was determined by a conditional logistic regression analysis (considering the different cohorts as covariate). The analyses were performed using PLINK (version 1.07) [8].

Results

The distributions of genotypic and allelic frequencies of the five *UABSH3a* evaluated polymorphisms were in HWE at 5% significance level. Additionally, MAFs of the studied SNPs were similar to those reported by the HapMap project for the CEU population (http://hapmap.ncbi.nlm.nih.gov/) in both, Spanish and German cohorts. The LD structure of the five *UABSH3a* SNPs in the Spanish cohort is shown in (Figure S1). The Table 1 summarizes the results of the association analysis for the discovery cohort. The minor allele of the rs9976767 polymorphism exhibited a statistical significant association with SLE in the Spanish population (P_c = 9.9E-03, OR = 1.21, 95%CI = 1.07–1.37). In addition we observed a trend of association with the rs2277798 polymorphism (P = 0.099, P_c = 0.248, OR = 0.9, 95%CI = 0.79–1.02). The frequency of the minor alleles of the rs2277800, rs13048049 and rs17114930 *UBASH3a* polymorphisms were not statistically significantly different between SLE patients and healthy controls in the Spanish cohort.

Based on these observations, we evaluated the frequency of the rs9976767 and rs2277798 in a replication cohort from Germany (Table 2). Genotypic and allelic frequencies of both polymorphisms were in HWE. The frequency of the minor allele of both

SNPs: rs9976767 and rs2277798 were statistically significant different between SLE patients and healthy controls: rs9976767 (P_c = 0.02, OR = 1.28 95%CI = 1.04–1.57) and rs227798 (P_c = 0.01, OR = 0.75, 95%CI = 0.6–0.92). Lastly, we combine both the Spanish and German cohorts through a meta-analysis in order to increase the statistical power and to determine the combine OR (Table 3 and Figure 1). This analysis showed evidence of association of the minor allele of rs9976767 with higher SLE risk (P_c = 4.7E-03, OR = 1.23 95%CI = 1.11–1.37) and the rs2277798 with lower risk to SLE (P_c = 2.4–04, OR = 0.85, 95%CI = 0.76–0.95).

Finally, we prompted out to evaluate whether one of both polymorphisms is responsible for the associations detected using a logistic regression analysis. Pair-wise conditional analysis showed that the association of the rs2277798 SNP was explained by the rs9976767effect, because only the coefficient for the test of rs9976767 remained significant (model conditioned by rs2277798P = 0.76; model conditioned by rs9976767 P = 9E-03, Table 4).

Discussion

UBASH3a is implicated in the regulation of tyrosine phosphorylation levels within T cells and is involved in facilitates the apoptosis induced in these cells. *UBASH3a* binds to the apoptosis-inducing protein AIF, which has previously been shown to function as a key factor of caspase-independent apoptosis [9]. It has also been reported that SLE T cells, compared with control T cells, undergo an increased rate of apoptosis, which contribute to SLE pathogenesis [4]. Changes in the *UBASH3a* structure or expression levels can affect the binding with AIF leading to an alteration in the apoptosis level.

Herein, we described for the first time the influence of five *UBASH3a* genetic variants in SLE susceptibility. Interestingly, the

Table 3. Meta-analysis of two *UBASH3a* genetic variants within Spanish and German SLE populations.

SNP	$\frac{1}{2}$	Subgroup (N)	Genotype, N (%)			Alleles, N(%)		Allele test		
			1/1	1/2	2/2	1	2	*P*-value*	P_{FDR}**	OR [CI 95%]***
rs2277798	G/A	Controls (n = 1544)	609 (39.44)	713 (46.18)	222 (14.38)	1931 (62.5)	1157 (37.5)			
		SLE (n = 1266)	565 (44.63)	543 (42.89)	158 (12.48)	1673 (66.1)	859 (33.9)	0.0047	4.7E-03	0.85 [0.76–0.95]
rs9976767	A/G	Controls (n = 1544)	499 (32.32)	744 (48.19)	301 (19.49)	1742 (56.4)	13446 (43.6)			
		SLE (n = 1266)	336 (26.54)	631 (49.84)	299 (23.62)	1303 (51.5)	1229 (48.5)	1.2E-04	2,4E-04	1.23 [1.11–1.37]

*All P-values have been calculated for the allelic model. **Benjamini & Hochberg (1995) step-up FDR control. ***Odds ratio for the minor allele.

Table 4. Conditional logistic regression analysis for two *UBASH3a* SNPs located in SLE considering the two European populations as covariate.

Group of analysis	SNP	MAF Cases	MAF Controls	p Value: add to rs9976767	rs9976767 p value: add to SNP	r2 with rs9976767	
						Spain	Germany
SLE							
	rs2277798	0.34	0.38	0.758	0.0087	0.45	0.41

rs9976767 polymorphism is located in the intronic region between the exons 5 and 6 while the other four studied SNPs (rs2277798, rs2277800, rs13048049 and rs17114930) are non-synonymous changes located in three different exons. The intronic regions flanking constitutive exons contain potential splicing regulatory sequences. Moreover, a study restricted to analysis of the canonical splice signals reported that 15% of point mutations disrupted splicing, a likely gross underestimate of the impact of splicing on human disease [10]. This suggests that the rs9976767 polymorphism could be affecting the expression of different *UBASH3a* isoforms consequently affecting the binding to AIF. Concerning to this we checked if there is any relation between the rs9976767 and expression of *UBASH3a* gene using expression quantitative trait loci (eQTL) databases. Interesting, there is a significant statistical correlation between the increase of *UBASH3a* expression in lymphoblastoid cell lines and the homozygotes for the minor allele of rs9976767 (rho = 0.483, P = 1.3E-05; Figure S2A) in one of the two groups of twins studied (this observation was done using Genevar 3.2.0 software) [11,12]. Furthermore the eQTL studies in asthma showed that the SNPs (rs9784215, rs3746923, rs2277797) with highest LOD score (LOD>4.5, P<1E-05) in the *UBAHS3a* locus are in moderate to high LD with rs9976767 (Figure S2B and C; this observation was done using mRNA by SNP Browser 1.0.1 http://www.sph.umich.edu/csg/liang/asthma/) [13,14]. This evidence suggested that rs9976767 could have a functional role in the regulation of the expression of *UBASH3a*. However, and according with HapMap project (http://hapmap.ncbi.nlm.nih.gov/), this SNP tags other six variants in this region (rs7278547, rs11702374, rs9976479, rs3746924, rs3761378, rs7283281; r^2>0.95) and considering the present study and the previous GWAS [15,16] we have studied approximately 15% of the genetic variation of *UBASH3a* locus. In order to cover all the genetic variation of this gene, it is necessary to genotype 181 SNPs (calculated through an aggressive tagging with 2-marker haplotypes in Haploview 4.2 software using CEPH population from HapMap project). All these together suggest that the rs9976767 is a good functional candidate risk factor to SLE, but it could be more than one variant related to SLE.

No previous reports have associated the rs9976767 *UBASH3a* polymorphism with SLE. Nevertheless, it is worth noting that the rs9976767 SNP or its six tags variants were not included in previous genome wide association studies (GWAS) in Caucasian SLE cohorts [15,16]. Although the statistical power is 96% for our meta-analysis (calculate using a p value = 0.05:OR = 1.2: MAF = 0.4), the results found in our study should be replicated in different Caucasian cohorts and other populations. Furthermore there is a need to determine whether the statistical associations are related with the involvement of *UBASH3a* in the pathogenesis of SLE and other autoimmune diseases. Regarding to this, the *UBASH3a* gene seems to be a common genetic factor in

autoimmune diseases because different polymorphism of this locus has been associated with autoimmune diseases like T1D, CD, RA and vitiligo [6,17–21]. Our results showed that the minor allele of the rs9976767 *UBASH3a* polymorphism is a risk factor to SLE, as similarly observed with T1D [6]. Nevertheless, there is no evidence of association between this variant and other autoimmune diseases. This can be linked with the suggestion that common genetic factors in autoimmune diseases could match a regional level but differ in the specific genetic variant associated to each disease, like the associations observed with *IL2–IL21* and MHC loci [22]. Based on the concept of quantitative thresholds for immune-cell signalling, the effect of the rs976767 *UBAHS3a* variant could diversely affect the range of values for the stimulus-response selection of the immune cells in different autoimmune pathologies, making it more or less relevant in different diseases [3].

In conclusion, our study showed the first evidence of association of the *UBASH3a* gene with the genetic background of SLE. Together the functional role of the protein encoded by this gene, the reported data in the eQTLs databases and our results point to the *UBASH3a* gene as a new element in the pathogenic mechanism of autoimmune diseases.

Supporting Information

Figure S1 Pattern of linkage disequilibrium of the five studied SNPs and their location in the UBAHS3a gene. The values correspond to r2 calculated for the Spanish cohort. The rs2277798 polymorphism [G/A] is located in exon 1 of *UBASH3a* gene. It's a no-synonymous change in the position 18 of the protein (S[Ser]/G[Gly]). The rs2277800 polymorphism [C/T] is also located in exon 1 of *UBASH3a* gene and generate a change in the position 28 of the protein (L[Leu]/F[Phe]). In the other hand, the rs9976767 [A/G] is an intronic variant located between the exons 5 and 6 of the *UBASH3a* gene. Both variants rs13048049 [G/A] and rs17114930 [C/G] are no-synonymous changes in exons 7 and 11, respectively. The first one produce a change from arginine (R[Arg]) to glutamine (Q[Gln]) in position 286; while the rs17114930 polymorphism generates a change from aspartic acid (D[Asp]) to glutamic acid (E[Glu]) in position 428 in Caucasian population.

Figure S2 Results observed using different expression quantitative trait loci (eQTL) tools to evaluate if there is any relationship between the rs9976767 variant and the *UBASH3a* expression **(A) SNP-gene association plot** for the rs9976767 and the *UBASH3a* gene based on Spearman's rank correlation coefficient (rho) using the Genevar 3.2 software (http://www.sanger.ac.uk/resources/software/genevar/) [1]. The eQTL analysis was performed in lymphoblastoid cell lines from peripheral blood sample (n = 74). The plot corresponds to one of the two twins groups studied [2]. **(B) Linkage disequilibrium (LD) plot** performed in Haploview 4.2 [3]. LD plot between rs9976767 and the rs9784215, rs3746923, rs2277797 SNPs which exhibited the highest LOD score (LOD>4.5, P<1E-05) in the *UBAHS3a* locus showed in **(C) Snapshot of observed eQTLs related with *UBASH3a* gene** from the mRNA by SNP Browser 1.0.1 software (http://www.sph.umich.edu/csg/liang/asthma/) based on eQTL studies in asthma [4,5]. The LOD scores and P values for those SNPs are: rs9784215, LOD = 4.909 P = 2E-06; rs3746923, LOD = 4.905 P = 2E-06; rs2277797, LOD = 4.68 P = 3.4E-06. They are signalled as red dots in the LOD plot. 1. Yang TP, Beazley C, Montgomery SB, Dimas AS, Gutierrez-Arcelus M, et al. (2010) Genevar: a database and Java application for the analysis and visualization of SNP-gene associations in eQTL studies. Bioinformatics 26: 2474-2476. 2. Nica AC, Parts L, Glass D, Nisbet J, Barrett A, et al. (2011) The architecture of gene regulatory variation across multiple human tissues: the MuTHER study. PLoS Genet 7: e1002003. 3. Barrett JC, Fry B, Maller J, Daly MJ (2005) Haploview: analysis and visualization of LD and haplotype maps. Bioinformatics 21: 263-265. 4. Dixon AL, Liang L, Moffatt MF, Chen W, Heath S, et al. (2007) A genome-wide association study of global gene expression. Nat Genet 39: 1202-1207. 5. Moffatt MF, Kabesch M, Liang L, Dixon AL, Strachan D, et al. (2007) Genetic variants regulating ORMDL3 expression contribute to the risk of childhood asthma. Nature 448: 470-473.

Acknowledgments

We thank to GemaRobledo, Sofia Vargas and Sonia Garcia for their excellent technical assistance. we thank to all donors, patients and controls. We thank BancoNacional de ADN (University of Salamanca, Spain) who supplied part of the control DNA samples.

Author Contributions

Colection of the samples and clinical information: NOC JMS FJGH EDG MAGG TW HJA MFGE. Review of the manuscript: ES NOC JMS FJGH EDG MAGG TW HJA MFGE. Conceived and designed the experiments: LMDG ES JM. Performed the experiments: LMDG ES. Analyzed the data: LMDG. Contributed reagents/materials/analysis tools: LMDG ES NOC JMS FJGH EDG MAGG TW HJA MFGE JM. Wrote the paper: LMDG JM.

References

1. Tsygankov AY (2009) TULA-family proteins: an odd couple. Cell Mol Life Sci 66: 2949-2952.
2. Zenewicz LA, Abraham C, Flavell RA, Cho JH (2010) Unraveling the genetics of autoimmunity. Cell 140: 791-797.
3. Cho JH, Gregersen PK (2011) Genomics and the multifactorial nature of human autoimmune disease. N Engl J Med. 2011/10/28 ed. 1612-1623.
4. Guerra SG, Vyse TJ, Cunninghame Graham DS (2012) The genetics of lupus: a functional perspective. Arthritis Res Ther 14: 211.
5. Hochberg MC (1997) Updating the American College of Rheumatology revised criteria for the classification of systemic lupus erythematosus. Arthritis Rheum 40: 1725.
6. Grant SF, Qu HQ, Bradfield JP, Marchand L, Kim CE, et al. (2009) Follow-up analysis of genome-wide association data identifies novel loci for type 1 diabetes. Diabetes 58: 290-295.
7. Benjamini Y HY (1995) Controlling the false discovery rate: a practical and powerful approach to multiple testing. J R Statist Soc B 57: 289-300.
8. Purcell S, Neale B, Todd-Brown K, Thomas L, Ferreira MA, et al. (2007) PLINK: a tool set for whole-genome association and population-based linkage analyses. Am J Hum Genet 81: 559-575.
9. Collingwood TS, Smirnova EV, Bogush M, Carpino N, Annan RS, et al. (2007) T-cell ubiquitin ligand affects cell death through a functional interaction with apoptosis-inducing factor, a key factor of caspase-independent apoptosis. J Biol Chem 282: 30920-30928.
10. Yeo GW, Van Nostrand EL, Liang TY (2007) Discovery and analysis of evolutionarily conserved intronic splicing regulatory elements. PLoS Genet 3: e85.
11. Nica AC, Parts L, Glass D, Nisbet J, Barrett A, et al. (2011) The architecture of gene regulatory variation across multiple human tissues: the MuTHER study. PLoS Genet 7: e1002003.
12. Yang TP, Beazley C, Montgomery SB, Dimas AS, Gutierrez-Arcelus M, et al. (2010) Genevar: a database and Java application for the analysis and visualization of SNP-gene associations in eQTL studies. Bioinformatics 26: 2474-2476.
13. Dixon AL, Liang L, Moffatt MF, Chen W, Heath S, et al. (2007) A genome-wide association study of global gene expression. Nat Genet 39: 1202-1207.
14. Moffatt MF, Kabesch M, Liang L, Dixon AL, Strachan D, et al. (2007) Genetic variants regulating ORMDL3 expression contribute to the risk of childhood asthma. Nature 448: 470-473.
15. Harley JB, Alarcon-Riquelme ME, Criswell LA, Jacob CO, Kimberly RP, et al. (2008) Genome-wide association scan in women with systemic lupus erythematosus identifies susceptibility variants in ITGAM, PXK, KIAA1542 and other loci. Nat Genet 40: 204-210.
16. Kozyrev SV, Abelson AK, Wojcik J, Zaghlool A, Linga Reddy MV, et al. (2008) Functional variants in the B-cell gene BANK1 are associated with systemic lupus erythematosus. Nat Genet 40: 211-216.
17. Concannon P, Onengut-Gumuscu S, Todd JA, Smyth DJ, Pociot F, et al. (2008) A human type 1 diabetes susceptibility locus maps to chromosome 21q22.3. Diabetes 57: 2858-2861.
18. Jin Y, Birlea SA, Fain PR, Gowan K, Riccardi SL, et al. (2010) Variant of TYR and autoimmunity susceptibility loci in generalized vitiligo. N Engl J Med 362: 1686-1697.
19. Smyth DJ, Plagnol V, Walker NM, Cooper JD, Downes K, et al. (2008) Shared and distinct genetic variants in type 1 diabetes and celiac disease. N Engl J Med 359: 2767-2777.
20. Stahl EA, Raychaudhuri S, Remmers EF, Xie G, Eyre S, et al. (2010) Genome-wide association study meta-analysis identifies seven new rheumatoid arthritis risk loci. Nat Genet 42: 508-514.
21. Zhernakova A, Stahl EA, Trynka G, Raychaudhuri S, Festen EA, et al. (2011) Meta-analysis of genome-wide association studies in celiac disease and rheumatoid arthritis identifies fourteen non-HLA shared loci. PLoS Genet 7: e1002004.
22. Diaz-Gallo LM, Martin J (2012) Common genes in autoimmune diseases: a link between immune-mediated diseases. Expert Rev Clin Immunol 8: 107-109.

Metabolic Alterations and Increased Liver mTOR Expression Precede the Development of Autoimmune Disease in a Murine Model of Lupus Erythematosus

Laia Vilà[1], Núria Roglans[2,3], Miguel Baena[1], Emma Barroso[1], Marta Alegret[2,3], Manuel Merlos[2,3], Juan C. Laguna[2,3]*

1 Department of Pharmacology and Therapeutic Chemistry, School of Pharmacy, University of Barcelona, Barcelona, Spain, 2 Institute of Biomedicine, University of Barcelona, Barcelona, Spain, 3 CIBER (Centro de Investigación Biomédica en Red) of Physiopathology of Obesity and Nutrition, Barcelona, Spain

Abstract

Although metabolic syndrome (MS) and systemic lupus erythematosus (SLE) are often associated, a common link has not been identified. Using the BWF1 mouse, which develops MS and SLE, we sought a molecular connection to explain the prevalence of these two diseases in the same individuals. We determined SLE- markers (plasma anti-ds-DNA antibodies, splenic regulatory T cells (Tregs) and cytokines, proteinuria and renal histology) and MS-markers (plasma glucose, non-esterified fatty acids, triglycerides, insulin and leptin, liver triglycerides, visceral adipose tissue, liver and adipose tissue expression of 86 insulin signaling-related genes) in 8-, 16-, 24-, and 36-week old BWF1 and control New-Zealand-White female mice. Up to week 16, BWF1 mice showed MS-markers (hyperleptinemia, hyperinsulinemia, fatty liver and visceral adipose tissue) that disappeared at week 36, when plasma anti-dsDNA antibodies, lupus nephritis and a pro-autoimmune cytokine profile were detected. BWF1 mice had hyperleptinemia and high splenic Tregs till week 16, thereby pointing to leptin resistance, as confirmed by the lack of increased liver P-Tyr-STAT-3. Hyperinsulinemia was associated with a down-regulation of insulin related-genes only in adipose tissue, whereas expression of liver mammalian target of rapamicyn (mTOR) was increased. Although leptin resistance presented early in BWF1 mice can slow-down the progression of autoimmunity, our results suggest that sustained insulin stimulation of organs, such as liver and probably kidneys, facilitates the over-expression and activity of mTOR and the development of SLE.

Editor: Vassiliki A. Boussiotis, Beth Israel Deaconess Medical Center, Harvard Medical School, United States of America

Funding: This study was supported by grants from the Fundació Privada Catalana de Nutrició i Lípids, project CENIT-GENIUSPHARMA, and the Spanish Society of Atherosclerosis. Laia Vilà and Miguel Baena were supported by Research and Teaching Grants from the University of Barcelona. We have been nominated as a Consolidated Research Group by the Autonomous Government of Catalonia (SGR09-00413). The funders had no role in study design, data collection and analysis, decision to publish, or preparation of the manuscript.

Competing Interests: The authors have declared that no competing interests exist.

* E-mail: jclagunae@ub.edu

Introduction

From the second half of the twentieth century onwards, there has been a growth in the prevalence of two apparently unrelated pathologic conditions, namely metabolic and autoimmune diseases, especially in affluent western societies [1–5]. This occurrence has coincided with a drastic change in life style, involving massive adoption of sedentary practices associated with dietary habits skewed towards the consumption of high caloric density, nutrient poor foods, which promote a marked positive energy balance in the general population [6,7].

These life style changes constitute a risk factor for predisposition to metabolic diseases (obesity, insulin resistance, metabolic syndrome, etc.) and their cardiovascular manifestations, such as angina pectoris and myocardial infarction [6,8]. In the past 25 years the prevalence of some of the risk factors for cardiovascular disease (i.e. cigarette smoking, dyslipaemia, etc.) has gradually declined; however, the prevalence of obesity, metabolic syndrome and diabetes mellitus has dramatically increased as a result of unhealthy changes in dietary habits and life style [3,7]. Besides, a clear risk factor (excluding the increased concentration of chemicals in the environment of urban areas) related to the increased prevalence of autoimmune diseases has not been identified to date.

Systemic lupus erythematosus (SLE) is an heterogeneous autoimmune disease that affects multiple organs, and its highest prevalence is reported in Italy, Spain, Martinique and the UK Afro-Caribbean population [5,7]. The disease progresses through four broad stages, which are in the following order: the presence of autoantibodies against a variety of ubiquitous self-antigens; the deposition of autoantibodies and immune complexes in tissues; the development of tissue inflammation; and tissue damage and fibrosis. There is a clear predominance of SLE in females, with female-to-male ratios between 9:1 and 13:1. There has been a marked increase in five-year survival from less than 50% in the 1950s to more than 90% in the 1990s as a result of improved therapeutics. Those who die early in the course of SLE have active disease and a high incidence of infection associated with treatment with large doses of corticosteroids, while most patients who die later in the course of the disease, the most common situation nowadays, die from myocardial infarction [9,10].

Patients with SLE are five to six times more likely to have a significant coronary event than the general population [9]. Epidemiological studies point to an association of metabolic syndrome (MS) and SLE, indicating that traditional risk factors for cardiovascular disease clustered in the MS, such as hypertension, insulin resistance, hepatic steatosis, diabetes mellitus and obesity, have a significant role in the development of premature atherosclerosis in patients with SLE [11,12]. There is growing epidemiological evidence that obesity increases the risk of autoimmnune diseases [13], but it is unknown whether these pathological conditions share common molecular pathways.

The New Zealand Black (NZB) mouse is characterized by mild SLE-like symptoms. F1 progeny from NZB mice and the non-autoimmune New Zealand White (NZW) strain, called BWF1,

exhibit an earlier onset and a high incidence of SLE manifestations, showing many features of human SLE, including a complex genetic origin, a bias for the female sex, immune complex glomerulonephritis, and the presence of antinuclear antibodies [14]. In a seminal article published by Ryan et al. [15], it was shown that, like humans, the BWF1 mouse model presents several characteristics of the MS, including hypertension, central obesity, insulin resistance, hepatic steatosis and hyperleptinemia.

Here we studied the temporal evolution of SLE and MS manifestations in the murine BWF1 model, with the aim to identify possible molecular connections that could help to explain the high prevalence of these two diseases in the same individuals. We show that MS symptoms appear before those of SLE and propose a possible interconnection of both diseases through

A)

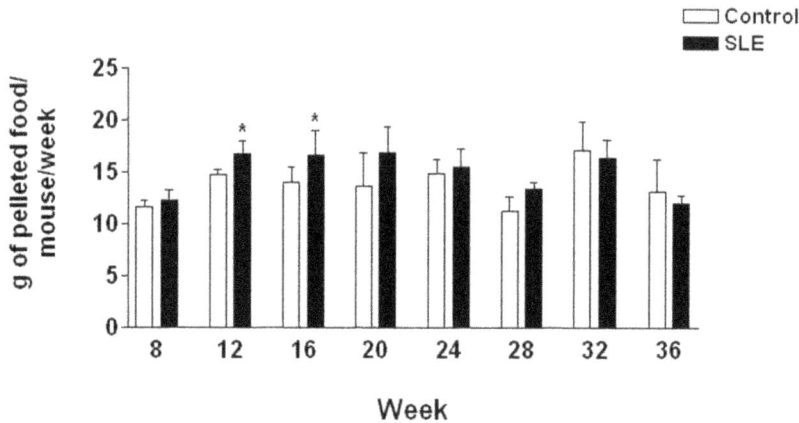

B)

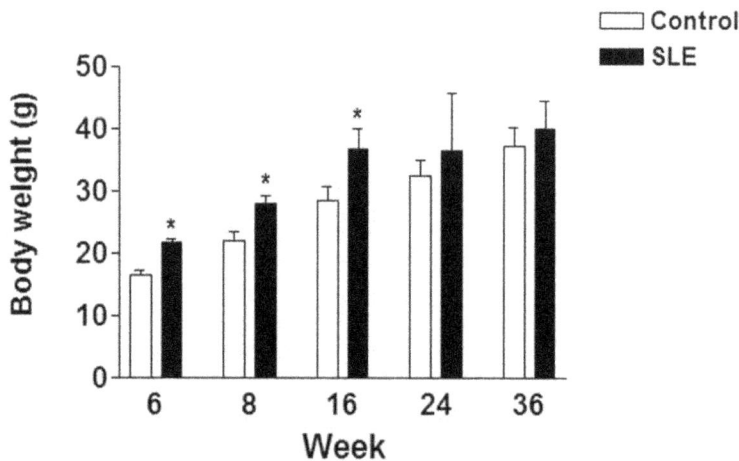

Figure 1. A. Bar diagram showing solid food consumption, expressed as the mean±sd of g of pelleted diet consumed per day and animal, at different times (weeks) for control and SLE mice (8 animals per group). B. Body weight, expressed as the mean±sd in g at the beginning of the study (week 6) and for control and SLE mice (8 animals per group) at the weeks of sacrifice. * P<0.05.

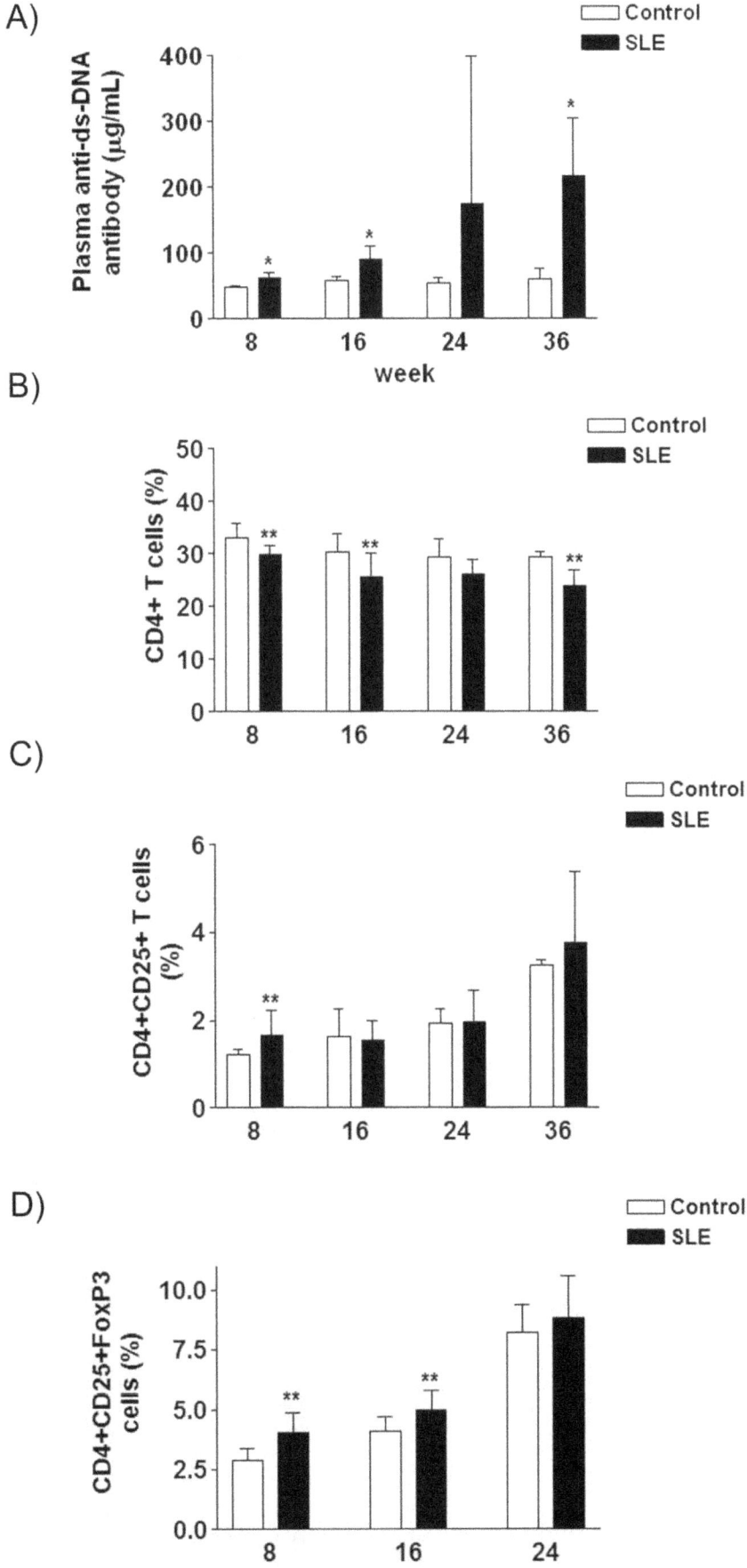

Figure 2. A. Bar diagram showing plasma anti-ds-DNA antibody concentrations expressed as the mean±sd of 8 animals, for control and SLE mice (8 animals per group) at the weeks of sacrifice. B–D. Percentages of CD4+- (**B**), CD4+CD25+- (**C**), and CD4+CD25+FoxP3-T cells (**D**) in spleen lymphocytes, expressed as the mean±sd of 8 animals, for control and SLE mice (8 animals per group) at the weeks of sacrifice. * $P<0.05$, ** $P<0.01$.

hyperinsulinemia and mammalian target of rapamicyn (mTOR) up-regulation.

Materials and Methods

Animals and Experimental Design

Thirty-two female F1 progeny from New Zealand Black/White mice characterized by SLE-like symptoms (SLE) and 32 New Zealand White female mice used as a control (CT) were provided by Charles River Laboratories (Barcelona, Spain). All mice were maintained with access to water and food *ad libitum* and under constant humidity and temperature with a light/dark cycle of 12 hours. After 8, 16, 24 and 36 weeks the mice were killed under isoflurane anesthesia between 9–10 a.m. During the study, we periodically measured solid food consumption and the body weight.

For each group, four mice were transferred to metabolic cages and kept 24 h for urine collection. Urinary protein excretion (proteinuria) was determined by Albustix[R] (Bayer, Barcelona, Spain) once every 4 weeks starting from 8 week of the study, always using the same animals.

When the animals were killed, blood was collected in 5% EDTA-tubes for measurement of serum anti-double stranded DNA (anti-dsDNA) antibody levels, lipids, glucose, creatinine, insulin and leptin concentrations. Kidneys were harvested for histological studies; spleens were also harvested and washed with PBS-FBS 10% (10% heat inactivated fetal bovine serum) and 1% antibiotic solution for isolation and culture of splenocytes. Hepatic and adipose tissues were excised, weighed and immediately frozen in liquid N_2.

All procedures were conducted in accordance with the guidelines established by the University of Barcelona's Bioethics Committee, as stated in Law 5/1995 (21st July) drawn up by the Generalitat de Catalunya.

Plasma Analysis

Blood samples were centrifuged to obtain plasma and then stored at $-20°C$ until needed. Plasma triglyceride, glucose concentrations and creatinine levels were measured using the colorimetric tests from SPINREACT (Girona, Spain) (ref. 1001312, 1001192 and K-4001, respectively). Non-esterified fatty acids (NEFA) were measured using a colorimetric test from Wako Chemicals GmbH (Neuss, West Germany). Plasma insulin and leptin concentrations were determined with the Insulin RIA kit (RI-13K) and Leptin RIA kit (RL-83K) from Linco Research (Missouri, USA), respectively.

Plasma anti-dsDNA antibody concentration was measured by an ELISA kit from Alpha Diagnostic International (Texas, USA), following the manufacturer's instructions.

Hepatic Triglyceride Contents

Liver triglyceride levels were measured as described previously [16] and were determined using the same colorimetric test from SPINREACT (Girona, Spain) as described above.

Fatty Acid Oxidation Activity

Hepatic fatty acid β-oxidation activity was determined as described previously [17], using 30 μg of post nuclear supernatant from each sample.

Western Blot Analysis

150 mg of hepatic and adipose tissue from each animal were homogenized in a buffer containing 150 mM NaCl, 1 mM EDTA, 1 mM EGTA, 1% Igepal, 100 mM NaF, 1 mM each of PMSF, Nappi, sodium ortovanadate and 20 mM Tris-HCl pH 7.5 buffer to obtain the total protein fraction by centrifugation. This fraction was stored at $-80°C$ until needed. The protein concentration was determined by the Bradford method [18].

30 μg of total protein (15 μg for IRS-1 experiments) were subjected to 10% SDS-polyacrylamide gel electrophoresis. Proteins were then transferred to Immobilon polyvinylidene diflouride transfer membranes (Millipore, Bedford, MA) and blocked for 1 h at room temperature with 5% non-fat milk solution in TBS-0.1% Tween-20. Membranes were then incubated with the primary polyclonal antibody raised against total-AKT, IRS-1, and RPS6K (dilution 1:1000) in adipose tissue samples and PPARγ, mTOR, RPS6K and p-Tyr-STAT-3 (dilution 1:1000) in liver samples in TBS-0.1% Tween-20 with 5% non-fat milk at 4°C overnight. After several washes, the membranes were incubated with horseradish peroxidase-conjugated anti-rabbit IgG (1:3000 dilutions). Detection was achieved using the ECL chemiluminescence kit for HRP (GE Healthcare Bio-Sciences AB, Uppsala, Sweden). To confirm the uniformity of protein loading in each lane, the blots were incubated with β-actin protein. The size of the proteins detected was estimated using protein molecular-mass standards (BioRad Laboratories SA, Barcelona, Spain). All antibodies were obtained from Cell Signaling Technology Inc. (Danvers, USA).

PCR- Arrays

Six total RNA pools from liver and six total RNA pools from adipose tissue were prepared, three for CT mice and three for SLE counterparts. Each pool was prepared with the same amount of RNA from two mice, with a total of 6 mice in each condition. Briefly, total RNA was isolated using TRIzol reagent (Invitrogen-Life Technologies, New York, USA) following the manufacturer's instructions and was then purified using RNeasy kit columns (Qiagen Iberia S.L., Madrid, Spain). Single stranded cDNA and PCR arrays were performed using the RT^2 Profiler™ PCR Array Mouse Insulin Signaling Pathway (PAMM-030A) from SaBiosciences (Madison, USA) and following the manufacturer's guidelines. Array data processing and analysis were performed by using a Web portal from SaBiosciences (Madison, USA).

Renal Histology

Kidney specimens were fixed in 10% formaldehyde and embedded in paraffin. Four μm sections were stained with haematoxylin and eosin (H&E). Inflammatory cell infiltration and glomerular hypercellularity were evaluated semi-quantitatively by a renal pathologist blinded to group assignment (arbitrary score 0 to 3+, where 0 = no change; 1+ = mid; 2+ = moderate and 3+ = severe).

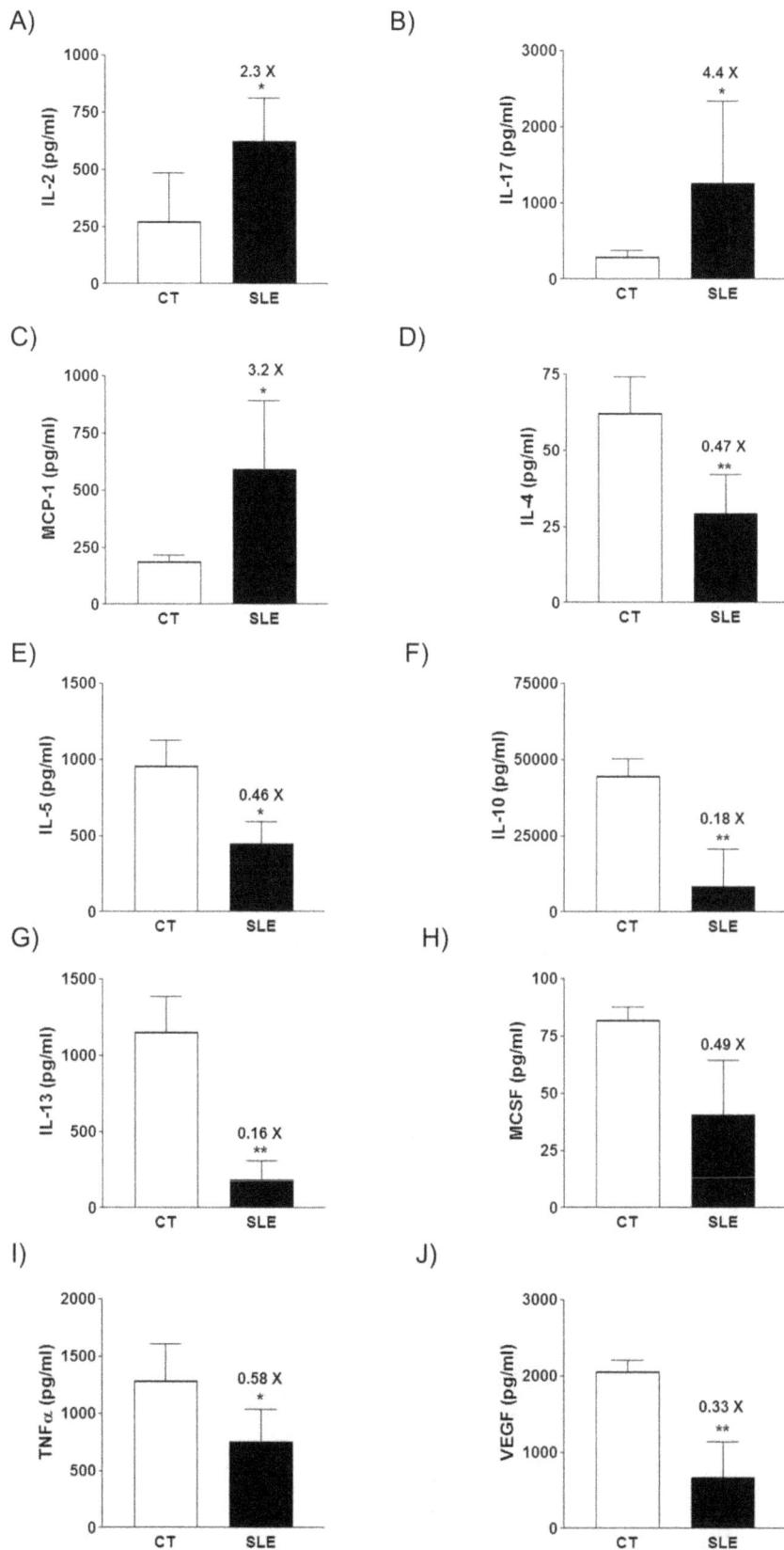

Figure 3. Bar diagrams showing IL-2 (A), IL-17 (B), MCP-1 (C), IL-4 (D), IL-5 (E), IL-10 (F), IL-13 (G), M-CSF (H), TNFα (I), and VEGF (J) concentrations in the supernatant of stimulated cultured splenocytes (see Material and Methods), expressed as the mean±sd of 8 cultures from separate animals, for control and SLE mice at week 36. * $P<0.05$, ** $P<0.01$.

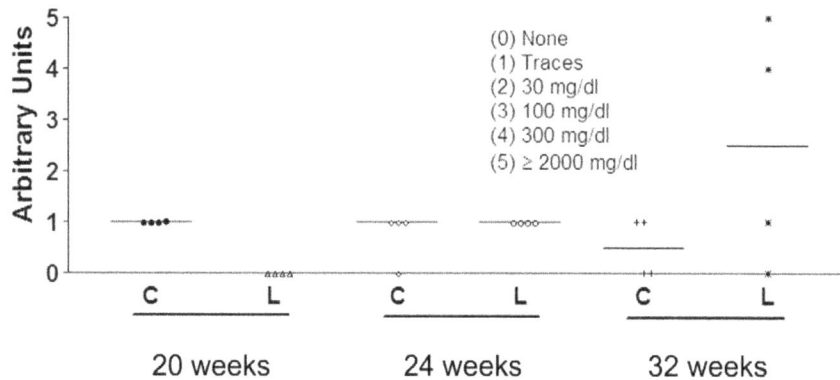

Figure 4. Plot of individual 24 h proteinuria values, expressed as arbitrary units, for control (C) and BWF1 mice (L) at weeks 20, 24 and 32.

Isolation of Splenocytes

The isolated spleen from each mouse was pressed through a sterile 40 μm nylon cell strainer (Sigma-Aldrich, St. Louis, CA, USA) to make a single cell suspension. After centrifugation at $538 \times g$ for 10 min at $4°C$, red blood cells in the pellet were lysed by osmotic shock with PBS 1X and distilled water. In order to restore tonicity, PBS 10X was added and the solution was vortexed and centrifuged at $538 \times g$ for 10 min at $4°C$. The pellet was then resuspended with PBS-FBS10%. The cells were then counted and viability was determined by the trypan blue exclusion method.

Labeling of Isolated Splenocytes and Flow Cytometry

5×10^5 isolated spleen cells were distributed into FACS tubes with 1 ml of PBS-FBS 2% and cold 1% NaN_3. After centrifugation at $538 \times g$ for 5 min at $4°C$, the pelleted cells were resuspended and stained with 10 μl of anti-mouse antibodies conjugated by fluorescent dyes (mouse anti-CD4 antibody PE conjugated, mouse anti CD25 FITC conjugated and human anti-CD7 antibody used as a control (eBiosciences, St. Diego, CA, USA). They were then incubated at $4°C$ for 20 min. After one wash with cold PBS, stained cells were centrifuged and permeabilized using 1X Permeabilizing Solution (ref. 00–5521, eBiosciences, St. Diego, CA, USA) and then incubated for 30 min at $4°C$ with 15 μl of anti-mouse/rat foxp3 antibody conjugated with APC. Cells were fixed using 500 μl of 0.5% paraformaldehyde solution (p-formaldehyde 2.5 g and NaCl 4.2 g) and 10.000 cells were analyzed by flow cytometry. Results were expressed as the percentage of surface CD4 and CD25 markers and foxp3 in total lymphocytes.

Measurement of Cytokine Production

The resuspended splenocytes (2×10^6 cells/ml) were stimulated in 2.5 μg/ml anti CD3 mAb-coated plates and incubated for three days at $37°C$ under 5% CO_2 and 95% air. Cells were harvested from 6-well culture plates and the supernatant medium was stored at $-20°C$. The amounts of cytokines in splenocytes culture media were measured by commercial semi-quantitative cytokine antibody array (Quantibody[R] Mouse Cytokine Array I, QAM-CYT-1, from Ray Biotech, Inc., Atlanta, GA, USA) following the manufacture's protocol. 100 μl of sample was used for each condition.

Statistical Analysis

The results are expressed as the mean of n values ± standard deviation. Plasma samples were assayed in duplicate. Significant differences were established by the unpaired t-test, using the computer program GraphPad InStat (GraphPad Software V2.03). When the variance was not homogeneous, a non-parametric test was performed (Mann-Whitney). The level of statistical significance was set at $P < 0.05$.

Results

Food Consumption and Body Weight Evolution

CT and BWF1 (SLE) mice showed a healthy appearance throughout the study. No death from unexpected causes or due to ethical euthanasia was recorded in either group. From the beginning of the study up to week 16, SLE mice consumed a higher amount (x1.18 fold, Figure 1A) of solid food than CT mice. Accordingly, during the same time period SLE mice showed a higher body weight (x1.18 fold, Figure 1B) than CT animals.

Markers of Systemic Lupus Erythematosus

The plasma anti-ds-DNA antibody concentration rose steadily in SLE mice in comparison with CT animals, from a ×1.3 fold increase at week 8 to a ×3.5 fold increase at week 36 (Figure 2A). SLE mice consistently showed a modest reduction (between ×0.81–×0.90 fold vs CT values) in the percentage of CD4+ T cells in spleen lymphocytes (Figure 2B). Despite this reduction, the percentage of CD4+CD25+ T cells was increased at week 8 (x1.4 fold vs CT values, Figure 2C), and the percentage of CD4+CD25+FoxP3 T cells increased in SLE mice at week 8 (x1.4 fold vs CT values) and 16 (x1.16 fold vs CT values) (Figure 2D).

Cytokine production by splenocytes was measured at week 8, 16, 24 and 36. The concentration of almost every cytokine in the supernatant of splenocytes from both SLE and CT mice increased throughout the study, except for granulocyte macrophage-colony stimulating factor (GM-CSF), interleukin (IL) -3, IL-12, IL-17, keratinocyte-derived cytokine (KC), and monocyte chemotactic protein-1 (MCP-1) (data not shown). At week 36, the concentrations of IL-2 (x2.3 fold, Figure 3A), IL-17 (x4.4 fold, Figure 3B), and MCP-1 (x3.2 fold, Figure 3C) were higher in samples from SLE mice than CT ones, while the concentrations of IL-4 (x0.47 fold, Figure 3D), IL-5 (x0.46 fold, Figure 3E), IL-10 (x0.18 fold, Figure 3F), IL-13 (x0.16 fold, Figure 3G), monocyte/macrophages colony stimulating factor (M-CSF) (x0.49 fold, Figure 3H), tumor necrosis factor α (TNFα) (x0.58 fold, Figure 3I), and vascular endothelial growth factor (VEGF) (x0.33 fold, Figure 3J) were lower in samples from SLE mice.

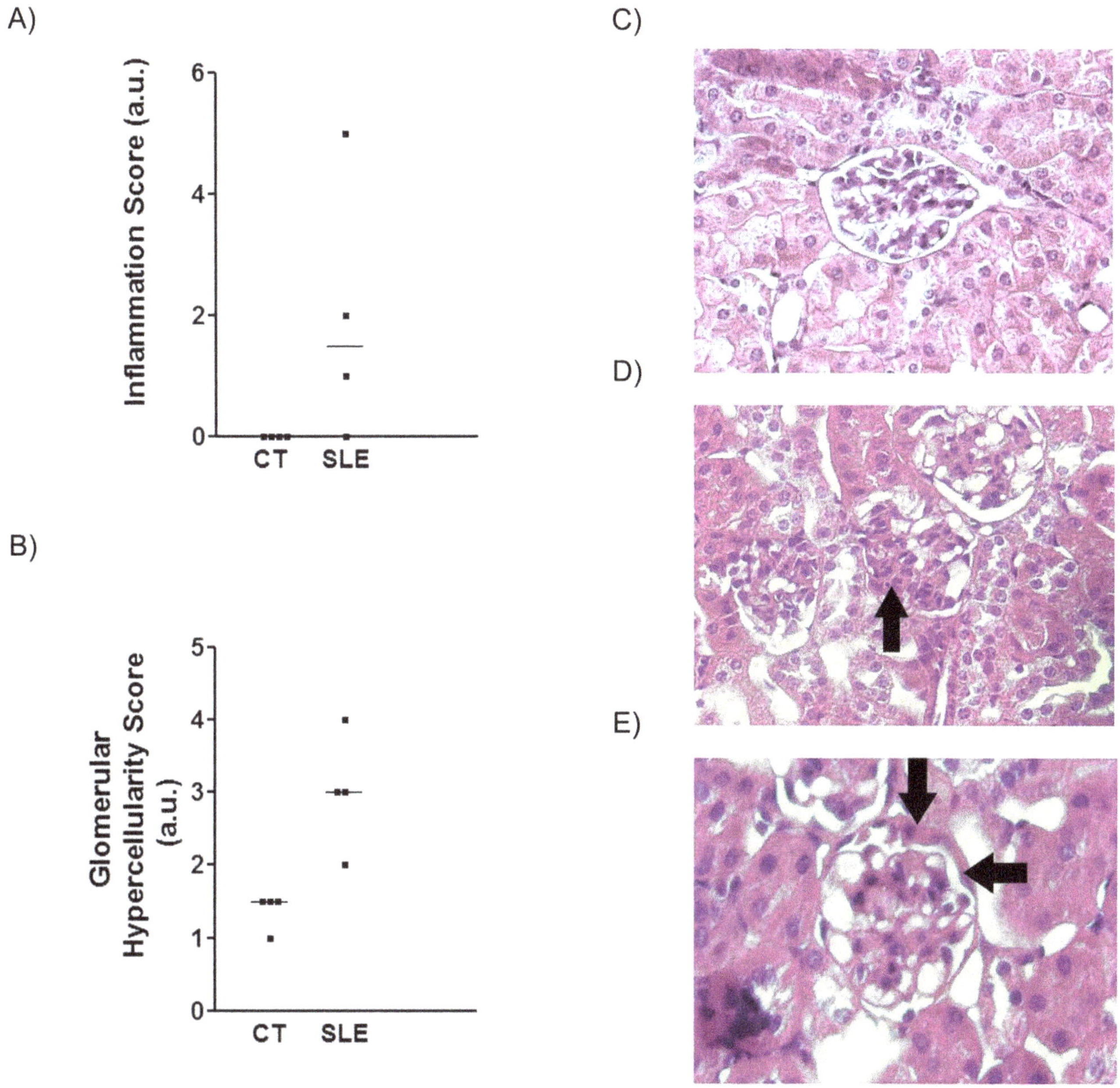

A)

B)

C)

D)

E)

Figure 5. BFWF1 mice, aged 36 weeks, showed increased kidney pathology. Hystological analysis of individual inflammatory (**A**) and glomerular hypercellularity scores (**B**) for CT and SLE mice, evaluated as described in the Material and Methods section. Representative photographs of renal sections from control (CT) (**C**) and BWF1 (SLE) (**D,E**) mice at the age of 36 weeks (H&E staining, light microscopy, original magnification ×40). Arrows indicate mesangial glomerular proliferation (**D**) and cellular extracapillary half-moon (**E**).

Renal function abruptly worsened in SLE mice by the end of the study. While plasma creatinine concentrations did not vary along the study (data not shown), 24 h proteinuria was higher in SLE than in CT mice by week 32 (Figure 4). In agreement, analysis of H&E-stained kidney sections obtained at week 36 showed a higher inflammation and glomerular hypercellularity score in tissue samples from SLE than from CT mice (Figure 5).

Markers of Metabolic Syndrome

SLE mice showed hepatic steatosis at weeks 8 and 16 (x1.5 fold *vs* CT for liver triglyceride content), which disappeared at later time points (Figure 6A), with no change in hepatic fatty acid β-oxidation activity (data not shown). Of the several plasma analytes

measured (triglycerides, NEFA, glucose, leptin and insulin) only leptin and insulin concentrations were changed in SLE vs CT mice (Figure 6B and 6C). SLE mice were hyperleptinemic at weeks 8 and 16 (x3.1 and ×2.1 fold *vs* CT, respectively), and hyperinsulinemic throughout the entire study (x2.2 fold *vs* CT, at week 16 the difference was not significant). Furthermore, the ratio between visceral adipose tissue and body weight was higher in SLE than in CT mice, although the difference progressively decreased throughout the study, from an increase of ×1.83 fold at week 8, to a ×1.17 fold at week 24, with no significant difference at the end of the study (week 36) (Figure 6D). Despite the hyperleptinemia, livers of 16-week-old SLE animals had no increased levels of P-Tyr-STAT3 protein (Figure 6E), a marker of leptin activity. As

A)

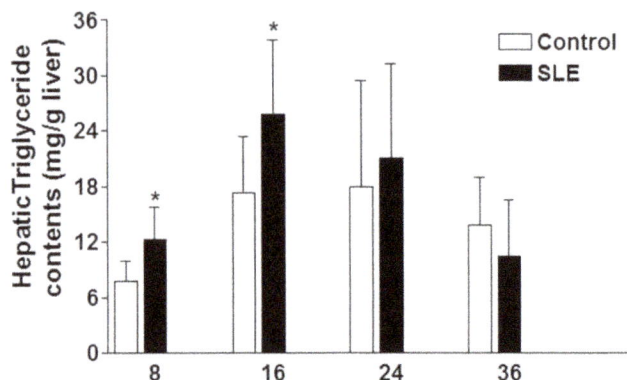

B)

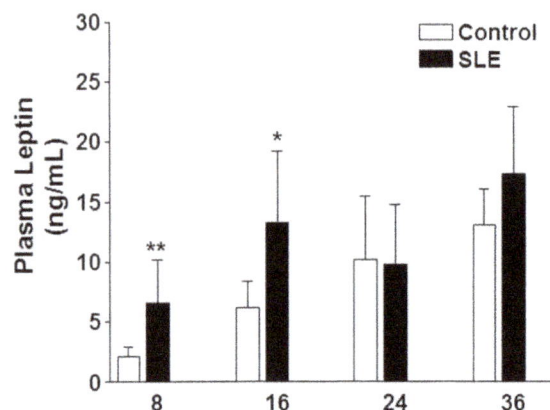

C)

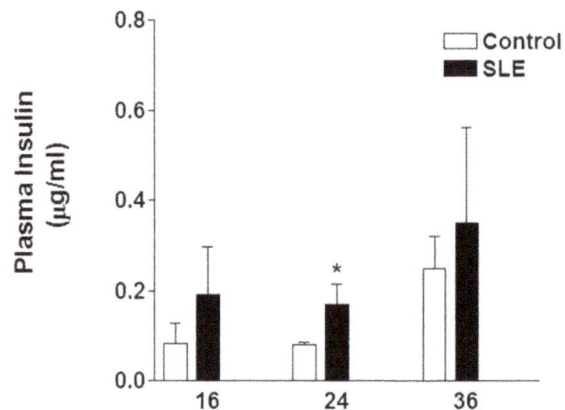

D)

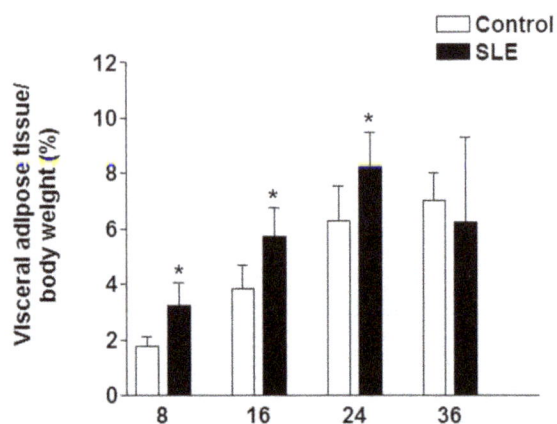

E)

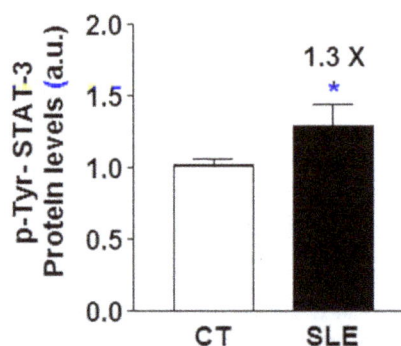

Figure 6. Bar diagrams showing hepatic triglyceride content (A), plasma leptin (B), and insulin concentrations (C), and percentage of adipose visceral tissue (D), expressed as the mean±sd of 8 animals, for control and SLE mice at the weeks of sacrifice. E. Bar diagrams showing the relative amount of P-Tyr-STAT-3 protein in liver tissue, expressed as the mean ± sd of values from 8 animals, from control (CT) and BWF1 (SLE) mice. The amount of protein loaded was confirmed by the Bradford method, and the uniformity of protein loading in each lane was assessed by determining the signal of β–actin as a control-loading protein.* $P<0.05$, ** $P<0.01$.

ADIPOSE TISSUE

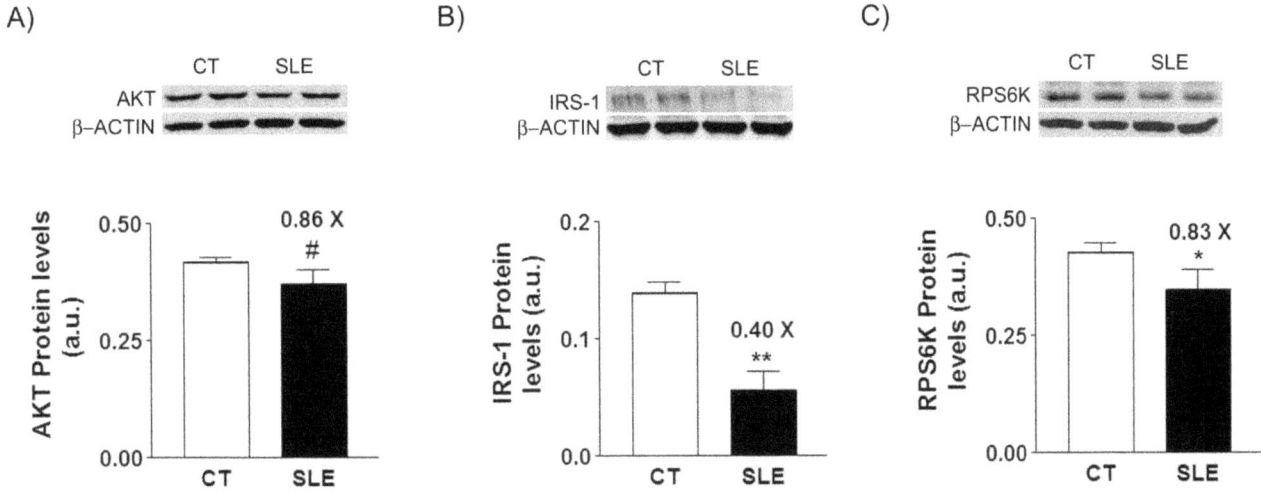

LIVER

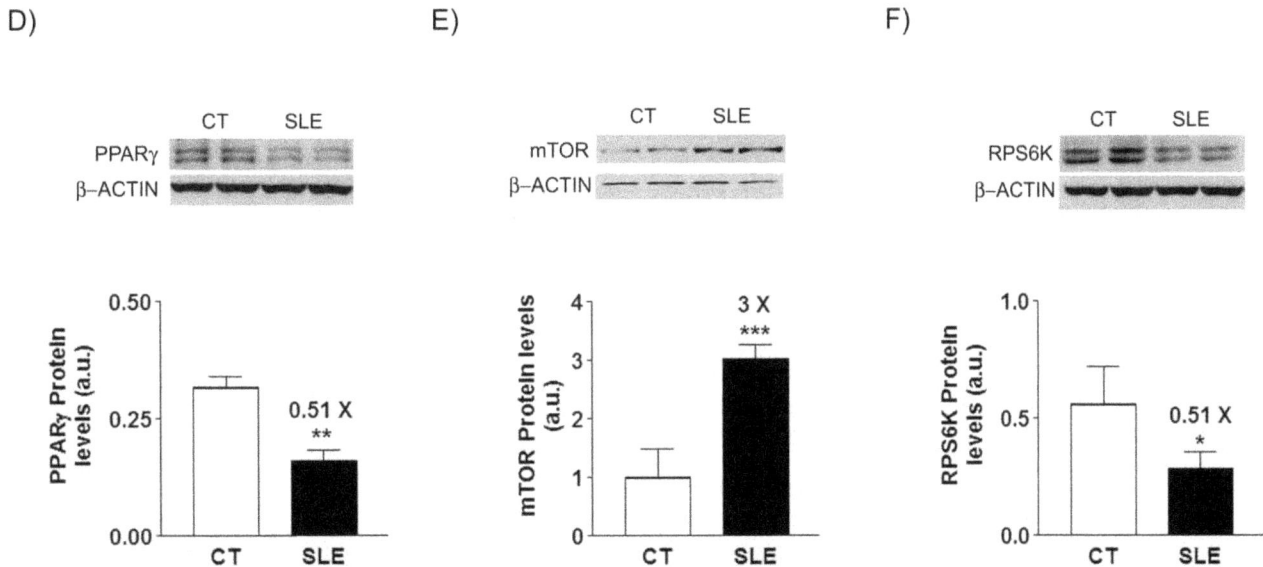

Figure 7. Bar diagrams showing the levels of AKT (A), IRS-1 (B) and RPS6K (C) protein in adipose tissue, and PPARγ (D), mTOR (E), and RPS6K (F) protein in liver tissue, expressed as the mean ± sd of values from 8 animals aged 16 weeks, for control (CT) and BWF1 (SLE) mice. The amount of protein loaded was confirmed by the Bradford method, and the uniformity of protein loading in each lane was assessed by determining the signal of β–actin as a control-loading protein. A representative autoradiography from a Western blot determination of two animals per group is shown. # $P = 0.05$, * $P<0.05$, ** $P<0.01$, *** $P<0.001$.

maximal differences in the MS between SLE and CT mice clustered around week 16, at this time point we used a commercial PCR Array to characterize the expression of 85 genes involved in insulin signaling in liver and visceral adipose tissue samples. In the liver, 12 genes were down-regulated and 1 gene was up-regulated in SLE vs CT mice, while in visceral adipose tissue, 23 genes were down-regulated and 1 gene was up-regulated in SLE vs CT mice (Tables 1 and 2). Of all these genes, only pck2 (phosphoenolpir-

uvate carboxykinase 2) and rps6k (ribosomal protein serine 6 kinase) were similarly down-regulated in both tissues. We selected some key genes in order to elucidate whether changes in mRNA were translated into similar alterations in protein levels. Thus, we determined the amount of total Akt (thymoma viral proto oncogen), IRS-1 (insulin receptor substrate-1), and RPS6K protein in visceral adipose tissue samples, as well as PPARγ(peroxisome proliferator activated receptor γ), FRAP1 (FK506 binding protein

Table 1. Genes whose expression was altered in livers from 16-week old SLE *vs* CT mice.

Gene	Name	Fold change	95% CI	P
Dok1	Docking protein 1	0.64	0.46–0.82	0.030
Dusp14	Dual specificity phosphatase 14	0.82	0.74–0.89	0.017
Eif2b1	Eukaryotic translation initiation factor 2B, subunit 1 (alpha)	0.23	0.00–0.67	0.019
Eif4ebp1	Eukaryotic translation initiation factor 4E binding protein 1	0.02	0.00–0.11	0.010
Frap1	FK506 binding protein 12-rapamycin associated protein 1	0.56	0.42–0.70	0.005
Gpd1	Glycerol-3-phosphate dehydrogenase 1 (soluble)	0.70	0.49–0.90	0.044
Hras1	Harvey rat sarcoma virus oncogene 1	4.78	3.80–5.77	0.000
Lep	Leptin	0.38	0.19–0.58	0.014
Pck2	Phosphoenolpyruvate carboxykinase 2 (mitochondrial)	0.54	0.36–0.72	0.022
PPARg	Peroxisome proliferator activated receptor gamma	0.57	0.46–0.68	0.002
Raf1	V-raf-leukemia viral oncogene 1	0.61	0.43–0.80	0.015
Rps6ka1	Ribosomal protein S6 kinase polypeptide 1	0.65	0.50–0.81	0.015
Klf10	Kruppel-like factor 10	0.43	0.25–0.61	0.015

12-rapamycin associated protein 1 or mTOR –mammalian target of rapamycin), and also RPS6K protein in liver samples. The expression of all these proteins was markedly reduced in samples from SLE *vs* CT (Figure 7), except in the case of mTOR (Figure 7e), which was increased ×3.04 fold in liver samples from SLE *vs* CT, in sharp contrast with the reduction in its specific mRNA levels.

Discussion

Here we used a murine model of SLE (the BWF1 mouse), which, like humans with this autoimmune disease, shows the classical manifestations of MS. Our results indicate that these metabolic alterations temporally precede the development of lupus symptoms in this model.

Thus, from the beginning of the study until week 16, SLE mice showed clear signs of metabolic alterations that temporally preceded the development of lupus symptoms, such as hyperphagia, hyperleptinemia, hyperinsulinemia, fatty liver and increased visceral adipose tissue. During this period, anti-dsDNA antibody plasma levels were low, and no clear signs of lupus disease were observed. By the end of the study, metabolic disturbances had almost disappeared, except for the increased levels of plasma

insulin. Coincident in time with the waning of metabolic alterations, anti-dsDNA antibody reached maximal levels and manifestations of lupus nephritis appeared, exemplified by proteinuria (week 32) and a higher inflammation score and glomerular hypercellularity in renal tissue samples from SLE mice (week 36). Also at week 36, the profile of cytokine production by stimulated splenocytes from these mice was consistent with autoimmunity promotion, with an increased production of type Th1 (IL-2) and Th17 (IL-17) cell cytokines, and fundamentally, a reduced production of type Th2 cell cytokines (IL-4, IL-5, IL-10, and IL-3) [19–22]. In a similar study using the same model, Alperovich et al. [23] reported the appearance of lupus-related signs earlier, and mortality was higher than in the present study. Thus, the authors reported a 69% survival rate at week 36, with high plasma anti-dsDNA antibody levels from week 20 and proteinuria from week 28. In our study, survival at week 36 was 100%, with animals showing a marked increase in plasma anti-dsDNA antibody levels at week 24 and proteinuria at week 32. Although we do not know the reason for this discrepancy in the severity of the evolution of lupus manifestations, in our case the metabolic disturbances preceded the appearance of the clinical symptoms of SLE. Once the autoimmune disease flourished, the deep alteration of whole body homeostasis may have obliterated the signs of diseased metabolism, such as the increase in triglyceride accretion in liver or adipose visceral tissue.

The development of autoimmune diseases is promoted by deficiency in a special set of regulatory T cells that are crucial in the maintenance of autologous tolerance and are characterized by the expression of CD4, CD25 and FoxP3 (CD4$^+$CD25$^+$FoxP3$^+$ Tregs) [24]. It has been described that leptin, an adipocytokine derived from body fat stores, reduces the proliferation of Tregs [25–27]. However, in our study SLE mice were hyperleptinemic at weeks 8 and 16, while at the same time points they showed increased proportions of natural or splenic Tregs. The observation that Tregs did not decrease suggests a deficit of leptin action on the proliferation of these cells.

Resistance to leptin action in the central nervous system and peripheral organs, such as the liver, has been reported in rodent experimental models and in humans [28,29]. Although Ryan et al. [15] described that hyperleptinemic BWF1 mice showed no signs of central leptin resistance, their results did not ruled out the possibility of peripheral leptin resistance. To explore this issue, we determined the amount of signal transducer and activator of transcription 3 (STAT3) protein phosphorylated on tyrosine (P-Tyr-STAT3), a marker of leptin receptor activation [30]. We did not detect differences in the amount of P-Tyr-STAT3 in liver samples of SLE or CT animals obtained at week 16 (Figure 6E). This observation confirms leptin resistance in peripheral tissues. It could be hypothesized that young SLE mice are protected from the development of the clinical symptoms of SLE by the increased production of Tregs, which occurs because of peripheral leptin resistance.

As SLE mice also showed mildly elevated plasma insulin concentrations during the entire study, we addressed whether these animals also developed insulin resistance in the liver or visceral adipose tissue. Using a commercial cDNA array specifically designed to determine the expression of genes involved in insulin signaling, we demonstrated a marked reduction in the expression of key genes directly participating in the transmission of this signal in the visceral adipose tissue of SLE mice at week 16. Of the 24 genes modified, 10 genes directly involved in insulin signaling (Akt1, Akt3, Frs3, Gab1, Igf1r, Irs1, Nck1, Pik3r2, Prkcz, and Slc2a1) were down-regulated. This finding points to insulin resistance in the visceral adipose tissue of SLE mice and suggests

Table 2. Genes whose expression was altered in visceral adipose tissue from 16-week old SLE *vs* CT mice.

Gene	Name	Fold change	95% CI	P
Acaca	Acetyl-Coenzyme A carboxylase alpha	0.07	0.00–0.27	0.029
Aebp1	AE binding protein 1	0.01	0.00–0.03	0.036
Akt1	Thymoma viral proto-oncogene 1	0.07	0.00–0.20	0.026
Akt3	Thymoma viral proto-oncogene 3	0.11	0.00–0.43	0.027
Araf	V-raf murine sarcoma 3611 viral oncogene homolog	0.18	0.00–0.46	0.046
Bcl2l1	Bcl2-like 1	0.10	0.00–0.37	0.010
Fbp1	Fructose bisphosphatase 1	0.47	0.24–0.70	0.027
Frs3	Fibroblast growth factor receptor substrate 3	0.10	0.00–0.35	0.034
Gab1	Growth factor receptor bound protein 2-associated protein 1	0.11	0.00–0.34	0.031
Grb10	Growth factor receptor bound protein 10	1.70	1.44–1.96	0.003
Igf1r	Insulin-like growth factor I receptor	0.05	0.02–0.09	0.010
Irs1	Insulin receptor substrate 1	0.33	0.10–0.57	0.028
Jun	Jun oncogene	0.07	0.00–0.17	0.028
Mapk1	Mitogen-activated protein kinase 1	0.29	0.04–0.54	0.048
Nck1	Non-catalytic region of tyrosine kinase adaptor protein 1	0.43	0.09–0.76	0.050
Pck2	Phosphoenolpyruvate carboxykinase 2 (mitochondrial)	0.16	0.00–0.32	0.004
Pik3r2	Phosphatidylinositol 3-kinase, regulatory subunit, polypeptide 2 (p85 beta)	0.07	0.00–0.24	0.023
Ppp1ca	Protein phosphatase 1, catalytic subunit, alpha isoform	0.08	0.00–0.26	0.015
Prkcz	Protein kinase C, zeta	0.26	0.00–0.55	0.004
Ptpn1	Protein tyrosine phosphatase, non-receptor type 1	0.04	0.00–0.13	0.001
Retn	Resistin	0.20	0.00–0.52	0.023
Rps6ka1	Ribosomal protein S6 kinase polypeptide 1	0.07	0.00–0.21	0.011
Slc27a4	Solute carrier family 27 (fatty acid transporter), member 4	0.09	0.00–0.27	0.045
Slc2a1	Solute carrier family 2 (facilitated glucose transporter), member 1	0.05	0.00–0.13	0.008

that this resistance is responsible for the increase in insulin plasma concentrations detected in these animals. The down-regulation of *Akt*, and *Irs1*, genes coding for two essential proteins in the intracellular transmission pathway of the insulin receptor [31], was confirmed at the protein level.

When we applied the same commercial cDNA array to hepatic samples, the expression of the above mentioned genes was not modified; instead, we detected a marked down-regulation of *Eif2b1*, *Eif4ebp1*, and *Rps6ka1* in the livers of 16-week-old SLE mice. Proteins coded by these genes are downstream of the signaling pathway of the mTORC1 complex, which is involved in cell growth, translation, and ribosomal protein synthesis [32]. Moreover, the mTORC1 complex is formed by two main components, the proteins Raptor and mTOR [32], the latter coded by *Frap1*, which was also down-regulated in the livers of SLE mice. When we attempted to confirm these results at the protein level, although liver Rps6ka1 protein (S6kinase) was reduced, the amount of mTOR protein was markedly increased. The reason for this discrepancy remains unknown. One can speculate that the mTORC1 system was over-stimulated in the livers of SLE mice. This may elicit a cellular compensatory response in an attempt to decrease the over-activity of the system by down-regulating the mRNA expression of its main components, Eif2b1, Eif4ebp1, and Rps6ka1 and mTOR itself.

Recent data points to an association between the increased prevalence of several types of cancer in type 2 diabetic patients and sustained hyperinsulinemia. In this situation, the continuous activity of insulin in non-resistant tissues promotes the activation of the mTORC1 system, thereby favoring cellular proliferation and tumor development [33]. Furthermore, it has been shown that lupus nephritis in rodent models and humans is directly related to the activation of the mTOR pathway in renal tissue [34,35]. Also, drugs that inhibit mTOR activity are effective in the treatment of SLE manifestations [4,5,23].

As a conclusion, our results indicate that, although metabolic alterations, mainly leptin resistance in the BWF1 mice, slow-down the progression of autoimmunity, the presence of hyperinsulinemia and the sustained insulin stimulation of organs that remain insulin-sensitive, such as the liver and potentially the kidneys, facilitates the overexpression and activity of the mTOR system and the appearance of the clinical symptoms of SLE. As the whole body homeostasis deteriorates, metabolic symptoms, except for increases in plasma insulin concentrations, decline and disappear, while classical SLE symptoms progressively develop. If these findings can be extrapolated to humans, subclinical insulin resistance, sustained over time, could be the key factor for the development of clinical SLE in subjects with an autoimmune-prone genetic background.

Acknowledgments

We appreciate the collaboration of the University of Barcelona Foreign Language Service in correcting the manuscript.

References

1. Feng PH (2007) Systemic lupus erythematosus: the face of Asia. Ann NY Acad Sci 1108: 114–120.
2. Peter S (2007) Trends in the incidence of type I diabetes mellitus worldwide. West Indian Med J 56: 264–269.
3. Rana JS, Nieuwdorp M, Jukema JW, JJ Kastelein (2007) Cardiovascular metabolic syndrome - an interplay of obesity, inflammation, diabetes and coronary heart disease. Diabetes Obes Metab 9: 218–232.
4. Rahman A, Isenberg DA (2008) Systemic Lupus Erythematosus. New Engl J Med 358: 929–939.
5. Manzi S (2009) Lupus update: Perspective and clinical pearls. Clev Clin J Med 76: 137–142.
6. Ordovas J (2007) Diet/genetic interactions and their effects on inflammatory markers. Nutr Rev 65: S203–S207.
7. Low YL, Tai ES (2007) Understanding diet-gene interactions: Lessons from studying nutrigenomics and cardiovascular disease. Mut Res 622: 7–13.
8. Chiuve SE, Willet WC (2007) The 2005 food guide pyramid: An oportunity lost? Nat Clin Pract Cardiovas Dis 4: 610–615.
9. Westerweel PE, Luyten RK, Koomans HA, Derksen RN, Verhaar MC (2007) Premature atherosclerotic cardiovascular disease in systemic lupus erythematosus. Arthritis Rheum 56: 1384–1396.
10. Sherer Y, Zinger H, Shoenfeld Y. (2010) Atherosclerosis in systemic lupus erythematosus. Autoimmunity 43: 98–102.
11. Haque S, Bruce IN (2005) Therapy insight: Systemic lupus erythematosus as a risk factor for cardiovascular disease. Nat Clin Pract Cardiovasc Dis 2: 423–430.
12. Mok CC (2006) Accelerated atherosclerosis, arterial thromboembolism, and preventive strategies in systemic lupus erythematosus. Scand J Rheumatol 35: 85–95.
13. Hersough L-G, Linneberg A (2007) The link between the epidemics of obesity and allergic diseases: does obesity induce decreased immune intolerance? Allergy 62: 1205–1213.
14. Furukawa S, Yoshimasu T (2005) Animal models of spontaneous and drug-induced cutaneous lupus erythematosus. Autoimmunity Rev 4: 345–350.
15. Ryan MJ, McLemore GR Jr, Hendrix ST (2006) Insulin resistance and obesity in a mouse model of systemic lupus erythematosus. Hypertension 48: 988–993.
16. Roglans N, Sanguino E, Peris C, Alegret M, Vázquez M, et al. (2002) Atorvastatin treatment induced peroxisome proliferator-activated receptor α expression and decreased plasma nonesterified fatty acids and liver triglyceride in fructose-fed rats. J Pharmacol Exp Ther 302: 232–239.
17. Lazarow PB (1981) Assay of peroxisomal β-oxidation of fatty acids. Meth Enzymol 72: 315–319.
18. Bradford MM (1976) A rapid sensitive method for the quantitation of microgram quantities of protein utilizing the principles of protein-dye binding. Anal Biochem 72: 248–254.
19. Sigal LH (2004) Basic Science for the clinician 33. Interleukins of current clinical relevance (part I). J Clin Rheumatol 10: 353–359.
20. Gutcher I, Becher B (2007) APC-derived cytokines and T cell polarization in autoimmune inflammation. J Clin Invest (117) 1119–1127.
21. Manjarrez-Orduño N, Quách TD, Sanz I (2009) B cells and immunological tolerance. J Invest Dermatol 129: 278–288.
22. Zhu J, Paul WE (2010) Heterogeneity and plasticity of T helper cells. Cell Res 20: 4–12.
23. Alperovich G, Rama I, Lloberas N, Franquesa M, Poveda R, et al. (2007) New immunosuppresor strategies in the treatment of murine lupus nephritis. Lupus 16: 18–24.
24. Bonelli M, Smolen JS, Scheinecker C (2010) Treg and lupus. Ann Rheum Dis 69: i65–i66.
25. Matarese G, Biagio P, La Cava A, F Perna, V Sanna et al. (2005) Leptin increase in multiple sclerosis associates with reduced number of CD4+CD25+ regulatory T cells. Proc Natl Acad Sci USA 102: 5150–5155.
26. De Rosa V, Procaccini C, Cali G, Pirozzi G, Fontana S, et al. (2007) A key role of leptin in the control of regulatory T cell proliferation. Immunity 26: 241–255.
27. Matarese G, Procaccini C, De Rosa V (2008) The intrincate interface between immune and metabolic regulation: a role for leptin in the pathogenesis of multiple sclerosis? J Leuk Biol 84: 893–899.
28. Myers MG, Cowley MA, Münzberg H (2008) Mechanisms of leptin action and leptin resistance. Annu Rev Physiol 70: 537–556.
29. Vilà L, Roglans N, Alegret M, Sánchez RM, Vázquez-Carrera M, et al. (2008) Suppressor of cytokine signaling-3 (SOCS-3) and a deficit of serine/threonine (Ser/Thr) phosphoproteins involved in leptin transduction mediate the effect of fructose on rat liver lipid metabolism. Hepatology 48: 1506–1516.
30. Roglans N, Vilà L, Alegret M, Sánchez RM, Vázquez-Carrera M, et al. (2007) Impairment of hepatic STAT-3 activation and reduction of PPARα activity in fructose-fed rats. Hepatology 45: 778–788.
31. Taguchi A, White MF (2008) Insulin-Like Signaling, Nutrient Homeostasis, and Life Span. Annu Rev Physiol 70: 191–212.
32. Yap TA, Garret MD, Walton MI, Raynaud F, de Bono JS, et al. (2008) Targeting the PI3K-AKT-mTOR pathway: progress, pitfalls, and promises. Curr Opin Pharmacol 8: 393–412.
33. Jalving M, Gietema JA, Lefrandt JD, de Jong S, Reyners AK, et al. (2010) Metformin: taking away the candy for cancer? Eur J Cancer 46: 2369–2380.
34. Reddy PS, Legault HM, Sypek JP, Collins MJ, Goad E, et al (2008) Mapping similarities in mTOR pathway perturbations in mouse lupus nephritis models and human lupus nephritis. Arthritis Res Ther 10: R127.
35. Stylianou K, Petrakis I, Mavroeidi V, Stratakis S, Vardaki E, et al. (2010) The PI3K/Akt/mTOR pathway is activated in murine lupus nephritis and downregulated by rapamycin. Nephrol Dial Transplant 26: 498–508.

Author Contributions

Conceived and designed the experiments: JCL MM. Performed the experiments: LV NR MB EB. Analyzed the data: JCL MA. Wrote the paper: JCL MA NR.

Construct and Criterion Validity of the Euro Qol-5D in Patients with Systemic Lupus Erythematosus

Su-li Wang[1], Bin Wu[2], Li-an Zhu[3], Lin Leng[3], Richard Bucala[3], Liang-jing Lu[1]*

1 Department of Rheumatology, Ren Ji Hospital, School of Medicine, Shanghai Jiao Tong University, Shanghai, China, 2 Clinical Outcomes and Economics Group, Department of pharmacy, Ren Ji Hospital, School of Medicine, Shanghai Jiao Tong University, Shanghai, China, 3 Department of Medicine, Section of Rheumatology, Yale University School of Medicine, The Anlyan Center, New Haven, Connecticut, United States of America

Abstract

Objective: To investigate the construct and criterion validity of the Euro Qol-5D (EQ-5D), which allows quality-adjusted life-years to be calculated, in patients with systemic lupus erythematosus (SLE).

Methods: Consecutive SLE patients who had been followed at the Renji Hospital, School of Medicine, Shanghai Jiao Tong University were recruited. Cross-sectional correlations of the EQ-5D with equivalent domains in disease-specific health-related quality of life (HRQoL), LupusQol, Systemic Lupus Erythematosus Disease Activity Index (SLEDAI) measures, the Systemic Lupus International Collaborating Clinics Damage Index (SDI), and patient characteristics were tested. Discriminant validity to assess the ability to distinguish between patients of different disease severity was assessed. There also were evaluations of ceiling and floor effects.

Results: 240 patients were recruited in total. The EQ-5D correlated moderately to strongly with all domains of the LupusQoL (r: 0.44–0.7) apart from intimate relationships (r = 0.25) and body image (r = 0.18). There was moderate negative correlation between EQ-5D and clinical assessment of disease, SLEDAI (r = −0.589) and SDI (r = −0.509). When compared with equivalent domains on LupusQoL, there was good construct validity in EQ-5D (r: 0.631–0.812). EQ-5D could also discriminate patients with varied disease severity (according SLEDAI and SDI). There was no floor effect in EQ-5D but the ceiling effect remains strong (34%).

Conclusion: Our results provide sufficient evidence that the EQ-5D displays construct and criterion validity for use in SLE patients. Disease-specific measures of HRQoL used alongside may be a better choice.

Editor: Masataka Kuwana, Keio University School of Medicine, Japan

Funding: This work was supported by grants from the National Natural Sciences Foundation of China (No. 81373209; No. 81072469; No. 30671946) and Shanghai Natural Sciences Foundation (No. 09ZR1417600). The funders had no role in study design, data collection and analysis,decision to publish, or preparation of the manuscript.

Competing Interests: The authors have declared that no competing interests exist.

* E-mail: lu_liangjing@medmail.com.cn

Introduction

Systemic lupus erythematosus (SLE) is a chronic inflammatory autoimmune disease characterised by the deposition of immune complexes in various tissues, which is found mainly in women during the childbearing years and is particularly common in Asian, and African American/Caribbean individuals [1–3]. Despite little conspicuous progress in the treatment of SLE, long-term survival has significantly improved [3]. At present, the health related quality of life (HRQoL) of patients with SLE is under increasing attention [4] as the HRQoL among SLE patients is worse than the general population, even compared with other rheumatic diseases [5]. As might be expected, a series of novel therapies are being developed for SLE [6]. For example, belimumab, a B cell modulator, is the first to demonstrate success in phase III studies and has received marketing authorization [7]. However, before widespread use in clinics, new therapies require evaluation for cost utility, which is of vital concern to policy makers.

Cost-utility analysis requiring quality adjusted life years (QALY) to measure the unit of health-gain is the most commonly used method [8] and compares interventions in terms of their cost per unit of effect. Where two or more interventions are found to achieve the same level of benefits, the one with the least cost is considered the most cost-effective alternative [8]. Generic preference-based measures, such as EQ-5D, SF-6D and HUI, have become widely used in economic evaluation, and have gained popularity to obtain health state value to calculate QALY over the last decade [9]. This development has arisen in part from their ease of use and their alleged generic properties. Assessment of HRQoL in patients with SLE also can be provided by disease-specific measures such as LupusQoL [10]; as they are designed for SLE, the results of these may be more specific. However, these disease-specific measures do not provide a single value for cost-utility analysis, which is the concern of the policy makers.

EQ-5D is a generic preference-based measure of health developed by a multidisciplinary group of researchers [11,12]. It has a structured health state descriptive system with five dimensions: mobility, self-care, usual activities, pain/discomfort and anxiety/depression. There are two types depending on the number of levels in each domain. The one with five levels, which was considered more friendly to users, was used in the present study. These five dimensions together define a total 5^5 health states formed by different combinations of levels. As a simple instrument, EQ-5D is widely used in various diseases. But the validity in SLE is not well established, especially in Chinese SLE patients. In this study, we collected and analyzed clinical data, HRQoL data, and socioeconomic data to examine the construct validity of the EQ-5D in patients with SLE.

Patients and Methods

This study was approved by the Institutional Review Board of Shanghai Jiao Tong University and the Ethics Committee of Renji Hospital. These committees specifically approved that written informed consent was not required because data were going to be analysed anonymously. Following feedback from participants in the pilot study, all participants granted oral consent after receiving comprehensive information about the study. Oral consent was documented by interviewers at the beginning of the patient interview.

Patients

Consecutive SLE patients were included, who were followed at the Renji Hospital, School of Medicine, Shanghai Jiao Tong University from March 2012 to May 2013. All patients fulfilled the 1997 revised American College of Rheumatology classification criteria for SLE [13], and had received stable therapy for at least 2 months.

Data collection

At baseline all patients underwent a clinical interview and examination to collect demographic information, including age, disease duration, age at protocol entry, clinical manifestations at

disease onset, cumulative clinical manifestations, education and marital status.

The clinical assessment included evaluation of disease activity using the Systemic Lupus Erythematosus Disease Activity Index(SLEDAI) [14] and cumulative damage using the Systemic Lupus International Collaborating Clinics (SLICC)/ACR Damage Index (SDI) [15]. The SLEDAI is a 24-item instrument for assessing SLE activity in nine organ systems, each item with a weighting from 1 to 8 depending on severity; the score ranges from 0 (no activity) to 105 (maximum activity) [14]. Clinical and laboratory data are required to complete the questionnaire. SLICC/ACR-DI (SDI) reports disease damage based on the evaluation of 12 organ systems. The dysfunction must be present for 6 consecutive months. The score ranges from 0 (no damage) to 46 (maximum damage), with higher scores signifying more damage.

All patients completed the generic preference-based measurement of health, EQ-5D-5L at baseline, each domain of which had 5 levels: no problems, slight problems, moderate problems, severe problems, and extreme problems. Scores for the five domains in EQ-5D were generated. Scoring algorithm estimated from the valuation survey undertaken by the UK Measurement and the Valuation of Health (MVH) group was used because of its widest popularity. The best possible score on the EQ-5D is 1 (equivalent to full health) and the worst possible score is −0.594 (presenting a state worse than death).

LupusQoL, a lupus-specific HRQoL questionnaire, which had been modified for applicability to Chinese SLE patients [16], also was completed. It consists of 34 items grouped in eight domains: physical health (PH), pain (PN), planning (PL), intimate relationships (IR), burden to others (BU), emotional health (EH), body image (BI) and fatigue (F) and has a five-point Likert response format, where 4 = never, 3 = occasionally, 2 = a good bit of the time, 1 = most of the time, and 0 = all of the time [10]. LupusQoL is scored for each domain as the mean domain score; the transformed scores range from 0 (worst) to 100 (best).

Table 1. Correlations of EQ-5D with SLE measures/patient characteristics (correlations are Spearman unless specified).

	Correlation R	P
LupusQoL		
Physical health	0.603	p<0.01
Pain	0.703	p<0.01
Planning	0.45	p<0.01
Intimate relationships	0.252	p<0.01
Burden to others	0.437	p<0.01
Emotional health	0.576	p<0.01
Body image	0.179	p<0.01
Fatigue	0.544	p<0.01
Disease activity/damage		
SLEDAI	−0.589	p<0.01
SDI	−0.509	p<0.01
Patient characteristics		
Age*	−0.141	p>0.01
Disease duration	−0.104	p>0.01
Education	0.238	p>0.01

SLEDAI: SLE Disease Activity Index; SDI: Systemic Lupus Collaborating Clinics Damage Index.
*Pearson correlation.

Table 2. Convergent validity of EQ-5D used in SLE patients.

EQ-5D domains	LupusQoL domains	Spearman's r
Self-care	Physical health	0.631
Usual activity	Physical health	0.747
Pain/Discomfort	Pain	0.812
Anxiety/Depression	Emotional health	0.767

We used both disease activity and damage to define disease severity of SLE, which were determined by SLEDAI and SLICC-DI [16].

Statistical Analyses

The data were analyzed cross-sectionally at baseline.

Convergent validity and discriminant validity were used to assess the construct validity of EQ-5D, which reflected the sensitivity and specificity of the measure. Convergent validity was assessed by measuring the extent of correlation of EQ-5D with the domains of the LupusQoL, SLEDAI (for activity), SDI (for damage), and characteristics of patients (age, disease duration and education). The extent of correlation between observed relationships of the concepts and the hypothesized concepts also were measured to assess the convergent validity. A strong correlation was defined as≥0.70, moderate to substantial as 0.30–0.70, and weak as <0.30 [17]. We expected that there would be moderate to strong correlations between EQ-5D and LupusQoL because the latter might be the closest measure to the gold standard of HRQoL in SLE patients [18]. Discriminant validity was used to assess whether the instrument could distinguish between patients of different disease severity. Patients were divided into two groups by a SLEDAI score cutoff of 4 or SLICC-DI score cutoff of 1 [19]. It was hypothesized that LupusQoL domains would be significantly altered in these two groups and an ordinary least-squares regression was used to test this possibility [18]. Effect sizes (Cohen's D) were calculated to quantify the magnitude of the differences in SD units by dividing the mean difference in EQ-5D by the standard deviation for both groups combined [18]. It was suggested that an effect size of 0.2 is small, 0.5 is moderate, and 0.7 is large [18].

Floor and ceiling effects were examined to explore potential to detect change. Ceiling effect exists if a large number of respondents occupy the best possible health state of a measure; a floor effect is just the opposite. If a ceiling effect exists, the ability of the measure to detect any further better states of health is inhibited and floor effect limits the ability to detect further worsening [20,21]. A ceiling/floor effect is considered to exist when >15% of respondents fall into the ceiling/floor [21]. The 5 domains of the EQ-5D with 5 levels and the overall score of EQ-5D were tested for ceiling or floor effects. When floor/ceiling effects were found to be serious, comparisons were made with responses to similar domains of LupusQoL.

We used SPSS software, version 10.0 to analyze data. Descriptive statistics were reported. The continuous variables were tested for normality; a non-parametric test (Mann-Whitney) was used for comparing continuous data.

Results

Among the 240 patients who participated in this study, complete data were available for 214 patients. 201(93.9%) patients were women; all are Chinese. At baseline the mean (SD) age and disease duration were 33.8 years (±9.2) and 4.8 years (±4.4), respectively. The mean (SD) SLEDAI and SDI were 2.9 (±3.9) (median 2, range 0–25) and 0.36(±0.9) (median 0, range 0–6).

Construct and criterion validity

There were positive correlations between EQ-5D score and all domains of LupusQoL (Table 1). The correlations were moderate to strong (r = 0.4–0.8) for all domains of LupusQoL except intimate relationships (r = 0.252) and body image (r = 0.179), which were weakly correlated to EQ-5D score. The correlations of the EQ-5D with the disease-specific measures were moderate for the SLEDAI score (r = −0.589) and SDI (r = −0.509) in the expected direction. There were no correlations between EQ-5D and patient characteristics such as age (r = −0.141) disease duration (r = −0.104) and education (r = 0.238).

The EQ-5D domains had good construct validity when compared with equivalent domains of LupusQoL (Table 2).

Table 3. Discriminant validity of EQ-5D used in SLE patients with disease activity and damage as the external anchors.

	EQ-5D, mean(SD)	P	Effect Size
Disease activity		<0.01	0.941
SLEDAI≤4	0.846(0.134)		
SLEDAI>4	0.619(0.261)		
Damage		<0.01	0.697
SDI≤1	0.843(0.137)		
SDI>1	0.663(0.260)		

SLEDAI: SLE Disease Activity Index; SDI: Systemic Lupus Collaborating Clinics Damage Index.
Ordinary least-squares regression was used.

Table 4. Ceiling effect and floor effect of EQ-5D used in SLE patients.

EQ-5D Subscale level	mobility	self-care	usual activities	pain/discomfort	anxiety/depression	EQ-5D Score	
1	30.8	47.9	45.2	47.2	22.8	1	34
2	42.1	25.1	25	36.9	41.3	−0.594	0
3	23.3	14.7	15.1	10.7	24.7		
4	2.8	11.9	13.7	4.2	7.5		
5	0.9	0.5	0.9	0.9	3.7		

Discriminant validity

The mean EQ-5D scores of patients with high disease activity (SLEDAI>4) was lower than those with low disease activity (0.619 vs. 0.846; EQ-5D: B coefficient −0.028, p<0.01; Table 3). Similarly, it was lower in patients with damage associated with SLE (SDI>1) (0.663vs.0.843; EQ-5D: B coefficient −0.107, p< 0.01; Table 3). The effect size (ES) of the difference in means suggested that the differences were moderate for SDI (ES = 0.697) and large for SLEDAI (ES = 0.941). It's suggested that EQ-5D could discriminate subjects with different disease severity, which was associated with different health states.

Ceiling effect and floor effect

There were no floor effects for the preference-based score and domains of EQ-5D. But serious ceiling effects were found to exist for both EQ-5D preference-based score and domain scores (34%; 22.8–47.9%), especially in the self-care domain. Almost half of the individuals (47.9%) responded with the ideal response "no problems" (Table 4). In the comparable domains of LupusQoL, patients at the ceiling of self-care, usual activity, pain/discomfort in EQ-5D also had a high median LupusQoL physical health score (90, IQR 81, 97) and pain score (92, IQR 75, 100).

Discussion

Data from studies assessing the HRQoL of SLE patients have shown that even with inactive disease, patients with SLE had a poorer HRQoL when compared to healthy subjects [22,23]. With patients enjoying a longer life span, interest in the HRQoL of SLE patients has gained growing attention. As the simplest generic preference-based measure, EQ-5D is widely used to make cost-utility analysis in various diseases, which is critical to policy-makers in health economics [24].

Our study provides evidence that EQ-5D is a valid measure for use in SLE. Because studies in China that directly elicit preferences from general population samples to derive value sets for the EQ-5D-5L are still under development, we used the UK value set in our study [12].

The present results include validity of EQ-5D against another well validated-tool LupusQoL. All domains have moderate to strong correlations with score of EQ-5D, except body image and intimate relationships, which are important aspects of HRQoL in SLE patients. This result reinforces the need to collect disease-specific measures of HRQoL alongside generic preference-based instruments. It also was found that the EQ-5D was differentiated between patients with different disease severity; this suggests it has the ability to distinguish patients with different health status, which plays an important role in clinical practice.

Serious ceiling effects are observed, especially in self-care and pain/discomfort, although EQ-5D-5L was established to reduce ceiling effects. This result indicates that health status above the highest level the instrument can measure is not accurately estimated. The health status distribution of patients in the study also should be taken into account. As an additional limitation, outpatients with inactive disease that were recruited into our study comprised a significant percentage and individuals with relatively better health status might also consist of a majority. Moreover, the high median score of the comparable domains of LupusQoL may also reflect these possibilities. Perhaps this limitation further contributed to the observed ceiling effect.

There is another limitation that must be considered: the population in our study included only Chinese patients. We will need to examine this scale in a more diverse population and include subjects from other ethnic backgrounds in order to understand it more comprehensively.

Conclusions

Sufficient data are available to indicate that the reliability and validity of EQ-5D among patients with SLE are acceptable. Disease-specific measures of HRQoL used alongside generic preference-based instruments are necessary to evaluate the actual health status. Further work remains to be done, including confirming its applicability in multi-ethnic SLE populations and exploring its precise value for clinical practice.

References

1. Mok CC, Mak A, Chu WP, To CH, Wong SN (2005) Long-term survival of southern Chinese patients with systemic lupus erythematosus: a prospective study of all age-groups. Medicine (Baltimore) 84: 218–224.
2. Cervera R, Khamashta MA, Font J, Sebastiani GD, Gil A, et al. (2003) Morbidity and mortality in systemic lupus erythematosus during a 10-year period: a comparison of early and late manifestations in a cohort of 1,000 patients. Medicine (Baltimore) 82: 299–308.
3. Alarcon GS, McGwin G Jr, Uribe A, Friedman AW, Roseman JM, et al. (2004) Systemic lupus erythematosus in a multiethnic lupus cohort (LUMINA). XVII. Predictors of self-reported health-related quality of life early in the disease course. Arthritis Rheum 51: 465–474.
4. Dua AB, Touma Z, Toloza S, Jolly M (2013) Top 10 recent developments in health-related quality of life in patients with systemic lupus erythematosus. Curr Rheumatol Rep 15: 380.
5. Jolly M (2005) How does quality of life of patients with systemic lupus erythematosus compare with that of other common chronic illnesses? J Rheumatol 32: 1706–1708.
6. Grech P, Khamashta M (2013) Targeted therapies in systemic lupus erythematosus. Lupus 22: 978–986.
7. FDA approves Benlysta to treat lupus Series (2011) FDA approves Benlysta to treat lupus [cited 2011 December 3]; Available: http://www.fda.gov/ NewsEvents/Newsroom/PressAnnouncements/ucm246489.htm.
8. Rudmik L, Drummond M (2013) Health economic evaluation: important principles and methodology. Laryngoscope 123: 1341–1347.
9. Kularatna S, Whitty JA, Johnson NW, Scuffham PA (2013) Health state valuation in low- and middle-income countries: a systematic review of the literature. Value Health 16: 1091–1099.
10. McElhone K, Abbott J, Shelmerdine J, Bruce IN, Ahmad Y, et al. (2007) Development and validation of a disease-specific health-related quality of life measure, the LupusQol, for adults with systemic lupus erythematosus. Arthritis Rheum 57: 972–979.
11. Sullivan PW, Ghushchyan V (2006) Preference-Based EQ-5D index scores for chronic conditions in the United States. Med Decis Making 26: 410–420.
12. Group E (1990) EuroQol—a new facility for the measurement of health-related quality of life. Health Policy 16: 199–208.
13. Hochberg MC (1997) Updating the American College of Rheumatology revised criteria for the classification of systemic lupus erythematosus. Arthritis Rheum 40: 1725.
14. Gladman DD, Ibanez D, Urowitz MB (2002) Systemic lupus erythematosus disease activity index 2000. J Rheumatol 29: 288–291.
15. Gladman DD, Urowitz MB, Goldsmith CH, Fortin P, Ginzler E, et al. (1997) The reliability of the Systemic Lupus International Collaborating Clinics/ American College of Rheumatology Damage Index in patients with systemic lupus erythematosus. Arthritis Rheum 40: 809–813.
16. Wang SL, Wu B, Leng L, Bucala R, Lu LJ (2013) Validity of LupusQoL-China for the assessment of health related quality of life in Chinese patients with systemic lupus erythematosus. PLoS One 8: e63795.
17. Aday LA, Cornelius LJ (1996) Designing and conducting health surveys. San Francisco, California: Jossey-Bass. 126 p.
18. Harrison MJ, Ahmad Y, Haque S, Dale N, Teh LS, et al. (2012) Construct and criterion validity of the short form-6D utility measure in patients with systemic lupus erythematosus. J Rheumatol 39: 735–742.
19. Jolly M, Pickard AS, Wilke C, Mikolaitis RA, Teh LS, et al. (2010) Lupus-specific health outcome measure for US patients: the LupusQoL-US version. Ann Rheum Dis 69: 29–33.
20. Veenhof C, Bijlsma JW, van den Ende CH, van Dijk GM, Pisters MF, et al. (2006) Psychometric evaluation of osteoarthritis questionnaires: a systematic review of the literature. Arthritis Rheum 55: 480–492.
21. McHorney CA, Tarlov AR (1995) Individual-patient monitoring in clinical practice: are available health status surveys adequate? Qual Life Res 4: 293–307.
22. Kuriya B, Gladman DD, Ibanez D, Urowitz MB (2008) Quality of life over time in patients with systemic lupus erythematosus. Arthritis Rheum 59: 181–185.
23. Waldheim E, Elkan AC, Pettersson S, Vollenhoven R, Bergman S, et al. (2013) Health-related quality of life, fatigue and mood in patients with SLE and high levels of pain compared to controls and patients with low levels of pain. Lupus 22: 1118–1127.
24. Whitehurst DG, Bryan S, Lewis M (2011) Systematic review and empirical comparison of contemporaneous EQ-5D and SF-6D group mean scores. Med Decis Making 31: E34–44.

Acknowledgments

We gratefully acknowledge the EuroQol Group for kindly providing EQ-5D (5L) to us. We also gratefully acknowledge Dr. Lee-Suan Teh, Mary Gawlicki and Translation Corporation Inc for providing us the LupusQoL(Chinese Traditional).

Author Contributions

Conceived and designed the experiments: SlW BW LjL. Performed the experiments: SlW LaZ LjL. Analyzed the data: SlW BW LaZ LL RB LjL. Contributed reagents/materials/analysis tools: SlW LaZ LjL. Wrote the paper: SlW LjL LL RB.

Galectin-9 Ameliorates Clinical Severity of MRL/lpr Lupus-Prone Mice by Inducing Plasma Cell Apoptosis Independently of Tim-3

Masahiro Moritoki[1]♀, Takeshi Kadowaki[2,3]♀, Toshiro Niki[2], Daisuke Nakano[4], Genichiro Soma[3], Hirohito Mori[5], Hideki Kobara[5], Tsutomu Masaki[5], Masakazu Kohno[1], Mitsuomi Hirashima[2,5]*

1 Department of Cardiorenal and Cerebrovascular Medicine, Faculty of Medicine, Kagawa University, Kagawa, Japan, 2 Department of Immunology and Immunopathology, Faculty of Medicine, Kagawa University, Kagawa, Japan, 3 Department of Holistic Immunology, Kagawa University, Kagawa, Japan, 4 Department of Pharmacology, Faculty of Medicine, Kagawa University, Kagawa, Japan, 5 Department of Gastroenterology and Neurology, Faculty of Medicine, Kagawa University, Kagawa, Japan

Abstract

Galectin-9 ameliorates various murine autoimmune disease models by regulating T cells and macrophages, although it is not known what role it may have in B cells. The present experiment shows that galectin-9 ameliorates a variety of clinical symptoms, such as proteinuria, arthritis, and hematocrit in MRL/lpr lupus-prone mice. As previously reported, galectin-9 reduces the frequency of Th1, Th17, and activated CD8$^+$ T cells. Although anti-dsDNA antibody was increased in MRL/lpr lupus-prone mice, galectin-9 suppressed anti-dsDNA antibody production, at least partly, by decreasing the number of plasma cells. Galectin-9 seemed to decrease the number of plasma cells by inducing plasma cell apoptosis, and not by suppressing BAFF production. Although about 20% of CD19$^{-/low}$ CD138$^+$ plasma cells expressed Tim-3 in MRL/lpr lupus-prone mice, Tim-3 may not be directly involved in the galectin-9-induced apoptosis, because anti-Tim-3 blocking antibody did not block galectin-9-induced apoptosis. This is the first report of plasma cell apoptosis being induced by galectin-9. Collectively, it is likely that galectin-9 attenuates the clinical severity of MRL lupus-prone mice by regulating T cell function and inducing plasma cell apoptosis.

Editor: Pierre Bobé, Institut Jacques Monod, France

Funding: This work was supported, in part, by Scientific Research (C) 2010 - (22590360) and Scientific Research (A) 2011 - (23256004) from the Japan Society for Promotion of Science. The funders had no role in study design, data collection and analysis, decision to publish, or preparation of the manuscript.

Competing Interests: The authors have declared that no competing interests exist.

* E-mail: mitsuomi@kms.ac.jp

♀ These authors contributed equally to this work.

Introduction

Systemic lupus erythematosus (SLE) is a systemic autoimmune disease characterized by autoantibody production against self-antigens. Among SLE complications, lupus nephritis is the most serious and a major predictor of poor prognosis [1]. Until recently, glucocorticoids, aspirin and antimalarials were approved for treatment of SLE. B-cell stimulatory factors promote the loss of B-cell tolerance and drive autoantibody production. B cell activation mediated by B-cell activator factor belonging to the TNF family (BAFF) and a proliferation-inducing ligand (APRIL) have been implicated in SLE pathogenesis [2,3,4]. This suggests that B cell regulation, in addition to T cell regulation, is required for SLE treatment [2].

Gal-9 is a β-galactoside binding lectin that exhibits therapeutic effects in autoimmune disease models, such as autoimmune arthritis, experimental allergic encephalomyelitis, and Type 1 diabetes mellitus [5,6,7]. Such therapeutic effects of Gal-9 seem to be ascribed to the decrease of Th1 and Th17 effector cells expressing Tim-3 [8]. It has also been found that the decrease of Th1 and Th17 effector cells is likely induced by programmed cell death of effector cells through a Gal-9/Tim-3 interaction [8]. In contrast, Gal-9 expands Foxp3$^+$ regulatory T cells (Tregs) in vivo and in vitro [5]. Furthermore, Gal-9 ameliorates immune complex (IC)-induced inflammation by suppressing IC-induced macrophage activation and C5a generation [9]. Collectively, Gal-9 seems to regulate a variety of immune cells to ameliorate autoimmune inflammation. Nevertheless, little is known about the effects of Gal-9 on B cell autoantibody production, although it is clear that B cells and B cell-derived autoantibody are associated with the pathogenesis of autoimmune disorders.

The purpose of the present study is to test whether Gal-9 ameliorates lupus signs and suppresses anti-dsDNA antibody production by inducing plasma cell apoptosis.

Materials and Methods

Mice

MRL/lpr lupus-prone and MRL/lpr$^{+/+}$ mice were purchased from Japan SLC (Shizuoka, Japan). All mice were housed in plastic boxes in groups of 3 to 4 under a 12:12 light cycle with food and water provided *ad libitum*.

The study protocol was approved by the Animal Care and Use Committee of Kagawa University, and mice used in this research

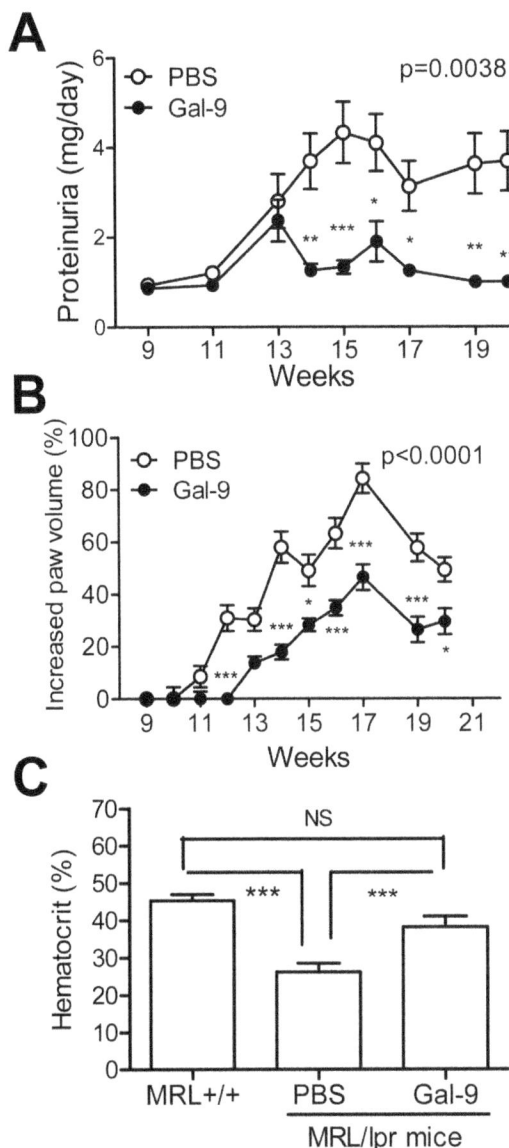

Figure 1. **Effects of Gal-9 on lupus nephritis in MRL/lpr mice.** (A) Comparison of proteinuria between PBS-treated (PBS) and Gal-9-treated (Gal-9) MRL/lpr lupus-prone mice. Gal-9 and PBS were injected intraperitoneally into 9-week-old MRL/lpr lupus-prone mice 3-times/week until they were 20 weeks of age. Mean and SEM of PBS treated mice (n = 10) and Gal-9 treated mice (n = 8) are shown. (*, P<0.05; **, P<0.01, ***, P<0.001). (B) Comparison of increase of paw volume between PBS and Gal-9-treated mice. Gal-9 or PBS was intraperitoneally injected to 9-week-old MRL/lpr lupus-prone mice 3-times/week until 20-weeks-old. Mean and SEM of PBS-treated (n = 10) and Gal-9-treated mice (n = 8) are shown. (*, P<0.05, ***, P<0.001). (C) Comparison of hematocrit between MRL$^{+/+}$ (MRL/lpr$^{+/+}$) mice and MRL/lpr (MRL/lpr$^{-/-}$ lupus-prone) mice in 20-week-old mice following treatment with PBS or human Gal-9. (***, P<0.001).

received humane care to minimize suffering in accordance with international and national guidelines of humane laboratory animal care. Mice were sacrificed by CO_2 narcosis unless otherwise specified.

Experimental Protocol

All Gal-9 preparations used in the present experiment were >95% pure by SDS-PAGE with less than 0.001 endotoxin units/µg, as assessed by a limulus turbimetric kinetic assay using a Toxinometer ET-2000 (Wako, Osaka, Japan). Nine-week-old MRL/lpr lupus-prone mice were injected intraperitoneally with human stable Gal-9 with no linker peptide (30 µg/mouse, 3-times/week) or PBS as a control, to assess the therapeutic effects of Gal-9. Proteinuria, paw volume, and hematocrit were monitored until mice were 20 weeks of age.

Eight-week-old mice were treated with Gal-9 for 4 weeks to assess the effects of Gal-9 on the level of anti-dsDNA antibody and the frequency of splenic T and B cell subpopulations.

Laboratory Methods

Proteinuria was measured using the BCA Protein Assay Reagent Kit (Takara Bio Inc., Otsu, Japan). Clinical signs of arthritis (i.e., paw swelling) were monitored during the course of disease by water displacement plethysmometry. Paw swelling was expressed as increased paw volume. Hematocrit values were collected from the tail vein (70 µl) in 1 mm heparinized tubes. The tubes were spun and hematocrit was determined using a Hawksley Micro-haematocrit reader (Lancing, Sussex, UK).

Flow Cytometric Analysis

Spleen cells were obtained from PBS or Gal-9 treated MRL/lpr lupus-prone mice. Single-cell suspensions were prepared, and red blood cells removed using lysis buffer (BioLegend, San Diego, CA, USA). One million splenocytes were incubated for 30 min on ice in staining buffer with the relevant fluorochrome-labeled monoclonal antibodies. For intracellular cytokine and Foxp3 staining, the cells were fixed and permeabilized with Cytofix/Cytoperm solution (BD Biosciences, San Jose, CA, USA) and Foxp3 Fix/Perm Buffer Set (BioLegend) according to the manufacturer's instructions. The following anti-mouse antibodies were used: IFNγ-FITC, CD4-PE, CD3-PerCP, Tim3-PE, (all from eBioscience, San Diego, CA, USA), CD138-PE (BD Biosciences), and Foxp3-Alexa488, IL-17A-PerCP, CD25-APC, CD8-Alexa488, CD44-APC, CD19-APC, NK1.1-PE, and GL-3-APC (all from BioLegend). All data were analyzed with a FACSCalibur flow cytometer (BD Biosciences) and Flowjo software (Tree Star, Ashland, OR, USA).

Apoptosis

Plasma cells were purified from spleen in MRL/lpr lupus-prone mice using MACS CD138$^+$ Plasma Cell Isolation Kit (Miltenyi Biotec) as recommended by the manufacturer. The cell population contained >98% CD138$^+$ cells. The isolated plasma cells were used for apoptosis assay. The single cell suspensions were incubated for 5 h with 30 nM Gal-9 in 96 well flat-bottom plates in humidified incubators in the presence of 5% CO2. After the incubation period was over, the cells were stained for Annexin V (BioLegend) with or without 7AAD and analyzed immediately by flow cytometry.

We further assessed the effects of lactose (30 mM), sucrose (30 mM), Tim-3 mAb (10 µg/ml, eBioscience), and rat IgG2a (10 µg/ml, eBioscience) on Gal-9-induced apoptosis. All data were acquired with a FACSCalibur (BD Biosciences) and analyzed with FlowJo software (Tree Star).

ELISA

The serum levels of anti-dsDNA antibody, total IgG and BAFF were measured with mouse anti-dsDNA antibody ELISA kit

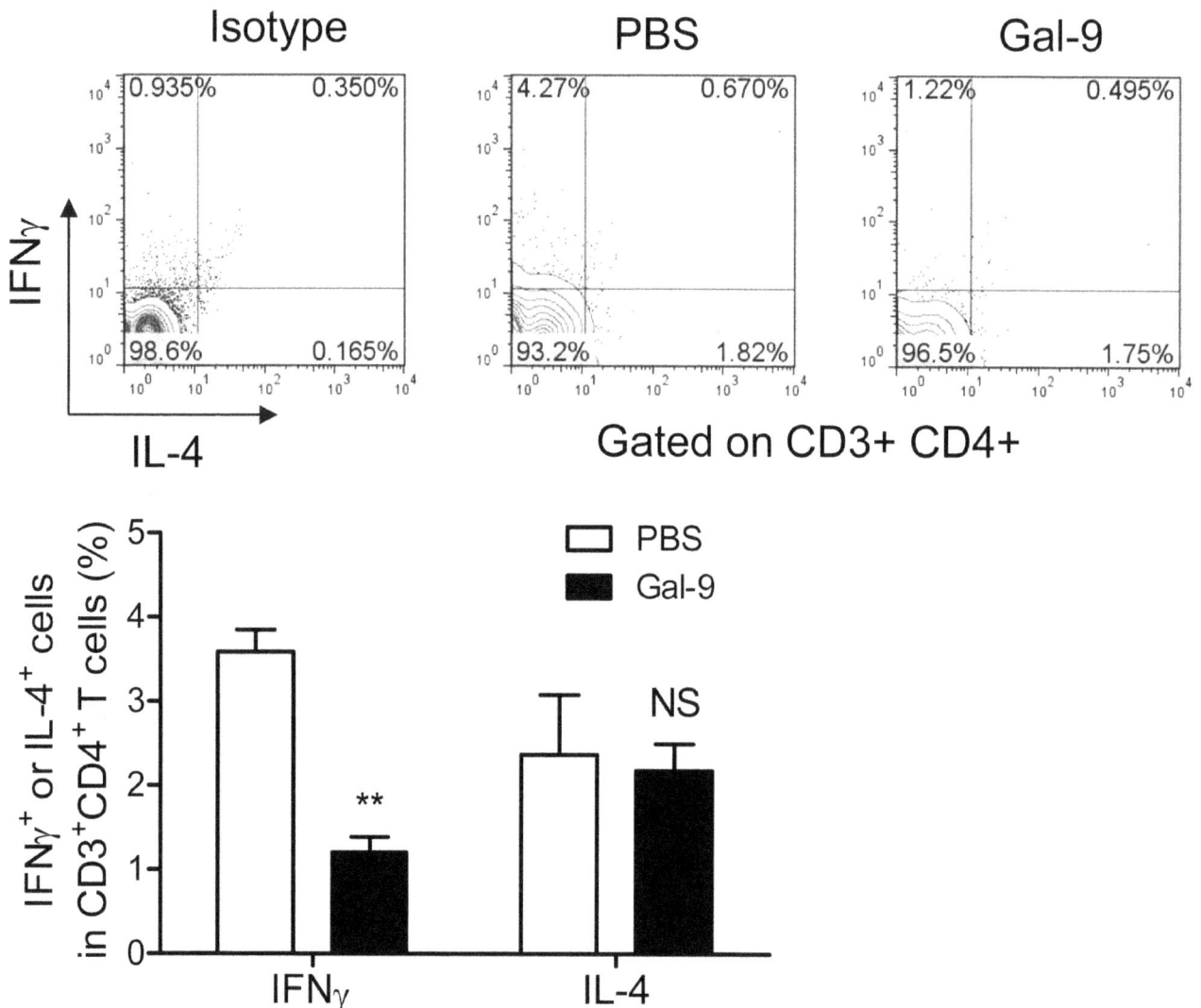

Figure 2. Effects of Gal-9 on splenic Th1 and Th2 subsets in MRL/lpr mice. Comparison of IFNγ⁺ Th1 and IL-4⁺ Th2 frequency between PBS-treated (n = 4) and Gal-9-treated (n = 4) mice (***, P<0.001). Representative data of flow cytometric profiles are shown.

(Shibayagi, Gunma, Japan), mouse IgG ELISA kit (Immunology Consultants Laboratory, Inc., Portland, OR, USA) and mouse BAFF Immunoassay kit (R&D Systems, Minneapolis, MN, USA) according to the manufacturer's instructions, respectively.

Statistical Analysis

Student's paired or unpaired t-tests and one- or two-way ANOVA were used for statistical comparisons. All statistical analyses were performed with Prism 5 software (Graphpad Software, La Jolla, CA).

Results

Galectin-9 Ameliorates Clinical Severity of MRL/lpr Lupus-prone Mice

We first evaluated the therapeutic effects of Gal-9 by treating 9-week-old MRL/lpr lupus-prone mice with Gal-9. Gal-9 significantly suppressed the level of proteinuria (**Figure 1A**). Since it is well known that MRL/lpr lupus-prone mice develop autoimmune arthritis and hemolytic anemia [11,12], we also examined the

effects of Gal-9 on these diseases. Gal-9 clearly retarded the onset of arthritis and suppressed the increase of paw volume (**Figure 1B**). Hematocrits of 20-week-old MRL/lpr lupus-prone mice were significantly lower than that of MRL/lpr⁺/⁺ mice. When MRL/lpr lupus-prone mice were treated with Gal-9, hematocrit increased significantly (**Figure 1C**). These results suggest that Gal-9 helps to ameliorate disease onset in MRL/lpr lupus-prone mice.

Regulatory Effects of Gal-9 on T Cells

It has been shown that Gal-9 induces apoptosis of Th1 and Th17 cells [6,13,14,15]. Similarly, Gal-9 induces apoptosis of activated CD8⁺ T cells [16,17]. Therefore, we treated 8-week-old MRL/lpr lupus-prone mice with Gal-9 to assess its effects on splenic effector T cells. MRL/lpr lupus-prone mice were sacrificed at 4 weeks after Gal-9 treatment (12-week-old). FACS analysis was first done to establish the frequency of splenic effector CD4 and CD8 T cells. We found that Gal-9 decreased the frequency of Th1 (IFNγ⁺ IL-4⁻ CD3⁺ CD4⁺ cells) significantly, while Th2 (IL-4⁺ IFNγ⁻ CD3⁺ CD4⁺ cells) were unchanged in Gal-9-treated

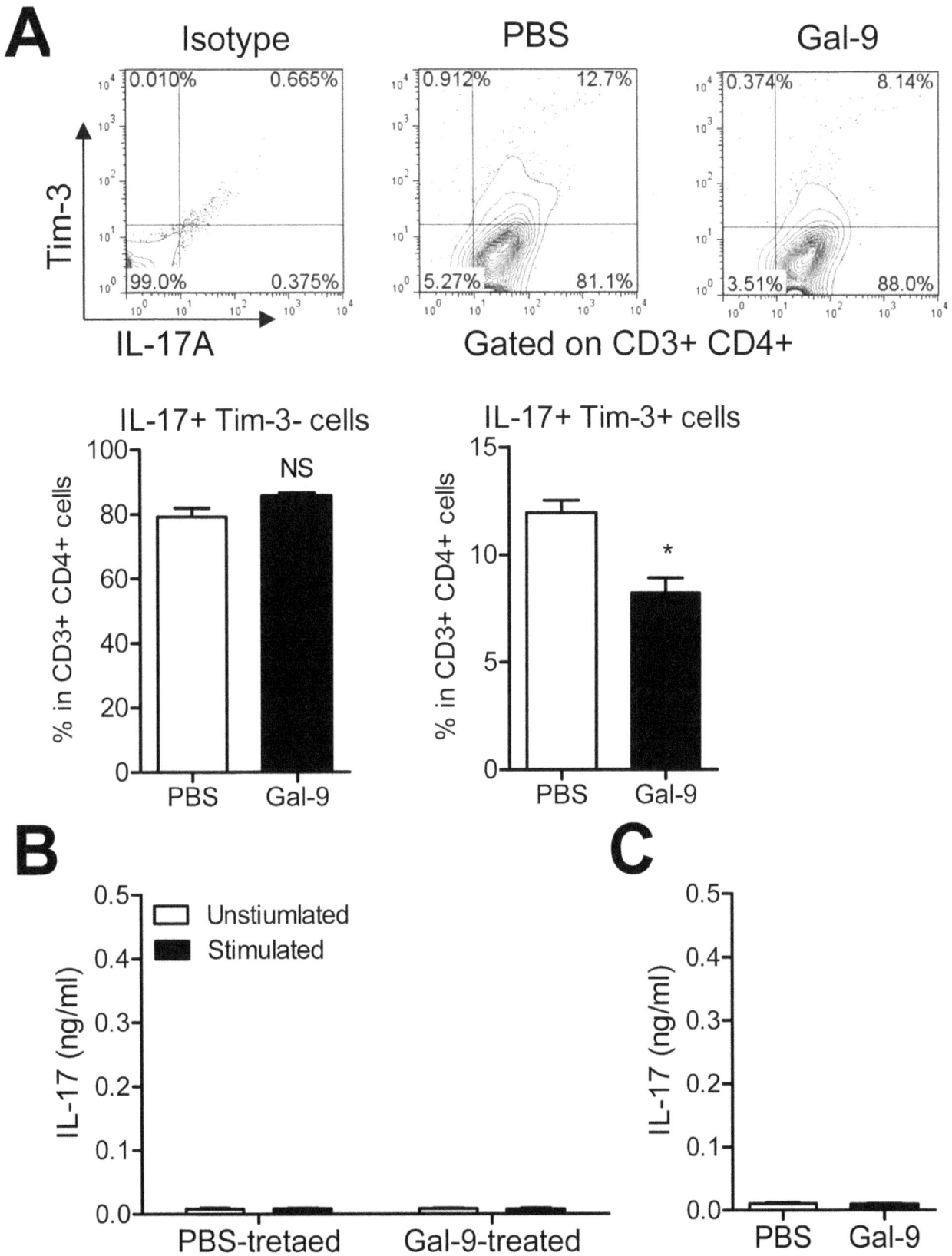

Figure 3. Gal-9 decreases splenic Th17 cells. (**A**) Comparison of frequency of Tim-3⁺ IL17A⁺ Th17 between PBS-treated (n = 4) and Gal-9-treated (n = 4) mice (**, P<0.01). Representative data of flow cytometric profiles are shown. (**B**) Spleen cells of MRL/lpr mice do not release IL-17. Spleen cells from PBS-treated (n = 4) and Gal-9-treated (n = 4) mice were cultured for 6 h with or without PMA+ionomycin. (**C**) Negligible level of IL-17 in plasma of MRL/lpr mice. PBS-treated (n = 4) and Gal-9-treated (n = 4) mice.

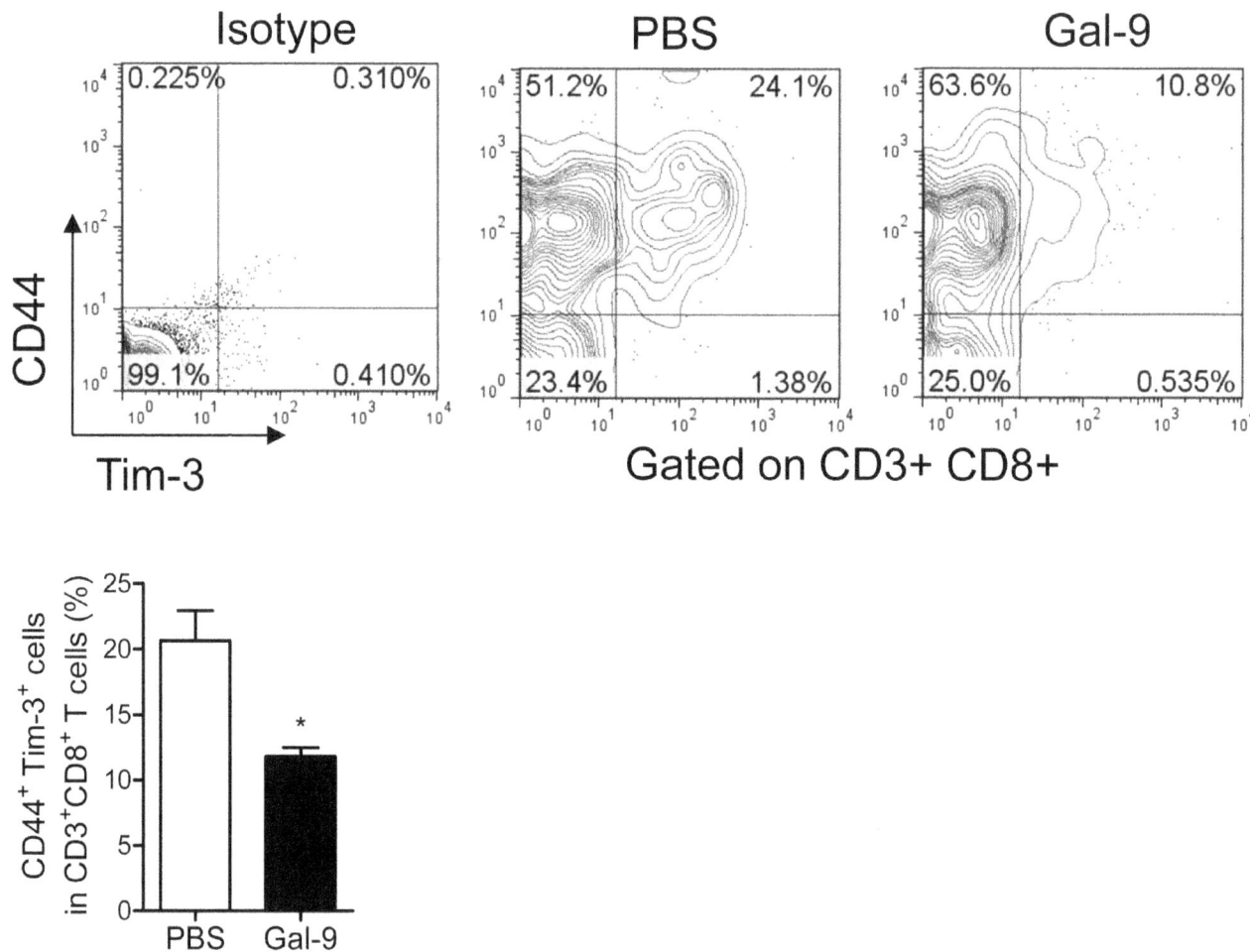

Figure 4. Gal-9 decreases splenic Tim-3$^+$ CD44$^+$ CD8 T cells. Comparison of the percentage of Tim-3$^+$ CD44$^+$ CD8$^+$ T cells between PBS-treated (n = 4) and Gal-9-treated (n = 4) mice (*, P<0.05). Representative data of flow cytometric profiles are shown.

MRL/lpr lupus-prone mice (**Figure 2**). In contrast, Gal-9 did not reduce γδT cells and NKT cells, and did not increase Foxp3$^+$ CD4 T cells (**data not shown**).

Surprisingly, most of CD4$^+$ T cells expressed IL-17 in the cytoplasm, and there was no significant difference in the frequency of total IL-17$^+$ Tim-3$^-$ CD4 T cells between PBS- and Gal-9-treated MRL/lpr lupus-prone mice (**Figure 3A**). In contrast, the frequency of Tim-3$^+$ IL-17$^+$ CD4 T cells, probably Th17, was decreased by Gal-9 treatment similar to Th1.

We assessed ELISA assay to compare the level of IL-17 in the culture supernatants of spleen CD4 T cells from PBS- and Gal-9-treated mice with or without PMA+ionomycin stimulation. Surprisingly, the levels of IL-17 in the culture supernatants were negligible even after the stimulation, and there was no significant difference in IL-17 levels between PBS- and Gal-9-treated MRL/lpr lupus-prone mice, suggesting that release of IL-17 was impaired in most CD4 T cells of MRL/lpr lupus-prone mice (**Figure 3B**). We also assessed ELISA assay for IL-17 levels in plasma of PBS-treated and Gal-9-treated MRL/lpr lupus prone mice. Expectedly, ELISA assay revealed that plasma IL-17 level was negligible in both PBS- and Gal-9-treated MRL/lpr lupus-prone mice (**Figure 3C**).

Moreover, most Tim-3$^+$ CD8 T cells in MRL/lpr lupus-prone mice co-expressed CD44, an activated cell marker, and CD44$^+$ Tim-3$^+$ CD8 T cells decreased significantly in Gal-9-treated mice,

suggesting that Gal-9 preferentially decreases Tim-3+ CD8 T cells (**Figure 4**). These results suggest that Gal-9 attenuates disease severity in MRL/lpr lupus-prone mice, at least partly, by regulating Tim-3 expressing effector Th1, Th17, and activated CD8 T cells.

Gal-9 Suppresses Anti-dsDNA Antibody Production

We hypothesized that Gal-9 suppresses autoantibody production in MRL/lpr lupus-prone mice, because Gal-9 improved hematocrit of MRL/lpr lupus-prone mice. MRL/lpr lupus-prone mice (8-week-old) were treated with Gal-9, since their anti-dsDNA antibody levels began to increase. Gal-9 treatment significantly suppressed anti-dsDNA antibody production in MRL/lpr lupus-prone mice (**Figure 5A**). Moreover, ANOVA analysis confirmed that the level of anti-dsDNA antibody in Gal-9-treated MRL/lpr lupus-prone mice did not increase, whereas the level in PBS-treated mice significantly increased (**Figure 5B**). Next, we performed experiments to ask whether Gal-9 also suppresses the levels of total IgG. In contrast, there was no significant difference in the levels of total IgG between PBS- and Gal-9-treated MRL/lpr lupus-prone mice (**Figure 5C and D**).

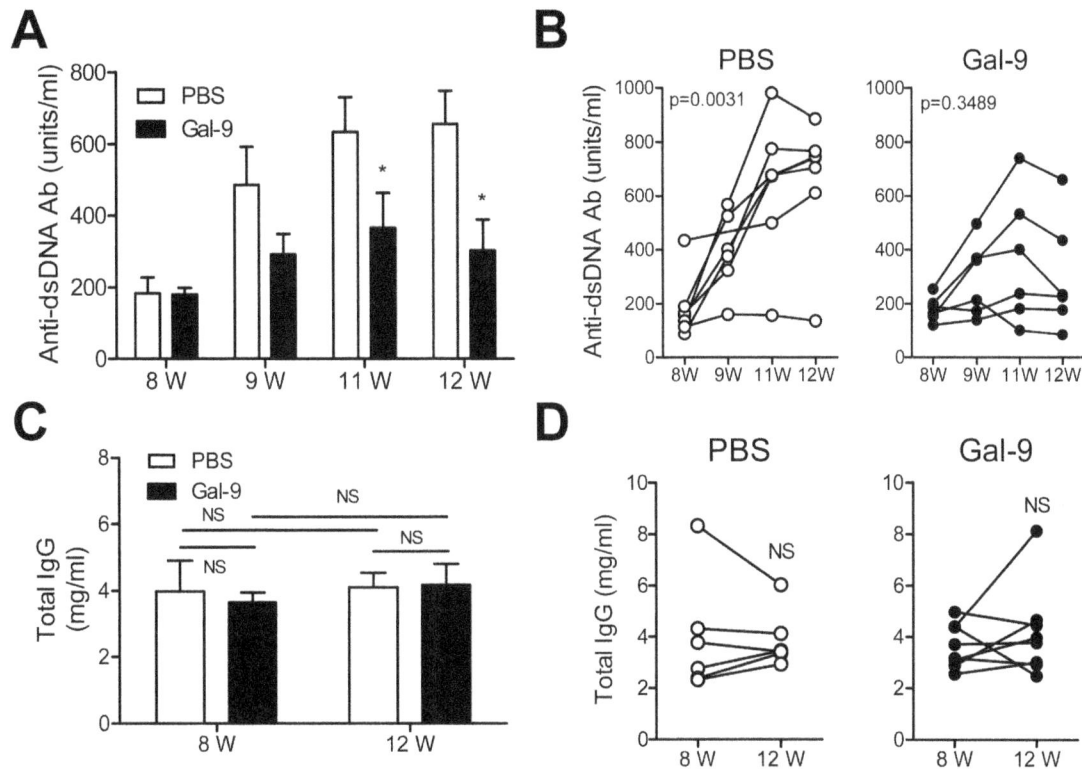

Figure 5. Effects of Gal-9 on the level of total IgG and anti-dsDNA antibody. (A) Comparison of anti-dsDNA antibody levels at 8, 9, 11, and 12 weeks of age between PBS-treated (n = 7) and Gal-9-treated (n = 6) mice. Human Gal-9 and PBS were injected intraperitoneally into 8-week-old mice 3-times/week for 4 weeks. (*, P<0.05) **(B)** Comparison of anti-dsDNA antibody levels in 8- to 12-week-old PBS-treated (n = 7) and Gal-9-treated (n = 6) mice. **(C)** Comparison of total IgG levels between PBS-treated (n = 7) and Gal-9-treated (n = 8) mice at 12 weeks of age. Human Gal-9 and PBS were injected intraperitoneally into 8-week-old mice 3-times/week for 4 weeks. (NS, not significant) **(D)** Comparison of total IgG levels in 8- and 12-week-old PBS-treated (n = 7) and Gal-9-treated (n = 8) mice. (NS, not significant).

Gal-9 Decreases the Frequency of CD19$^{-/low}$ CD138$^+$ Plasma Cells

The above results raised the possibility that Gal-9 suppresses anti-dsDNA antibody production through B cell regulation. FACS analysis revealed that the frequency of CD19$^+$ B cells was increased in 12-week-old Gal-9-treated MRL/lpr lupus-prone mice (**Figure 6A**). In contrast, Gal-9 significantly reduced the frequency of splenic plasma cells (CD19$^{-/low}$ CD138$^+$) but not plasmablasts (CD19$^+$ CD138$^+$) (**Figure 6A**). It was thus suggested Gal-9 preferentially decreases plasma cells in MRL/lpr lupus-prone mice.

Since BAFF levels are up regulated in SLE patients and MRL/lpr lupus-prone mice to induce plasma cell differentiation [18,19,20,21], we assessed the effects of Gal-9 on serum level of BAFF. ELISA analysis unexpectedly revealed that Gal-9 does not reduce BAFF level (**Figure 6B**). These results suggest that Gal-9 does not decrease plasma cells by downregulating BAFF production, at least in this model.

Gal-9 Induces Plasma Cell Apoptosis

Because Gal-9 induces apoptosis of Th1, Th17, and CD8 T cells through Gal-9/Tim-3 interaction, we first asked whether plasma cells express Tim-3, and intriguingly found that about 20% of plasma cells (CD19$^-$ CD138$^+$) in MRL/lpr lupus-prone mice express Tim-3 (**Figure. 7A**). In order to ask whether Gal-9 induces plasma cell apoptosis, CD19$^-$ CD138$^+$ cells were prepared by MACS. Gal-9 significantly increased the frequency of Annexin V$^+$ apoptotic plasma cells (**Figure 7B**). The apoptosis

was significantly suppressed by lactose, whereas anti-Tim-3 antibody unexpectedly did not (**Figure 7B**). Further experiments revealed that Gal-9 induced both early apoptosis (Annexin V$^+$7AAD$^-$) and late apoptosis (Annexin V$^+$7AAD$^+$) of plasma cells (**Figure 7C**). Further experiments, however, revealed that Gal-9 induced Tim-3$^+$ plasma cell apoptosis than Tim-3$^-$ plasma cells (**Figure 7D**). Taken together, Tim-3 may not be directly involved in the apoptosis, and Tim-3 may be associated with vulnerability to Gal-9-mediated plasma cell apoptosis, at least, in MRL/lpr lupus-prone mice.

Discussion

We found that in MRL/lpr lupus-prone mice, Gal-9 attenuates the severity of various symptoms, such as lupus nephritis, arthritis, and hemolytic anemia. It has been shown that Gal-9 induces apoptosis of Th1 and Th17 cells through Gal-9/Tim-3 interactions [8]. Our recent studies revealed that Gal-9 downregulates Th17 cell differentiation whereas it upregulates differentiation of Foxp3$^+$ Tregs, independently of Tim-3 [5]. The beneficial effects of Gal-9 on lupus symptoms in MRL/lpr lupus-prone mice seem partially ascribed to Gal-9-induced decrease of Tim-3$^+$ Th1 and Th17 cells because imbalance of Th17 and Th1 cells in SLE and Th17 and Tregs are critical for SLE pathogenesis. Interestingly, Gal-9 failed to expand Foxp3$^+$ Tregs in MRL/lpr lupus-prone mice, suggesting that this is attributed to T cell abnormality in MRL/lpr lupus-prone mice [24].

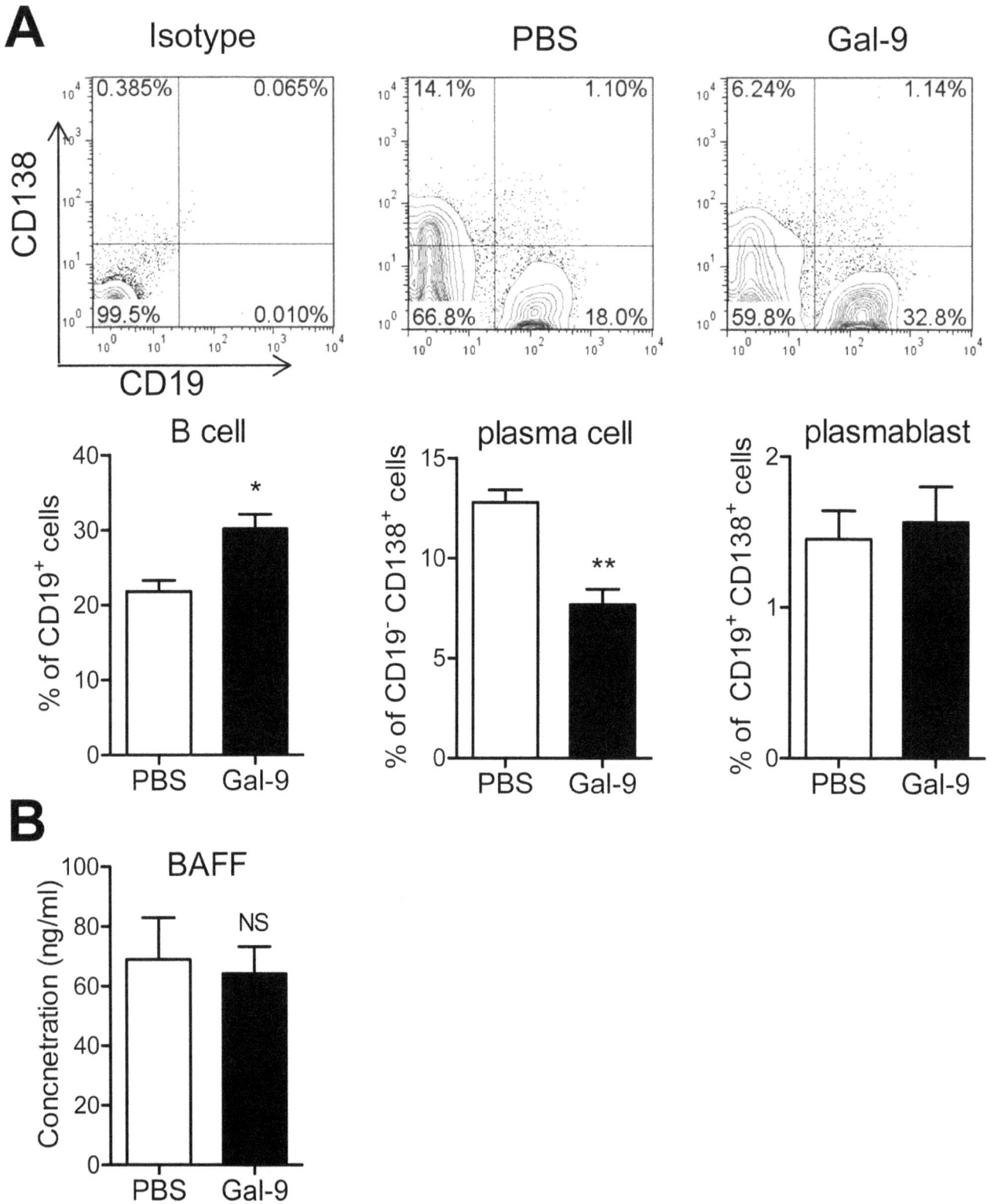

Figure 6. Gal-9 decreases spleen plasma cells in MRL/lpr mice. (**A**) Comparison of the percentage of B cells, plasma cells, and plasmablasts in the spleen of 12-week-old PBS-treated (n = 4) and Gal-9-treated (n = 4) mice. (*, P<0.05, **, P<0.01). Representative data of flow cytometric profiles are shown. (**B**) Comparisons of the level of BAFF between PBS-treated (n = 7) and Gal-9-treated (n = 8) mice at 12-weeks. (NS, not significant).D.

In the present experiments, we also found that CD4$^+$ T cells from MRL/lpr lupus-prone mice did not release IL-17 even by PMA stimulation though most of them surprisingly expressed IL-17 in the cytoplasm, suggesting T cell abnormality in the mice.

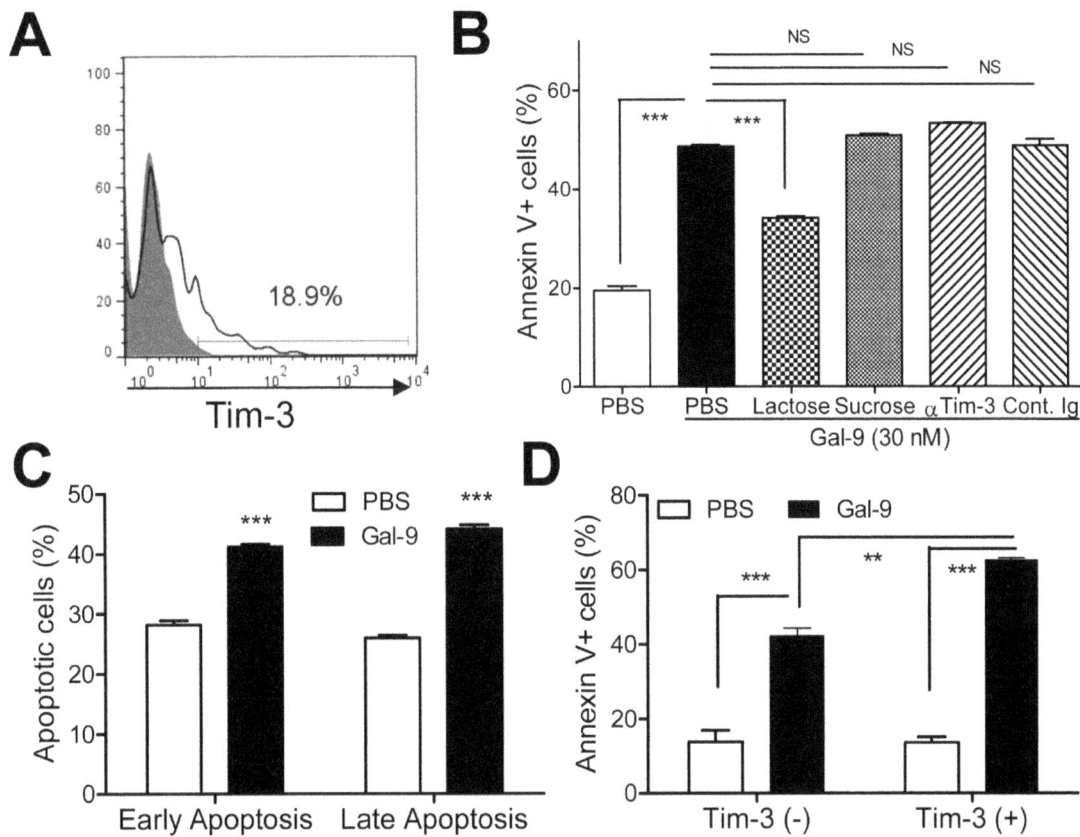

Figure 7. Gal-9 Induces plasma cell apoptosis independently of Tim-3. (A) Plasma cells express Tim-3. Tim-3 expression on $CD19^{-/low}$ $CD138^{+}$ cells of spleen cells from 12-week-old MRL/lpr lupus-prone mice was assessed. The results shown are representative data from one of four independent experiments. Filled histogram represents isotype-matched control. **(B)** Induction of plasma cell apoptosis by Gal-9. Plasma cells were treated with 30 nM Gal-9 for 5 h in the presence or absence of lactose, in quadruplicate. (***, P<0.001; NS, not significant). **(C)** Gal-9 induces both early (Annexin $V^{+}7AAD^{-}$) and late (Annexin $V^{+}7AAD^{+}$) apoptosis of plasma cells from MRL/lpr mice. Plasma cells were treated with 30 nM Gal-9 for 5 h in quadruplicate. (***, P<0.001). **(D)** Susceptibility of Tim-3^{+} plasma cells to Gal-9. Plasma cells were treated with Gal-9 for 5 h. The frequency of Annexin V^{+} cells was assessed in quadruplicate. (***, P<0.001; **, P<0.01; NS, not significant).

Oppositely, Hou et al recently reported that only less than 1% of cells in CD4 T cells of MRL/lpr mice expressed IL-17 in the cytoplasm [25]. Although heterogeneity in MRL/lpr mice according to the source may be one explanation for the above discrepancy, further studies are, of course, required to ascertain it.

Gal-9 also induces apoptosis of $CD8^{+}$ alloreactive T cells in allografts and viral infections [15,26,27,28]. The fact that Gal-9 also reduces Tim-3^{+} $CD44^{+}$ $CD8^{+}$ T cells in MRL/lpr lupus-prone mice suggests that Tim-3^{+} $CD44^{+}$ $CD8^{+}$ T cells are also associated with lupus pathogenesis in MRL/lpr lupus-prone mice, since infiltrating $CD4^{+}$ and $CD8^{+}$ T cells in lupus kidney indicate that they have the potential to mediate kidney injury [29].

In the present experiments, we show that Gal-9 suppresses anti-dsDNA antibody levels in MRL/lpr lupus-prone mice though the level of total IgG was not changed by Gal-9. Although Gal-9 treatment increased $CD19^{+}$ cells in MRL/lpr lupus-prone mice, it reduced $CD19^{-}$ $CD138^{+}$ plasma cells but not $CD19^{+}$ $CD138^{+}$ plasmablasts. This plasma cell reduction may result in the suppression of anti-dsDNA antibody production.

Recently it was shown that Belimumab, a specific inhibitor of BAFF, and atacicept (TACI-immunoglobulin), a receptor molecule for APRIL, effectively ameliorates clinical symptoms in SLE patients [30,31,32]. Although family receptors for BAFF and APRIL vary in their expression patterns and levels across different B-cell subsets, biologic action of BAFF and APRIL may be

primarily on memory and/or plasma cells [33,34]. Moreover, the innate immune system initiates and perpetuates autoimmunity [35]. A small number of patients, undergoing type I IFN therapy for cancer or viral infections, developed SLE. Similarly, IFN-α accelerates SLE in some murine models and is associated with increased BAFF serum levels. Blockade of TNF-α induces increased levels of BAFF via upregulation of type I IFNs and has been associated with development of anti-nuclear antibodies in up to 50% of patients with clinical SLE [37]. B cell depletion in patients treated with anti-CD20 also results in high levels of BAFF, likely an attempt to maintain B cell homeostasis [38].

However, Gal-9 treatment fails to reduce BAFF levels, although it attenuates disease severity. Instead, Gal-9 induces plasma cell apoptosis, suggesting Gal-9 induced plasma cell apoptosis is, at least, partly involved in the suppression of anti-dsDNA antibody production. Of course, It can be raised an alternative explanation that Gal-9 block maturation of $CD19^{+}$ B cells to $CD19^{-}$ plasma cells, because of increased $CD19^{+}$ B cells and decreased plasma cells in MRL/lpr mice. Furthermore, we cannot, however, exclude the possibility of involvement of Gal-9 in the biological function of BAFF. It remains to be clarified whether Gal-9 inhibits binding between BAFF and BAFF receptors, Gal-9 downregulates BAFF receptors on B cells, and suppresses BAFF/BAFF receptor-induced signal transduction.

Furthermore, plasma cells in the spleen of MRL/lpr lupus-prone mice express Tim-3, and the Tim-3$^+$ plasma cells are more susceptible to Gal-9-induced apoptosis than the Tim-3$^-$ plasma cells. Curiously, a blocking Tim-3 antibody does not abrogate the Gal-9-induced apoptosis. These observations raise several questions. Firstly, as far as we know, this is the first example of Tim-3 expression in the cells of B cell linage. It is, thus, urgently required to ascertain whether Tim-3 expression on plasma cells is limited in MRL/lpr lupus-prone mice or plasma cells in general, including in WT mice and in humans. The second question is whether there are any functional differences between Tim-3$^+$ and Tim-3$^-$ plasma cells. Tim-3 expression is associated with exhausted phenotypes in virus-infected T-cells and those T-cells are also known to be susceptible to Gal-9-induced apoptosis [40]. The third question is how Tim-3 expression renders plasma cells susceptible to Gal-9, even though Tim-3 may not be the direct target molecule for Gal-9-induced apoptosis. Last, it will be intriguing to clarify whether Gal-9 is also involved in the regulation of B cell development other than plasma cells, including germinal center B cells as they regulate Th17 and Foxp3+ regulatory T cells [7]. Further in-depth studies will be, thus, required to answer the above questions to understand the exact molecular mechanisms of Gal-9-induced regulation of antibody production.

In conclusion, Gal-9 ameliorates clinical severity of MRL/lpr lupus-prone mice by decreasing the level of anti-dsDNA antibody in addition to T cell regulation. The suppressive mechanism was supposed to be the result of induction of apoptosis of plasma cells but not of decrease of BAFF production. Although some CD19$^{-/low}$ CD138$^+$ plasma cells in MRL/lpr lupus-prone mice express Tim-3, Gal-9 induced plasma cell apoptosis independently of Tim-3. This suggests that Gal-9 may be a novel candidate for SLE therapy, which would involve an orchestrated mode of action on T cells [41,42], macrophages [43,44] and plasma cells.

Author Contributions

Conceived and designed the experiments: MM TK TN DN GS HM HK TM MK MH. Performed the experiments: MM TK TN MH. Analyzed the data: MM TK TN MH. Contributed reagents/materials/analysis tools: TK TN DN GS HM HK TM MK MH. Wrote the paper: MM TK TN MH.

References

1. Anaya JM, Canas C, Mantilla RD, Pineda-Tamayo R, Tobon GJ, et al. (2011) Lupus nephritis in Colombians: contrasts and comparisons with other populations. Clin Rev Allergy Immunol 40: 199–207.
2. Davidson A (2012) The Rationale for BAFF Inhibition in Systemic Lupus Erythematosus. Curr Rheumatol Rep 14: 295–302.
3. Liu Z, Davidson A (2011) BAFF and selection of autoreactive B cells. Trends Immunol 32: 388–394.
4. Liu Z, Davidson A (2011) BAFF inhibition: a new class of drugs for the treatment of autoimmunity. Exp Cell Res 317: 1270–1277.
5. Seki M, Oomizu S, Sakata KM, Sakata A, Arikawa T, et al. (2008) Galectin-9 suppresses the generation of Th17, promotes the induction of regulatory T cells, and regulates experimental autoimmune arthritis. Clin Immunol 127: 78–88.
6. Oomizu S, Arikawa T, Niki T, Kadowaki T, Ueno M, et al. (2012) Galectin-9 suppresses Th17 cell development in an IL-2-dependent but Tim-3-independent manner. Clin Immunol 143: 51–58.
7. Kanzaki M, Wada J, Sugiyama K, Nakatsuka A, Teshigawara S, et al. (2012) Galectin-9 and T cell immunoglobulin mucin-3 pathway is a therapeutic target for type 1 diabetes. Endocrinology 153: 612–620.
8. Wiersma VR, de Bruyn M, Helfrich W, Bremer E (2011) Therapeutic potential of Galectin-9 in human disease. Med Res Rev July 26. doi:10 1002/med.20249.
9. Arikawa T, Watanabe K, Seki M, Matsukawa A, Oomizu S, et al. (2009) Galectin-9 ameliorates immune complex-induced arthritis by regulating Fc gamma R expression on macrophages. Clin Immunol 133 (2009) 382–392.
10. Nishi N, Itoh A, Fujiyama A, Yoshida N, Araya S, et al. (2005) Development of highly stable galectins: truncation of the linker peptide confers protease-resistance on tandem-repeat type galectins. FEBS Lett 579: 2058–2064.
11. Koopman WJ, Gay S (1988) The MRL-lpr/lpr mouse. A model for the study of rheumatoid arthritis, Scand J Rheumatol Suppl 75: 284–289.
12. Fagiolo E, Toriani-Terenzi C (2003) Mechanisms of immunological tolerance loss versus erythrocyte self-antigens and autoimmune hemolytic anemia, Autoimmunity 36: 199–204.
13. Lee J, Park EJ, Noh JW, Hwang JW, Bae EK, et al. (2012) Underexpression of TIM-3 and blunted galectin-9-induced apoptosis of CD4+ T cells in rheumatoid arthritis. Inflammation 35: 633–637.
14. Wang F, Xu J, Liao Y, Wang Y, Liu C, et al. (2011) Tim-3 ligand galectin-9 reduces IL-17 level and accelerates Klebsiella pneumoniae infection. Cell Immunol 269: 22–28.
15. Sakai K, Kawata E, Ashihara E, Nakagawa Y, Yamauchi A, et al. (2011) Galectin-9 ameliorates acute GVH disease through the induction of T-cell apoptosis. Eur J Immunol 41: 67–75.
16. Tsuchiyama Y, Wada J, Zhang H, Morita Y, Hiragushi K, et al. (2000) Efficacy of galectins in the amelioration of nephrotoxic serum nephritis in Wistar Kyoto rats. Kidney Int 58: 1941–1952.
17. Wang F, He W, Zhou H, Yuan J, Wu K, et al. (2007) The Tim-3 ligand galectin-9 negatively regulates CD8+ alloreactive T cell and prolongs survival of skin graft. Cell Immunol 250: 68–74.
18. Dillon SR, Harder B, Lewis KB, Moore MD, Liu H, et al.(2010) B-lymphocyte stimulator/a proliferation-inducing ligand heterotrimers are elevated in the sera of patients with autoimmune disease and are neutralized by atacicept and B-cell maturation antigen-immunoglobulin. Arthritis Res Ther 12: R48.
19. Koyama T, Tsukamoto H, Miyagi Y, Himeji D, Otsuka J, et al. (2005) Raised serum APRIL levels in patients with systemic lupus erythematosus. Ann Rheum Dis 64: 1065–1067.
20. Gross JA, Johnston J, Mudri S, Enselman R, Dillon SR, et al. (2000) TACI and BCMA are receptors for a TNF homologue implicated in B-cell autoimmune disease. Nature 404: 995–999.
21. Mackay F, Sierro F, Grey ST, Gordon TP (2005) The BAFF/APRIL system: an important player in systemic rheumatic diseases. Curr Dir Autoimmun 8: 243–265.
22. Shah K, Lee WW, Lee SH, Kim SH, Kang SW, et al. (2010) Dysregulated balance of Th17 and Th1 cells in systemic lupus erythematosus. Arthritis Res Ther 12: R53.
23. Kleczynska W, Jakiela B, Plutecka H, Milewski M, Sanak M, et al. (2011) Imbalance between Th17 and regulatory T-cells in systemic lupus erythematosus. Folia Histochem Cytobiol 49: 646–653.
24. Yang J, Chu Y, Yang X, Gao D, Zhu L, et al. (2009) Th17 and natural Treg cell population dynamics in systemic lupus erythematosus. Arthritis Rheum 60: 1472–1483.
25. Hou LF, He SJ, Li X, Yang Y, He PL, et al. (2011) Oral administration of artemisinin analogue SM 934 ameliorates lupus syndromes in MRL/lpr mice by inhibiting Th1 and Th17 cell responses. Arthritis Rheum 63: 2445–2455.
26. Wang F, He W, Zhou H, Yuan J, Wu K, et al. (2007) The Tim-3 ligand galectin-9 negatively regulates CD8+ alloreactive T cell and prolongs survival of skin graft. Cell Immunol 250: 68–74.
27. Reddy PB, Sehrawat S, Suryawanshi A, Rajasagi NK, Mulik S, et al. (2011) Influence of galectin-9/Tim-3 interaction on herpes simplex virus-1 latency. J Immunol 187: 5745–5755.
28. Sehrawat S, Reddy PB, Rajasagi N, Suryanshi A, Hirashima M, et al., (2010) Galectin-9/TIM-3 interaction regulates virus-specific primary and memory CD8 T cell response. PLoS Pathog 6: e1000882.
29. Winchester R, Wiesendanger M, Zhang HZ, Steshenko V, Peterson K, et al. (2012) Immunologic characteristics of intrarenal T cells: trafficking of expanded CD8+ T cell beta-chain clonotypes in progressive lupus nephritis. Arthritis Rheum 64: 1589–1600.
30. Manzi S, Sanchez-Guerrero J, Merrill JT, Furie R, Gladman D, et al. (2012) Effects of belimumab, a B lymphocyte stimulator-specific inhibitor, on disease activity across multiple organ domains in patients with systemic lupus erythematosus: combined results from two phase III trials. Ann Rheum Dis May 11.
31. Fiorina P, Sayegh MH (2009) B cell-targeted therapies in autoimmunity: rationale and progress. F1000 Biol Rep May 28;1:39. doi: 10.3410/B1-39.
32. Dall'Era M, Chakravarty E, Wallace D, Genovese M, Weisman M, et al. (2007) Reduced B lymphocyte and immunoglobulin levels after atacicept treatment in patients with systemic lupus erythematosus: results of a multicenter, phase Ib, double-blind, placebo-controlled, dose-escalating trial. Arthritis Rheum 56: 4142–4150.
33. Chu VT, Enghard P, Riemekasten G, Berek C (2007) In vitro and in vivo activation induces BAFF and APRIL expression in B cells. J Immunol 179: 5947–5957.
34. Belnoue E, Pihlgren M, McGaha TL, Tougne C, Rochat AF (2008) APRIL is critical for plasmablast survival in the bone marrow and poorly expressed by early-life bone marrow stromal cells. Blood 111: 2755–2764.
35. WilsonLE, Widman D, Dikman SH, Gorevic PD (2002) Autoimmune disease complicating antiviral therapy for hepatitis C virus infection. Semin Arthritis Rheum 32: 163–173.

36. Mathian A, Weinberg A, Gallegos M, Bancherau J, Koutouzov S (2005) IFN-alpha induces early lethal lupus in preautoimmune (New Zealand Black x New Zealand White) F1 but not in BALB/c mice. J Immunol 174: 2499–2506.

37. Mohan AK, Edwards ET, Cote TR, Siegel JN, Braun MM (2002) Drug-induced systemic lupus erythematosus and TNF-alpha blockers. Lancet 360: 646.

38. Nagel A, Podstawa E, Eickmann M, Muller HH, Hertl M, et al. (2009) Rituximab mediates a strong elevation of B-cell-activating factor associated with increased pathogen-specific IgG but not autoantibodies in pemphigus vulgaris. J Invest Dermatol 129: 2202–2210.

39. Jones RB, Ndhlovu LC, Barbour JD, Sheth PM, Jha AR, et al. (2008) Tim-3 expression defines a novel population of dysfunctional T cells with highly elevated frequencies in progressive HIV-1 infection. J Exp Med 205: 2763–79.

40. Reddy PB, Sehrawat S, Suryawanshi A, Rajasagi NK, Mulik S, et al. (2011) Influence of galectin-9/Tim-3 interaction on herpes simplex virus-1 latency. J Immunol 187: 5745–55.

41. Pan HF, Zhang N, Li WX, Tao JH, Ye DQ (2010) TIM-3 as a new therapeutic target in systemic lupus erythematosus. Mol Biol Rep 37: 395–398.

42. Wang Y, Meng J, Wang X, Liu S, Shu Q, et al. (2008) Expression of human TIM-1 and TIM-3 on lymphocytes from systemic lupus erythematosus patients. Scand J Immunol 67: 63–70.

43. Kadowaki T, Arikawa T, Shinonaga R, Oomizu S, Inagawa H, et al. (2012) Galectin-9 signaling prolongs survival in murine lung-cancer by inducing macrophages to differentiate into plasmacytoid dendritic cell-like macrophages. Clin Immunol 142: 296–307.

44. Arikawa T, Saita N, Oomizu S, Ueno M, Matsukawa A, et al. (2010) Galectin-9 expands immunosuppressive macrophages to ameliorate T-cell-mediated lung inflammation. Eur J Immunol 40: 548–558.

Multiple Sites of the Cleavage of 21- and 25-Mer Encephalytogenic Oligopeptides Corresponding to Human Myelin Basic Protein (MBP) by Specific Anti-MBP Antibodies from Patients with Systemic Lupus Erythematosus

Anna M. Timofeeva[1], Pavel S. Dmitrenok[2], Ludmila P. Konenkova[3], Valentina N. Buneva[1,4], Georgy A. Nevinsky[1,4]*

1 Institute of Chemical Biology and Fundamental Medicine, Siberian Division of Russian Academy of Sciences, Novosibirsk, Russia, 2 Pacific Institute of Bioorganic Chemistry, Far East Division, Russian Academy of Sciences, Vladivostok, Russia, 3 Institute of Clinical Immunology, Siberian Division of Russian Medical Academy of Sciences, Novosibirsk, Russia, 4 Novosibirsk State University, Novosibirsk, Russia

Abstract

IgGs from patients with multiple sclerosis and systemic lupus erythematosus (SLE) purified on MBP-Sepharose in contrast to canonical proteases hydrolyze effectively only myelin basic protein (MBP), but not many other tested proteins. Here we have shown for the first time that anti-MBP SLE IgGs hydrolyze nonspecific tri- and tetrapeptides with an extreme low efficiency and cannot effectively hydrolyze longer 20-mer nonspecific oligopeptides corresponding to antigenic determinants (AGDs) of HIV-1 integrase. At the same time, anti-MBP SLE IgGs efficiently hydrolyze oligopeptides corresponding to AGDs of MBP. All sites of IgG-mediated proteolysis of 21-and 25-mer encephalytogenic oligopeptides corresponding to two known AGDs of MBP were found by a combination of reverse-phase chromatography, TLC, and MALDI spectrometry. Several clustered major, moderate, and minor sites of cleavage were revealed in the case of 21- and 25-mer oligopeptides. The active sites of anti-MBP abzymes are localised on their light chains, while heavy chains are responsible for the affinity of protein substrates. Interactions of intact globular proteins with both light and heavy chains of abzymes provide high affinity to MBP and specificity of this protein hydrolysis. The affinity of anti-MBP abzymes for intact MBP is approximately 1000-fold higher than for the oligopeptides. The data suggest that all oligopeptides interact mainly with the light chains of different monoclonal abzymes of total pool of IgGs, which possesses a lower affinity for substrates, and therefore, depending on the oligopeptide sequences, their hydrolysis may be less specific than globular protein and can occur in several sites.

Editor: Vladimir N. Uversky, University of South Florida College of Medicine, United States of America

Funding: This research was made possible in part by grants from the Presidium of the Russian Academy of Sciences (Molecular and Cellular Biology Program, 6.7; Fundamental Sciences to Medicine, 5.13), Russian Foundation for Basic Research (10-04-00281), and funds from the Siberian Division of the Russian Academy of Sciences. The funders had no role in study design, data collection and analysis, decision to publish, or preparation of the manuscript.

Competing Interests: The authors have declared that no competing interests exist.

* E-mail: nevinsky@niboch.nsc.ru

Introduction

It is known, that the occurrence of auto-Abs in increased concentration is a distinctive feature of various autoimmune diseases (ADs) (reviewed in [1–8]). It was shown that small fractions of auto-Abs can possess different catalytic activities [1–8]. Catalytically active artificial antibodies (Abs) or abzymes (Abzs) against transition chemical states of different reactions were studied intensively (reviewed in [1]). Healthy humans and patients with many diseases with insignificant autoimmune reactions usually lack abzymes or develop Abzs with very low catalytic activities, with these activities being often on a borderline of the sensitivity of detection methods (reviewed in [2–8]). Natural abzymes hydrolyzing DNA, RNA, polysaccharides, oligopeptides (OPs), and proteins are described from the sera of patients with several autoimmune (systemic lupus erythematosus, Hashimoto's

thyroiditis, polyarthritis, multiple sclerosis, asthma, rheumatoid arthritis, etc.) and viral diseases with a pronounced immune system disturbance (viral hepatitis, AIDS, and tick-borne encephalitis) (reviewed in [2–10]). Abzymes may play a significant positive and/ or negative role in broadening Ab properties, forming specific pathogenic patterns and clinical settings in different autoimmune conditions [1–10].

Multiple sclerosis (MS) and systemic lupus erythematosus (SLE) are well known ADs. MS is a chronic demyelinating disease of the central nervous system. Its etiology remains unclear, and the most widely accepted theory of MS pathogenesis assigns the main role in the destruction of myelin to the inflammation related to autoimmune reactions [11]. Several recent findings imply an important role of B cells and auto-Abs against myelin autoantigens including myelin basic protein (MBP) in the pathogenesis of MS [11–13].

SLE is a systemic autoimmune polyetiologic diffuse disease characterized by disorganization of conjunctive tissues with the paramount damage to skin and visceral capillaries [14]. The polyetiologic and polysyndromic character of SLE leads to highly variable manifestations of this disease in terms of many biochemical, immunological, and clinical indices. SLE is usually considered to be related to patient's autoimmunization with DNA, since the sera of such patients usually contain DNA and anti-DNA Abs in high concentrations [15]. At the same time, in comparison with healthy donors, an increased concentration of auto-Abs was observed for various antigens (% of patients): DNA (60), cardiolipin (48), thyroglobulin (42), microsomal fraction of thyrocytes (48), and rheumatoid factor (23) [5].

It should be mentioned, that SLE and MS demonstrated some similarity in the development of the same medical, biochemical and immunological indexes. MS is a chronic disease of the central nervous system leading to the manifestation of different nervous and psychiatric disturbances. However, neuropsychiatric involvement occurs in about 50% of SLE patients and carries a poor prognosis (reviewed in [11]). SLE predominantly affects the central nervous system, and within its cerebral complications it has a particular propensity-perhaps more than any other systemic inflammatory disease– to cause psychiatric disorders [11]. Peripheral nervous system involvement is much less common. The distinctive production of diverse auto-Abs seems to be related to defective clearance of apoptotic cells. Antibody-mediated neural cell injury and rheological disturbances represent the two principal suggested mechanisms of tissue injury [11]. Interplay between these processes, underlying genetic factors, their modification by hormones, complicated by a number of secondary factors, may explain the wide spectrum of features encountered in this disease. Some indicators of disease common to SLE and MS were observed [11].

For diagnostics of MS, thirteen Poser's medical indices are often used [16], but clinically definite MS diagnosis is usually based on the tomographic detection of specific plaques in the brain, which appear on late stages of not only this disease, but also in SLE patients. Similarly to SLE, the high-affinity anti-DNA Abs has been recently identified as a major component of the intrathecal IgGs in MS patient's brains and cells of the cerebrospinal fluid [17]. It was recently shown that titers of Abs against human myelin basic protein in SLE patients 4.2-fold higher than in healthy individuals, but 2.1-fold lower than in patients with MS [9]. In addition, abzymes from the sera of patients with SLE and MS possess by the same catalytic activities (see below).

It was shown that SLE IgGs and IgMs effectively hydrolyzed DNA, RNA, and polysaccharides [18–22]. Similarly to SLE, homogeneous IgGs from the sera and the cerebrospinal fluid of MS patients were active in the hydrolysis of DNA, RNA, and polysaccharides [23–25]. Whereas only 18 and 53% of MS patients contained increased concentrations of Abs to native and denatured DNA, respectively, as compared with healthy donors, DNase abzymes were found in ~80–90% of MS patients [23–24]. Since DNase abzymes of MS patients [4] similarly to SLE patients [26] are cytotoxic and induce apoptosis, they can play an important role in SLE and MS pathogenesis.

It has been recently shown that MBP-hydrolyzing activity is an intrinsic property of IgGs, IgMs, and IgAs from the sera of MS patients [27–30] and the specific sites of the neural antigen cleaved by abzymes have been established [31]. Recognition and degradation of MBP peptides by serum auto-Abs was confirmed as a novel biomarker for MS [31]. In MS, anti-MBP abzymes with

protease activity can attack MBP of the myelin-proteolipid sheath of axons. The established MS drug Copaxone appears to be a specific inhibitor of MBP-hydrolyzing activity of the abzymes [31]. Consequently, MBP-hydrolyzing abzymes may play an important negative role in MS pathogenesis. At the same time, the similarity in some immunological indexes between MS and SLE can speak in favour of that anti-MBP Abs with proteolytic activity can occur in SLE patients. Recently, it was shown that electrophoretically and immunologically homogeneous IgGs (approximately 86% of SLE patients) purified using several affinity resins including Sepharose with immobilized MBP (MBP-Sepharose) specifically hydrolyze only MBP but not many other tested proteins [9]. Several rigid criteria were applied to show that the MBP-hydrolyzing activity is an intrinsic property of SLE IgGs but not from healthy donors. It was shown, that the immune systems of individual SLE similarly to MS patients can generate a variety of anti-MBP abzymes with different proteolytic properties, which can attack MBP of myelin-proteolipid shell of axons and play an important role in pathogenesis not only MS but also SLE patients.

Anti-MBP abzymes from the sera of MS patients hydrolyze MBP at several sites localized within four known immunodominant regions of MBP [31]. In addition, it was shown that anti-MBP abzymes from the sera of SLE patients hydrolyze MBP at the same four immunodominant sites of MBP [9]. Four peptides corresponding to known immunodominant regions of MBP are encephalytogenic and can play a negative role in the MS and SLE pathogenesis [31].

Taking this into account, it was interesting to study the Ab-dependent hydrolysis of MBP specific sequences in more detail. In this paper, we have analyzed site-specific degradation of two oligopeptides (21- and 25-mer) corresponding to two AGDs of MBP using combination of reverse-phase chromatography (RPhC), thin-layer chromatography (TLC), MALDI spectrometry, affinity chromatography, and enzymic kinetics.

Results

Abzyme characterization

In this work, electrophoretically and immunologically homogeneous polyclonal IgGs (pIgGs) were purified from the sera SLE and MS patients as well as healthy donors by sequential chromatography of the serum proteins on Protein G-Sepharose under conditions that remove non-specifically bound proteins, followed by gel filtration under the conditions that destroy immune complexes as in [9]. Electrophoretical and immunological homogeneity of the pIgGs was confirmed respectively by SDS-PAGE with silver staining and by Western blotting similarly to [9,27–30]. To analyze an "average" situation, we have prepared a mixture of equal amounts of homogeneous pIgGs from the sera of ten SLE (sle-IgG$_{mix}$), ten MS (ms-IgG$_{mix}$) patients, and ten healthy donors (hd-IgG$_{mix}$). Then sle-IgG$_{mix}$, ms-IgG$_{mix}$, and hd-IgG$_{mix}$ preparations having affinity for hMBP were separated by affinity chromatography on MBP-Sepharose as in [9]. The fractions of IgG$_{mix}$ eluted from MBP-Sepharose with 3 M NaCl were used in this study. To exclude possible artefacts due to traces of contaminating proteases, these fractions were separated by SDS-PAGE and their proteolytic activity was detected after the extraction of proteins from the excised gel slices as in [9]; only sle-IgG$_{mix}$ and ms-IgG$_{mix}$ preparations were active, when hd-IgG$_{mix}$ was catalytically inactive. The detection of MBP-hydrolyzing activity of these Abs similarly to [9] in the gel region corresponding only to IgGs (150 kDa) together with the absence of any other band of the activity or protein, provided a direct evidence that all pIgG preparations used are not contaminated

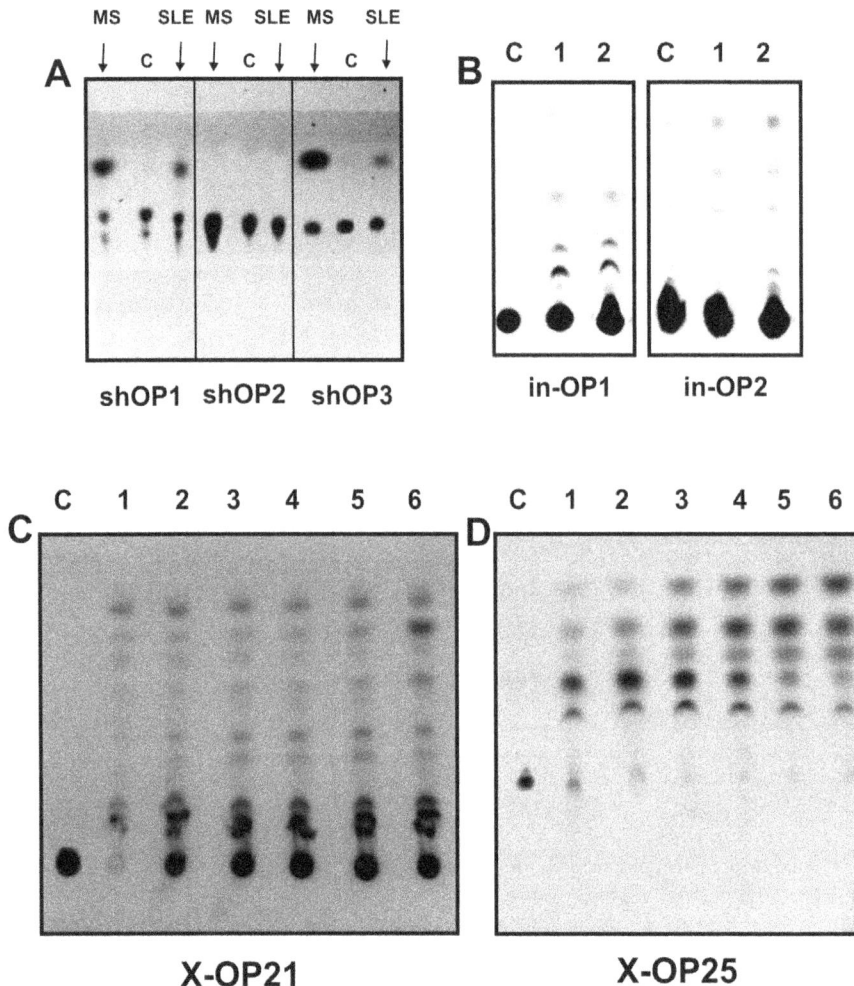

Figure 1. TLC analysis of the hydrolysis of different OPs. A, Boc-Val-Leu-Lys-MCA (shOP1), Pro-Phe-Arg-MCA (shOP2), and Boc-Ile-Glu-Gly-Arg-MCA (shOP3) (5 mM) were incubated for 24 h without Abs (lanesC) and in the presence of 0.05 mg/ml MS IgG$_{mix}$ or SLE IgG$_{mix}$ preparations (lanes shown on the panel) demonstrating comparable relative activities in the hydrolysis of intact MBP. B, Nonspecific in-OP1 and in-OP2 were incubated for 24 h without Abs (lanes 1) and in the presence of 0.05 mg/ml SLE IgG$_{mix}$ (lanes 2); lanes C correspond to in-OP1 and in-OP2 before incubation. C, Specific X-OP21 (C) and X-OP25 oligopeptides were incubated for 7 h with hd-IgG$_{mix}$ (lane C) and in the presence of 0.02 mg/ml sle-IgG$_{mix}$. These OPs were used in different concentrations (mM): 0.05 (lanes 1), 0.1 (lanes 2), 0.2 (lanes 3), 0.3 (lanes 4), 0.4 (lanes 5), and 0.5 (lanes 6).

with canonical proteases. In addition, similarly to [9] it was shown that, in contrast to canonical proteases, the SLE and MS IgG$_{mix}$ purified on MBP-Sepharose specifically hydrolyzed only MBP but not many other tested proteins.

Ab-dependent hydrolysis of oligopeptides

It was shown previously, that thyroglobulin-directed proteolytic IgGs effectively hydrolyzed not only thyroglobulin but also Pro-Phe-Arg-methylcoumarinamide (MCA) at the Arg-MCA bond with a significantly lower affinity [32]. Polyclonal IgG preparations from patients with rheumatoid arthritis also displayed Pro-Phe-Arg-MCA-hydrolyzing activity [32]. Anti-integrase IgGs and IgMs from HIV-infected patients hydrolyze not only globular HIV-1 integrase but also different specific and nonspecific tri- and tetraoligopeptides [33,34]. Therefore, first we have analyzed the efficiency of hydrolysis of nonspecific tri- and tetrapeptides using sle-IgG$_{mix}$ and ms-IgG$_{mix}$ purified by affinity chromatography on MBP-Sepharose. It was shown that anti-MBP sle-IgG$_{mix}$ and ms-IgG$_{mix}$ cannot hydrolyse short peptide Pro-Phe-Arg-MCA (sh-OP1), but after 24–48 h of the incubation they cleavage Boc-Val-

Leu-Lys-MCA (sh-OP1) and Boc-Ile-Glu-Gly-Arg-MCA (sh-OX3) with very low efficiency (Fig. 1A). The relative rate of the MCA formation was approximately 4-5- (sh-OP2) and 20-25-fold (sh-OX3) higher in the presence of ms-IgG$_{mix}$ than that for sle-IgG$_{mix}$. Similar situation was observed for longer nonspecific 20-mer oligopeptides in-OP1 and in-OP2 (Fig 1B) corresponding to viral integrase, that, as revealed by a MALDI analysis, contain several sites of IN cleavage in the case of anti-IN IgGs from HIV-infected patients [33,34]. Nonspecific in-OP1 and in-OP2 oligopeptides corresponding to HIV integrase were slightly hydrolyzed nonspecifically after 24 of the incubation, but there was no detectable difference in the fluorescence intensities of the spots after the incubation of these OPs without (lanes 2) and with sle-IgG$_{mix}$ (lanes 3) (Fig. 1B). Consequently, if sle-IgG$_{mix}$ can hydrolyze nonspecific in-OP1 and in-OP2, this hydrolysis is a very negligible.

First, we have shown that all ten individual SLE IgG preparations before purification on MBP-Sepharose produced, according to TLC, the same products of specific (corresponding to MBP) X-OP21 and X-OP25 oligopeptides cleavage, but every preparation was characterized by a specific ratio of formation of

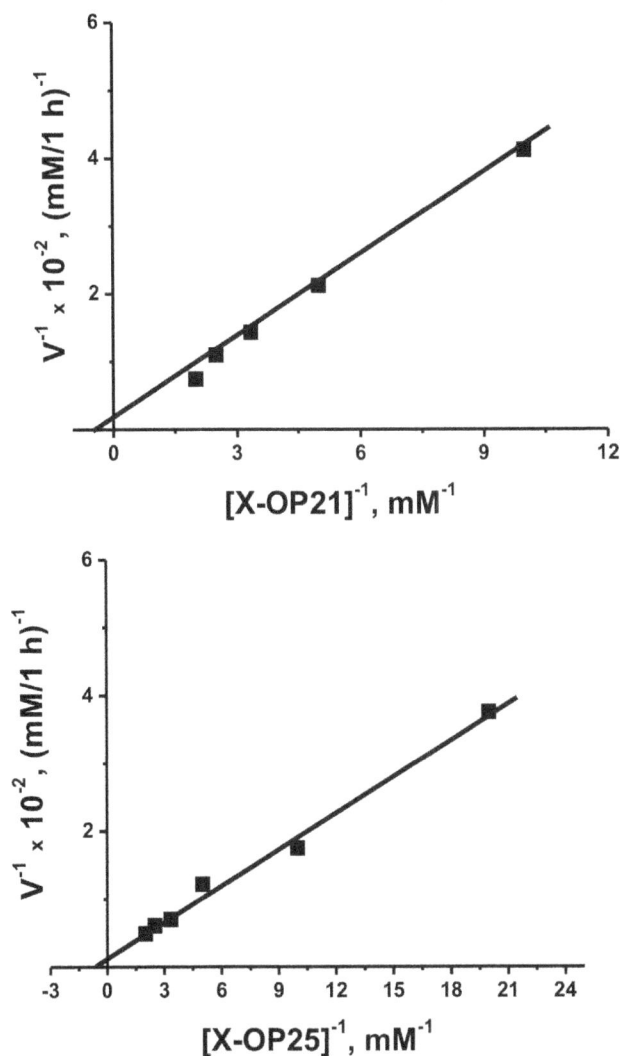

Figure 2. Determination of the K_m and V_{max} values for OP21 (A) and OP25 (B) in the reaction catalyzed by sle-IgG$_{mix}$ (0.1 μM) using a Lineweaver–Burk plot. The reactions were performed as described in Materials and Methods. The average error in the initial rate determination from two experiments for each substrate concentration did not exceed 7–10%.

different cleavage products. In addition, using TLC it was shown when sle-IgG$_{mix}$ and ms-IgG$_{mix}$ after purification on MBP-Sepharose produce the same X-OP hydrolysis products, but at remarkably different ratios. To analyze in more detail an "average" situation concerning hydrolysis of X-OP21 and X-OP25 by SLE anti-MBP IgGs we have used sle-IgG$_{mix}$; Figs 1C and 1D demonstrate efficient hydrolysis of these specific encephalytogenic OPs by sle-IgG$_{mix}$.

Thus, anti-MBP IgGs from SLE patients can efficiently hydrolyze not only globular molecules of MBP (not many other tested proteins) [9], but also specific OPs corresponding to AGDs of MBP. Interestingly, sle-IgG$_{mix}$-dependent proteolysis of both specific OP21 and OP25 leads to the formation of several products corresponding to 5-10 fluorescent spots (Fig. 1).

The dependency of the initial rate on the X-OP21 and X-OP25 concentrations in the reaction catalyzed by sle-IgG$_{mix}$ was consistent with Michaelis–Menten kinetics (for example, Fig. 2). The K_m and apparent k_{cat} values for X-OP21 (2.8±0.3 mM;

1.1±0.1min^{-1}) and X-OP25 (1.6±0.2 mM; 1.4±0.2 min^{-1}) were estimated.

MALDI spectrometry analysis of specific peptides hydrolysis

Fig. 1 demonstrates that hydrolysis of specific X-OP21 and X-OP25 by anti-MBP sle-IgG$_{mix}$ produces several fluorescent oligopeptides, the relative amounts of which increase with the increase in the concentration of these OPs. TLC alone cannot unambiguously determine the sequences of these products, since their TLC mobility depends on many factors including the amino acid content, relative hydrophobicity, the nature of the terminal amino acids, etc. To identify major sites of IgG-mediated proteolysis of these OPs, we analyzed products of peptide cleavage by a combination of RPhC, TLC, and MALDI massspectrometry.

First, we have analyzed the products of nearly complete X-OP21 hydrolysis after 7 h of incubation (Fig. 3). Seven major and several very small peaks corresponding to fluorescent products of X-OP21 hydrolysis were revealed by RPhC (Fig. 3A). The products of all peaks were analyzed by TLC (Fig. 3B) and by massspectrometry (Figs 3C and 3D). One can see that only the 4th and 7th RPhC peaks according to TLC contain a single predominant product of the hydrolysis. According to TLC and massspectrometry major peak 2 contains seven products of the cleavage (n = 6, 7, 8, 9, 10, 12, and 13) and initial non-cleaved X-OP21 having comparable affinity to RPhC-resin (Fig. 3A), but different mobility at TLC (Fig. 3B). Badly separated 4th and 5th peaks (Fig. 3A) contained mainly 4- and 5-mers (Fig. 3D), while 7th peak 2- and 3-mer X-OPs.

Fig. 4A demonstrates the data of RPhC of the cleavage products corresponding to X-OP21 after its complete hydrolysis (12 h). In this case there was observed only four major and many very small peaks. According to TLC (Fig. 4B, lane 2) and massspectrometry (Fig. 4C), peak 2 contained mainly three products: 6-, 7-, and 8-mer X-OPs. Peak 3 corresponded to 4-mer (Fig. 4D), while 4th peak to 2-mer X-OP (Fig. 4E). Thus, long products of the hydrolysis finally can be hydrolyzed by SLE-Abs to short X-dimer and X-tetramer. In addition, after a long incubation small amount of a free X-fluorescent compound and X-monomer were revealed (peak 1, Figs 4A and 4B) using TLC and massspectrometry. It should be mentioned that massspectrometry analysis of products of X-OP21 hydrolysis after 3 h of incubation has shown that three OPs with low TLC mobility (Fig. 1C) correspond to 10-, 12-, and 13-mer X-OPs.

Nine brightly expressed and several additional very small peaks corresponding to fluorescent products of X-OP25 medium hydrolysis were revealed by RPhC (Fig. 5A). After RPhC the same products of the hydrolysis were identified by TLC and by massspectrometry in several peaks (Fig. 5). It means that some individual products of X-OP25 hydrolysis can be eluted from the sorbent by different concentrations of acetonitrile. The reaction mixture contains Tris-HCl and trifluoroacetic acid, which components can interact with positively and negatively charged amino acid residues of products of the X-OP25 hydrolysis. In addition, one cannot exclude that some of OPs can form interpeptide complexes. An existence of multiple forms of the X-OP products can lead to the elution of these forms of the same X-OPs from the sorbent by different concentration of acetonitrile.

Using the combination of RPhC, TLC, and MALDI-TOF analysis of the products of the X-OP25 hydrolysis were identified. For example, the highest peak 4 according to TLC (Fig 5B, lane 4) and massspectrometry (Fig. 5C) contained several X-OPs: 5-mer>>25-mer>3-mer≥2-mer≥1-mer≥4-mer>8-mer. PanelD demonstrates the spectrum of initial X-OP25 and the signals of

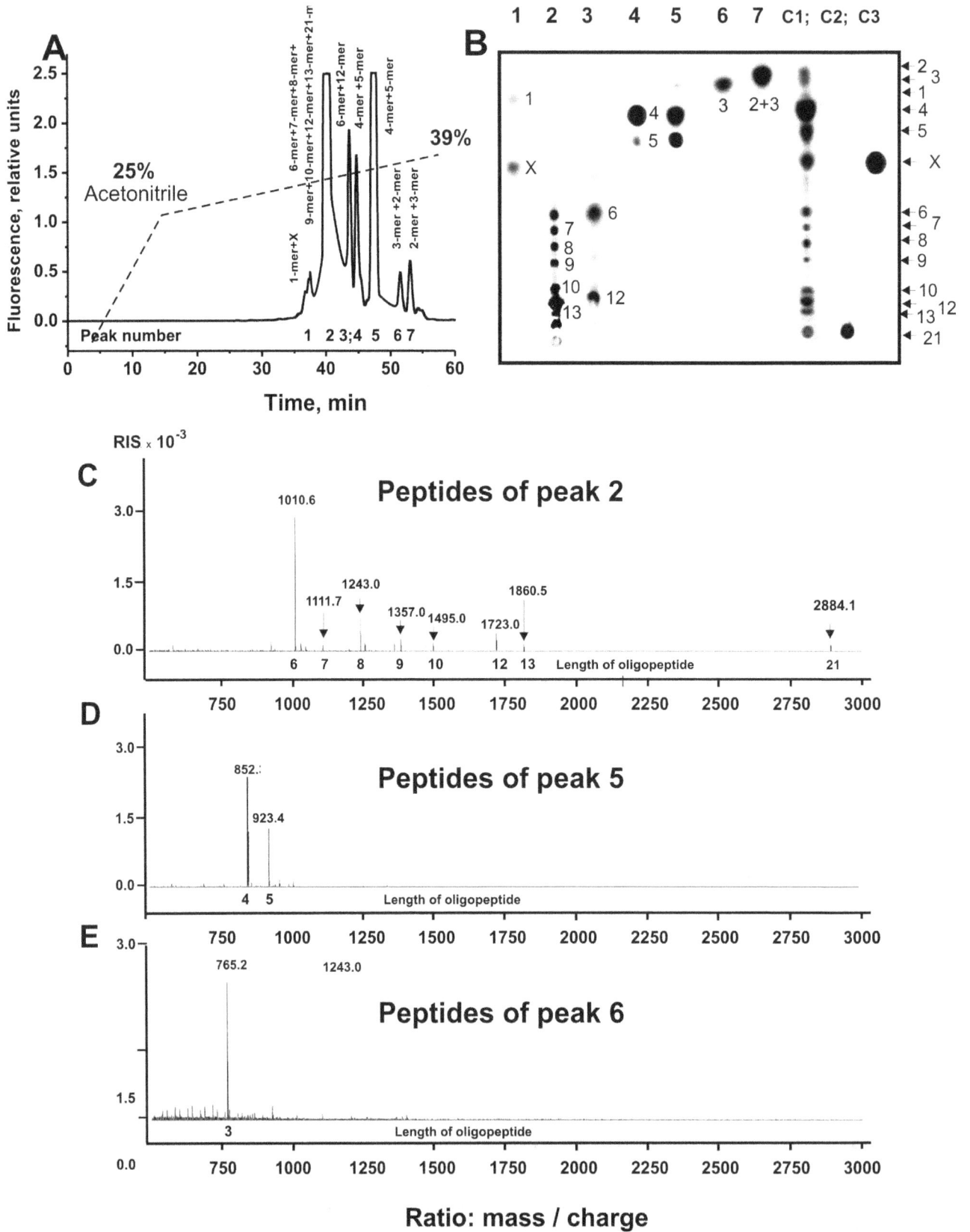

Figure 3. Profile of RPhC of SLE IgG$_{mix}$-dependent products of X-OP21 relatively deep hydrolysis (A) and analysis of X-OP products of the hydrolysis corresponding to different peaks after RPhC by TLC (B) or massspectrometry (C–E): (–), relative fluorescence (A).
Numbers of lines in panel B coincide with numbers of peaks on panel A; lanes C1, C2, and C3 correspond to the products of reaction mixture before their separation by RPhC, X-OP25 incubated in the absence of IgGs, and a free fluorescent compound X, respectively. The arrows (and numerals on

panel B) indicate the positions of OPs of different length and compound X. Panels C, D, and E demonstrate the MALDI spectrum signals corresponding to the products eluted under RPhC in peaks 2, 5 and 6, respectively. See Materials and Methods for other details.

peptides corresponding to major OPs of peak 9. The signals of all products of X-OP25 hydrolysis before their separation by RPhC are given on panel E. It was shown that at the beginning of the reaction (1-3 h of the incubation) 18-mer OP is a major product of the X-OP25 cleavage, while the formation of long products containing 8, 9, 12, and 21 amino acid residues occurs with significantly lower rate.

As it was shown above, the relative content of different length X-OPs in the final reaction mixtures depend upon concentrations of X-OP21, X-OP25 (Fig. 1), and IgGs as well as time of the incubation. An approximate relative content of different products of in the final reaction mixtures was estimated taking into account a relative total fluorescence of the spots with different mobility after TLC (Figs 3B and 5B). The data for X-OP21 is given in Table 1. Since several products of different length in the case of X-OP25 demonstrated comparable mobility and were badly separated (Fig. 5B), their relative content was estimated approximately as a sum of several products (Table 2).

Discussion

Autoantibody-mediated tissue destruction is among the main features of organ-specific autoimmunity. It was recently shown that, anti-MBP IgGs from the sera of patients with MS [27–31] and SLE [9] efficiently hydrolyze globular MBP but not many other tested proteins. No activity was found for IgG fraction of healthy donors in the hydrolysis of MBP or different OPs (Fig. 1) [27–31]. The sites of MBP cleavage by MS IgGs determined by mass spectrometry were localized within four known immunodominant regions of MBP [31]. SLE IgGs hydrolyzed MBP within the same immunodominant regions of MBP [9]. It should be mentioned that for the identification of these sites only the largest peptides generated by Ab-dependent hydrolysis of intact MBP after short times of the incubation were used [31]. At the same time, we have seen that long incubation of MBP with MS and SLE IgGs (48–72 h), especially with abzymes possessing high proteolytic activity, led to the formation of short and very short fragments. Similar situation was observed for anti-IN abzymes from HIV-infected patients in the hydrolysis of viral integrase [33,34]. It means that the total pools of various IgGs can contain different subfractions of anti-protein abzymes, which are capable to hydrolyze a target protein in many sites but with different rates. Theoretically, a mammalian immune system can produce up to 10^6 variants of Abs against a single antigen including abzymes and various Abzs can be different in their specificity toward their substrates. To understand possible general features of production and mechanisms of the action of different monoclonal abzymes in the total IgG pool leading finally to the formation of short OPs only, it was interesting and useful to analyze not only the major cleavage sites but also various minor ones.

In the case of MS IgGs, the major sites of Ab-dependent cleavage of globular MBP within the sequences corresponding to OP21 and OP25 were identified earlier [31]; they are shown on Fig. 6B and 6E. Interestingly, one cleavage site of OP21 coincides with one of two possible trypsin-dependent sites of this OP hydrolysis (Fig. 6A). In the case of OP25 there are five potential sites of its hydrolysis by trypsin (Fig. D), but globular MBP was digested by MS IgGs only at one of these sites (Fig. 6E) [31].

In this article for a more exact identification of the major and minor sites of the MBP cleavage by SLE IgGs we have used

several nonspecific and two specific OPs corresponding to two cleavage sequences of MBP (X-OP21 and X-OP25; Fig. 6). It was shown, that anti-MBP sle-IgG$_{mix}$ hydrolyze efficiently only specific X-OP21 and X-OP25, while cannot efficiently hydrolyze different nonspecific short and long OPs. To identify major sites of abzyme-dependent proteolysis of X-OP21 and X-OP25, we analyzed these peptide cleavage products by a combination of RPhC, TLC, and MALDI spectrometry. Using conditions of a deep Ab-dependent degradation of these OPs several major and minor cleavage sites were identified (Figs 6C and 6F).

As one can see from Fig. 1, the relative amounts of different products of X-OP21 and X-OP25 cleavage significantly depend upon the concentration of these OPs. We have estimated the relative amount of the products after a medium (for example, Fig. 1C) and deep hydrolysis of OPs hydrolysis (Figs 3 and 5; Tables 1 and 2). It should be mentioned, that at the beginning of the X-OP21 cleavage reaction (1-3 h of the incubation) three fluorescent spots corresponding to three OPs (X-OP12> XOP13≥X-OP10) were revealed (Fig. 1C). Overall, in the case of hydrolysis of X-OP21 five major sites of cleavage corresponding to 4-, 5-, 10-, 12-, and 13-mer X-OPs were identified (Fig. 6C). In addition, a remarkable accumulation of the free fluorescent X-compound was observed. The rate of X-OP21 cleavage leading to a formation of 6-mer and 8-mer X-OPs was significantly lower. The relative content of 1-, 2-, 3-, 7-, and 9-mer X-OPs did not exceed 1–3% (Table 1).

§The relative content of different products after a medium hydrolysis of X-OP25 was performed taking into account the data of TLC analysis (Fig. 5B); a range of the values from three repeats is given.

Three major sites of cleavage (10-, 12-, and 13-mer X-OPs) are localized in one cluster. One of them (12 -mer OP, cleavage of R-H bond) coincides with the cleavage site identified recently for 21-mer sequence of intact MBP (it coincides with trypsin-dependent site) in the case of IgGs from MS patients (Fig. 6B; [31]), while two other were new sites. After short time of the incubation in parallel with the formation of long OPs several shorter X-OPs was observed (Fig. 1C). Deeper incomplete hydrolysis of X-OP21 (7 h) results in the degradation of long 10-18-mer X-OPs and the formation of several additional products of the cleavage including major OPs: 4-mer>5-mer>8-mer (Fig. 3B, Table 1). After practically complete hydrolysis of the initial X-OP21 the reaction mixture contained only six products of the cleavage: 4-mer>2-mer>7-mer>6 mer≥8-mer X-OPs (Fig. 4B). Taken together, one can say that cleavage sites corresponding to the formation of 13-mer, 10-mer, 5-mer and especially 12-mer and 4-mer X-OPs may be considered as major sites of the cleavage. Several sites correspond to a remarkably lower efficiency of the hydrolysis (6- and 8-mer OPs), and finally there are several sites of very low rate of the hydrolysis (1-, 2, 3,-7,-, 9-mer X-OPs). All sites of IgG-dependent hydrolysis of X-OP21 are shown on Fig. 6C. Interestingly, eight amino acid residues of YLASASTM sequence correspond to a specific cluster of seven sites of very weak, medium and strong cleavage (Fig. 6C).

Similar situation was observed for X-OP25. After 3 h of the hydrolysis of X-OP25 a fast formation of 5-mer, 4-mer, and 18-mer OPs was observed. After a deep hydrolysis the same 5-, 4-, and 18-mer OPs were major products (Fig. 5B, Table 2). Taken together, only three sites of X-OP25 may be considered as major (5-, 4-, and 18-mer OPs), while other sites correspond to a

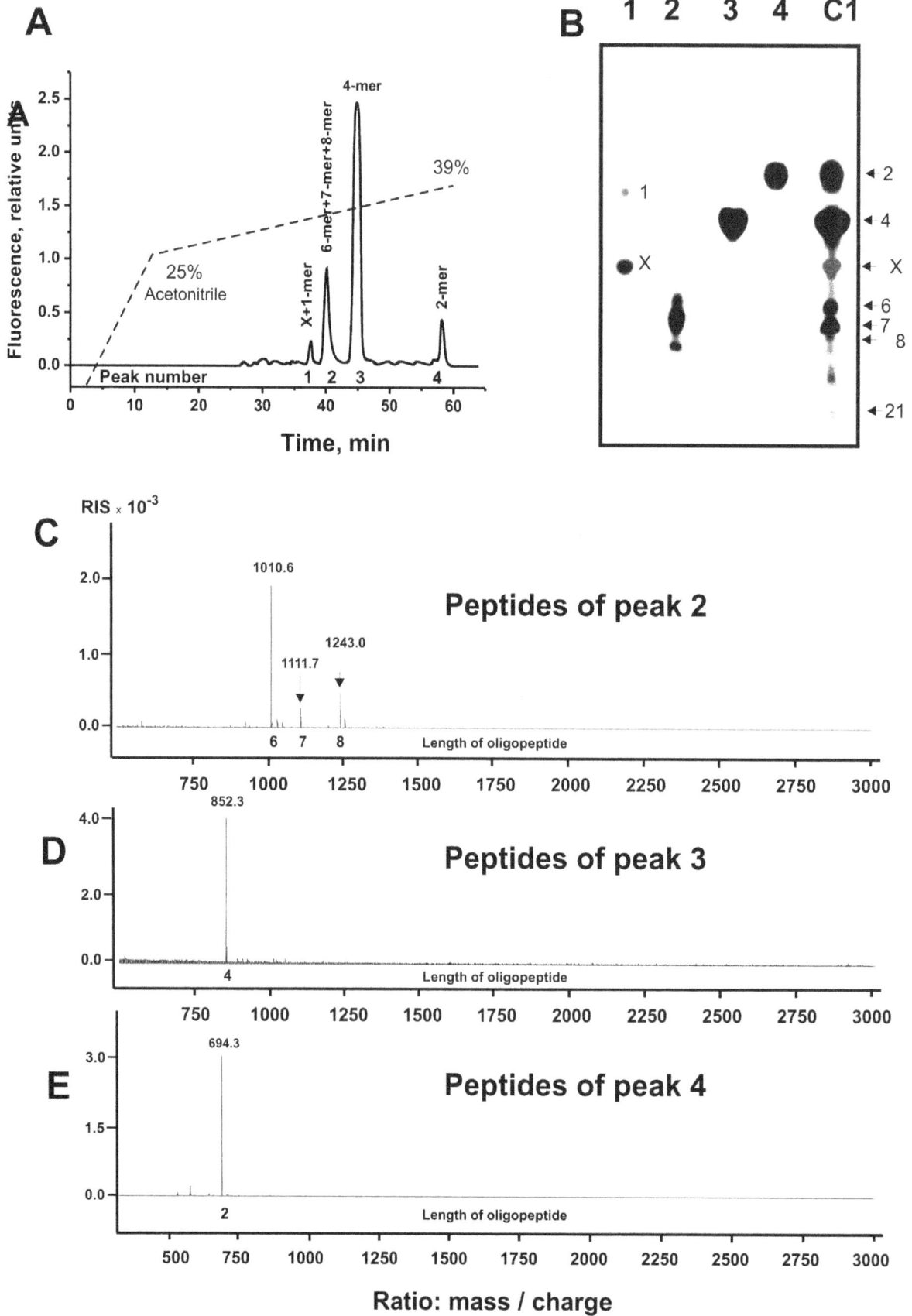

Figure 4. Profile of RPhC of sle-IgG$_{mix}$-dependent products of a complete hydrolysis of X-OP21 (A) and analysis of the products corresponding to different peaks after RPhC by TLC (B) or massspectrometry (C–E): (–), relative fluorescence (A). Numbers of lines in panel B coincide with numbers of peaks on panel A; lane C1 corresponds to the products of reaction mixture before their separation by RPhC. The arrows (and numerals on panel B) indicate the positions of OPs of different length and compound X. Panels C, D, and E demonstrate the MALDI spectra corresponding to the products of the hydrolysis eluted under RPhC in peaks 2, 3, and 4, respectively (Fig. 4A). See Materials and Methods for other details.

moderate of a low efficiency of the X-OP25 digestion (Fig 6F). Only one cleavage site of intact globular MBP in the case of MS IgGs was determined and it corresponds to the formation of 10-mer OPs and coincides with trypsin-dependent site (Fig. 6E). However, we did not find X-OP10 among products of X-OP25 cleavage by SLE anti-MBP IgGs; a remarkable digestion was observed at three neighboring sites (8-, 9- and 12-mer OPs) (Fig. 6F, Table 2). The 10-mer sequence AQGTLSKIFK contains eight clustered sites of the cleavage (Fig. 6D).

The first question is why in the case of SLE anti-MBP IgGs there are more major cleavage sites of sequences corresponding to X-OP21 and X-OP25 than those for MS abzymes in the case of intact MBP as substrate. It was recently shown that incubation of many individual IgGs with iodoacetamide (a specific inhibitor of thiol proteases) or pepstatin A (a specific inhibitor of acidic proteases) has moderate effect (5-15%) on SLE Ab-dependent hydrolysis of MBP [9]; the same was demonstrated for MS IgGs, IgAs and IgMs [27-31]. However, PMSF, AEBSF (specific inhibitors of serine proteases), and EDTA (an inhibitor of metalloproteases) significantly suppressed the proteolytic activity of SLE and MS pIgGs in the case of MBP and OPs as substrates [9]. In contrast to MS IgGs, abzymes from SLE patients are more sensitive to EDTA like canonical metalloproteases and less sensitive to specific inhibitors of serine-like proteases [9]. The cleavage sites of Me^{2+}- dependent fractions of the total pool of SLE anti-MBP abzymes may be different from those of serine-like proteolytic IgG fraction dominating in the sera of MS patients.

Then, for the revealing of the SLE Ab-dependent cleavage sites we have used X-OPs, while the cleavage sites in the case of MS IgGs were identified using digestion of intact globular MBP [31]. In this connection it should be mentioned, that catalytic centers of proteolytic abzymes (including MS and SLE anti-MBP IgGs [9,27]) are usually located on the light chain, while the heavy chain is more often responsible for specific antigen recognition and increased antigen affinity for Abs [1-8]. Intact proteins usually interact with both light and heavy chains of abzymes, thus ensuring the specificity of the target protein recognition and its cleavage. Specific binding of globular protein with the heavy chains of abzymes can determine what fragment of protein sequences may be localized in the active centers of the light chains. At the same time, short oligopeptides may interact mostly with the light chain, which possesses a lower affinity for substrates. For example, the affinity of SLE pIgGs for hMBP ($K_m = 0.6$–2.7 μM [9]) is comparable with that for MS IgGs ($K_m = 0.9$–5.0 μM [30]) and corresponds to the typical affinity of abzymes for different protein antigens ($K_m = 0.038$–30 μM) [1–8]. At the same time, the affinity of SLE anti-MBP IgGs for X-OP21 and X-OP25 ($K_m = 1.6$–2.8 mM; Fig. 2) approximately three orders of magnitude lower that to MBP. Therefore depending on the sequence, IgG-dependent hydrolysis of OPs may in principle be less specific or completely nonspecific in comparison with intact globular MBP.

The second question is whether the minor sites of OPs cleavage have any biological significance. In this connection it should be mentioned that sle-IgG$_{mix}$ cannot effectively hydrolyze short nonspecific tri- or tetrapeptides and long OPs (Fig. 1). In addition,

between products of the hydrolysis of X-OP21 and X-OP25 there is only a limited number of shorter X-OPs, which do not cover all possible sites of these OPs digestion. Notably, light chains of IgGs from patients with different diseases can hydrolyze not only intact specific protein substrates, but also different tri- and tetrapeptides demonstrating significantly lower affinities; the K_m for Pro-Phe-Arg-MCA were determined in the case of IgGs from Hashimoto thyroiditis (18 μM, $k_{cat} = 6.3 \times 10^{-2}$ min^{-1} [35]). The affinity (K_m) of these very short OPs for intact IgGs and for monoclonal light chains corresponding to Abs against different proteins are to some extent comparable: anti-VIP (0.012 mM, $k_{cat} = 6.8 \times 10^{-3}$ min^{-1} [36]), anti-prothrombin abzymes (0.1 mM, $k_{cat} = 2.6 \times 10^{-2}$ min^{-1} [37]), proteolytic Bence Jones proteins (different MCA-peptides; 0.015–0.29 mM, $k_{cat} = (2.1$–$9) \times 10^{-2}$ min^{-1} [38]). These data support the hypothesis that all short peptides interact mainly with light chains of intact Abs.

It was shown that anti-integrase IgGs from HIV-infected patients efficiently hydrolyze specific 17-20-mer peptides corresponding to AGDs of viral integrase, nonspecific tri- and tetrapeptides, and 17-25-mer nonspecific OPs of human myelin basic protein AGDs, suggesting poor discriminatory properties of the sites for substrate binding and hydrolysis located on the light chains of anti-IN IgGs from HIV-infected patients [33]. Taken together, all data support the hypothesis that short peptides can interact directly with the light chains of intact Abs.

Protein-binding sites of light chains of SLE anti-MBP IgGs are much more selective, but these abzymes also can with very low efficiency hydrolyzed short nonspecific MCA-peptides. Therefore, one cannot exclude that the observed multiple sites of the hydrolysis of specific OPs at some sites may be to some extent nonspecific. However, using MALDI mass spectrometry we have recently identified 40sites of integrase cleavage by anti-IN IgGs from HIV infected patients [33], which are localized within seven known immunodominant regions of IN. Interestingly, all these cleavage sites were clustered within the AGDs. For example, three clusters of cleavage sites were located within the long AGD3. A block of 12 closely spaced cleavage sites corresponded to the N-terminal part of AGD4. Similar situation was observed in the case of X-OP21 and X-OP25 degradation by SLE IgGs; several sites of the major and minor cleavage are clustered (Fig. 6).

On one hand, it cannot be excluded that the digestion of the X-OP21 and X-OP25 at different sites is catalyzed by different monoclonal Abzs present in the total pool of polyclonal anti-MBP abzymes. Depending on their affinity, specificity, and relative activity, different monoclonal abzymes may participate at different stages of MBP degradation; faster cleavage may lead to the formation of several major products, while significantly slower cleavage, to the minor ones. However, it is possible that single abzymes can cleave MBP at multiple sites in a sequential series of cleavage reactions. For example, several different monoclonal light chains (corresponding to SLE) obtained using phage display specifically hydrolyze only myelin basic protein, but are very different in their site specificity (A. M. Bezuglova and G. A. Nevinsky, personal communication). Some monoclonal light chains efficiently hydrolyze only OPs corresponding to one of four known AGDs of MBP. However, we have found monoclonal

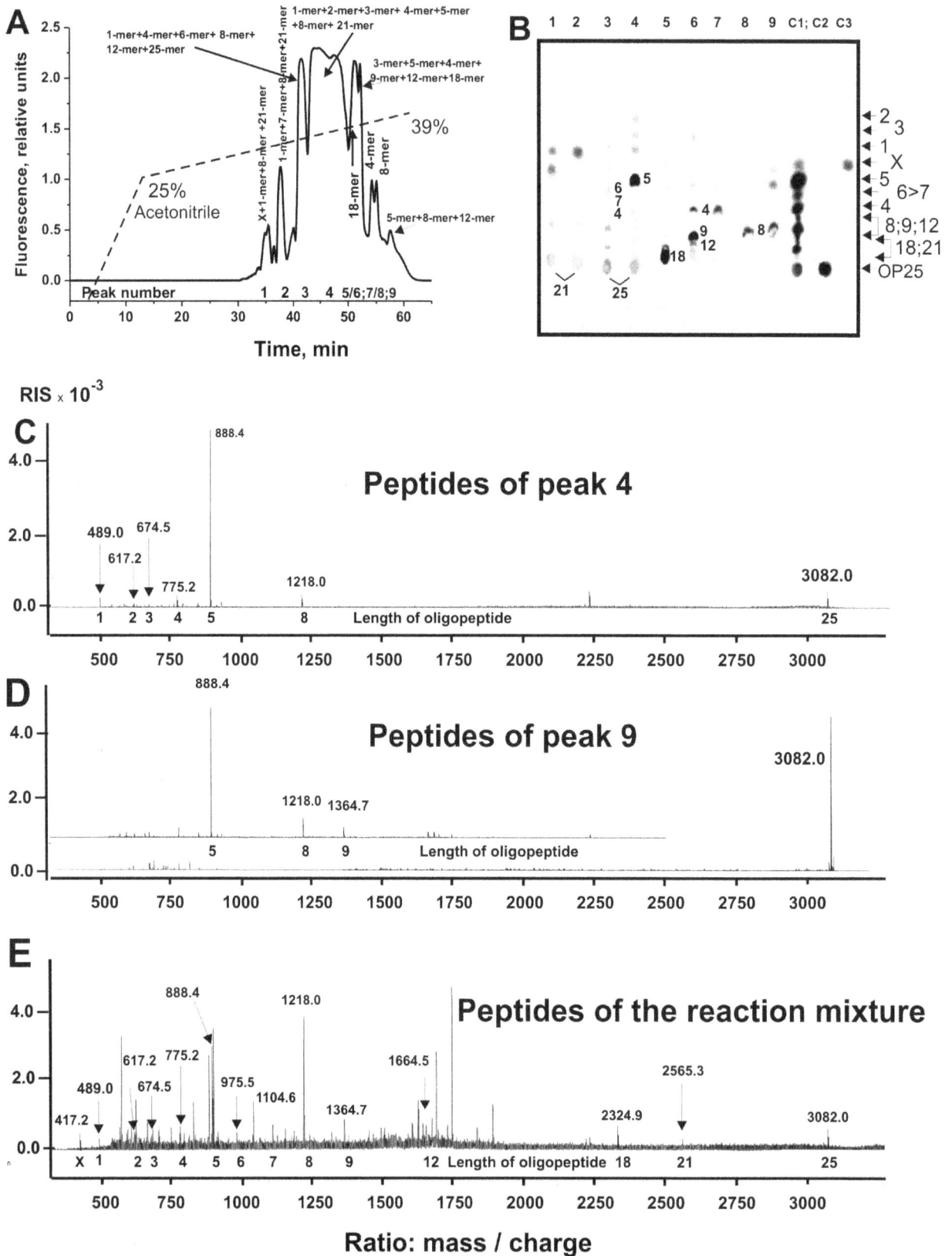

Figure 5. Profile of RPhC of sle-IgG$_{mix}$-dependent products of X-OP25 relatively deep hydrolysis (A) and analysis of the products of the hydrolysis corresponding to different peaks after RPhC by TLC (B) or massspectrometry (C–E): (–), relative fluorescence (A). Numbers of lines in panel **B** coincide with numbers of peaks on panel **A**; lanes C1, C2 and C3 correspond to the products of reaction mixture before their separation by RPhC, X-OP25 incubated in the absence of IgGs, and a free fluorescent compound X, respectively. The arrows (and numerals on panel **B**) indicate the positions of OPs of different length and compound X. Panel **C** demonstrates the MALDI spectrum of the products

corresponding to peak 4, while panel D to peak 9 (Fig. 5A) and the intact X-OP25 before its hydrolysis, respectively. MALDI spectrum of all products of X-OP25 hydrolysis after 24 h of its incubation corresponding to non-fractionated reaction mixture is given on panel **E**. The length of the X-OPs is given on the bottom. See Materials and Methods for other details.

light chain preparations hydrolyzing OPs corresponding to two, three and even four AGDs of MBP with comparable rates. The deep hydrolysis of intact MBP led to the formation of many short peptides. Thus, one cannot exclude that monoclonal anti-MBP abzymes in the total Ab pool can also be significantly different in their site specificity. Altogether, it seems reasonable to suggest that the observed multiplicity of the specific OPs cleavage sites may be explained both by differences in the site specificity of many monoclonal abzymes and by the existence of single abzymes possessing low site specificity in the MBP hydrolysis.

In addition, the sera of MS and SLE patients are characterized by increased concentration of free light chains of IgGs [39]. Therefore, one can not exclude that free light chains can also be important for the hydrolysis of MBP at minor sites of cleavage.

Taken together, we have shown for the first time an enormous multiplicity of MBP cleavage sites for abzymes from patients with SLE.

Materials and Methods

Chemicals, donors, and patients

Human MBP was from the Department of Biotechnology, Research Center of Molecular Diagnostics and Therapy (Moscow); all other chemicals including Protein G-Sepharose were from Sigma or Pharmacia. MBP-Sepharose was prepared by immobilizing human MBP on BrCN-activated Sepharose according to the standard manufacturer's protocol. Sera of 14 patients (27–60 yr old; men and women) with clinically definite SLE were used to study proteolytic abzymes. The SLE diagnosis was confirmed and its reliability was checked according to the criteria developed by the American Rheumatoid Association. For comparison we have used the sera of 10 healthy donors and of 12 patients (16–55 yr old; men and women) with clinically definite MS according to the Poser criteria [16]. The blood sampling protocol conformed to the local human ethics committee guidelines (Ethics committee of Novosibirsk State Medical University, Novosibirsk, Russia; Institutional ethics committee specifically approved this study) including written consent of patients and healthy donors to present of their blood for scientific purposes in accordance with Helsinki ethics committee guidelines.

Antibody purification and analysis

Electrophoretically and immunologically homogeneous pIgGs from healthy volunteers, SLE, and MS patients were prepared by sequential affinity chromatography of the serum proteins on protein G-Sepharose and FPLC gel filtration on a Superdex 200 HR 10/30 column as in [9]. SDS-PAGE analysis of Abs for homogeneity was performed in 12% or 4–15% gradient gels (0.1%

Table 1. The data of RPhC, TLC, and MALDI analysis of molecular masses of fluorescent oligopeptides forming after incubation of X-OP21 with sle-IgG$_{mix}$.

Num-ber of AA	Sites of cleavage of X-OP21 (OPs found by massspectrometry in the reaction mixture and peaks after RPhC)	Mol. mass, Da (ratio mass/charge, H$^+$-form)		Peak number after RPhC (Fig. 3A)	Lane number after TLC, (Fig. 3B)	Relative content at a incomplete hydrolysis of OP,%§
		Calculated	Experimental			
0	X*	417	416.75	1;C1**	1***	8-11 **
1	X- Y	58.94	581.0	1;C1	1	≤1.0
2	X- YL	694.1	694.3	6(7);C1	7(6)	1–2
3	X- YLA	765.17	765.2	6(7);C1	6(7)	2–3
4	X- YLAS	852.25	852.4	4(5);C1	4(5)	33–37
5	X- YLASA	923.33	923.4	5(4);C1	5(4)	11–15
6	X- YLASAS	1011.5	1010.6	2(3);C1	2(3)	3–6
7	X- YLASAST	1111.51	1112.7	2(4);C1	2	2–3
8	X- YLASASTM	1242.71	1243.0	2;C1	2	5–6
9	X- YLASASTMD	1356.79	1357.0	2;C1	2	1–2
10	X- YLASASTMDH	1494.43	1495.0	2;C1	2	3–4
12	X- YLASASTMDHAR	1722.7	1723.0	2(3);C1	2(3)	7–11
13	X- YLASASTMDHARH	1860.34	1860.5	2;C1	2	3–4
21	YLASASTMDHARHGFLPRRHR	2884.07	2884.1	2;C1	2	4–5

*Free fluorescent compound; all analyzed OPs contained fluorescent X-component.
**The same products of the hydrolysis separated by RPhC (Fig. 3A) were revealed in several peaks by MALDI spectrometry; the main peaks are marked in bold, while additional peaks containing low amount of the same OPs are shown in parentheses. C1 reflects the presence of signal corresponding to the analyzed product in spectrum of total reaction mixture.
***The same several products of the hydrolysis corresponding to each peak after RPhC (Fig. 3A) were revealed not only by MALDI spectrometry, but also by TLC (Fig. 3B).
§The relative content of different products after incomplete hydrolysis of X-OP21 was performed taking into account the data of TLC analysis (Fig. 3B); a range of the values from three repeats is given.

Sequence of human MBP

AAQKRPSQRSKH**YLASASTMDHARHGFLPR**RDTGILDS

LGRFFGSDRGAPKRGSGKDGHHAARTTHYGSLPQKAQ

GHRPQDENPVVHFFKNIVTPRTPPPSQGKGRGLS

LSRFSWGAEGQKPGFGYGGRASDYKSAHKGLKGH

D**AQGTLSKIFKLGGRDSRSGSPMARR**

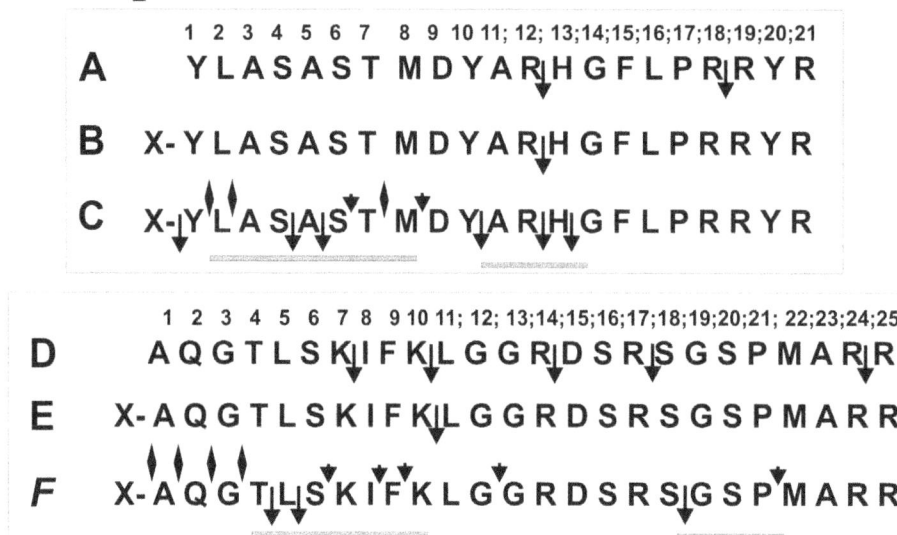

Figure 6. Complete sequence of human MBP (on the top) and all sites of cleavage of X-OP21 (C) and X-OP25 (F) determined using a combination of RPhC, TLC, and massspectrometry of detectable major and minor products of these OPs hydrolysis by sle-IgG$_{mix}$. The positions of OP21 and OP25 sequences in the human MBP sequence are shown in bold. Panels **A** and **D** show all possible sites of these OPs cleavage by trypsin, while panels **B** and **E** demonstrate the major cleavage sites of MBP, which were found previously in the case of hydrolysis of globular intact MBP by MS IgGs [31]. All sites corresponding to major and moderate products of the cleavage are shown by long and short arrows respectively, while to minor ones by diamonds (panels **C** and **F**).

SDS); the polypeptides were visualized by silver and Coomassie R250 staining [9].

We have prepared three mixtures of equal amounts of homogeneous IgGs from the sera of ten SLE (sle-IgG$_{mix}$), ten MS (ms-IgG$_{mix}$) patients, and ten healthy donors (hd-IgG$_{mix}$). The sle-IgG$_{mix}$, ms-IgG$_{mix}$, and hd-IgG$_{mix}$ preparations were chromatographed on Sepharose bearing immobilized MBP similarly to [9]. The column (3 ml; 0.7 mg MBP per ml of Sepharose) was equilibrated with 50 mM Tris-HCl (pH 7.5) containing 50 mM NaCl; the protein was applied, and the column was washed with the same buffer to zero optical density. IgGs were eluted from MBP-Sepharose with the same buffer containing different concentrations of NaCl (0.1–3 M) and then with 2–3 M MgCl$_2$. Fractions after chromatography were dialyzed against 50 mM Tris-HCl (pH 7.5) containing 50 mM NaCl and concentrated using Amicon-50. All 5 major fractions of sle-IgG$_{mix}$ and ms-IgG$_{mix}$ eluted from MBP-Sepharose with different concentrations of NaCl (0.1–3.0 M) and MgCl$_2$ (2–3 M) were active, while fractions of hd-IgG$_{mix}$ preparation were inactive in the hydrolysis of MBP. In order to protect the Ab preparations from bacterial contamination IgGs after all stages of purification were sterilized by filtration through a Millex filter (pore size 0.2 µm). In this study

we have used sle-IgG$_{mix}$ and ms-IgG$_{mix}$ fractions eluted from MBP-Sepharose with 3 M NaCl demonstrating comparable activities in the hydrolysis of intact MBP. These fractions of Abs were marked in the following text as sle-IgG$_{mix}$ and ms-IgG$_{mix}$.

Ab proteolytic activity assay

The reaction mixture (10–100 µl) for analysis of OP-hydrolyzing activity of IgGs containing 20 mM Tris-HCl (pH 7.5), 3 mM NaCl, 0.05–1.0 mM one of two specific or various nonspecific OPs, and 0.001–0.02 mg/ml of IgGs (purified on BMP-Sepharose), was incubated for 1–24 h at 30°C. Specific X-OP21 (X-YLASASTMDHARHGFLPRRHR) and X-OP25 (X-AQGTLS-KIFKLGGRDSRSGSPMARR) corresponding to two of four known IgG-dependent specific cleavage sites of hMBP [31] were used. In the case of X-OP21 only 18 N-terminal residues correspond to the antigenic determinant; this OP contains three additional C-terminal amino acid residues. As controls, we have used OPs corresponding to specific cleavage sites of two known AGDs of HIV-1 integrase, which were identified in the case of abzymes from HIV-infected patients: 20-mer X-EHEKYHSN-WRAMASDFNLPP (in-OP1) and 20-mer X-VESMNKELK-

Table 2. The data of RPhC, TLC, and MALDI analysis of molecular masses of fluorescent ligopeptides forming after incubation of X-OP25 with sle-IgG$_{mix}$.

Num-ber of AA	Sites of cleavage of X-OP25 (OPs found by massspectrometry in the reaction mixture and peaks after RPhC)	Mol. mass, Da (ratio mass/charge, H$^+$-form)		Peak number after RPhC (Fig. 5A)	Lane number after TLC, (Fig. 5B)	Relative content of different products after a medium hydrolysis of X-OP25,%§
		Calculated	Experimental			
0	X*	417.0	417.2	1;C1**	1***	≤1
1	X- A	488.84	489.0	1;2;C1	1;2(3)	≤1
2	X- AQ	616.97	617.2	4;C1	4	≤1
3	X- AQG	674.02	674.5	4 (6);C1	4(6)	≤1
4	X- AQGT	775.13	775.2	6;7(3.4) C1	6;7(3;4)	16–20
5	X- AQGTL	888.29	888.4	4(9);C1	4(9)	32–36
6	X-AQGTLS	975.36	975.5	2;3;C1	2;3	Together 6–7; 6>>7
7	X-AQGTLSK	1104.54	1104.6	2; C1	2	
8	X-AQGTLSKI	1217.7	1218.0	8;9(1;2;3); C1	8;9(1;2;3)	Together 13–17
9	X-AQGTLSKIF	1364.87	1364.9	6 (9);C1	6 (9)	
12	X-AQGTLSKIFKLG	1664.26	1664.5	3;6;C1	3;6	
18	X-AQGTLSKIFKLGGRDSRS	2323.94	2324.9	5(6);C1	5(6)	16–19
21	X-AQGTLSKIFKLGGRD SRSGSP	2565.18	2565.3	1;2; C1	1;2	Together 10–15
25	X-AQGTLSKIFKLGGRDS RSGSPMARR	3081.84	3082.0	3;4;C1	3;4	

*Free fluorescent compound; all analyzed OPs contained fluorescent X-component.
**The same products of the hydrolysis separated by RPhC (Fig. 5A) were revealed in several peaks by MALDI spectrometry; the main peaks are marked in bold, while additional peaks are shown in parentheses. C1 reflects the presence of signal corresponding to the analyzed product in the spectrum of total reaction mixture.
***The same several products of the hydrolysis corresponding to each peak after RPhC (Fig. 5A) were revealed not only by MALDI spectrometry, but also by TLC (Fig. 5B)

KIIGQVRDQAE (in-OP2) [33,34]. All mentioned OPs contained fluorescent residue 6-O-(Carboxymethyl)fluorescein ethyl ester (X) on its N-terminus. In addition, three short fluorogenic peptidyl-4-methylcoumaryl-7-amides (MCA) were used as nonspecific controls: Boc-Val-Leu-Lys-MCA (shOP1), Pro-Phe-Arg-MCA (shOP2), Boc-Ile-Glu-Gly-Arg-MCA (shOP3).

The cleavage products of different OPs were separated by TLC on Kieselgel F60 plates using acetic acid – n-butanol – H$_2$O (1:4:5) system. The plates were dried and photographed. To quantify the intensities of the fluorescent spots after TLC, X-OP21, X-OP25, and other OPs incubated without IgGs (or with hd-IgG$_{mix}$) was used as controls. Photographs of the plates were imaged by scanning and quantified using GelPro v3.1 software.

In some experiments the cleavage products of specific X-OP21 and X-OP25 were first separated by reverse-phase chromatography on Nucleosil C-18 column (4.6×250 mm) using 0.05% trifluoroacetic acid and gradient of acetonitrile concentration (0 - 80%). The relative amount of various cleavage products was calculated by the fluorescence. Excitation was performed at 320 nm and fluorescence emission detected at 490 nm. The fractions corresponding to different peaks were collected, evaporated to minimal volume and products of the hydrolysis were analyzed by TLC (see above) and by MALDI spectrometry (see below).

MALDI-TOF analysis Ab-dependent hydrolysis of OPs

In all cases the products of OP hydrolysis were analysed by MALDI-TOF mass spectrometry using a ReflexIII system (Bruker, Germany) equipped with a 337-nm nitrogen laser (VSL-337ND, Laser Science, Newton, MA), 3 ns pulse duration. Saturated solution of cyano-4-hydroxycinnamic acid in a mixture of 0.1%

acetonitrile and trifluoroacetic acid (1:2) was used as the matrix. To 1 μl of the reaction mixture containing hydrolyzed OPs before or after their separation by RPhC or TLC, 1 μl of 0.2% trifluoroacetic acid and 2 μl of the matrix were added, and 1 μl of the final mixture was spotted on the MALDI plate, air-dried, and used for the analysis. Calibration of the MALDI spectra was performed using the protein and OP standards I and II (Bruker Daltonic, Germany) in the external and internal calibration mode.

Determination of the kinetic parameters

The reaction mixtures contained the standard components and different concentrations of OPs. All measurements (initial rates) were taken under the conditions of the pseudo-first order of the reaction within the linear regions of the time courses(<40% of OP hydrolysis). The cleavage products were analyzed by TLC. The activity of IgG$_{mix}$ was determined as a decrease in the percentage of initial X-OPs converted to shorter X-OPs, corrected for the distribution of the fluorescence label between these spots in the control (incubation of X-OPs in the absence of Abs) and taking into account the concentration of each OP in every reaction mixture. The K_M and V_{max} (apparent k_{cat} = V_{max}/[Abs]) values were calculated from the dependencies of V versus [OP] by least-squares non-linear fitting using Microcal Origin v5.0 software and presented as linear transformations using a Lineweaver–Burk plot [40]. Errors in the values were within 10–15%. The results are reported as mean±S.E. of at least three independent experiments.

Acknowledgments

This research was made possible in part by grants from the Presidium of the Russian Academy of Sciences (Molecular and Cellular Biology Program, 6.7; Fundamental Sciences to Medicine, 5.13), Russian

Foundation for Basic Research (10-04-00281), and funds from the Siberian Division of the Russian Academy of Sciences.

Author Contributions

Idea of study: GAN. Performed the experiments: AT PD LPK. Analyzed the data: VNB GAN. Contributed reagents/materials/analysis tools: LPK VNB. Wrote the paper: GAN.

References

1. Keinan E ed (2005) Catalytic antibodies: Weinheim, Germany: Wiley-VCH Verlag GmbH and Co. KgaA. p. 1–586

2. Nevinsky GA, Buneva VN (2002) Human catalytic RNA- and DNA-hydrolyzing antibodies. J Immunol Methods 269: 235–249.

3. Nevinsky GA, Favorova OO, Buneva VN (2002) Natural Catalytic Antibodies-New Characters in the Protein Repertoire. In: Golemis E editor. Protein-protein interactions; a molecular cloning manual. New York: Cold Spring Harbor Lab. Press, pp. 1–523.

4. Nevinsky GA, Buneva VN (2003) Catalytic antibodies in healthy humans and patients with autoimmune and viral pathologies. J Cell Mol Med 7: 265–276.

5. Nevinsky GA, Buneva VN (2005) Natural catalytic antibodies-abzymes. In: Keinan E editor. Catalytic antibodies. Weinheim, Germany: VCH-Wiley press. pp. 503–567.

6. Nevinsky GA, Buneva VN (2010) Natural catalytic antibodies in norm, autoimmune, viral, and bacterial diseases. **ScientificWorldJournal** 10: 1203–1233.

7. Nevinsky GA (2010) Natural catalytic antibodies in norm and in autoimmune diseases. In: Brenner KJ editor. Autoimmune Diseases: Symptoms, Diagnosis and Treatment. USA: Nova Science Publishers, Inc. pp. 1–107.

8. Nevinsky GA (2011) Natural catalytic antibodies in norm and in HIV-infected patients. In: Fyson Hanania Kasenga editor. Understanding HIV/AIDS Management and Care–Pandemic Approaches the 21st Century. InTech. pp. 151–192.

9. Bezuglova AM, Konenkova LP, Doronin BM, Buneva VN, Nevinsky GA (2011) Affinity and catalytic heterogeneity and metal-dependence of polyclonal myelin basic protein-hydrolyzing IgGs from sera of patients with systemic lupus erythematosus. **J Mol Recognit** 24: 960–974.

10. Parkhomenko TA, Buneva VN, Tyshkevich OB, Generalov II, Doronin BM, et al. (2010) DNA-hydrolyzing activity of IgG antibodies from the sera of patients with tick-borne encephalitis. **Biochimie** 92: 545–554.

11. O'Connor KC, Bar-Or A, Hafler DA (2001) Neuroimmunology of multiple sclerosis. J Clin Immunol 21: 81–92.

12. Archelos JJ, Storch MK, Hartung HP (2000) The role of B cells and autoantibodies in multiple sclerosis. Ann Neurol 47: 694–706.

13. Hemmer B, Archelos JJ, Hartung HP (2002) New concepts in the immunopathogenesis of multiple sclerosis. Nat Rev Neurosci 3: 291–301.

14. Hhachn BCh (1996) Systemic lupus erythematosus. In: Braunvald EE, Isselbakher KD, Petersdorf RG, Wilson DD, Martin DB, Fauchi AS, editors. Moscow: Internal diseases, Medicine. pp. 407–419.

15. Pisetsky D (2001) Immune response to DNA in systemic lupus erythematosus. Isr Med Ass J 3: 850–853.

16. Poser CM (1984) The diagnosis of multiple sclerosis, NY: Thieme-Stratton; pp. 3–13.

17. Williamson RA, Burgoon MP, Owens GP, Ghausi O, Leclerc E, et al. (2001) Anti-DNA antibodies are a major component of the intrathecal B cell response in multiple sclerosis. Proc Natl Acad Sci USA 98: 1793–1798.

18. Shuster AM, Gololobov GV, Kvashuk OA, Bogomolova AE, Smirnov IV, et al. (1992) DNA hydrolyzing autoantibodies. Science 256: 665–667.

19. Andrievskaya OA, Buneva VN, Naumov VA, Nevinsky GA (2000) Catalytic heterogeneity of polyclonal RNA-hydrolyzing IgM from sera of patients with lupus erythematosus. Med Sci Monit 6: 460–470.

20. Andrievskaya OA, Buneva VN, Baranovskii AG, Gal'vita AV, Naumov VA, et al. (2000) Catalytic diversity of polyclonal RNA-hydrolyzing IgG antibodies from from sera of patients with lupus erythematosus. Med Sci Monit 6: 460–470.

21. Savel'ev AN, Eneyskaya EV, Shabalin K A, Filatov MV, Neustroev KN (1999) Antibodies with amylolytic activity. Prot Pept Lett 6: 179–183.

22. Savel'ev AN, Kulminskaya AA, Ivanen DR, Nevinsky GA, Neustroev KN (2004) Human antibodies with amylolytic activity. Trends in Glycoscience and Glycotechnology 16: 17–31.

23. Baranovskii AG, Kanyshkova TG, Mogelnitskii AS, Naumov VA, Buneva VN, et al. (1998) Polyclonal antibodies from blood and cerebrospinal fluid of patients with multiple sclerosis effectively hydrolyze DNA and RNA. Biochemistry (Moscow) 63: 1239–1248.

24. Baranovskii AG, Ershova NA, Buneva VN, Kanyshkova TG, Mogelnitskii AS, et al. (2001) Catalytic heterogeneity of polyclonal DNA-hydrolyzing antibodies from the sera of patients with multiple sclerosis. Immunol Let 76: 163–167.

25. Saveliev AN, Ivanen DR, Kulminskaya AA, Ershova NA, Kanyshkova TG, et al. (2003) Amylolytic activity of IgM and IgG antibodies from patients with multiple sclerosis. Immunol Lett 86: 291–297.

26. Kozyr AV, Kolesnikov A, Aleksandrova ES, Sashchenko LP, Gnuchev NV, et al. (1998) Novel functional activities of anti-DNA autoantibodies from sera of patients with lymphoproliferative and autoimmune diseases. **Appl Biochem Biotechnol** 75: 45–61.

27. Polosukhina DI, Kanyshkova T, Doronin BM, Tyshkevich OB, Buneva VN, et al. (2004) Hydrolysis of myelin basic protein by polyclonal catalytic IgGs from the sera of patients with multiple sclerosis. J Cell Mol Med 8: 359–368.

28. Polosukhina DI, Buneva VN, Doronin BM, Tyshkevich OB, Boiko AN, et al. (2005) Hydrolysis of myelin basic protein by IgM and IgA antibodies from the sera of patients with multiple sclerosis. Med Sci Monit 11: BR266–BR272

29. Polosukhina DI, Kanyshkova TG, Doronin BM, Tyshkevich OB, Buneva VN, et al. (2006) Metal-dependent hydrolysis of myelin basic protein by IgGs from the sera of patients with multiple sclerosis. Immunol Lett 103: 75–81.

30. Legostaeva GA, Polosukhina DI, Bezuglova AM, Doronin BM, Buneva VN, et al. (2010) Affinity and catalytic heterogeneity of polyclonal myelin basic protein-hydrolyzing IgGs from sera of patients with multiple sclerosis. **J Cell Mol Med** 14: 699–709.

31. Ponomarenko NA, Durova OM, Vorobiev II, Belogurov AA, Kurkova IN, et al. (2006) Autoantibodies to myelin basic protein catalyze site-specific degradation of their antigen. Proc Natl Acad Sci USA 103: 281–286.

32. Paul S, Li L, Kalaga R, O'Dell J, Dannenbring RE, et al. (1997) Chacterization of thyroglobulin-directed and polyreactive catalytic antibodies in autoimmune disease. J Immunol 159: 1530–1536.

33. Odintsova ES, Baranova SV, Dmitrenok PS, Rasskazov VA, Calmels C, et al. (2011) Antibodies to HIV integrase catalyze site-specific degradation of their antigen. **Int Immunol** 23: 601–612.

34. Odintsova ES, Baranova SV, Dmitrenok PS, Calmels C, Parissi V, et al. (2012) Anti-integrase abzymes from the sera of HIV-infected patients specifically hydrolyze integrase but nonspecifically cleave short oligopeptides. **J Mol Recognit** 25: 193–207.

35. Li L, Paul S, Tyutyulkova S, Kazatchkine MD, Kaveri S (1995) Catalytic activity of anti-thyroglobulin antibodies. J Immunol 154: 3328–3332.

36. Gao QS, Sun M, Tyutyulkova S, Webster D, Rees A, et al. (1994) Molecular cloning of a proteolytic antibody light chain. **J Biol Chem** 269: 32389–32393.

37. Thiagarajan P, Dannenbring R, Matsuura K, Tramontano A, Gololobov G, et al. (2000) Monoclonal antibody light chain with prothrombinase activity. Biochemistry 39: 6459–6465.

38. Paul S, Li L, Kalaga R, Wilkins-Stevens P, Stevens FJ, et al. (1995) Natural catalytic antibodies: peptide-hydrolyzing activities of Bence Jones proteins and VL fragment. **J Biol Chem** 270: 15257–15261.

39. Boiko AN, Favorova OO (1995) Multiple sclerosis: molecular and cellular mechanisms. **Mol Biol (Mosk)** 29: 727–749.

40. Fersht A (1985) Enzyme Structure and Mechanism. 2nd ed., N.Y.: W. H. Freeman Co.

14

Mesangial Cell-Binding Activity of Serum Immunoglobulin G in Patients with Lupus Nephritis

Desmond Y. H. Yap, Susan Yung, Qing Zhang, Colin Tang, Tak Mao Chan*

Division of Nephrology, Department of Medicine, Queen Mary Hospital, The University of Hong Kong, Hong Kong

Abstract

In vitro data showed that immunoglobulin G (IgG) from patients with lupus nephritis (LN) could bind to cultured human mesangial cells (HMC). The clinical relevance of such binding was unknown. Binding of IgG and subclasses was measured in 189 serial serum samples from 23 patients with Class III/IV±V LN (48 during renal flares, 141 during low level disease activity (LLDA)). 64 patients with non-lupus glomerular diseases (NLGD) and 23 healthy individuals were used as controls. HMC-binding was measured with cellular ELISA and expressed as OD index. HMC-binding index of total IgG was 0.12 ± 0.09, 0.36 ± 0.25, 0.59 ± 0.37 and 0.74 ± 0.42 in healthy subjects, NLGD, LN patients during LLDA, and LN flares respectively ($P=0.046$, LN flare vs. LLDA; $P<0.001$, for healthy controls or NLGD vs. LN during flare or LLDA). Binding of serum IgG_1 to HMC was 0.05 ± 0.05, 0.15 ± 0.11, 0.41 ± 0.38 and 0.55 ± 0.40 for the corresponding groups respectively ($P=0.007$, LN flare vs. remission; $P<0.001$, for healthy controls or NLGD vs. LN during flare or remission). IgG_2, IgG_3 and IgG_4 from patients and controls did not show significant binding to HMC. Total IgG and IgG_1 HMC-binding index correlated with anti-dsDNA level ($r=0.26$ and 0.39 respectively, $P<0.001$ for both), and inversely with C3 ($r=-0.17$ and -0.45, $P<0.05$ for both). Sensitivity/specificity of total IgG or IgG_1 binding to HMC in predicting renal flares were 81.3%/39.7% (ROC AUC 0.61, $P=0.03$) and 83.8%/41.8% (AUC 0.63, $P=0.009$) respectively. HMC-binding by IgG_1, but not total IgG, correlated with mesangial immune deposition in LN renal biopsies under electron microscopy. Our results showed that binding of serum total IgG and IgG_1 in LN patients correlates with disease activity. The correlation between IgG_1 HMC-binding and mesangial immune deposition suggests a potential pathogenic significance.

Editor: Irun R. Cohen, Weizmann Institute of Science, Israel

Funding: This project was supported by the Hong Kong Society of Nephrology Research Grant 2009 awarded to Desmond Y. H. YAP and the endowment fund of the Yu Chiu Kwong Professorship in Medicine at University of Hong Kong awarded to T. M. Chan. S. Yung is supported by the Wai Hung Charitable Foundation. The funders had no role in study design, data collection and analysis, decision to publish, or preparation of the manuscript.

Competing Interests: The authors have declared that no competing interests exist.

* Email: dtmchan@hku.hk

Introduction

Lupus nephritis (LN) is a severe manifestation in patients with systemic lupus erythematosus (SLE), and is an important cause of renal failure in some racial groups such as Asians [1,2]. The treatments to date are based on non-selective immunosuppression. The pathogenic mechanisms are multifactorial and complex, but increased understanding of the pathogenic mechanisms could lead to improvements in disease activity monitoring and treatment. SLE is a prototype autoimmune disease and is characterized by the production of different autoantibodies, resulting in immune-mediated injury to various organs including the kidneys [3,4]. The pathogenic importance of anti-dsDNA antibodies is exemplified by in vitro studies demonstrating their presence in renal eluates obtained from patients and mice with LN [5–7], and by clinical observations demonstrating a correlation between anti-dsDNA antibody titre and disease activity [8].

Mesangial cells have a central location in the glomerulus. Not only do mesangial cells provide structural support to adjacent capillary loops but it is well established that they also participate actively in disease mechanisms through the production of inflammatory and fibrotic growth factors [9,10]. Immunoglobulin deposition in the mesangial area, mesangial cell proliferation, and increase in mesangial matrix are constant features in renal biopsies

of active LN [3,11]. Our group has previously reported that anti-dsDNA isolated from patients with LN can bind to human mesangial cells (HMC) and such binding correlates with clinical activity in selected LN patients and could contribute to intra-renal disease pathogenesis [12,13]. We also observed a correlation between anti-dsDNA and total IgG levels. In this study, we investigated whether the binding activity of total serum IgG and its subclasses to HMC might have clinical correlations in patients with LN, which have implications on the use of such binding as a biomarker for disease monitoring and further exploration into its pathogenic importance.

Materials and Methods

Patients

This study and the consent procedures were approved by the Institutional Review Board of the University of Hong Kong/ Hospital Authority Hong Kong West Cluster (HKU/HA HKW IRB). All included subjects have signed consent for the use of the serum samples in this study and the consent forms are kept in patients' case records. Patients attending follow-up at the SLE Clinic of Queen Mary Hospital, Hong Kong, with biopsy-proven Class III/IV±V LN and two or more episodes of renal flare during the period 2001 to 2013 were included. Histological

Table 1. Characteristics of 23 patients with Class III/IV±V lupus nephritis who had two or more episodes of renal flare during follow-up and included in the present study.

Age (year)	39.4±11.2
Female/Male	14/9
Duration of follow up (month)	138.2±80.5
Previous immunosuppressive exposure	
Prednisolone	23 (100%)
Cyclophosphamide	17 (73.9%)
Mycophenolate mofetil	18 (78.3%)
Azathioprine	19 (82.6%)
Calcineurin inhibitors	8 (34.8%)
Laboratory parameters at first renal flare	
Serum creatinine level (μmol/L)	111.8±56.4
Urine protein (g/D)	3.1±3.4
Anti-dsDNA level (iu/mL)	238.7±249.3
C3 level (mg/dL)	64.4±38.1

findings of LN were reported in accordance with the International Society of Nephrology/Renal Pathology Society (ISN/RPS) 2003 classification [14,15]. Standard treatment for active LN included corticosteroids combined with either cyclophosphamide or mycophenolate mofetil (MMF) as induction immunosuppression, followed by low-dose corticosteroids with either azathioprine or MMF as long-term maintenance immunosuppression. Disease activity was categorized as "active" or "low level disease activity" (LLDA) on the basis of both clinical and serologic parameters. "Active" disease had SLE Disease Activity Index (SLEDAI) score >10 with ≥4 points in the renal domain, and "low level disease activity" status was defined by SLEDAI score <4 with no points in the renal domain [16]. Patients with non-lupus glomerular diseases (NLGD) and healthy subjects (age- and sex-matched) were included as controls. The NLGD group included patients with IgA nephropathy, minimal change nephropathy, membranous nephropathy and ANCA-associated glomerulonephritis, and serum samples were obtained at presentation when the diagnoses were established by renal biopsy.

Laboratory methods

Archived serum samples from LN patients collected at baseline (i.e. at initiation of induction therapy) then serially at 3-month intervals with informed consent were retrieved. Single serum samples were obtained from patients with non-lupus glomerular diseases and healthy subjects.

HMC-binding activity of IgG in serum samples was measured using a cellular ELISA as previously described [12]. Briefly, HMC were seeded into 96-well microtitre plates at a density of 10,000 cells/cm^2. Cells were cultured in RPMI 1640 medium supplemented with 15% FCS and medium changed every 3 days. At 90% confluence HMC were growth arrested for 72 h, washed with PBS then fixed with 1% paraformaldehyde in PBS for 15 min. Cells were washed thrice with PBS in between steps, and all incubations were for 1 h at 37°C. HMC were blocked with 3% BSA followed by normal IgG (100 μg/ml) to block Fc receptor-mediated binding. HMC were incubated with serum samples (diluted 1:100, 100 μl) in triplicate, then incubated with anti-human IgG F(ab) conjugated with alkaline phosphatase. Degree of IgG binding to HMC was detected by incubation with para-

nitrophenol phosphate at room temperature and with optical density measurement at A$_{405/420}$ when pre-established positive control sample showed an optical density of 1.5. The positive control was pooled serum from a patient with high HMC-binding activity. Seropositivity for HMC binding was denoted by results that exceed mean+3SD of results from healthy subjects. Circulating anti-dsDNA antibody titre was measured using a commercial ELISA (Microplate autoimmune anti-DNA quantitative ELISA) according to the manufacturer's instructions (BioRad, Hong Kong). Samples giving a value >60 IU/ml were considered positive. Kidney biopsies were performed within one week when renal flares were suspected clinically, and were reviewed by the same pathologist. The amount of mesangial deposits was semi-quantitated by electron microscopy (EM) in the following scale: 0 = no deposit; 1 = scanty deposits; 2 = moderate deposits; 3 = numerous deposits.

Data analysis and statistics

Continuous variables were expressed as mean±SD and analyzed by student's t-test, unless otherwise specified. Categorical variable were expressed as frequencies and percentages, and analyzed with Chi-square test where appropriate. Correlation of HMC-binding activity with clinical parameters was assessed by the Spearman's method. The sensitivity/specificity, positive and negative predictive value (PPV and NPV) of HMC-binding activity in predicting renal flares was calculated, and the Area Under Curve (AUC) of the Receiver Operator Characteristics (ROC) curves was determined. Statistical analysis was performed by Graphpad Prism 5 (La Jolla, California, USA) and two-tailed P $values<0.05$ was considered statistically significant.

Results

Patient characteristics

Twenty-three Chinese patients with biopsy-proven Class III/IV±V LN and who had experienced at least two episodes of renal flares during follow-up of 138.2±80.5 months were included (Table 1). A total of 276 serum samples were analyzed, with 189 samples from LN patients (48 during active renal flare and 141 during LLDA, 64 samples from patients with non-lupus glomer-

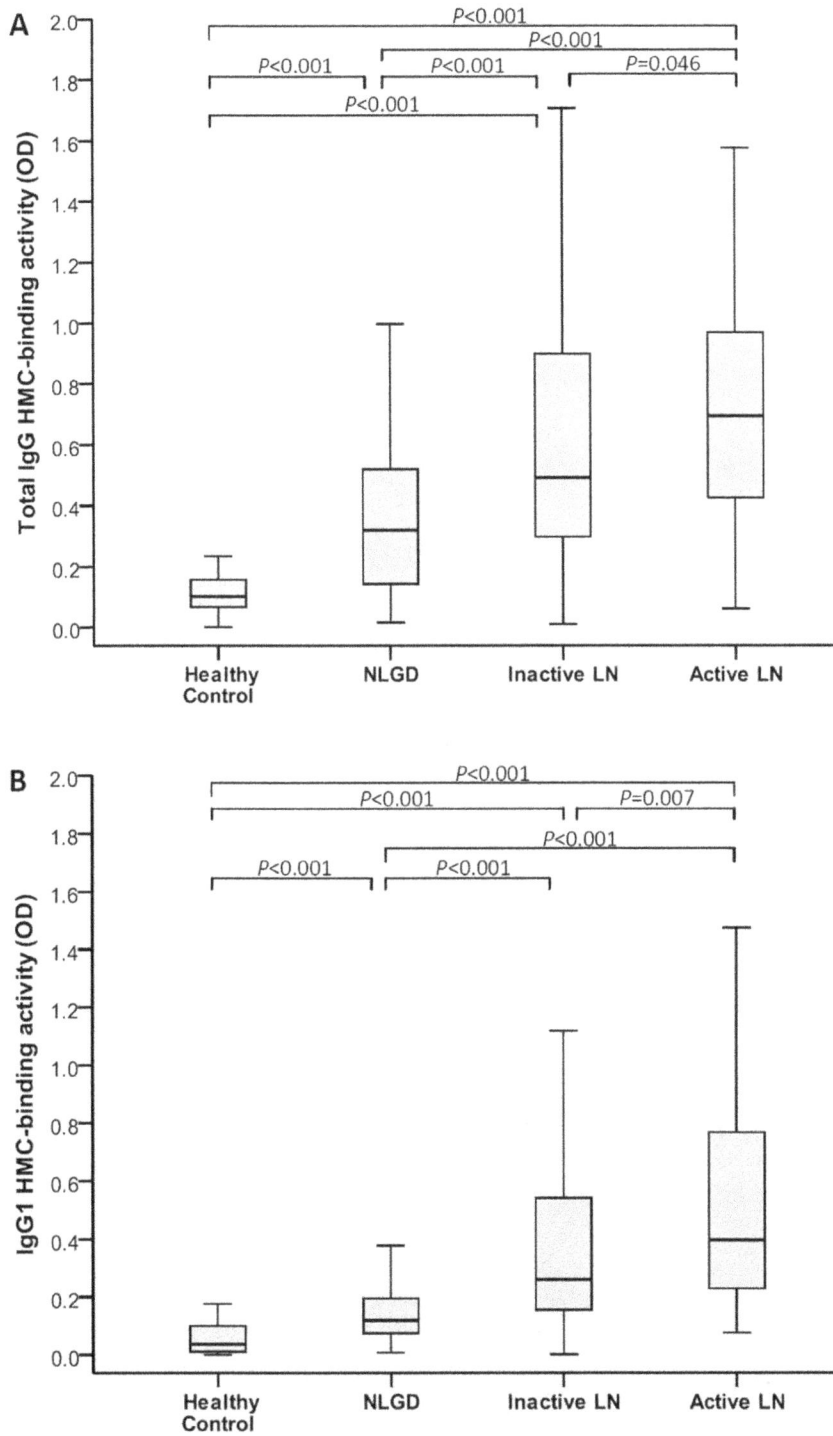

Figure 1. Mesangial cell-binding by (A) total IgG and (B) IgG$_1$ in serum samples of patients with inactive or active lupus nephritis, non-lupus glomerular diseases, and patients with inactive or active lupus nephritis, non-lupus glomerular diseases, and healthy controls.

ular diseases (NLGD), and 23 samples from healthy subjects respectively.

HMC-binding activity of serum total IgG and its subclasses in LN patients

Binding index of serum total IgG to HMC was 0.12 ± 0.09, 0.36 ± 0.25, 0.59 ± 0.37 and 0.74 ± 0.42 for healthy controls,

NLGD, LN patients during LLDA, and active LN respectively ($P = 0.046$, LN flare vs. LLDA; $P<0.001$, healthy controls or NLGD vs. active or inactive LN; $P<0.001$, NLGD vs. active or inactive LN) (Figure 1, A). Binding index of serum IgG$_1$ to HMC was 0.05 ± 0.05, 0.15 ± 0.11, 0.41 ± 0.38 and 0.55 ± 0.40 for healthy controls, NLGD, LN patients in LLDA, and active LN respectively ($P = 0.007$, LN flare vs. LLDA; $P<0.001$, healthy controls or

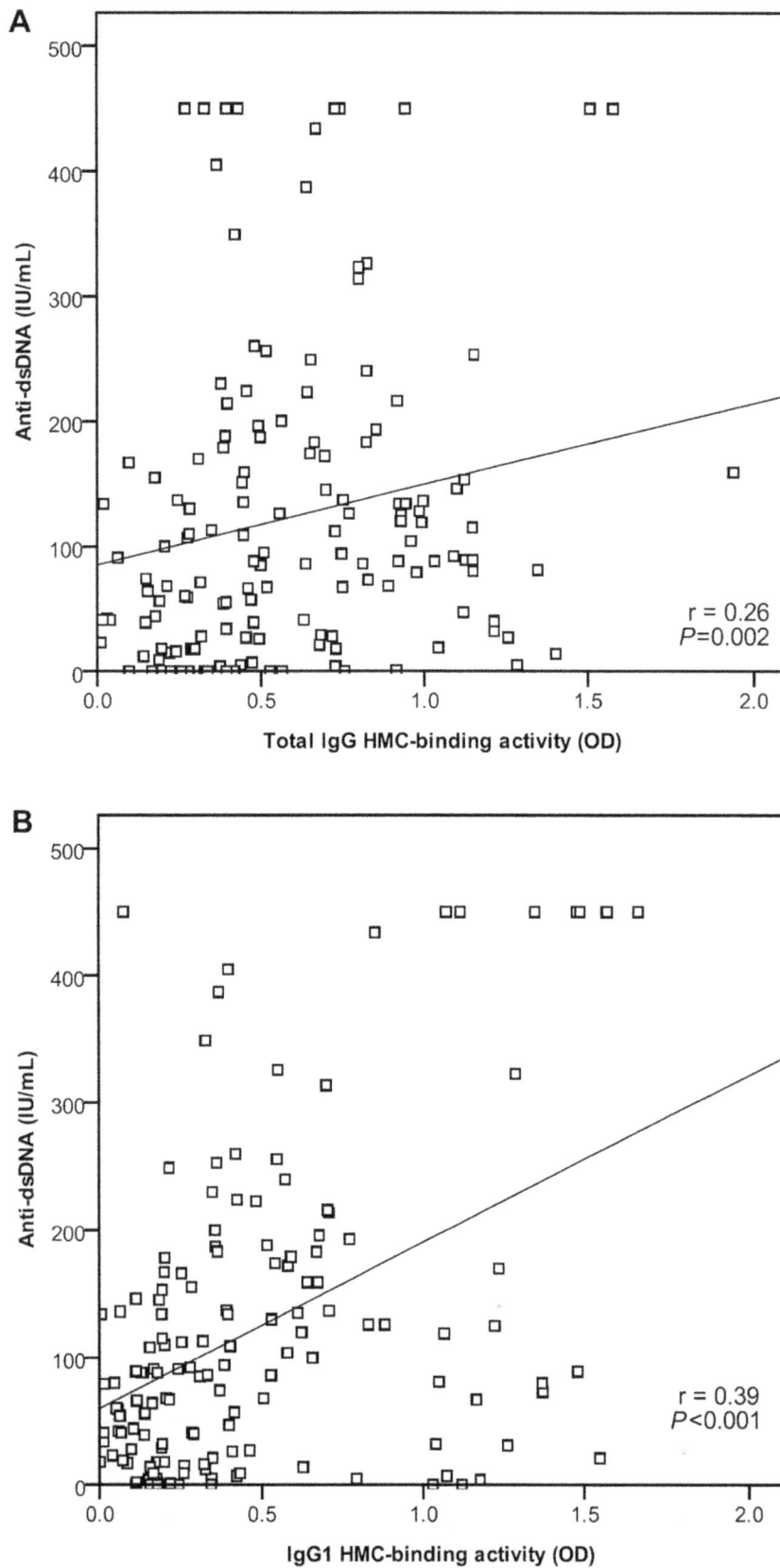

Figure 2. Correlation between mesangial cell-binding by (A) total IgG and (B) IgG₁ with anti-dsDNA level in 23 patients with Class III/IV±V lupus nephritis.

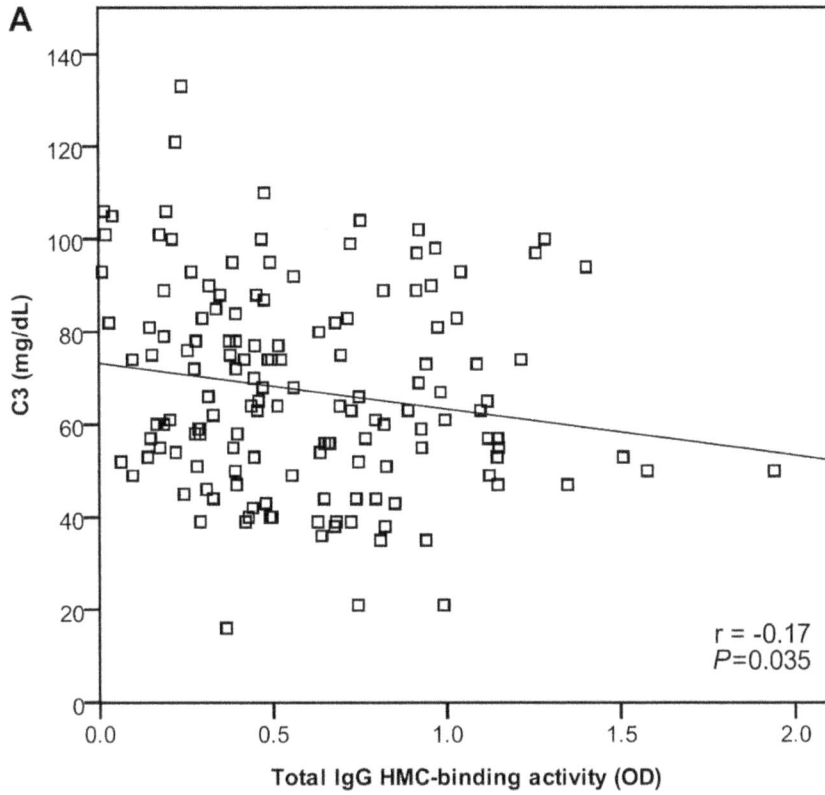

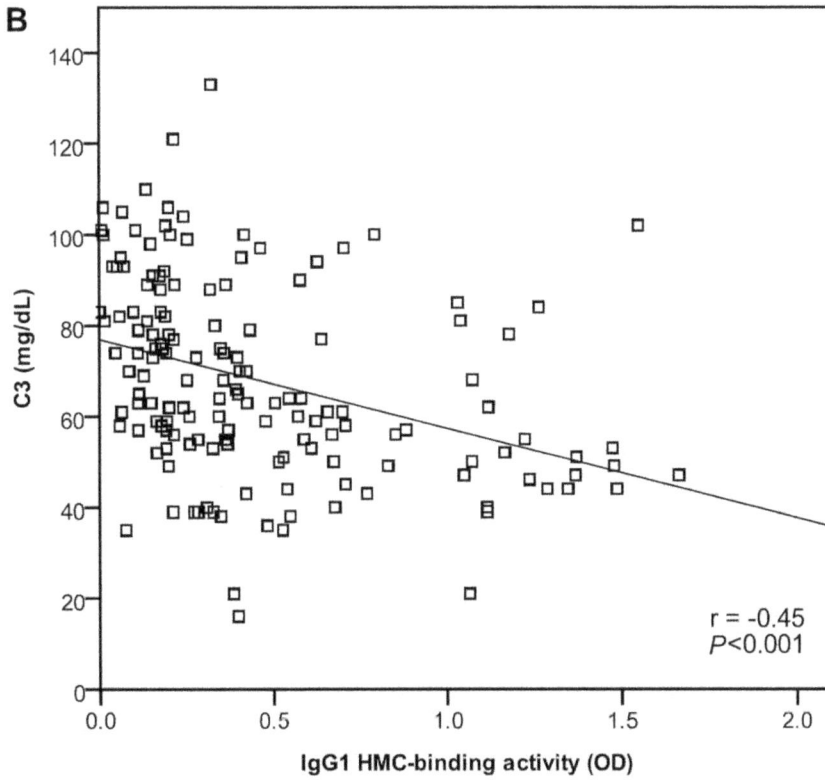

Figure 3. Negative correlation between mesangial cell-binding by (A) total IgG and (B) IgG₁ with C3 level in 23 patients with Class III/IV±V lupus nephritis.

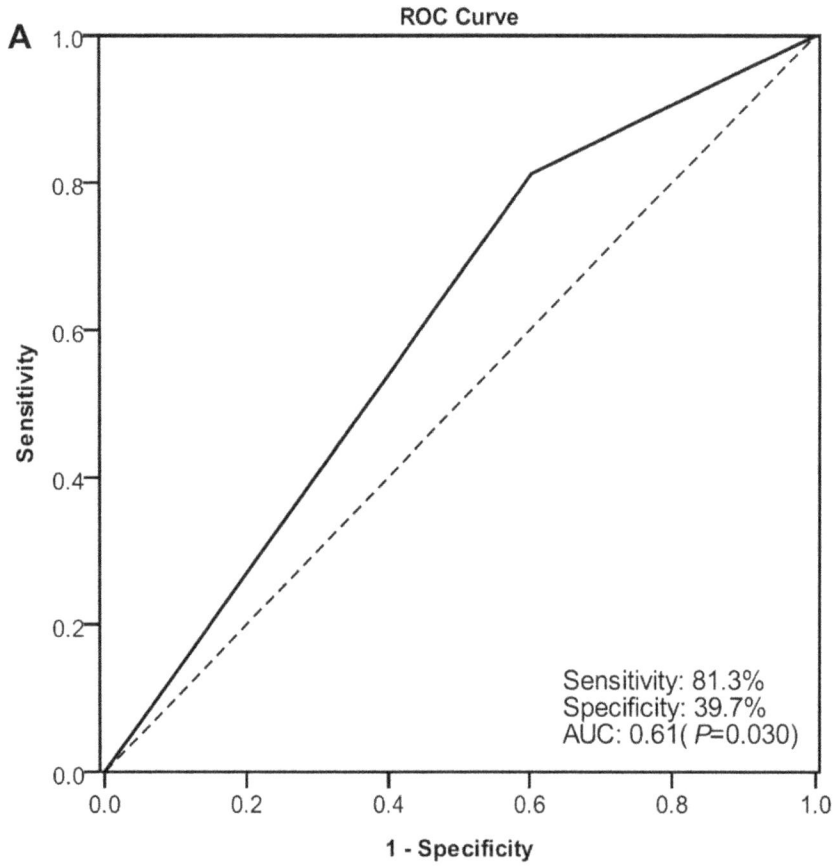

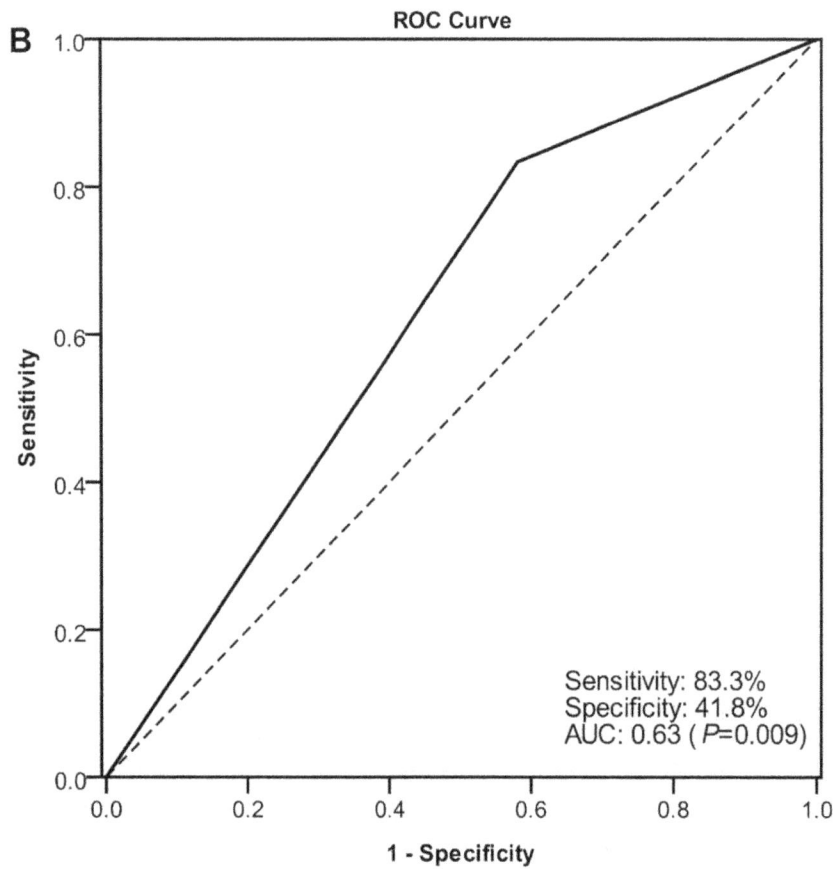

Figure 4. Receiver Operator Characteristics (ROC) curve for sensitivity/specificity in renal flare prediction using the level of mesangial cell-binding by (A) total IgG and (B) IgG$_1$ in serum samples of 23 patients with Class III/IV±V lupus nephritis.

NLGD vs. active or inactive LN; $P<0.001$, NLGD vs. active or inactive LN) (Figure 1, B). There was no significant binding of serum IgG$_2$, IgG$_3$ or IgG$_4$ to HMC, which also did not vary between healthy controls, NLGD patients, and LN patients during flare or LLDA.

HMC binding by serum IgG and IgG$_1$ and clinical parameters

Total serum IgG and serum IgG$_1$ HMC-binding index both correlated positively with anti-dsDNA levels ($r = 0.26$ and 0.39 respectively, $P<0.001$ for both) (Figure 2, A&B). In contrast, both showed a negative correlation with C3 levels ($r = -0.17$ and -0.45 respectively, $P<0.05$ for both) (Figure 3, A&B). HMC-binding by IgG and IgG$_1$ was not related to the level of serum creatinine, serum albumin, or proteinuria at the time of blood sample collection ($P = 0.735$, 0.546 and 0.700 respectively for total IgG HMC-binding; $P = 0.628$, 0.443 and 0.170 for IgG$_1$ HMC-binding).

Overall sensitivity/specificity of total IgG or IgG$_1$ HMC-binding index in the prediction of renal flares (with or without systemic flares) was $81.3\%/39.7\%$ (AUC 0.61, $P = 0.030$) and $83.8\%/41.8\%$ (AUC 0.63, $P = 0.009$) respectively (Figure 4, A&B). The overall PPV and NPV of total IgG or IgG1 HMC-binding index in prediction of renal flares (with or without systemic flares) were $31.5\%/86.2\%$ and $32.8\%/88.1\%$ respectively. The sensitivity/specificity of total IgG or IgG$_1$ HMC-binding index to predict renal flares with concomitant systemic flares were $80.0\%/35.1\%$ (PPV: 12.1%; NPV: 94.1%) and $83.3\%/36.1\%$ (PPV: 12.7%; NPV: 95.1%), and $79.6\%/38.6\%$ (PPV: 28.2%; NPV: 86.2%) and $83.3\%/40.8\%$ (PPV: 28.7%; NPV: 89.6%) for renal flares without systemic flares. Two patients (8.7%) showed positive total IgG and IgG$_1$ binding to HMC during active renal flare when their anti-dsDNA and C3 levels remained within normal limits. Seropositivity of HMC-binding IgG$_1$ precedes renal flares by 43.8 ± 62.9 days.

HMC binding by serum IgG and IgG$_1$ and mesangial immune deposition assessed by electron microscopy

Total IgG HMC-binding seropositivity was not related to the degree of mesangial immune deposition ($P = 0.733$). In contrast, patients seropositive for IgG$_1$ HMC-binding were more likely to show increased mesangial immune deposition at grades 2 or 3 (i.e. moderate to numerous) ($P = 0.016$). HMC-binding index of IgG$_1$, but not total IgG, also correlated positively with the mesangial deposition score ($r = 0.776$ and $P<0.001$ for IgG$_1$; $r = 0.263$ and $P = 0.363$ for total IgG).

Discussion

SLE is characterized by the production of various autoantibodies [4]. Previous studies have reported that different autoantibodies can bind to different renal components including podocytes, mesangial cells, endothelial cells, and renal tubular epithelial cells, and it has been speculated that such binding could have a pathogenic role in immune-mediated kidney injury [10,12,13,17–19]. Mesangial cells are located strategically at the centre of glomeruli and are juxtaposed to the capillary loops [9]. Mesangial immunoglobulin deposition and mesangial cell proliferation are cardinal histological features in LN [3,11]. Our previous investigations showed that anti-dsDNA antibodies from patients

with LN could bind to HMC and trigger cellular responses involved in inflammation and fibrosis, and that such binding correlated with total serum IgG level (10,12). The present study sought to investigate the potential clinical correlations of the in vitro findings.

Our results showed a clear relationship between disease activity and HMC-binding by total serum IgG and IgG$_1$ in LN, and the degree of binding was significantly increased in LN compared with healthy subjects and patients with non-lupus glomerular diseases. Also, the positive correlation of IgG HMC-binding with anti-dsDNA level, and negative relationship with C3 level, prompted us to investigate whether HMC-binding index might serve as a biomarker for disease activity monitoring. In this context, previous studies have also found that active LN patients had significantly stronger IgG binding to isolated rat glomeruli in an in vitro assay when compared to SLE patients without nephritis [20]. That HMC-binding index of total IgG or IgG$_1$ was not related to serum creatinine, serum albumin, or proteinuria was not a disadvantage since these clinical parameters represent a summative outcome of both active disease and prior chronic damage and are also subject to modulating factors distinct from the lupus disease process such as hypertensive renal damage. Conventional serological parameters C3 and anti-dsDNA levels have been reported to show sensitivity and specificity of 49–79% and 51–74% respectively in the detection of disease flares [21–27]. The present results from samples collected serially in LN patients showed that in the majority of cases increased HMC-binding by IgG and IgG$_1$ was associated with increased disease activity, so that these parameters had sensitivities of over 80% in the predication of renal flares. However, seropositivity for HMC-binding by itself could be present in patients during remission and thus was non-specific for active disease. Notwithstanding its lack of specificity, assessment of HMC-binding index may be of value in the small proportion of patients in whom conventional serological parameters such as anti-DNA and C3 levels do not correlate with disease activity, as was demonstrated in two of the 23 patients studied, when both anti-DNA and C3 were still within the normal range at disease flare but serum HMC-binding IgG was positive.

The present results also have implications on pathogenic mechanisms in LN. Among the different IgG subclasses from LN patients tested, only IgG$_1$ showed significant binding to HMC. Furthermore, HMC-binding by IgG$_1$ correlated with clinical disease activity and also the degree of mesangial immune deposition as assessed by electron microscopy. In this context, previous studies have suggested that IgG$_1$ might be more pathogenic compared with other IgG subclasses in LN, attributed to its ability to fix complements [28,29]. Further studies are required to investigate the downstream cellular processes that follow the binding of HMC by IgG$_1$, and whether intervention or interruption of such binding could present a novel therapeutic approach.

Conclusions

The degree of mesangial cell binding by circulating IgG and IgG$_1$ in serum samples of patients with LN correlates with disease activity, and thus may complement anti-dsDNA and C3 as biomarkers for disease monitoring. Its relationship with mesangial immunoglobulin deposition in LN kidney tissue also suggests a pathogenic role.

Author Contributions

Conceived and designed the experiments: DY SY TMC. Performed the experiments: QZ. Analyzed the data: CT. Contributed reagents/materials/analysis tools: SY. Wrote the paper: DY TMC.

References

1. Bomback AS, Appel GB (2010) Updates on the treatment of lupus nephritis. J Am Soc Nephrol 21: 2028–2035.
2. Saxena R, Mahajan T, Mohan C (2011) Lupus nephritis: current update. Arthritis Res Ther 13: 240.
3. Golbus J, McCune WJ (1994) Lupus nephritis. Classification, prognosis, immunopathogenesis, and treatment. Rheum Dis Clin North Am 20: 213–242.
4. Tan EM, Schur PH, Carr RI, Kunkel HG (1966) Deoxybonucleic acid (DNA) and antibodies to DNA in the serum of patients with systemic lupus erythematosus. J Clin Invest 45: 1732–1740.
5. Winfield JB, Faiferman I, Koffler D (1977) Avidity of anti-DNA antibodies in serum and IgG glomerular eluates from patients with systemic lupus erythematosus. Association of high avidity antinative DNA antibody with glomerulonephritis. J Clin Invest 59: 90–96.
6. Kalunian KC, Panosian-Sahakian N, Ebling FM, Cohen AH, Louie JS, et al. (1989) Idiotypic characteristics of immunoglobulins associated with systemic lupus erythematosus. Studies of antibodies deposited in glomeruli of humans. Arthritis Rheum 32: 513–522.
7. Termaat RM, Assmann KJ, van Son JP, Dijkman HB, Koene RA, et al. (1993) Antigen-specificity of antibodies bound to glomeruli of mice with systemic lupus erythematosus-like syndromes. Lab Invest 68: 164–173.
8. Rovin BH, Zhang X (2009) Biomarkers for lupus nephritis: the quest continues. Clin J Am Soc Nephrol 4: 1858–1865.
9. Schlondorff D, Banas B (2009) The mesangial cell revisited: no cell is an island. J Am Soc Nephrol 20: 1179–1187.
10. Yung S, Chan TM (2012) Autoantibodies and resident renal cells in the pathogenesis of lupus nephritis: getting to know the unknown. Clin Dev Immunol 2012: 139365.
11. Mery JP, Morel-Maroger L, Boelaert J (1975) Immunoglobulin and complement deposits in lupus glomerulonephritis. Proc Eur Dial Transplant Assoc 11: 506–511.
12. Chan TM, Leung JK, Ho SK, Yung S (2002) Mesangial cell-binding anti-DNA antibodies in patients with systemic lupus erythematosus. J Am Soc Nephrol 13: 1219–1229.
13. Yung S, Cheung KF, Zhang Q, Chan TM (2010) Anti-dsDNA antibodies bind to mesangial annexin II in lupus nephritis. J Am Soc Nephrol 21: 1912–1927.
14. Tan EM, Cohen AS, Fries JF, Masi AT, McShane DJ, et al. (1982) The 1982 revised criteria for the classification of systemic lupus erythematosus. Arthritis Rheum 25: 1271–1277.
15. Weening JJ, D'Agati VD, Schwartz MM, Seshan SV, Alpers CE, et al. (2004) The classification of glomerulonephritis in systemic lupus erythematosus revisited. J Am Soc Nephrol 15: 241–250.
16. Bombardier C, Gladman DD, Urowitz MB, Caron D, Chang CH (1992) Derivation of the SLEDAI. A disease activity index for lupus patients. The Committee on Prognosis Studies in SLE. Arthritis Rheum 35: 630–640.
17. Chan TM, Cheng IK (1997) Identification of endothelial cell membrane proteins that bind anti-DNA antibodies from patients with systemic lupus erythematosus by direct or indirect mechanisms. J Autoimmun 10: 433–439.
18. Yung S, Tsang RC, Sun Y, Leung JK, Chan TM (2005) Effect of human anti-DNA antibodies on proximal renal tubular epithelial cell cytokine expression: implications on tubulointerstitial inflammation in lupus nephritis. J Am Soc Nephrol 16: 3281–3294.
19. Yung S, Cheung KF, Zhang Q, Chan TM (2013) Mediators of inflammation and their effect on resident renal cells: implications in lupus nephritis. Clin Dev Immunol 2013: 317682.
20. Budhai L, Oh K, Davidson A (1996) An in vitro assay for detection of glomerular binding IgG autoantibodies in patients with systemic lupus erythematosus. J Clin Invest 98: 1585–1593.
21. Rovin BH, Birmingham DJ, Nagaraja HN, Yu CY, Hebert LA (2007) Biomarker discovery in human SLE nephritis. Bull NYU Hosp Jt Dis 65: 187–193.
22. Moroni G, Radice A, Giammarresi G, Quaglini S, Gallelli B, et al. (2009) Are laboratory tests useful for monitoring the activity of lupus nephritis? A 6-year prospective study in a cohort of 228 patients with lupus nephritis. Ann Rheum Dis 68: 234–237.
23. Esdaile JM, Abrahamowicz M, Joseph L, MacKenzie T, Li Y, et al. (1996) Laboratory tests as predictors of disease exacerbations in systemic lupus erythematosus. Why some tests fail. Arthritis Rheum 39: 370–378.
24. Esdaile JM, Joseph L, Abrahamowicz M, Li Y, Danoff D, et al. (1996) Routine immunologic tests in systemic lupus erythematosus: is there a need for more studies? J Rheumatol 23: 1891–1896.
25. Coremans IE, Spronk PE, Bootsma H, Daha MR, van der Voort EA, et al. (1995) Changes in antibodies to C1q predict renal relapses in systemic lupus erythematosus. Am J Kidney Dis 26: 595–601.
26. Ho A, Barr SG, Magder LS, Petri M (2001) A decrease in complement is associated with increased renal and hematologic activity in patients with systemic lupus erythematosus. Arthritis Rheum 44: 2350–2357.
27. Ho A, Magder LS, Barr SG, Petri M (2001) Decreases in anti-double-stranded DNA levels are associated with concurrent flares in patients with systemic lupus erythematosus. Arthritis Rheum 44: 2342–2349.
28. Rothfield NF, Stollar BD (1967) The relation of immunoglobulin class, pattern of anti-nuclear antibody, and complement-fixing antibodies to DNA in sera from patients with systemic lupus erythematosus. J Clin Invest 46: 1785–1794.
29. Imai H, Hamai K, Komatsuda A, Ohtani H, Miura AB (1997) IgG subclasses in patients with membranoproliferative glomerulonephritis, membranous nephropathy, and lupus nephritis. Kidney Int 51: 270–276.

15

Phagocytosis is the Main CR3-Mediated Function Affected by the Lupus-Associated Variant of CD11b in Human Myeloid Cells

Liliane Fossati-Jimack[1]⑨, Guang Sheng Ling[1]⑨, Andrea Cortini[1], Marta Szajna[1], Talat H. Malik[1], Jacqueline U. McDonald[2], Matthew C. Pickering[1], H. Terence Cook[1], Philip R. Taylor[2], Marina Botto[1]*

1 Centre for Complement and Inflammation Research, Division of Immunology and Inflammation, Department of Medicine, Imperial College, London, United Kingdom, **2** Cardiff Institute of Infection and Immunity, Cardiff University School of Medicine, Cardiff, United Kingdom

Abstract

The CD11b/CD18 integrin (complement receptor 3, CR3) is a surface receptor on monocytes, neutrophils, macrophages and dendritic cells that plays a crucial role in several immunological processes including leukocyte extravasation and phagocytosis. The minor allele of a non-synonymous CR3 polymorphism (rs1143679, conversation of arginine to histidine at position 77: R77H) represents one of the strongest genetic risk factor in human systemic lupus erythematosus, with heterozygosity (77R/H) being the most common disease associated genotype. Homozygosity for the 77H allele has been reported to reduce adhesion and phagocytosis in human monocytes and monocyte-derived macrophages, respectively, without affecting surface expression of CD11b. Herein we comprehensively assessed the influence of R77H on different CR3-mediated activities in monocytes, neutrophils, macrophages and dendritic cells. R77H did not alter surface expression of CD11b including its active form in any of these cell types. Using two different iC3b-coated targets we found that the uptake by heterozygous 77R/H macrophages, monocytes and neutrophils was significantly reduced compared to 77R/R cells. Allele-specific transduced immortalized macrophage cell lines demonstrated that the minor allele, 77H, was responsible for the impaired phagocytosis. R77H did not affect neutrophil adhesion, neutrophil transmigration in vivo or Toll-like receptor 7/8-mediated cytokine release by monocytes or dendritic cells with or without CR3 pre-engagement by iC3b-coated targets. Our findings demonstrate that the reduction in CR3-mediated phagocytosis associated with the 77H CD11b variant is not macrophage-restricted but demonstrable in other CR3-expressing professional phagocytic cells. The association between 77H and susceptibility to systemic lupus erythematosus most likely relates to impaired waste disposal, a key component of lupus pathogenesis.

Editor: Masataka Kuwana, Keio University School of Medicine, Japan

Funding: This work was supported by the Wellcome Trust (grant number 088517)http://www.wellcome.ac.uk/. The funders had no role in study design, data collection and analysis, decision to publish, or preparation of the manuscript.

Competing Interests: The authors have declared that no competing interests exist.

* E-mail: m.botto@imperial.ac.uk

⑨ These authors contributed equally to this work.

Introduction

Complement receptor type 3 (CR3, also known as Mac-1, CD11b/CD18, αMβ2) is a heterodimeric transmembrane receptor found on most immune cells including dendritic cells (DCs), monocytes/macrophages, neutrophils and NK cells. A wide range of ligands have been described for CR3, including complement activation fragments (C3b/iC3b) [1], intravascular adhesion molecule-1 (ICAM-1, CD154 [2]), fibrinogen [3], high mobility group box protein 1 (HMGB-1) [4] and lipopolysaccharide (LPS) [5]. CR3 has been shown to contribute to cell activation, chemotaxis, cytotoxicity, phagocytosis [6,7] and tolerance induction [8].

Genome-wide association studies (GWAS) have shown that an allelic variant of the alpha-chain, encoded by the *ITGAM* gene, is associated with risk of developing systemic lupus erythematosus (SLE) [9–11]. The strongest association between *ITGAM* and risk of SLE is with the minor allele of a non-synonymous SNP,

rs1143679 (odds ratio 1.4–2.17), which converts the arginine at amino acid position 77 to a histidine (R77H, minor allele frequency of ~10% in European American individuals) [9–11]. This variant does not appear to increase the risk for other autoimmune conditions, except for systemic sclerosis [12,13], for which the association is much weaker [14]. Although the possibility of other independent rare causal variant(s) within the *ITGAM* gene cannot be ruled out with certainty, imputation-based association results have confirmed that rs1143679 remains the most promising candidate for causal association with SLE [13]. The rs1143679 SNP encodes the Mart alloantigen that can cause alloimmune neutropenia in neonates [15]. Interestingly some anti-Mart antibodies are able to interfere with Mac-1-dependent adhesive properties of neutrophils and monocytes and to prime neutrophils for the production of reactive oxygen species [15].

Structurally CD11b consists of five extracellular domains and a small cytoplasmic domain. The extracellular part of the protein is composed of seven 60 amino acid repeats that fold into a seven bladed beta-propeller and an inserted (I) domain of 200 amino acids between beta-sheets 2 and 3 of the beta-propeller. Ligand binding appears to take place in the I domain [16]. The R77H polymorphism is within the beta-propeller domain and currently it is unclear how it may affect ligand binding, particularly as the full crystal structure of CR3 has not yet been resolved.

Two recent studies have reported that the lupus-associated minor CD11b allele (77H) impairs phagocytosis and adhesion [17,18]. The first study used only transfected cell lines expressing the 77H and 77R variants, whilst the second study also analysed ex-vivo human 77H/H cells and demonstrated functional perturbations in monocytes/macrophages carrying the SLE-associated allele. To define the in vivo significance of R77H we elected to study the risk allele in heterozygosity as this is the genotype of the vast majority of SLE patients [9–11] and to assess several CR3-mediated activities in the major human CR3 expressing cell types: monocytes, macrophages, neutrophils and DCs. Using this systematic and comprehensive approach we found that the lupus-associated 77H allele impairs the phagocytosis of iC3b-coated particles but does not appear to affect other CR3-mediated functions including neutrophil adhesion and in vivo transmigration. CR3 activation through iC3b-coated targets inhibited to a certain degree the TLR7/8-mediated pro-inflammatory cytokine release by 77R/H monocytes but, unlike the report by Rhodes et al [18] with 77H/H monocytes, this effect was not influenced by R77H. Our data demonstrate that the 77H allele selectively influences CR3-mediated phagocytosis. The removal of cell debris (waste disposal) without causing either inflammation or triggering an autoimmune response is an important physiological activity. Abnormalities in waste disposal pathways have been associated with lupus pathogenesis [19,20]. The robust genetic association between the 77H allele and lupus susceptibility together with our data demonstrating a reduction in phagocytosis by 77R/H-expressing phagocytic cells strengthen the hypothesis that abnormalities in waste disposal pathways play a key role in lupus pathogenesis.

Materials and Methods

Donors and samples

Peripheral blood samples were obtained by venepuncture of healthy adult volunteers after obtaining informed written consent in accordance with the Declaration of Helsinki. The study was approved by the Hammersmith and Queen Charlotte's & Chelsea Research Ethics Committee (REC 2000/6000). DNA was obtained using a buccal kit according to the manufacturer instruction (Qiagen Ltd, UK). The rs1143679 variant of ITGAM was genotyped by direct sequencing of the PCR amplicon (forward primer: $5'$AGTGCGACTACAGCACAGGCTCAT$3'$ and reverse: $5'$GAGACAAGGAGGTCTGACGGTGAA$3'$). All the volunteers were healthy with no history of autoimmune conditions.

Human cell isolation

All blood samples were treated in a similar manner and processed promptly. All ex-vivo assays were performed using freshly isolated cells from sex- and ethnicity-matched individuals, one individual homozygous for the common allele (77R/R) paired with one 77H/H or 77R/H subject. Human neutrophils (PMNs) were isolated by dextran sedimentation and discontinuous plasma-Optiprep gradients [21] followed by negative selection using a custom antibody cocktail containing antibodies to CD36, CD2, CD3, CD19, CD56, glycophorin A and beads (Stemcell Technologies, Vancouver, Canada) as previously described [22]. Cell purity was consistently >95% as verified by flow cytometry

(CD16^{hi}CD14^{neg}CD11b$^+$) and cytospin. Monocytes were obtained by density gradient separation coupled with a negative selection kit for human monocytes as recommended by the manufacturer (Miltenyi Biotec GmbH, Germany). Monocyte-derived macrophages (for simplicity abbreviated as macrophages) were generated by culturing the cells for two days in RPMI-1640 medium supplemented with 10% fetal calf serum (FCS), 2 mM L-glutamine, 1% penicillin/streptomycin (Life Technologies, Grand Island, NY) and 20 ng/ml recombinant human macrophage colony stimulating factor (M-CSF) (PeproTech, Rocky Hill, NJ) as described previously [23]. Monocyte-derived dendritic cells (DCs) were generated by culturing monocytes for 5–6 days in RPMI 1640 medium, 10% FCS, 1% penicillin/streptomycin, 2 mM L-glutamine, 100 ng/ml recombinant human granulocyte-macrophage colony stimulating factor (GM-CSF) (PeproTech) and 50 ng/ml recombinant human IL-4 (PeproTech). Every 2–3 days, 50% of the culture media was exchanged with fresh media.

Murine cells

C57BL/6 mice were obtained from Harlan UK. CD11b-deficient mice (Itgam$^{-/-}$) [24] were from Jackson Laboratory (Bar Harbor, ME, USA) and were backcrossed on the C57BL/6 genetic background for 10 generations. All animals were handled in accordance with institutional guidelines and procedures approved by the UK Home Office in accordance with the Animals (Scientific Procedures) Act 1986. Conditional-Hoxb8 immortalized myeloid precursors were generated from C57BL/6 and Itgam$^{-/-}$ mice as previously described using a retrovirus encoding an estrogen receptor binding domain Hoxb8 fusion protein [25]. The Itgam$^{-/-}$ myeloid precursors were further transduced with pMXs-IZ vector containing the human CD11b variants. The cDNA of the 77R CD11b allele was obtained from OriGene Technologies (Rockville, MD, USA, SC315229, NM-000632.2), whilst the lupus susceptible allele (77H) was obtained by site-directed mutagenesis by changing the G at position 230 to an A (R77H). Both alleles were checked by sequencing. As control an empty vector was added to conditional-Hoxb8 immortalized myeloid precursors generated from C57BL/6 Itgam$^{-/-}$ cells. The different Hoxb8 immortalized myeloid precursors were differentiated in vitro into murine neutrophils or macrophage cell lines by removing estrogen and resuspending the cells in the appropriate differentiation medium [Opti-MEM, 10% v/v FCS, 2 mM L-Glutamine, 1% Penicillin/Streptomycin and 30 μM-mercaptoethanol supplemented with 20 ng/ml recombinant murine stem cell factor (SCF) (PeproTech) and recombinant murine granulocyte colony stimulating factor (G-CSF) (PeproTech) for the neutrophils; RPMI 1640, 10% v/v FCS, 2 mM L-Glutamine, Penicillin/Streptomycin, and 20 ng/ml recombinant murine M-CSF (PeproTech) for the macrophages] as previously reported [25,26]. By day 4, neutrophils routinely represented ~98% of the cells and were identified by flow cytometry as Ly-6B.2^{high}CD117^{low} cells and on cytospins by their typical nuclear morphology. By day 5, 90–98% of the macrophages expressed high levels of F4/80 [27]. Cell surface expression of the heterodimer (murine CD18/human CD11b) was assessed by flow cytometry using the following antibodies: anti-human CD11b (ICRF44) or anti-mouse CD11b (M1–70), the latter cross-reacts with human CD11b.

Flow cytometry

Murine and human leukocytes were stained using standard protocols in the presence of a saturating concentration of 2.4G2 mAb. The following antibodies were used: anti-mouse CD11b (M1–70), anti-mouse Ly-6B.2 (7/4), anti-mouse CD117 (2B8), anti-mouse F4/80 (BM8), anti-human CD11b (ICRF44 and D12), anti-human CD11b (active epitope) (CBRM1/5), anti-human CD14 (61D3), anti-human CD16 (3G8), anti-human CD62L (DREG56). Antibodies were purchased from BD Biosciences Pharmingen (San Diego, CA) or eBioscience (San Diego, CA). In some assays PMNs were stimulated with 25 nM phorbol myristate acetate (PMA; Sigma) for 5, 10 and 15 min prior to the staining. Data were acquired using a FACSCalibur (Becton-Dickinson, Mountain View, CA) and analyzed using FlowJo software, version 7.6 (TreeStar, Ashland, OR).

Phagocytosis assays

CD11b-mediated phagocytosis was performed using human and murine cells and using three types of iC3b-coated particles: mouse apoptotic thymocytes, guinea pig red blood cells (gRBCs) and fluoresbrite® carboxylate YG 1.5 µm microspheres. Apoptotic thymocytes and gRBCs (TCS Biosciences, Buckingham, UK) were washed three times in PBS/1%BSA and then resuspended to 1%v/v in PBS. These cell suspensions were incubated with pHrodo^{TM} Dye Succinimidyl Ester (1 µg/ml, Life Technologies, Grand Island, NY) for 30 minutes at room temperature. After three washes the cells were opsonised with mouse C5-deficient serum at 37°C for 30 mins (gRBCs-miC3b) and resuspended to 1%v/v in culture medium. Fluoresbrite® carboxylate microspheres (Polysciences Inc, Warrington, PA) were resuspended (1/200) in Krebs' Ringers PBS-Glucose buffer with human iC3b (20 µg/ml, Complement Technology Inc, USA) and incubated at 37°C for 30 mins. Human iC3b-coated beads were then washed with PBS/1%BSA/EDTA and resuspended in culture medium (1/400). For all experimental protocols the level of iC3b-opsonisation was checked by flow cytometry using a biotinylated polyclonal antibody that recognises human and mouse C3 fragments (Clone: 6C9, Cedarlane Labs, Ontario, Canada) followed by streptavidin-PE (BD Biosciences Pharmingen). In each phagocytic assay complement-opsonised particles were fed at a 10:1 ratio to DCs (0.7×10^5 cells/well), macrophages (1×10^5 cells/well), PMNs (2×10^5 cells/well) or monocytes (2×10^5 cells/well) in U-bottom wells. Cells were collected at different time points as indicated in the result section and the uptake quantified by flow cytometry. Phagocytosis was calculated as % of cells that had internalised the iC3b-coated particles. Non-opsonised particles were used as negative controls. In selective experiments phagocytosis was visualised using ImageStream (Amnis, Seattle, WA). The data obtained were analyzed using the ImageStream Data Exploration and Analysis Software (IDEAS, Amnis). Single focused cells were gated by area aspect ratio followed by gradient root mean square of the brightfield image.

PMN – functional assays

Freshly isolated PMNs were assessed in several functional assays:

i) **Rosetting.** Guinea pig RBCs were labelled with carboxyfluorescein diacetatesuccinimidyl ester (CFSE) as described previously [28]. Different amounts of mouse or human iC3b was deposited on the gRBCs by using increasing dilution of mouse or human C5-deficient serum respectively. Freshly isolated PMNs were washed and resupended in 1 mM Mg^{2+}/1 mM Ca^{2+} buffer and incubated with gRBCs-iC3b for 30 min at 4°C with gentle shaking. Rosetting was assessed by flow cytometry and on slide (at least 200 PMNs analysed). PMN binding ≥3 RBCs was recorded as a single rosette.

ii) **Adhesion assays.** Adhesion was measured by coating Immunolon plates with fibrinogen (10 µg/ml). Plates were blocked with PBS 1% BSA for 3 hr at room temperature. Freshly isolated PMNs were then added (2×10^5 cells/well) and incubated for 90 min at 37°C. Cells were gently washed with Opti-MEM medium and adhesion assessed by staining the adherent cells with crystal violet.

iii) **Oxidative burst.** Production of reactive oxygen species (ROS) was studied by loading PMNs (10^5 cells/ml) with 2′, 7′-dichlorodihydrofluorescin diacetate (DCFH-DA) (Sigma) (5 µM) for 30 min at 37°C. After stimulation with PMA (25 nM) for 30 min at 37°C, the increase in ROS production was measured by flow cytometry.

iv) **Neutrophil extracellular traps (NETs).** PMNs seeded at 10^5 cells/well in complete medium (DMEM 10% v/v FCS, 2 mM L-Glutamine, Penicillin/Streptomycin without phenol red) were stimulated with 25 nM PMA (final concentration) for 3 hours. Quantification was performed as described previously [29].

v) **In vitro chemotaxis assay.** Chemotaxis assays were performed as before [25]. Briefly, transwells (3 µm polycarbonate membrane, 6.5-mm-diameter wells; Costar, Corning, NY, USA), pre-treated with 2% (w/v) gelatin (porcine skin type A; Sigma) were seeded with mouse microvascular endothelial cells (3×10^4/transwell) (kindly donated by Prof F. Marelli-Berg, Imperial College London) [30] or human umbilical vein endothelial cells (HUVEC) (3×10^4/transwell). After overnight culture, transwells were washed, recombinant murine macrophage inflammatory protein (MIP)-2 (PeproTech) was added to the bottom chamber at a final concentration of 1 nM and 5×10^5 neutrophils (murine neutrophil cell lines or freshly isolated human PMNs) were added to the top chamber. At different time points (from 30 to 120 minutes) cells were collected from the bottom chamber for analysis. The number and the viability of migrated cells were assessed by flow cytometry by adding counting beads (Life Technologies) and by staining the cells with propidium iodide.

vi) **In vivo adoptive transfer model.** *In-vitro*-differentiated *Itgam$^{-/-}$* murine neutrophils reconstituted with one of the human CD11b variants (mCD18/hCD11b-77R or mCD18/hCD11b-77H) were labelled with either 1 µM Cell Trace dodecyldimethylamine oxide succinimidyl ester (DDAO) (Life Technologies) or 250 nM CFSE (Life Technologies). DDAO- and CFSE-labelled neutrophils (5×10^6 of each type) were mixed in a 1:1 ratio in PBS and injected i.v. into C57BL/6 mice. This was immediately followed by an i.p. injection of 4% thioglycollate broth (0.4 ml/mice, Sigma) or 330 nM MIP-2 (0.2 ml/mice, PeproTech). PBS injection was used as control. Two hrs after MIP-2 injection and 4 hours after the thioglycollate injection, the mice were sacrificed and the peritoneal cells were recovered by lavage with 5 ml of cold 5 mM EDTA in HBSS. Total cell counts and differential analyses were performed by flow cytometry.

Cytokine assays

Monocytes (2×10^5 cells/well) and DCs (0.7×10^5 cells/well) were incubated with iC3b-coated particles alone (gRBCs-miC3b or hiC3b-coated beads). Non-opsonised particles and medium were used as controls. In separate wells cells were pre-incubated for 1 hr with hiC3b-coated beads and then stimulated with R848 (Life

Technologies) (2 µg/ml or 10 µg/ml accordingly to the cell type). Supernatants were collected after 24 hrs and frozen until analysis. Cytokine levels were measured with a bead multiplex assay (eBioscience) according to the manufacturer's instructions. IL-1β, IL-6, IL-10, IP-10, TNF-α were measured. Results were analysed in two ways: i) the difference in cytokine production (expressed as absolute value) between samples pre-incubated with coated particles to samples pre-incubated with uncoated particle or medium (as indicated in the figure legends) and ii) as % of change induced by iC3b coated particle compared to medium or uncoated particle. Both analyses gave statistically similar findings.

Statistics

Data are expressed as mean+/−SEM. Statistical analysis was performed using GraphPad Prism version 3.0 (GraphPad Software, San Diego, CA). Unless otherwise stated, data from *in vitro* assays were analysed by two-tailed Student's t-test for paired samples. One-way analysis of variance with Bonferroni's multiple comparison tests were applied for analysis of multiple groups. Differences were considered significant for p values<0.05.

Results

The lupus CD11b variant (77H) does not affect CD11b cell surface expression

Due to the rarity of the minor allele (77H), the vast majority of SLE patients are heterozygous (77R/H) and not homozygous for the risk allele [11]. As a consequence, we elected to compare healthy subjects that were homozygous for the non-risk allele (77R/R) with healthy individuals carrying the risk allele in heterozygosity (77R/H). However, for each assay we also extended the analysis to three individuals that were homozygous for the risk allele (77H/H). We did not detect any obvious differences in these assays between 77R/H and the three 77H/H samples. Therefore in representing our data we pooled the findings obtained from the homozygous 77H/H and heterozygous 77R/H individuals (77R/H-77H/H).

We initially assessed whether the 77H variant influenced CD11b cell surface expression on resting cells. We measured CD11b expression on PMNs, monocytes, macrophages and DCs by flow cytometry using the ICRF44 antibody. Though the CD11b expression varied among individuals there was no genotype-specific difference (figure 1A). Similarly the analysis of the active high affinity state of CD11b with the CBRM1/5 antibody failed to reveal any significant difference between the 77R/H and the 77R individuals (figure 1B). We also assessed how quickly the two CD11b variants changed conformational state in response to stimuli by performing a time course experiment with PMNs activated with PMA (25 nM). The response of 77R/H PMNs was similar to that of 77R/R PMNs (figure S1).

The CD11b risk allele leads to a defective uptake of complement-coated particles without altering the binding affinity for iC3b

CR3 is known to mediate phagocytosis of complement opsonised microorganisms. We investigated whether the SLE-associated allele affected this CR3-mediated function using two different particles: gRBCs-miC3b and hiC3b-coated beads. The use of gRBCs opsonised with mouse iC3b is likely to reduce the strength of the receptor-ligand interaction allowing the detection of subtle abnormalities, whilst the use of hiC3b-coated beads minimises the confounding contribution of other phagocytic mechanisms as the particles do not have other molecules expressed on their surface and cannot release intracellular components. gRBCs-miC3b were labelled with pHrodo that changes colour when the particles are fused with the lysosome allowing us to selectively quantify engulfed particles. In the assay with hiC3b-coated bead ImageStream was used to confirm that the vast majority (approximately 98%) of the positive cells had engulfed at least one bead (data not shown). Using both iC3b-coated particles we found that phagocytosis by 77R/H cells (macrophages, PMNs and monocytes) was significantly less compared to the uptake by the corresponding 77R/R cells (figure 2 and figure S2). The mean values were statistically significant if the data were analysed as either as percentage phagocytosis (figure 2) or as percentage difference to 77R/R cells standardised to 100% in each assay (macrophages after 30 min: 77R/R 100 vs 77R/H-77H/H 80.5+/−5.8, p=0.0054, 13 pairs; PMN after 15 minutes: 77R/R 100 vs 77R/H-77H/H 83.9+/−4.5, p=0.0039, 13 pairs; monocytes after 18 hrs: 77R/R 100 vs 77R/H-77H/H 90.0+/−3.6, p=0.0315, 7 pairs). However, no genotype-specific defect in phagocytosis was detected using DCs (% of phagocytosis after 1 hour: 100 in 77R/R vs 161.0+/−28.0 in 77R/H-77H/H individuals, p=0.0608, 9 pairs).

Although *in silico* models indicate that the iC3b binding takes place in the I domain and the 77R/H polymorphism is unlikely to affect this binding site, we explored whether the differences observed in phagocytosis were the result of different binding to CR3. To address this issue in the most physiological *ex-vivo* setting we used the traditional rosetting binding assay. Using this assay we confirmed that the R77H polymorphism does not alter the binding affinity for iC3b, at least on PMNs (figure 3). We also analysed the adhesion of 77R/R and 77R/H-77H/H PMNs to plates coated with fibrinogen and detected no differences between the two genotypes (data not shown).

To circumvent all the technical limitations of using *ex-vivo* human cells and to confirm that the impaired phagocytosis was indeed specific to the R77H polymorphism and not due to another independent variant(s) within the *ITGAM* gene or a gene closely linked (e.g. *ITGAX*), we generated conditional-Hoxb8 immortalized myeloid precursors from CD11b-deficient mice and transduced them with either the 77R or 77H human CD11b variant. The CD11b-transfected precursors were then matured into fully differentiated macrophages or PMNs using the appropriate conditional media [25,27]. Importantly, the immortalized cell lines had similar cell surface expression of the hybrid CR3 molecule (mCD18/hCD11b-77R or mCD18/hCD11b-77H) (figure S3A). We then performed the same phagocytic and binding assays applied to the human cells. The uptake of pHrodo loaded gRBCs-miC3b by (mCD18/hCD11b-77H)-expressing macrophages was significantly reduced compared to the engulfment by (mCD18/hCD11b-77R)-expressing macrophages (p=0.0256), mirroring the data obtained with the human cells (figure S3B). A similar phagocytic defect was observed using opsonised apoptotic cells, whilst the clearance of non-opsonised cells was not affected by the expression of CD11b suggesting the engagement of other receptors (figure S3C). Consistent with the findings with *ex-vivo* human PMNs no differences were detected in the percentage of gRBC-hiC3b bound to the immortalised neutrophil cell lines expressing the hybrid CR3 molecules (figure S3D).

In vivo and in vitro migration of neutrophils is not affected by the 77R/H CD11b polymorphism

Given the technical hurdle of comparing resting neutrophils isolated from different individuals we elected to use the immortalised neutrophil cell lines to investigate whether the 77H

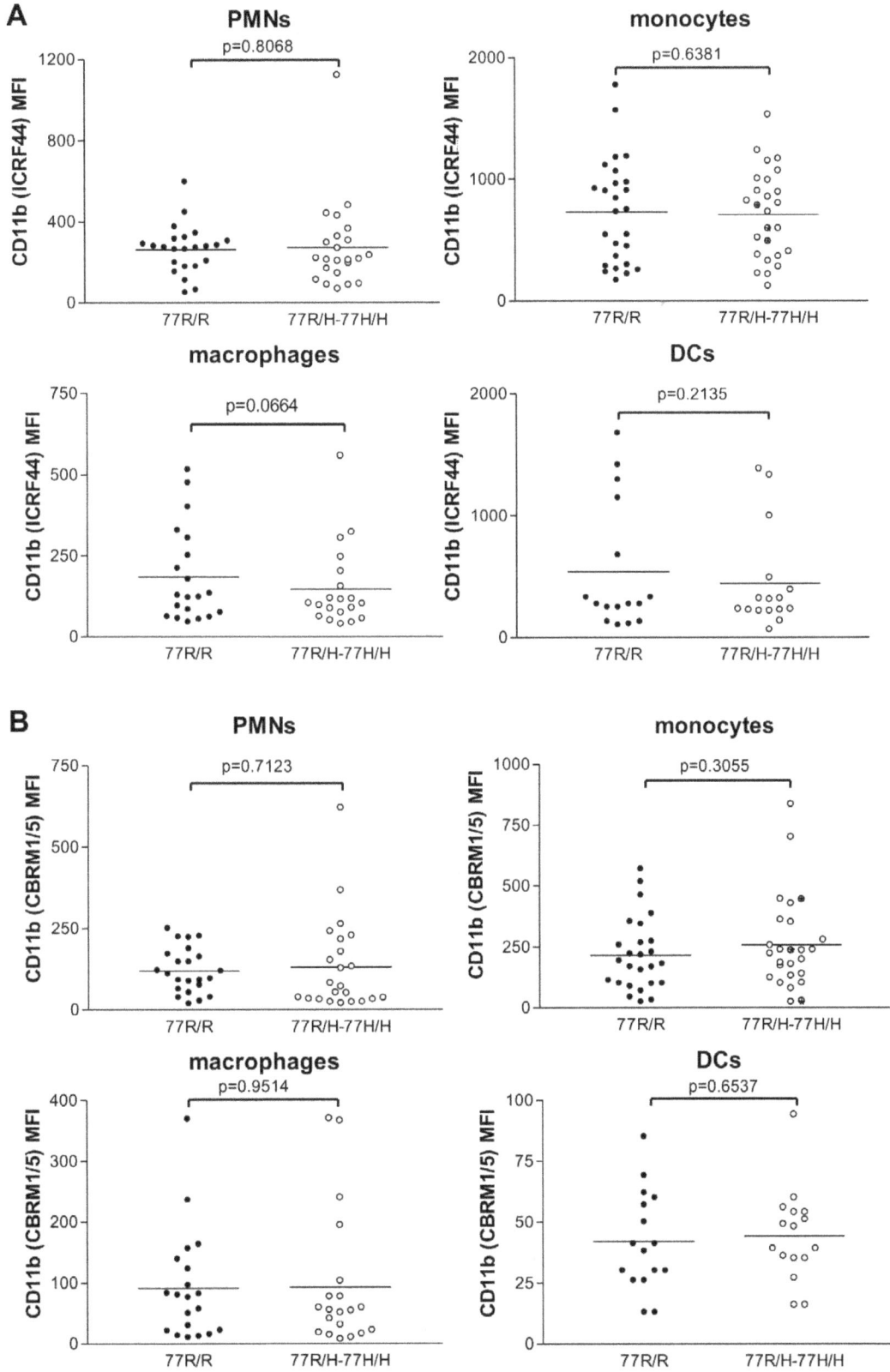

Figure 1. Cell surface expression of CD11b on different cell populations. The expression was quantified by flow cytometry using ICRF44 (A) and CBRM1/5 (B) antibodies. The latter only recognises the headpiece of CD11b in its active state. Data are presented in mean fluorescence intensity (MFI), closed symbols 77R/R donors, open symbols 77R/H-77H/H donors. The two groups were not statistically different. Bars indicate means.

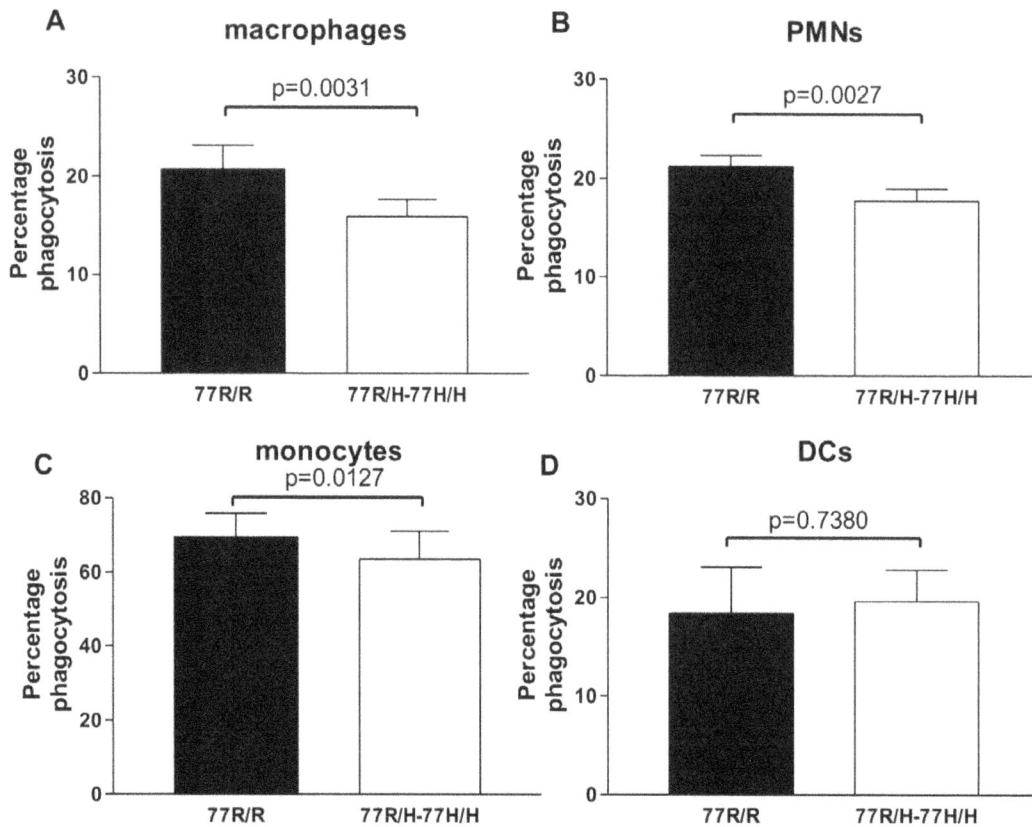

Figure 2. Phagocytosis of hiC3b-coated fluorescent beads. The uptake by macrophages (A), PMNs (B), monocytes (C) and DCs (D) was quantified by flow cytometry and the data are represented as percentage of phagocytosis. Data are expressed as mean+/−SEM. Filled columns 77R/R individuals, open columns 77R/H-77H/H individuals. Paired T test was applied and the p values are indicated.

variant altered the ability of PMNs to migrate through an endothelium layer. We initially measured the migration through a mouse endothelium layer in response to MIP-2 using a transwell assay and found no differences between the CD11b-deficient *in vitro*-derived neutrophils reconstituted with either of the two hybrid CR3 molecules (figure 4A). As previously reported [25], the

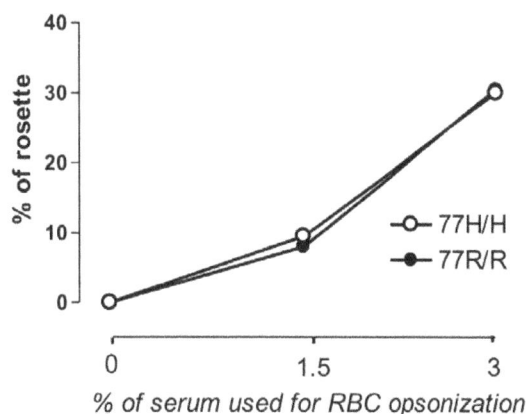

Figure 3. Rosetting assay. Percentage of rosettes formed by CFSE-labelled RBC-hiC3b with freshly isolated PMNs from donors carrying the susceptible allele (77H/H, open symbol) or the common allele (77R/R, closed symbol). One representative assay out of 3 independent experiments.

CD11b-deficient PMNs, used as negative controls, showed an accelerated migration compared to the wild type PMNs. In keeping with these findings we observed no genotype-specific differences in the number of freshly isolated human neutrophils migrating through a HUVEC layer in response to MIP-2 (figure 4B). As the transmigration assays were performed under static conditions, we adopted a previously described peritonitis model [25] to evaluate the behaviour of the cells *in vivo*. The *in vitro* differentiated PMN cell lines expressing the 77H or 77R CD11b variant were labelled with DDAO or CFSE and co-injected i.v. at a 1:1 ratio into wild type C57BL/6 mice. Immediately after the adoptive transfer, inflammation was induced in the peritoneum either with thioglycollate or MIP-2 injected i.p. and the number of DDAO- and CFSE-labelled neutrophils elicited into the peritoneum assessed by flow cytometry at different time points. Using this *in vivo* migration assay we found that the same number of (mCD18/hCD11b-77R)- and (mCD18/hCD11b-77H)-expressing PMNs accumulated in the peritoneum irrespective of the inflammatory stimuli applied (figure 4C, 4D). As predicted the presence of the hybrid CR3 molecule, regardless of the CD11b variant transduced, decreased the number of PMNs in the peritoneum compared to that of the PMN cell line lacking CD11b (data not shown) confirming that an interaction between the hybrid mCD18/hCD11b molecule and mouse endothelium had occurred. No labelled neutrophils were recovered from the peritoneal lavage of animals injected with PBS. We also explored other typical PMN functions: R77H polymorphism failed to alter the oxidative burst and netosis of PMNs after stimulation with PMA (data not shown).

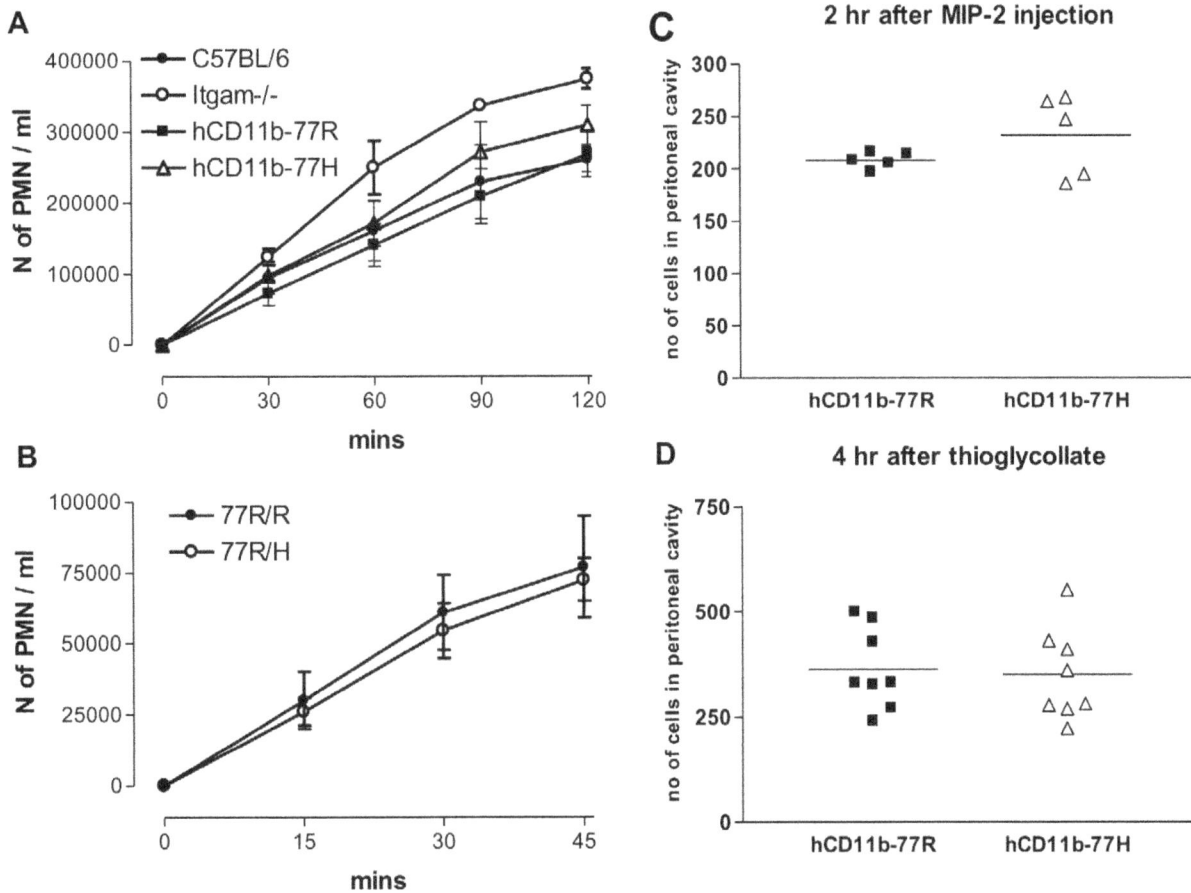

Figure 4. *In vitro* and *in vivo* PMN migration. (A) Migration of neutrophil cell lines through transwells seeded with mouse endothelial cells. PMNs migrated into the bottom chamber in response to MIP-2 were counted at different time points as indicated. Pooled results from at least 4 independent experiments are presented as mean ± SEM. *Itgam−/−* and wild type C57BL/6 neutrophil cell lines were used as controls. CD11b-deficient PMNs, known to have weaker endothelial interactions, migrated faster than the C57BL/6 and the hCD11b expressing cell lines (p<0.001 at 60 mns and p<0.05 at 90 mns). Statistical analysis by Bonferroni's multiple comparison test. (B) Time course of the migration of freshly isolated human 77R/R or 77R/H neutrophils through a HUVEC layer in response to MIP-2. Pooled results from at least 4 independent experiments are presented as mean ± SEM. (C, D) In vivo peritoneal migration of hCD11b-77R and hCD11b-77H PMN cells lines following i.p. injection of MIP-2 (C) and thioglycollate (D). The two hCD11b expressing PMN lines were labelled with DDAO or CFSE and adoptive transferred at a 1:1 ratio into C57BL/6 mice. Absolute numbers of labelled PMNs recovered from the peritoneum are shown. Data of one out of at least 3 independent experiments are presented. Bars indicate means.

Modulation of cytokine secretion

There is evidence in the literature that CR3 can alter the cytokine production by TLR-stimulated monocytes/macrophages and DCs [31–35]. More recently the R77H CD11b polymorphism has been shown to induce a different inhibitor effect on the TLR7/8-mediated pro-inflammatory cytokine release by monocytes [18]. We initially measured the cytokine secretion (IL-6, IL-10, TNF-α, IP-10 and IL-1β) by monocytes and DCs after TLR7/8 stimulation. The CD11b genotype did not influence the cytokine response (figure 5A and 5B). We also analysed the cytokine production after overnight stimulation with beads or hiC3b-coated beads. Neither of them induced detectable cytokines demonstrating no endotoxin contamination (data not shown). We then investigated whether the 77R/H monocytes and DCs down-regulated less efficiently the pro-inflammatory response induced by TLR7/8 activation as recently reported [18]. To this end, we compared the cytokine production with/without pre-incubation with hiC3b-coated beads and analysed the difference between the two samples. In DCs the pre-incubation with hiC3b-coated beads induced a strong up-regulation of IL-10 and TNF-α with a modest

down-modulation of IL-6 (figure 5D). The effect on IP-10 was barely detectable. In monocytes, the pre-incubation with hiC3b-coated particles resulted in a small increase of IL-10, a decrease in TNF-α, whilst IL-6 and IP-10 remained largely unchanged. The changes in IL-1β secretion were variable (figure 5C). More importantly, in both cell types we found no statistically significant differences between the two CD11b variants in the cytokine modulation by iC3b-coated particles after TLR7/8 stimulation. In selected experiments we also used iC3b-gRBCs to mirror more closely the experimental conditions used by Rhodes et al [18]. Although we observed a slightly different cytokine pattern with a stronger effect on IL-1β secretion, we failed to identify a genotype-specific difference in monocyte cytokine responses (figure S4). Similarly CR3 ligation by hiC3b-coated particles modified the TLR9-mediated pro-inflammatory cytokine released by monocytes but the effect was not modulated by the CD11b genotype (data not shown).

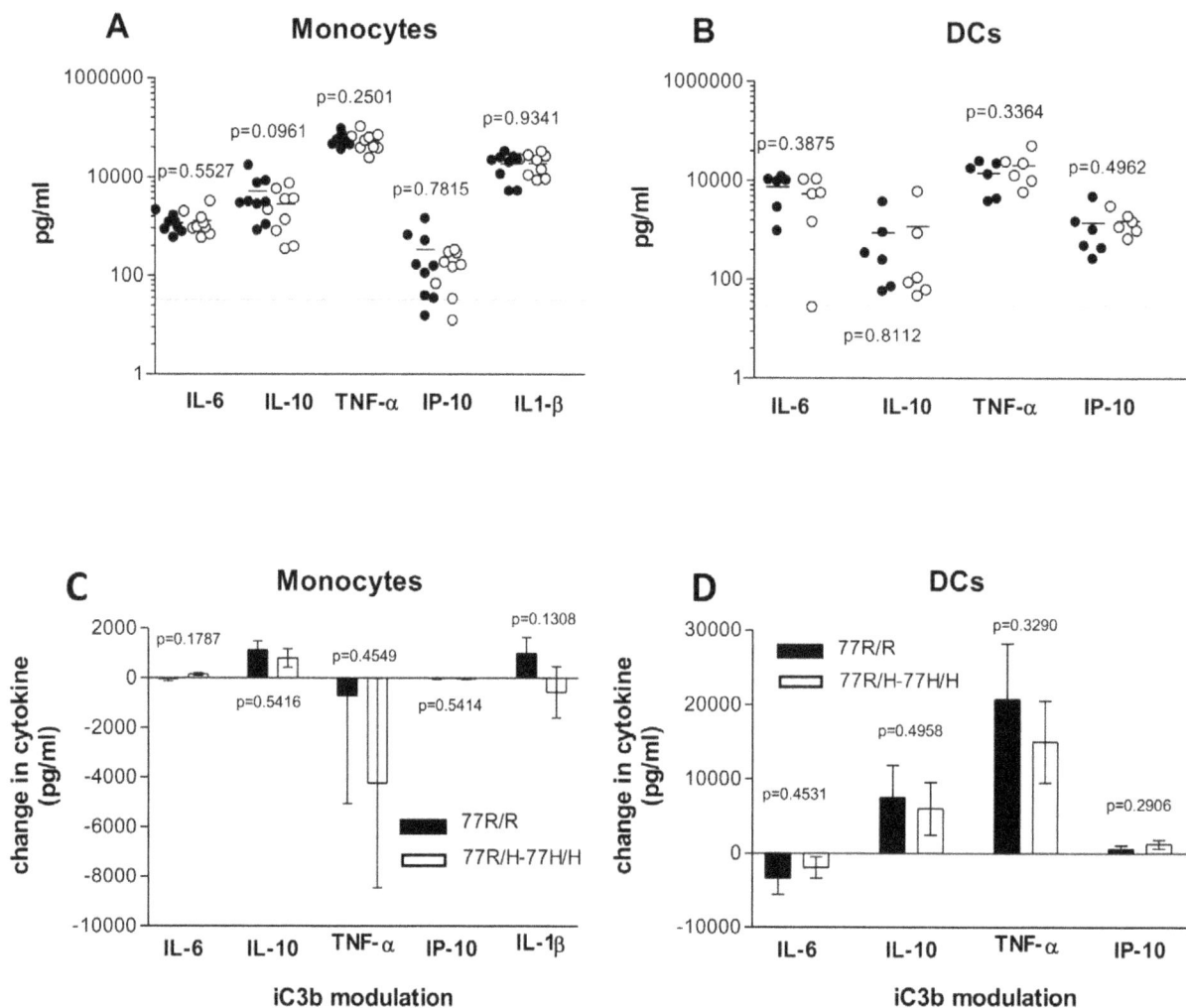

Figure 5. Cytokine response. Monocytes (A), DCs (B) were stimulated with 2 μg/ml and 10 μg/ml of TLR7/8 ligand (R848) respectively for 24 h. Cytokines quantified using a bead multiplex assay. Closed symbols: 77R/R cells, open symbols: 77R/H-77H/H cells. Each dot represents a single individual, bars denote means. No significant differences between the two CD11b genotypes. Statistical analysis by paired t test. (C, D) Modulation of TLR7/8-induced cytokine release by hiC3b-coated beads. Monocytes (C), DCs (D) were fed with hiC3b-coated beads one hour prior to R848 stimulation. The cytokine changes between the samples with and without CR3 pre-engagement with iC3b are shown with the p values indicated. Data are expressed as mean+/−SEM. The cytokine responses of 77R/R cells (black column) and 77R/H-77H/H cells (white columns) were not statistically different in paired assays. IL, interleukin; TNF-α, tumour necrosis factor alpha; IP-10, Interferon gamma-induced protein 10.

Discussion

Several genes that exert their effect through relatively common allelic variants have been shown to be associated with SLE by GWA studies [9,10,36–41] One of most prominent susceptibility factors for SLE was found to be a SNP (rs1143679) which confers the R77H amino acid substitution in CD11b. The functional effects of this variant remains elusive. By using a broad approach (*ex-vivo* human cells and immortalized PMN and macrophage lines expressing the hCD11b variants) and by analysing the main human CR3 expressing cells (monocytes, neutrophils, macrophages and DCs) herein we demonstrate that in these cells the lupus susceptibility allele (77H) impairs only the uptake of hiC3b-coated targets without altering other CR3-mediated functions including TLR7/8-induced cytokine secretion and neutrophil extravasation. These findings highlight the importance of minor functional changes in genes controlling waste disposal mechanisms in lupus pathogenesis.

Two recent reports have suggested that the CD11b lupus risk allele causes an impaired adhesion/phagocytosis and abnormal cytokine modulation after TLR7/8 stimulation in monocytes [17,18]. In both studies the function of the risk allele was compared to the non-risk allele using transfected cell lines or homozygous individuals. However, as the lupus risk allele has a frequency of only 9–11% in populations of European and African descent [9–11], with a much lower frequency (<0.01) in Asian Populations [39], the vast majority of the SLE patients are heterozygous for the rs1143679 SNP: approximately 27% are 77R/H compared to ~3% 77H/H. Assuming a codominant model the odds ratio was significantly increased for both the 77R/H (1.63) and the 77H/H (4.64) genotypes [11]. Therefore in our study we have deliberately elected to analyse healthy 77R/H individuals as they mirror more closely the disease population. In all the assays with *ex-vivo* human cells we have also included in the analysis 3 homozygous 77H/H individuals whose cells consistently behaved like the 77R/H cells showing that a single 77H allele was sufficient to induce the cellular abnormalities detected. Therefore, though we recognise that by adopting this approach some subtle differences between the two CD11b variants might have been overlooked, we think that our data mirror more realistically the modest magnitude of risk carried by the 77H Cd11b variant.

It has been postulated that lupus patients might have higher surface expression of CD11b resulting in an increased cellular infiltrate and amplified inflammation [41–43]. Consistent with the findings reported by Rhodes et al [18] we failed to detect any obvious difference between 77R/R and 77R/H-77H/H individuals in the surface expression of CD11b including its active form assessed by the CBRM1/5 antibody.

The position of the 77R/H polymorphism in the beta-propeller domain predicts that it is unlikely to affect the iC3b binding site [11,44]. In keeping with this prediction we found no defects in the binding of 77H PMNs to iC3b-RBC in the rosetting assay [15,18]. We observed, however, a significant reduction in the uptake of iC3b-coated targets (gRBC and beads) by neutrophils indicating that phagocytosis is not simply a function of ligand/receptor interaction, but entails several subsequent events in which CR3 may play a role. Not surprisingly the impaired phagocytosis was also detected in 77R/H monocytes and macrophages but not in immature DCs. We confirmed the specificity of the effect for the 77H variant using stably genetically-modified *in vitro*-derived macrophage lines lacking CD11b or expressing variant-specific CD11b molecules. Using the allele-specific macrophage cell lines we were able to show that the lupus-associated 77H allele impaired also the phagocytosis of iC3b-coated apoptotic cells, a defect seen in macrophages from lupus patients [45,46]. Overall our data not only provide further support to previous reports linking the 77H variant to impaired phagocytosis [17,18] but significantly expand previous observations by demonstrating that the impaired phagocytosis associated with the 77H CD11b variant is not macrophage-restricted.

CR3 is known to bind a large range of ligands and to contribute to leukocyte extravasation. Previous reports [17,18] have shown that the lupus CD11b allele reduces cell adhesion to several CR3 ligands, including ICAM-1, under static and/or flow conditions. However, these data, obtained in part with transfected cells [17], are hard to reconcile with the clinical observations of hypercellularity present in injured tissue. To circumvent some of the limitations of the previous assays we applied a novel *in vivo* adoptive transfer approach [25]. We found no genotype-specific difference in the migration of PMNs under two distinct inflammatory stimuli casting doubts on some of the previous findings [17,18] and demonstrating that the 77H allele is unlikely to affect this CR3-mediated pathway.

There is a growing body of evidence demonstrating that engagement of CD11b can mediate both positive and negative regulation of TLR signalling with contradictory results accordingly to the experimental conditions applied [31,32,34,47–49]. Under our experimental conditions we could not replicate the genotype-specific difference in the cytokine responses induced by TLR7/8 stimulation after CR3 ligation recently reported by Rhodes et al. in monocytes [18]. In our assay pre-incubation of monocytes with hiC3b-coated beads had a less striking effect on the TLR7/8-induced cytokine release compared to that reported [18] with just an appreciable, though variable, inhibitory effect on TNF-α production. However, regardless of the degree of cytokine inhibition, the 77H variant did not affect the cytokine response. Though we recognise that the use of 77R/H cells could have masked a potential difference, most likely the explanation for the discrepancy between the studies lies in the different hiC3b-coated targets used. We deliberately avoided using sheep RBCs for two

main reasons: i) sheep RBCs require opsonisation with rabbit anti-sheep erythrocyte IgM and human serum, both potential source of contaminants causing non-specific interactions/effects; ii) RBCs can release several molecules including haemoglobin that is known to bind to CD163 on monocytes/macrophages dampening the inflammatory response [50–52]. Consistent with the explanation that, at least to a certain degree, the CR3-mediated inhibitor effect on the TLR7/8-induced pro-inflammatory cytokine was due to the use of the RBCs, we observed a much stronger IL-1β inhibition when we pre-incubated the monocytes with gRBC-iC3b. However, we used guinea pig red blood cells that do not require opsonisation with IgM for complement activation and our cytokine pattern did not entirely replicate the one reported by Rhodes et al. Interestingly in DCs we observed a marked synergistic positive effect on IL-10 and TNF-α secretion that was again comparable between 77R/R and 77R/H cells. Therefore CR3 may well act as an important regulator of several TLR signalling pathways including the TLR7/8 but the effect does not appears to be influenced by the R77H amino acid substitution.

In summary our observations demonstrate that the CD11b lupus-associated variant leads to an impaired phagocytosis of complement-opsonised targets, including apoptotic cells, by monocytes/macrophages and PMNs. A reduced clearance of iC3b-coated targets might lead to increased tissue damage and inflammation, providing a plausible explanation for the genetic linkage identified by GWA studies. CR3 may also interact with the Fc receptors on the surface of neutrophils/macrophages modulating the effect of immune complex binding and this cross-talk warrants further analysis. However, one should not ignore the fact that CR3 is also expressed on NK and a subset of B cells, cell types that have recently shown to contribute to SLE pathogenesis [53–55] and the effect of the lupus CD11b allele on these cells remains to be examined.

Supporting Information

Figure S1   Fold increase expression of CD11b on PMNs after PMA stimulation. Cell surface expression of CD11b was assessed by flow cytometry using two antibodies: ICRF44 and CBRM1/5 (active state). Closed symbols indicate the 77R/R donors, open symbols the 77R/H-77H/H donors. Data were normalised to the MFI of the respective unstimulated PMN. Pooled results from 3 experiments are presented as mean of fold increase ± SEM.

Figure S2   Phagocytosis of gRBCs-miC3b. Uptake by macrophages (A) and PMNs (B) carrying one of the two CD11b variants (77R/R closed columns, 77R/H-77H/H open columns). gRBCs were labelled with pHrodo and the uptake was quantified by flow cytometry. The data are represented as percentage of phagocytosis (macrophages:18 pairs; PMN: 13 pairs). Data are expressed as mean+/−SEM. Statistical analysis by paired T test.

Figure S3   Assays with *Itgam*[−/−] cell lines reconstituted with a hybrid CR3 molecule (mCD18/hCD11b-77R or mCD18/hCD11b-77H). (A) Cell-surface expression of the hybrid molecules quantified by flow cytometry using an anti-human CD11b antibody (ICRF44). Data are presented for macrophages and PMNs. Dotted line: CD11b-deficient cells transduced with an empty vector; solid line: mCD18/hCD11b-77R cells; dashed line: mCD18/hCD11b-77H; shaded histogram: cells derived from wild type C57BL/6 mice. (B) Engulfment of pHrodo-loaded gRBC opsonised with miC3b. The percentage of phagocytosis was determined by flow cytometry at one hour time point. A significant difference between the two macrophage lines expressing the hybrid CR3 molecule was detected (p = 0.0256). The parental CD11b-deficient macrophages were used as negative control to confirm the specificity for CR3 of the assay. Bars indicate means. (C) Phagocytosis of opsonised (black column) or non opsonised (empty column) pHrodo labelled murine apoptotic thymocytes. The percentage of phagocytosis was determined by flow cytometry at one hour time point. Pooled data of 5 independent experiments. Data were normalised to the C57BL/ 6 cell line and are expressed as mean+/−SEM. Statistical analysis by paired T test. (D) Rosetting assay with CFSE-labelled gRBC-hiC3b. Percentage of neutrophils bound to CFSE-labelled gRBCs was measured by flow cytometry. Square symbols: mCD18/ hCD11b-77R; triangle symbols: mCD18/hCD11b-77H; circle symbols: wild type C57BL/6 neutrophils.

Figure S4 Cytokine response. Modulation of TLR7/8-induced cytokine release by iC3b-gRBC. Monocytes were fed with iC3b-gRBC or gRBC one hour prior to R848 stimulation.

The cytokine changes between the samples with and without CR3 pre-engagement are shown with the p values indicated. Data are expressed as mean+/−SEM. The cytokine responses of 77R/R cells (black column) and 77R/H-77H/H cells (white columns) were not statistically different in paired assays. IL, interleukin; TNF-α, tumour necrosis factor alpha; IP-10, Interferon gamma-induced protein 10.

Acknowledgments

We thank M Patel and K Vernon for their technical help. We are also grateful to M Whyte for advice on isolating human PMNs and to F. Marelli-Berg for providing the mouse microvascular endothelial cells.

Author Contributions

Critically reviewed manuscript: PRT HTC MCP.. Conceived and designed the experiments: MB HTC PRT LFJ GSL. Performed the experiments: LFJ GSL AC MS JUM THM. Analyzed the data: LFJ GSL MB AC MCP. Contributed reagents/materials/analysis tools: MCP PRT JUM. Wrote the paper: LFJ MB GSL.

References

1. Beller DI, Springer TA, Schreiber RD (1982) Anti-Mac-1 selectively inhibits the mouse and human type three complement receptor. J Exp Med 156: 1000–1009.
2. Diamond MS, Staunton DE, de Fougerolles AR, Stacker SA, Garcia-Aguilar J, et al. (1990) ICAM-1 (CD54): a counter-receptor for Mac-1 (CD11b/CD18). J Cell Biol 111: 3129–3139.
3. Wright SD, Weitz JI, Huang AJ, Levin SM, Silverstein SC, et al. (1988) Complement receptor type three (CD11b/CD18) of human polymorphonuclear leukocytes recognizes fibrinogen. Proc Natl Acad Sci U S A 85: 7734–7738.
4. Orlova VV, Choi EY, Xie CP, Chavakis E, Bierhaus A, et al. (2007) A novel pathway of HMGB1-mediated inflammatory cell recruitment that requires Mac-1-integrin. Embo Journal 26: 1129–1139.
5. Wright SD, Jong MT (1986) Adhesion-promoting receptors on human macrophages recognize Escherichia coli by binding to lipopolysaccharide. J Exp Med 164: 1876–1888.
6. Arnaout MA (1990) Leukocyte adhesion molecules deficiency: its structural basis, pathophysiology and implications for modulating the inflammatory response. Immunol Rev 114: 145–180.
7. Springer TA (1990) Adhesion receptors of the immune system. Nature 346: 425–434.
8. Ehirchiou D, Xiong Y, Xu G, Chen W, Shi Y, et al. (2007) CD11b facilitates the development of peripheral tolerance by suppressing Th17 differentiation. J Exp Med 204: 1519–1524.
9. Harley JB, Alarcon-Riquelme ME, Criswell LA, Jacob CO, Kimberly RP, et al. (2008) Genome-wide association scan in women with systemic lupus erythematosus identifies susceptibility variants in ITGAM, PXK, KIAA1542 and other loci. Nat Genet 40: 204–210.
10. Hom G, Graham RR, Modrek B, Taylor KE, Ortmann W, et al. (2008) Association of systemic lupus erythematosus with C8orf13-BLK and ITGAM-ITGAX. N Engl J Med 358: 900–909.
11. Nath SK, Han S, Kim-Howard X, Kelly JA, Viswanathan P, et al. (2008) A nonsynonymous functional variant in integrin-alpha(M) (encoded by ITGAM) is associated with systemic lupus erythematosus. Nat Genet 40: 152–154.
12. Anaya JM, Kim-Howard X, Prahalad S, Chernavsky A, Canas C, et al. (2012) Evaluation of genetic association between an ITGAM non-synonymous SNP (rs1143679) and multiple autoimmune diseases. Autoimmun Rev 11: 276–280.
13. Han S, Kim-Howard X, Deshmukh H, Kamatani Y, Viswanathan P, et al. (2009) Evaluation of imputation-based association in and around the integrin-alpha-M (ITGAM) gene and replication of robust association between a non-synonymous functional variant within ITGAM and systemic lupus erythematosus (SLE). Hum Mol Genet 18: 1171–1180.
14. Coustet B, Agarwal SK, Gourh P, Guedj M, Mayes MD, et al. (2011) Association Study of ITGAM, ITGAX, and CD58 Autoimmune Risk Loci in Systemic Sclerosis: Results from 2 Large European Caucasian Cohorts. Journal of Rheumatology 38: 1033–1038.
15. Sachs UJ, Chavakis T, Fung L, Lohrenz A, Bux J, et al. (2004) Human alloantibody anti-Mart interferes with Mac-1-dependent leukocyte adhesion. Blood 104: 727–734.
16. Diamond MS, Garcia-Aguilar J, Bickford JK, Corbi AL, Springer TA (1993) The I domain is a major recognition site on the leukocyte integrin Mac-1 (CD11b/CD18) for four distinct adhesion ligands. J Cell Biol 120: 1031–1043.
17. MacPherson M, Lek HS, Prescott A, Fagerholm SC (2011) A systemic lupus erythematosus-associated R77H substitution in the CD11b chain of the Mac-1 integrin compromises leukocyte adhesion and phagocytosis. J Biol Chem 286: 17303–17310.
18. Rhodes B, Furnrohr BG, Roberts AL, Tzircotis G, Schett G, et al. (2012) The rs1143679 (R77H) lupus associated variant of ITGAM (CD11b) impairs complement receptor 3 mediated functions in human monocytes. Ann Rheum Dis.
19. Walport MJ (2000) Lupus, DNase and defective disposal of cellular debris. Nat Genet 25: 135–136.
20. Munoz LE, Gaipl US, Franz S, Sheriff A, Voll RE, et al. (2005) SLE–a disease of clearance deficiency? Rheumatology (Oxford) 44: 1101–1107.
21. Haslett C, Guthrie LA, Kopaniak MM, Johnston RB, Jr., Henson PM (1985) Modulation of multiple neutrophil functions by preparative methods or trace concentrations of bacterial lipopolysaccharide. Am J Pathol 119: 101–110.
22. Wardle DJ, Burgon J, Sabroe I, Bingle CD, Whyte MK, et al. (2011) Effective caspase inhibition blocks neutrophil apoptosis and reveals Mcl-1 as both a regulator and a target of neutrophil caspase activation. PLoS One 6: e15768.
23. Wang L, Gordon RA, Huynh L, Su XD, Min KHP, et al. (2010) Indirect Inhibition of Toll-like Receptor and Type I Interferon Responses by ITAM-Coupled Receptors and Integrins. Immunity 32: 518–530.
24. Coxon A, Rieu P, Barkalow FJ, Askari S, Sharpe AH, et al. (1996) A novel role for the beta 2 integrin CD11b/CD18 in neutrophil apoptosis: A homeostatic mechanism in inflammation. Immunity 5: 653–666.
25. McDonald JU, Cortini A, Rosas M, Fossati-Jimack L, Ling GS, et al. (2011) In vivo functional analysis and genetic modification of in vitro-derived mouse neutrophils. Faseb Journal 25: 1972–1982.
26. Wang GG, Calvo KR, Pasillas MP, Sykes DB, Hacker H, et al. (2006) Quantitative production of macrophages or neutrophils ex vivo using conditional Hoxb8. Nat Methods 3: 287–293.
27. Rosas M, Osorio F, Robinson MJ, Davies LC, Dierkes N, et al. (2011) Hoxb8 conditionally immortalised macrophage lines model inflammatory monocytic cells with important similarity to dendritic cells. European Journal of Immunology 41: 356–365.
28. Norsworthy PJ, Fossati-Jimack L, Cortes-Hernandez J, Taylor PR, Bygrave AE, et al. (2004) Murine CD93 (C1qRp) contributes to the removal of apoptotic cells in vivo but is not required for C1q-mediated enhancement of phagocytosis. Journal of Immunology 172: 3406–3414.
29. Garcia-Romo GS, Caielli S, Vega B, Connolly J, Allantaz F, et al. (2011) Netting neutrophils are major inducers of type I IFN production in pediatric systemic lupus erythematosus. Sci Transl Med 3: 73ra20.
30. Marelli-Berg FM, Peek E, Lidington EA, Stauss HJ, Lechler RI (2000) Isolation of endothelial cells from murine tissue. Journal of Immunological Methods 244: 205–215.
31. Hajishengallis G, Shakhatreh MA, Wang M, Liang S (2007) Complement receptor 3 blockade promotes IL-12-mediated clearance of Porphyromonas gingivalis and negates its virulence in vivo. Journal of Immunology 179: 2359–2367.
32. Huynh L, Wang L, Shi C, Park-Min KH, Ivashkiv LB (2012) ITAM-coupled receptors inhibit IFNAR signaling and alter macrophage responses to TLR4 and Listeria monocytogenes. Journal of Immunology 188: 3447–3457.
33. Behrens EM, Sriram U, Shivers DK, Gallucci M, Ma Z, et al. (2007) Complement receptor 3 ligation of dendritic cells suppresses their stimulatory capacity. Journal of Immunology 178: 6268–6279.
34. Han C, Jin J, Xu S, Liu H, Li N, et al. (2010) Integrin CD11b negatively regulates TLR-triggered inflammatory responses by activating Syk and promoting degradation of MyD88 and TRIF via Cbl-b. Nat Immunol 11: 734–742.

35. Skoberne M, Somersan S, Almodovar W, Truong T, Petrova K, et al. (2006) The apoptotic-cell receptor CR3, but not alphavbeta5, is a regulator of human dendritic-cell immunostimulatory function. Blood 108: 947–955.

36. Kozyrev SV, Abelson AK, Wojcik J, Zaghlool A, Linga Reddy MV, et al. (2008) Functional variants in the B-cell gene BANK1 are associated with systemic lupus erythematosus. Nat Genet 40: 211–216.

37. Graham RR, Cotsapas C, Davies L, Hackett R, Lessard CJ, et al. (2008) Genetic variants near TNFAIP3 on 6q23 are associated with systemic lupus erythematosus. Nat Genet 40: 1059–1061.

38. Gateva V, Sandling JK, Hom G, Taylor KE, Chung SA, et al. (2009) A large-scale replication study identifies TNIP1, PRDM1, JAZF1, UHRF1BP1 and IL10 as risk loci for systemic lupus erythematosus. Nat Genet 41: 1228–1233.

39. Han JW, Zheng HF, Cui Y, Sun LD, Ye DQ, et al. (2009) Genome-wide association study in a Chinese Han population identifies nine new susceptibility loci for systemic lupus erythematosus. Nat Genet 41: 1234–1237.

40. Yang W, Shen N, Ye DQ, Liu Q, Zhang Y, et al. (2010) Genome-wide association study in Asian populations identifies variants in ETS1 and WDFY4 associated with systemic lupus erythematosus. PLoS Genet 6: e1000841.

41. Buyon JP, Shadick N, Berkman R, Hopkins P, Dalton J, et al. (1988) Surface expression of Gp 165/95, the complement receptor CR3, as a marker of disease activity in systemic Lupus erythematosus. Clin Immunol Immunopathol 46: 141–149.

42. D'Agati VD, Appel GB, Estes D, Knowles DM, 2nd, Pirani CL (1986) Monoclonal antibody identification of infiltrating mononuclear leukocytes in lupus nephritis. Kidney International 30: 573–581.

43. Lhotta K, Neumayer HP, Joannidis M, Geissler D, Konig P (1991) Renal expression of intercellular adhesion molecule-1 in different forms of glomerulonephritis. Clin Sci (Lond) 81: 477–481.

44. Li Y, Zhang L (2003) The fourth blade within the beta-propeller is involved specifically in C3bi recognition by integrin alpha M beta 2. J Biol Chem 278: 34395–34402.

45. Tas SW, Quartier P, Botto M, Fossati-Jimack L (2006) Macrophages from patients with SLE and rheumatoid arthritis have defective adhesion in vitro, while only SLE macrophages have impaired uptake of apoptotic cells. Ann Rheum Dis 65: 216–221.

46. Baumann I, Kolowos W, Voll RE, Manger B, Gaipl U, et al. (2002) Impaired uptake of apoptotic cells into tingible body macrophages in germinal centers of patients with systemic lupus erythematosus. Arthritis Rheum 46: 191–201.

47. Cao C, Gao Y, Li Y, Antalis TM, Castellino FJ, et al. (2010) The efficacy of activated protein C in murine endotoxemia is dependent on integrin CD11b. J Clin Invest 120: 1971–1980.

48. Yoshida Y, Kang K, Berger M, Chen G, Gilliam AC, et al. (1998) Monocyte induction of IL-10 and down-regulation of IL-12 by iC3b deposited in ultraviolet-exposed human skin. Journal of Immunology 161: 5873–5879.

49. Marth T, Kelsall BL (1997) Regulation of interleukin-12 by complement receptor 3 signaling. J Exp Med 185: 1987–1995.

50. Moestrup SK, Moller HJ (2004) CD163: a regulated hemoglobin scavenger receptor with a role in the anti-inflammatory response. Ann Med 36: 347–354.

51. Schaer CA, Vallelian F, Imhof A, Schoedon G, Schaer DJ (2007) CD163-expressing monocytes constitute an endotoxin-sensitive Hb clearance compartment within the vascular system. J Leukoc Biol 82: 106–110.

52. Schaer DJ, Schaer CA, Buehler PW, Boykins RA, Schoedon G, et al. (2006) CD163 is the macrophage scavenger receptor for native and chemically modified hemoglobins in the absence of haptoglobin. Blood 107: 373–380.

53. Green MR, Kennell AS, Larche MJ, Seifert MH, Isenberg DA, et al. (2007) Natural killer T cells in families of patients with systemic lupus erythematosus: their possible role in regulation of IGG production. Arthritis Rheum 56: 303–310.

54. Dai Z, Turtle CJ, Booth GC, Riddell SR, Gooley TA, et al. (2009) Normally occurring NKG2D+CD4+ T cells are immunosuppressive and inversely correlated with disease activity in juvenile-onset lupus. J Exp Med 206: 793–805.

55. Griffin DO, Rothstein TL (2011) A small CD11b(+) human B1 cell subpopulation stimulates T cells and is expanded in lupus. J Exp Med 208: 2591–2598.

Flare, Persistently Active Disease, and Serologically Active Clinically Quiescent Disease in Systemic Lupus Erythematosus

Fabrizio Conti, Fulvia Ceccarelli, Carlo Perricone*, Francesca Miranda, Simona Truglia, Laura Massaro, Viviana Antonella Pacucci, Virginia Conti, Izabella Bartosiewicz, Francesca Romana Spinelli, Cristiano Alessandri, Guido Valesini

Lupus Clinic, Reumatologia, Dipartimento di Medicina Interna e Specialità Mediche, Sapienza Università di Roma, Rome, Italy

Abstract

Objective: Several indices have been proposed to assess disease activity in patients with Systemic Lupus Erythematosus (SLE). Recent studies have showed a prevalence of flare between 28–35.3%, persistently active disease (PAD) between 46%–52% and serologically active clinically quiescent (SACQ) disease ranging from 6 to 15%. Our goal was to evaluate the flare, PAD and SACQ rate incidence in a cohort of SLE patients over a 2-year follow-up.

Methods: We evaluated 394 SLE patients. Flare was defined as an increase in SLEDAI-2K score of ≥4 from the previous visit; PAD was defined as a SLEDAI-2K score of ≥4, on >2 consecutive visits; SACQ was defined as at least a 2-year period without clinical activity and with persistent serologic activity.

Results: Among the 95 patients eligible for the analysis in 2009, 7 (7.3%) had ≥1 flare episode, whereas 9 (9.4%) had PAD. Similarly, among the 118 patients selected for the analysis in 2010, 6 (5%) had ≥1 flare episode, whereas 16 (13.5%) had PAD. Only 1/45 patient (2.2%) showed SACQ during the follow-up.

Conclusion: We showed a low incidence of flare, PAD and SACQ in Italian SLE patients compared with previous studies which could be partly explained by ethnic differences.

Editor: Stamatis-Nick Liossis, University of Patras Medical School, Greece

Funding: The authors have no support or funding to report.

Competing Interests: The authors have declared that no competing interests exist.

* E-mail: carlo.perricone@gmail.com

Introduction

Monitoring of disease activity is an important aspect in the management of patients affected by Systemic Lupus Erythematosus (SLE) as was recently pointed out in a core-set of recommendations proposed by the European League Against Rheumatism (EULAR) [1]. In clinical practice and in randomized controlled trials, several validated disease activity indices, derived from cohort or cross-sectional studies, have been widely applied [2,3]. The EULAR recommendations for monitoring patients with SLE suggest that at least one validated index should be used to assess disease activity at each visit [1].

Flare is one of the most commonly used outcome measures in the core-set of indices evaluated in clinical trials on SLE. By using the existing disease activity indices, several definitions of flare have been proposed. Thus, a critical question is how to best define SLE flare. One of the most used was proposed by Gladman and colleagues in 2000 [3]. They defined flare when the SLE disease activity index (SLEDAI) score increases 4 or more points from the previous visit [3]. The investigators of the "Safety of Estrogen in Lupus National Assessment" (SELENA) group introduced a distinction between "mild/moderate" and "severe" flare. The authors emphasized that such distinction could be made on the basis of the *intention to treat* the flare [4].

More recently, Nikpour and colleagues underlined that such definition of flare does not capture patients who have a disease course characterized by periods of persistently active disease (PAD), defined as a SLEDAI-2K score ≥4, excluding serology alone, on ≥2 consecutive visits [5]. The authors observed that periods of PAD were more common than flare episodes, a result that we further confirmed in a subsequent evaluation on an Italian SLE population [5,6].

"Serologically active clinically quiescent" (SACQ) disease was proposed as another outcome measure. This index identifies patients clinically quiescent despite persistent serologic activity, and appears to have a prevalence of 6–15% in SLE patients [7–9].

Thus, our goal was to evaluate the incidence of flare, PAD, and SACQ in a cohort of Italian SLE patients over a two-year follow-up.

Materials and Methods

SLE patients referred to the Lupus Clinic of the Rheumatology Unit, Sapienza University of Rome (Sapienza Lupus Cohort) were enrolled in a prospective study. SLE diagnosis was performed according to the revised 1997 American College of Rheumatology (ACR) criteria [10]. Two-hundred ninety four consecutive SLE patients were evaluated during a two-year follow-up (2009–2010). Patients provided a written informed consent at the time of the first visit. The local ethical committee of "*Policlinico Umberto I*", Rome, approved the study. At each visit, the patients underwent a complete physical examination, the clinical and laboratory data were collected in a standardized, computerized, and electronically-filled form, which included demographics, past medical history with date of diagnosis, co-morbidities, previous and concomitant treatments.

Disease activity was assessed with the SLEDAI-2K, while chronic damage was measured with the Systemic Lupus International Collaborating Clinics/ACR Damage Index score (SLICC) [11–13]. All the patients were observed at least twice per year, even though most of the patients were evaluated quarterly. Selected patients could be followed more often, according to the clinical condition.

Prospectively collected data were used to determine the incidence of flares and PAD in 2009 and 2010. According to Nikpour and colleagues, flare was considered as an increase in SLEDAI-2K score of ≥4 from the previous visit with a minimum interval of 2 months between visits; PAD as a SLEDAI-2K score ≥4, excluding serology alone, on ≥2 consecutive visits, with a minimum interval of 2 months between visits [5]. The proportion of patients with ≥1 flare episode(s) or PAD period(s) was determined. We recorded the organ systems involvement at the time of the flare or during a period of PAD.

SACQ was defined as a period of at least two years without clinical activity but with persistent serologic activity (SLEDAI-2K score 2 or 4, due to positive anti-dsDNA antibody titers and/or hypocomplementemia, at each clinic visit).

Therapy

The patients evaluated for flare and PAD did not have any restriction concerning medications given. The patients evaluated for SACQ were taking only anti-malarials, while those receiving corticosteroids or immunosuppressive medications were excluded [7].

Statistical Evaluation

We used version 13.0 of the SPSS statistical package. Normally distributed variables were summarized using the mean ± SD, and non-normally distributed variables by the median and range. Wilcoxon's matched pairs test and paired t-test were performed accordingly. Univariate comparisons between nominal variables were calculated using chi-square test or Fisher-test where appropriate. Two-tailed P values were reported, P values less than 0.05 were considered significant.

Results

Ninety-five and one-hundred eighteen SLE patients were eligible for the study in 2009 and 2010, respectively, as they underwent at least two visits per year. The main clinical and laboratory parameters are reported in Table 1. Patients selected for inclusion in the analysis were mostly women (94.7% in 2009 and 94.9% in 2010). No statistically significant differences were found between patients evaluated in 2009 and 2010 regarding the mean age (39.7±12.6 years and 41.8±11.3 years, respectively) and mean disease duration (124.7±97.6 months and 134.8±92.4 months, respectively).

The mean ± SD time interval between visits used to diagnose are and PAD in 2009 and 2010 was 3.6±0.6 months and 3.5±0.6 months, respectively.

Among the 95 patients selected for the analysis in 2009, 7 (7.3%) had 1 flare episode (only 1/7 showed 2 flare episodes), whereas 9 (9.4%) had PAD. Similarly, among the 118 patients selected for the analysis in 2010, 6 (5%) had 1 flare episode (none more than 1 episode), whereas 16 (13.5%) had PAD.

In 2009, 1 patient showed both flare and PAD. One patient had flare in 2009 and in 2010, while 5 patients showed PAD in both years.

Table 2 shows the clinical characteristics of patients with flare and the organ/system involved at the time of flare. In 2009, the most commonly involved organ/systems in patients with flare were immunologic and musculoskeletal (57.1% and 42.8%, respectively), while nervous system involvement was the most frequent manifestation in patients with flare in 2010 (66.6%). Specifically, 2 patients experienced psychosis, one patient organic brain syndrome, and one patient a new onset of cerebrovascular accident.

Notably, 5/7 patients (71.4%) in 2009 and 5/6 (83.4%) in 2010 of the patients who experienced flares were not on immunosuppressive drugs. The patients who experienced flares showed a significantly longer disease duration compared with those who did not experience flares in both years of observation (187.2±115.2 *versus* 128.4±84.6 months, P=0.02 in 2009; 188.4±100.08 *versus* 135.8±89.5 months, P=0.03 in 2010).

The clinical characteristics of the patients with PAD and the involved organ/systems are reported in table 3. Musculoskeletal involvement and immunological abnormalities were found in 50% of the patients with PAD in 2009, while in 2010 kidney and nervous system involvement were the most frequent manifestations (37.5% and 25%, respectively). As seen in the group with flare, the patients with PAD showed a significantly longer disease duration compared with those who did not have PAD in both years of observation (184.8±118.32 *versus* 122.6±88.6 months, P=0.02 in 2009; 188.4±100.08 *versus* 138.8±83.5 months, P=0.02, in 2010).

The occurrence of flare was associated with a history of nervous system involvement (P=0.001, OR=10.9, CI 2.1–56.8). The logistic regression analysis confirmed such association (P=0.008). The occurrence of PAD was associated with a history of arthritis, renal and nervous system involvement (P=0.007, OR=5.7, CI 1.4–22.9; P<0.001, OR=9.37, CI 2.6–33.7; P=0.002, OR=7.49, CI 1.7–32, respectively). The logistic regression analysis confirmed the association only with nervous system involvement (P=0.01).

Forty-five patients were eligible for the evaluation of SACQ. Only 1 patient (2.2%) had SACQ during the two-year follow-up. The patient (D.G.) was a 37-year-old female, with a disease duration of 144 months, who was taking hydroxychloroquine and, in the absence of clinical manifestations, showed persistent complement reduction and elevated anti-dsDNA antibodies (titer ≥1:40).

Discussion

In this prospective study, we showed that, in a large cohort of Italian patients affected by SLE, flares and PAD are relatively infrequent conditions. In fact, in 2009 flares were observed in 7% and PAD in 9.4% of our patients, while in 2010 flares were observed in 5% and PAD in 13.5% of our patients, respectively.

SLE is a prototype of systemic autoimmune diseases, characterized by heterogeneity of clinical features and presence of a wide autoantibodies profile. The great heterogeneity of SLE determined a still open debate, concerning the possibility that SLE is a single

Table 1. Clinical, serological and therapeutical features of SLE patients.

Characteristic	Patients evaluated in 2009 (N = 95)	Patients evaluated in 2010 (N = 118)
M/F	5/90	6/112
Age (years) mean±SD	39.7±12.6	41.8±11.3
Disease duration (months) mean±SD	124.7±97.6	134.8±92.4
Race		
Caucasian (N/%)	93/97.9	115/97.4
Asian (N/%)	2/2.1	3/2.6
Clinical Manifestations		
Renal disorder N (%)	19 (20.0)	27 (22.8)
Serositis N (%)	4 (4.2)	3 (2.5)
Cytopenia N (%)	21 (22.1)	27 (22.9)
NPSLE N (%)	12 (12.6)	15 (12.7)
Muscoloskeletal N (%)	24 (25.2)	24 (20.3)
Mucocutaneous N (%)	28 (29.5)	29 (24.6)
Immunological Manifestations		
ANA N (%)	92 (96.8)	112 (95)
Anti-dsDNA N (%)	38 (40)	40 (34)
Low C3 N (%)	39 (41.0)	39 (33)
Low C4 N (%)	45 (47.4)	47 (39.8)
SLEDAI (mean±SD)	1.72±2.19	1.84±2.25
SLICC (mean±SD)	0.51±0.82	0.48±0.89
Drugs		
Hydroxychloroquine N (%)	62 (65.3)	67 (56.8)
Mycophenolate mofetil N(%)	22 (23.1)	27 (22.9)
Cyclophosphamide N(%)	1 (1)	1 (0.8)
Methotrexate N(%)	6 (6.3)	9 (7.6)
Cyclosporine A N(%)	5 (5.2)	9 (7.6)
Azathioprine N(%)	16 (16.8)	18 (15.2)

SD: Standard Deviation; NP: NeuroPsychiatric; ANA: Anti-Nuclear Antibody; anti-dsDNA: anti-double strand DNA; SLEDAI: Systemic Lupus Erythematosus Disease Activity Index; SLICC: Systemic Lupus International Collaborating Clinics.
*As stated in 1997 ACR Classification criteria for SLE.

disease with varied phenotypes or a similar phenotype shared by a variety of different diseases with diverse pathogenic mechanisms [14].

SLE is characterized from heterogeneous degrees of severity as well as unpredictable disease flares and remissions. Several experimental trials are in progress to evaluate new biologic drugs to treat patients affected by SLE. However, the remitting and relapsing course of the disease and the heterogeneity of SLE features make the design and the interpretation of clinical trials difficult. Quantification of disease activity is mandatory to identify patients eligible to participate in clinical trials and, thereafter, to establish the efficacy of the drug examined.

Data published in the literature suggested that the disease activity in SLE patients could be evaluated by using laboratory markers and/or global indices. Conventional biomarkers for the assessment of disease activity include anti-dsDNA antibodies and serum complement levels. However, the "classical" markers of activity are not specific and accurate in differentiating between disease flares and other concomitant conditions, such as infections. Recent research has provided data about new potential biomarkers to guide clinical decision-making in the management of SLE patients [15].

Disease activity indices are helpful in the routine assessment of SLE patients, as suggested by recent EULAR recommendations for monitoring patients with SLE [1].

Several indices have been applied to evaluate disease activity, such as SLEDAI, European Consensus Lupus Activity Measurement (ECLAM) and British Isles Lupus Assessment Group index (BILAG) [16].

Recent randomized controlled trials for new biologic treatment in patients affected by SLE used a new composite assessment, called SLE Responder Index (SRI), that combines the SELENA-SLEDAI, BILAG and Physician Global Assessment (PGA). A responder according to the SRI is defined as having ≥4 point reduction from baseline in SELENA-SLEDAI score and no new BILAG A score and no more than one new BILAG B organ domain score compared with baseline and no worsening in PGA. When all three criteria are met, the patient is a responder at that time point according to the SRI [17].

Several definitions of flare were proposed and used in clinical trials and observational studies. Nevertheless, how to define the best SLE flare is still an open and critical question. Global scoring systems, such as the SLEDAI, are easy to perform and widely standardized. They are used to define flare; nonetheless they only

Table 2. Demographic characteristics of SLE patients with flare and the organ/systems involved at the time of flare.

Characteristic	Patients with flare in 2009 (N = 7)	Patients with flare in 2010 (N = 6)
M/F	0/7	1/5
Age (years) mean±SD	37.7±9.2	40.3±11.8
Disease duration (months) mean±SD	187.2±115.2	188.4±100.08
Systemic involvement*		
Renal disorder N(%)	1/14.3	0/0
Serositis N(%)	0/0	1/16.6
Cytopenia N(%)	0/0	1/16.6
NPSLE N(%)	2/28.6	4/66.6
Musculoskeletal N(%)	3/42.8	0/0
Mucocutaneous N(%)	1/14.3	1/16.6
Immunological abnormalities (besides ANA) N(%)	4/57.1	1/16.6
Prednisone dosage (mg/week) mean±SD**	73.9±123.7	66.0±67.03
Drugs		
Hydroxychloroquine N(%)	2/28.6	6/100
Mycophenolate mofetil N(%)	2/28.6	0/0
Cyclophosphamide N(%)	0/0	0/0
Methotrexate N(%)	0/0	0/0
Cyclosporine A N(%)	0/0	1/16.6
Azathioprine N(%)	0/0	0/0
SLEDAI (mean±SD)	6.8±3.02	8±1.26
SLICC (mean±SD)	0.57±1.13	1.2±0.8

SD: Standard Deviation; NP: NeuroPsychiatric; SLEDAI: Systemic Lupus Erythematosus Disease Activity Index; SLICC: Systemic Lupus International Collaborating Clinics.
*As stated in 1997 ACR Classification criteria for SLE.
**Prednisone equivalents.

take a snapshot of the patient rather than indicating the trend of the disease.

Thus, Nikpour et al. proposed a new outcome measure, the so-called "persistently active disease" (PAD), to define those patients not in remission but without flare. They addressed that these patients require the most frequent monitoring [5]. Their study published in 2009 showed a high prevalence of flare and PAD in a Canadian lupus cohort. At least 1 flare was registered in nearly one third of evaluated patients (specifically 35.3% in 2004 and 28% in 2005), while PAD was identified in almost half of the patients evaluated during the two-year follow-up (specifically, 52.3% in 2004 and 46.1% in 2005). The most commonly involved organ/systems were musculoskeletal, cutaneous, renal, immunologic, and the nervous system [5].

We have already reported a preliminary study on 63 SLE patients who were referred to the Sapienza Lupus Clinic followed during 1 year of follow-up (September 2008–September 2009) in which we observed a lower incidence of flare and PAD compared with the Canadian cohort (7.9% and 14.3%, respectively) [6]. In the present study, we extended the time and cohort size the preliminary data on Italian SLE patients. This two-year follow-up study confirmed a lower incidence of flare (7% in 2009 and 5% in 2010), and PAD (9.4% in 2009 and 13.5% in 2010), indicating a relatively infrequent occurrence of relapses and a good control of disease activity. Ethnic differences, i.e., the presence of one-third of African-American patients in the Canadian cohort, could explain the better outcome of our patients. Nonetheless, we observed a more frequent involvement of the central nervous system and less frequent of the skin during flares or PAD.

Neuropsychiatric involvement is frequent manifestations in SLE patients and could be found up to 80% of patients, includeing a wide range of neurological and psychiatric manifestations as well as cognitive impairment. Recently we found an association between cognitive dysfunction and disease activity in a cohort of 58 consecutive SLE patients [18].

Occurrence of flares and PAD in our SLE cohort was associated with longer disease duration. Moreover, most patients who experienced flares were not taking an immunosuppressive drug. Thus, longer disease duration and the absence of an immunosuppressive treatment should be considered risk factors for the worsening of disease activity.

In the logistic regression analysis NPSLE involvement was associated with both flare and PAD. This is in agreement with the definition of flare, as well as of PAD, probably due to the fact that in the SLEDAI, used in the formulation of both indices, neuropsychiatric manifestations account for the highest scores.

SACQ is another important outcome measure that was first suggested by Gladman et al. in 1979. They described a subset of patients who had persistent serologic activity (elevated anti-dsDNA antibody levels and/or hypocomplementemia) despite clinical quiescence [8]. Walz & LeBlanc reported 12% of SLE patients with SACQ [15], and even a lower percentage was found (6.1%) by Steiman and colleagues [7] who further found that 58.9% of patients with SACQ may experience flare at median 155 weeks of follow-up. Changes in complement and anti-dsDNA antibody serum levels drawn at routine clinic visits might not be predictive of flares in SACQ patients. Thus, it was suggested that the decision to treat patients with SACQ should be based on close clinical

Table 3. Demographic characteristics of SLE patients (N = 16) with PAD and organ/system involving during PAD.

Characteristic	Patients with PAD in 2009 (N = 6)	Patients with PAD in 2010 (N = 16)
M/F	1/5	1/15
Age (years) mean±SD	35.8±5.3	38.3±8.02
Disease duration (months) mean±SD	184.8±118.32	152.4±111.6
Systemic involvement*		
Renal disorder N(%)	2 (33.3)	6/37.5
Serositis N(%)	1/16.6	1/6.25
Cytopenia N(%)	1/16.6	2/12.5
NPSLE N(%)	1/16.6	4/25
Musculoskeletal N(%)	3/50	3/18.75
Mucocutaneous N(%)	0/0	2/12.5
Immunological abnormalities (besides ANA) N(%)	3/50	3/18.75
Prednisone dosage (mg/week) mean±SD**	38.3±6.05	67.3±86.3
Drugs		
Hydroxychloroquine N(%)	3/50	5/31.25
Mycophenolate mofetil N(%)	3/50	5/31.25
Cyclophosphamide N(%)	0/0	0/0
Methotrexate N(%)	2/33.3	2/12.5
Cyclosporine A N(%)	0/0	0/0
Azathioprine N(%)	1/16.6	3/18.75
SLEDAI (mean±SD)	5.8±1.86	5.96±1.94
SLICC (mean±SD)	0.33±0.56	0.71±1.437

SD: Standard Deviation; NP: NeuroPsychiatric; SLEDAI: Systemic Lupus Erythematosus Disease Activity Index; ECLAM: European Consensus Lupus Activity Measurement; SLICC: Systemic Lupus International Collaborating Clinics.
*As stated in 1997 ACR Classification criteria for SLE.
**Prednisone equivalents.

observation. In our population, only 1 (2.2%) of the 45 eligible patients showed SACQ. We identified a lower incidence of SACQ in SLE patients, but the importance of this index in the clinical assessment should be addressed in larger cohorts.

Conclusions

Our study showed a low incidence of flares, PAD and SACQ in Italian SLE patients compared with previous studies where the results could be only partly explained by ethnic differences. This may suggest that definition of disease activity is critical for SLE management, and that timing for immunosuppressive treatment suspension should be carefully evaluated. In this view, it is very important to improve, select and use indices of outcome in SLE in order to better assess and treat patients. Flares, PAD and SACQ could be considered useful parameters of clinical evaluation in SLE patients in monitoring disease progression and response to treatment.

Author Contributions

Conceived and designed the experiments: F. Conti F. Ceccarelli CP GV. Performed the experiments: F. Conti F. Ceccarelli CP GV FM ST LM FRS CA. Analyzed the data: F. Conti F. Ceccarelli CP VP VC IB GV. Contributed reagents/materials/analysis tools: F. Conti F. Ceccarelli CP GV. Wrote the paper: F. Conti F. Ceccarelli CP GV.

References

1. Mosca M, Tani C, Aringer M, Bombardieri S, Boumpas D, et al. (2010) European League Against Rheumatism recommendations for monitoring patients with systemic lupus erythematosus in clinical practice and in observational studies. Ann Rheum Dis 69: 1269–74.
2. Griffiths B, Mosca M, Gordon C (2005) Assessment of patients with systemic lupus erythematosus and the use of lupus disease activity indices. Best Pract Res Clin Rheumatol 19: 685–708.
3. Gladman DD, Urowitz MB, Kagal A, Hallett D (2000) Accurately describing changes in disease activity in Systemic Lupus Erythematosus. J Rheumatol 27: 377–9.
4. Petri M, Kim MY, Kalunian KC, Grossman J, Hahn BH, et al. (2005) Combined oral contraceptives in women with systemic lupus erythematosus. N Engl J Med 353: 2550–8.
5. Nikpour M, Urowitz MB, Ibañez D, Gladman DD (2009) Frequency and determinants of flare and persistently active disease in systemic lupus erythematosus. Arthritis Rheum 61: 1152–8.
6. Conti F, Ceccarelli F, Perricone C, Massaro L, Spinelli FR, et al. (2010) Low incidence of flare and persistent active disease in a cohort of Italian patients with systemic lupus erythematosus: comment on the article by Nikpour, et al. Arthritis Care Res (Hoboken) 62: 899–900.
7. Steiman AJ, Gladman DD, Ibañez D, Urowitz MB (2010) Prolonged serologically active clinically quiescent systemic lupus erythematosus: frequency and outcome. J Rheumatol 37: 1822–7.
8. Gladman DD, Urowitz MB, Keystone EC. (1979) Serologically active clinically quiescent systemic lupus erythematosus: a discordance between clinical and serologic features. Am J Med 66: 210–5.
9. Walz LeBlanc BA, Gladman DD, Urowitz MB (1994) Serologically active clinically quiescent systemic lupus erythematosus – predictors of clinical flares. J Rheumatol 21: 2239–41.
10. Hochberg MC (1997) Updating the American College of Rheumatology revised criteria for the classification of systemic lupus erythematosus. Arthritis Rheum 40: 1725.
11. Gladman DD, Ibañez D, Urowitz MB (2002) Systemic lupus erythematosus disease activity index 2000. J Rheumatol 29: 288–91.

12. Mosca M, Bencivelli W, Vitali C, Carrai P, Neri R, et al. (2000) The validity of the ECLAM index for the retrospective evaluation of disease activity in systemic lupus erythematosus. Lupus 9: 445–50.

13. Gladman DD, Urowitz MB, Goldsmith CH, Fortin P, Ginzler E, et al. (1997) The reliability of the Systemic Lupus International Collaborating Clinics/ American College of Rheumatology Damage Index in patients with systemic lupus erythematosus. Arthritis Rheum 40: 809–13.

14. Agmon-Levin N, Mosca M, Petri M, Shoenfeld Y (2012) Systemic lupus erythematosus one disease or many? Autoimmun Rev 11: 593–5.

15. Sciascia S, Ceberio L, Garcia-Fernandez C, Rocatello D, Karim Y, et al. (2012) Systemic lupus erythematosus and infections: Clinical importance of conventional and upcoming biomarkers. Autoimmune Rev: Apr. 1.

16. Romero-Diaz J, Isenberg D, Ramsey-Goldman R (2011) Measures of adult systemic lupus erythematosus: updated version of British Isles Lupus Assessment Group (BILAG 2004), European Consensus Lupus Activity Measurements (ECLAM), Systemic Lupus Activity Measure, Revised (SLAM-R), Systemic Lupus Activity Questionnaire for Population Studies (SLAQ), Systemic Lupus Erythematosus Disease Activity Index 2000 (SLEDAI-2K), and Systemic Lupus International Collaborating Clinics/American College of Rheumatology Damage Index (SDI). Arthritis Care Res 63 Suppl 11: S37–46.

17. Luijten KM, Tekstra J, Bijlsma JW, Bijl M (2012) The Systemic Lupus Erythematosus Responder Index (SRI); a new SLE disease activity assessment.Autoimmun Rev 11: 326–9.

18. Conti F, Alessandri C, Perricone C, Scrivo R, Rezai S, et al. (2012) Neurocognitive dysfunction in systemic lupus erythematosus: association with antiphospholipid antibodies, disease activity and chronic damage. PLoS One 7: e33824.

17

Mannose-Binding Lectin Blunts Macrophage Polarization and Ameliorates Lupus Nephritis

Yanxing Cai[1,9], **Weijuan Zhang**[1,9], **Sidong Xiong**[1,2]*

1 Department of Immunology and Institute for Immunobiology, Shanghai Medical College, Fudan University, Shanghai, People's Republic of China, **2** Institutes of Biology and Medical Sciences, Soochow University, Suzhou, People's Republic of China

Abstract

Background: Deficiency in clearance of self nuclear antigens, including DNA, is the hallmark of systemic lupus erythematosus (SLE), a chronic autoimmnue disease characterized by the production of various autoantibodies, immune complex deposition and severe organ damage. Our previous studies revealed that administration of syngeneic BALB/c mice with activated lymphocyte-derived DNA (ALD-DNA) could induce SLE disease. Mannose-binding lectin (MBL), a secreted pattern recognition receptor with binding activity to DNA, has been proved to be a modulator of inflammation, but whether MBL takes responsibility for DNA clearance, modulates the DNA-mediated immune responses, and is involved in the development of DNA-induced SLE disease remain poorly understood.

Methodology/Principal Findings: The levels of serum MBL significantly decreased in lupus mice induced by ALD-DNA and were negatively correlated with SLE disease. MBL blunted macrophage M2b polarization by inhibiting the MAPK and NF-κB signaling while enhancing the activation of CREB. Furthermore, MBL suppressed the ability of ALD-DNA–stimulated macrophages to polarize T cells toward Th1 cells and Th17 cells. Importantly, MBL supplement *in vivo* could ameliorate lupus nephritis.

Conclusion/Significance: These results suggest MBL supplement could alleviate SLE disease and might imply a potential therapeutic strategy for DNA-induced SLE, which would further our understanding of the protective role of MBL in SLE disease.

Editor: Deyu Fang, Northwestern University Feinberg School of Medicine, United States of America

Funding: This work was supported by grants from the National Natural Science Foundation of China (30890141, 81273300, 31100629, 31270863), Major State Basic Research Development Program of China (2013CB530501), Jiangsu "333" project of cultivation of high-level talents, Qing Lan Project of the Jiangsu higher education institutions, Jiangsu Provincial Innovative Research Team, Jiangsu "Pan-Deng" Project (BK2010004), Priority Academic Program Development of Jiangsu Higher Education Institutions (PAPD) and Program for Changjiang Scholars and Innovative Research Team in University (PCSIRT-IRT1075), Shanghai STC grant (10JC1401400). The funders had no role in study design, data collection and analysis, decision to publish, or preparation of the manuscript.

Competing Interests: The authors have declared that no competing interests exist.

* E-mail: sdxiongfd@126.com

9 These authors contributed equally to this work.

Introduction

Systemic lupus erythematosus (SLE) is a chronic autoimmune disease characterized by the production of various autoantibodes, complement activation, immune complex (IC) deposition and the subsequent inflammation that contribute to severe organ damage [1,2]. The precise etiology of SLE remains elusive; however, inefficient clearance of self nuclear antigens released from apoptotic cells has been implicated as an important factor leading to the initiation and development of SLE [3–5]. Accumulation of self nuclear antigens, including DNA and RNA, would trigger the autoimmune responses that eventually initiate the production of autoantibodies in SLE patients.

In our previous studies, a novel murine model of SLE was generated by immunizing the syngeneic female BALB/c mice with activated lymphocyte-derived DNA (ALD-DNA), which developed high titers of anti-dsDNA antibodies, IC deposition, proteinuria, and glomerular nephritis that closely resembled human SLE [6–8]. We further found that ALD-DNA could induce macrophage M2b polarization [9], which was consistent with previous reports on macrophage M2b polarization in lupus nephritis [10]. These findings suggest that ALD-DNA might serve as an important autoimmunogen to initiate the autoimmune responses that eventually lead to the pathogenesis of SLE. Therefore, recognition and elimination of the autoimmunogen such as ALD-DNA is essential to prevent and treat DNA-induced SLE and other autoimmune diseases.

During lymphocyte activation induced by infection, stress, and other danger signals, DNA was released from activated lymphocytes, but not always provoking the autoimmunity, indicating that free DNA could be removed by the intrinsic physiological mechanisms [11]. Clearance of DNA is important for maintaining immune homeostasis and preventing SLE disease. Therefore, it is essential to study the intrinsic physiological mechanisms of recognizing and eliminating DNA.

The complement system, which is one of the first defence in the innate immunity, is important for recognizing and eliminating invading microorganisms and clearance of cellular debris, apoptotic cells and immune complexes to maintain tissue homeostasis [12–14]. Inherited deficiency of complement components has been reported to be associated with the development of autoimmune diseases [15]. Mannose-binding lectin (MBL), one member of complement components, is a secreted pattern recognition receptor (PRR) and mainly produced by the liver during the acute phase response at early stages of infection [16–18]. In addition to the binding ability of MBL to the carbohydrates of microorganisms, accumulating data indicate that MBL can enhance the uptake of apoptotic cells and immune complexes by the interaction with its receptors on the cell surface, such as C1q phagocytic receptor C1qRp (CD93), cC1qR (CRT) and CR1 (CD35), which might play a protective role in the development of autoimmune diseases [19–25]. It has been reported that MBL deficiency or low serum MBL levels have been observed in SLE [26–28]. Previous studies indicate that MBL has the ability of recognizing DNA and is a modulator of inflammatory responses, but whether MBL takes responsibility for DNA clearance, modulates the DNA-mediated immune responses, and plays a protective role in DNA-induced SLE disease remain poorly understood [29–32].

In this present study, we examined the levels of serum MBL and found that they decreased in ALD-DNA–induced lupus mice and were negatively correlated with the levels of anti-dsDNA antibodies and urine protein in SLE mice. Furthermore, MBL could blunt ALD-DNA–induced macrophage M2b polarization by down-regulating the MAPK and NF-κB signaling while up-regulating CREB activation and suppress the ability of ALD-DNA–stimulated macrophages to promote T cell differentiation. MBL supplement in vivo could ameliorate ALD-DNA–induced lupus nephritis by decreasing anti-dsDNA antibodies production and IC deposition. These results might provide MBL as a potential therapeutic strategy for DNA-induced SLE and other autoimmune diseases.

Materials and Methods

Ethics Statement

All experiments carried out in this study were strictly performed in a manner to minimize suffering of laboratory mice. All animal procedures were performed according to the Guide for the Care and Use of Medical Laboratory Animals (Ministry of Health, P.R. China, 1998) and with the ethical approval of the Shanghai Medical Laboratory Animal Care and Use Committee (Permit number: SYXK 2010–0020) as well as the Ethical Committee of Fudan University (Permit number: 2010015).

Mice and Cells

Six-week-old female BALB/c mice were purchased from the Experimental Animal Center of Chinese Academy of Sciences (Shanghai, P. R. China) and housed in a pathogen-free environment. RAW264.7 cells were purchased from Chinese Academy of Sciences (Shanghai, P. R. China). Peritoneal macrophages were collected as described previously [33].

Plasmid and Purification of Mouse MBL

The full length of MBL cDNA was amplified from total RNA of murine liver using the primers 5′-ATG CTT CTG CTT CCA TTA CTC CCT GT-3′ and 5′-GGC TGG GAA CTC GCA GAC AGC C-3′. MBL cDNA was inserted into the pcDNA3.1 vector (Invitrogen) to generate pcDNA3.1-MBL plasmid (pMBL). The plasmid construct was confirmed by DNA sequencing. 293T cells were transfected with pMBL plasmid using Lipofectamine 2000 transfection reagent. 4 days after transfection, the super-

natants were collected for purification of mouse MBL protein. The purification of mouse MBL protein was performed as described previously [34].

DNA Preparation

ALD-DNA and UnALD-DNA were prepared with murine splenocytes which were generated from surgical resected spleens of six- to eight-week-old female BALB/c mice and cultured with or without Con A (Sigma-Aldrich) in vitro as previously described [7]. Briefly, for generation of ALD-DNA, splenocytes were seeded at 2×10^6 cells/ml in 75 cm^2/cell culture flask and cultured in the presence of Con A (5 μg/ml) for 6 days to induce apoptosis. The apoptotic cells were stained with FITC-labeled Annexin V (BD Biosciences) and propidium iodide (PI; Sigma-Aldrich), and sorted using a FACSAria (BD Biosciences). Genomic DNAs from syngeneic apoptotic splenocytes were treated with S1 nuclease (TaKaRa) and proteinase K (Sigma-Aldrich), and then purified using the DNeasy Blood & Tissue Kits (Qiagen) according to the manufacturer's instructions. UnALD-DNA was prepared with unactivated (resting) splenocytes and extracted using the same methods. To exclude contaminations with LPS, sterile endotoxin-free plastic ware and reagents were used for DNA preparation. DNA samples were also monitored for low level of endotoxin by the Limulus amoebocyte lysate assay (BioWhittaker) according to the manufacturer's instructions. The concentration of DNA was determined by detection of the absorbance (A) at 260 nm. The apoptotic DNA ladder of ALD-DNA was confirmed by agarose gel electrophoresis (AGE).

Generation of SLE Murine Model

To generate SLE murine model, 6- to 8-week-old syngeneic female BALB/c mice were divided into several groups of 8–10 mice and actively immunized by subcutaneous injection on the back with 0.2 ml of an emulsion containing ALD-DNA (50 μg/mouse) in phosphate-buffered saline (PBS) plus equal volume of complete Freund's adjuvant (CFA; Sigma-Aldrich) at week 0, and followed by two booster immunizations of ALD-DNA (50 μg/mouse) emulsified with IFA (Sigma-Aldrich) at week 2 and week 4 for total 3 times as previously described [7]. 8–10 mice in each group received an equal volume of PBS plus CFA or IFA, or UnALD-DNA (50 μg/mouse) plus CFA or IFA were used as controls. Mice were bled from retro-orbital sinus prior to immunization and at 2-week internals until 3 months after the initial immunization. 8 or 12 weeks later, mice were sacrificed and surgical resected spleens and kidneys were collected for further cellular function and tissue histology analysis.

Autoantibody and Proteinuria Examination

Anti-dsDNA antibodies in the mice serum were determined by ELISA assay as described previously [7]. In briefly, ELISA plates (Costar) were pre-treated with protamine sulphate (Sigma-Aldrich) and then coated with calf thymus dsDNA (Sigma-Aldrich). After incubation with mouse serum, the levels of anti-dsDNA Abs were detected with the horseradish peroxidase (HRP)-conjugated goat anti-mouse IgG (Southern Biotech). Tetramethylbenzidine (TMB) substrate was used to develop colors and absorbance at 450 nm was measured on a microplate reader (BIO-TEK ELX800). Proteinuria of the mice was measured with the BCA Protein Assay Kit (Thermo Scientific) according to the manufacturer's instructions.

Reagents and Pharmacological Inhibitor Treatment

The pharmacological reagents were obtained from Calbiochem (San Diego, CA) and were reconstituted in sterile DMSO and used at the following concentrations: NF-κB inhibitor PDTC (50 μM), MEK1/2 inhibitor U0126 (10 μM), p38 MAPK inhibitor SB203580 (20 μM), and JNK inhibitor SP600125 (50 μM). DMSO at 0.1% concentration was used as the vehicle control. In all experiments with inhibitors, a tested concentration was used after careful titration experiments assessing the viability of the macrophages, and the chosen concentrations are in agreement with published reports [7]. In addition, when a given inhibitor was tested, its efficacy in terms of inhibition of phosphorylation of the intended signaling molecule, as well as a nonintended signaling molecule, was also tested. In the experiments with inhibitors, the macrophages were treated with a given inhibitor for 1 h before ALD-DNA stimulation.

Measurement of Circulating DNA level

DNA was extracted from serum samples and then quantified using a PicoGreen DNA detection kit (Invitrogen) according to the manufacturer's instructions [8]. In briefly, DNA was extracted from 200 μl of serum samples using a QIAamp Blood Kit (Qiagen) using the blood and body fluid protocol as recommended by the manufacturer. After the removal of most proteins by digestion with proteinase K, the sample was applied to the QIAamp 96 plate. DNA was adsorbed onto the silica membrane during a brief centrifugation step, while any remaining protein, salt and other contaminants were completely removed by three consecutive washes. Membrane-bound DNA was then eluted in double deionized H_2O or Tris–EDTA buffer. A final elution volume of 200 μl was used. Quantification of DNA was carried out using a PicoGreen DNA detection kit (Invitrogen). Calf thymus DNA (100 mg/ml; Sigma-Aldrich) was used as the standard. The concentration of DNA in the standard curve ranged from 0 to 100 ng/ml. Briefly, 20 ml of final DNA eluated was mixed with 1 ml of Tris-EDTA (10 mmol/l Tris–HCl, 1 mmol/l EDTA, pH 7.5) diluted with PicoGreen reagent. Fluorescence intensity was measured on an F-2000 spectrofluorometer (Molecular Devices) at excitation wavelength of 480 nm and an emission of 520 nm. Standard curve used to determine the levels of circulating DNA in the samples was established by the linear relationship between the known concentrations of calf thymus DNA (Sigma-Aldrich) and the corresponding fluorescence intensities.

Cell Culture and Stimulation

RAW264.7 cells or peritoneal macrophages were cultured in Dulbecco's modified Eagle's medium (Invitrogen) supplemented with 10% fetal calf serum (Invitrogen) and 100 units/ml penicillin/streptomycin (Invitrogen) in a 5% CO_2 incubator at 37°C. MBL (10 μg/ml) was incubated with ALD-DNA (ALD-DNA/MBL) for 1 h before stimulating RAW264.7 cells or peritoneal macrophages. RAW264.7 cells or peritoneal macrophages were treated with PBS, ALD-DNA (50 μg/ml) or ALD-DNA/MBL (50 μg/ml) for 24 h.

ELISA Assay

The protein levels of TNF-α, MCP-1, IL-6 and IL-10 in the supernatants were assessed by ELISA assay with cytokine ELISA kits (eBioscience) according to the manufacturer's instructions. A standard curve was generated using known amounts of the respective purified recombinant mouse cytokines or chemokines.

Real-time PCR Analysis

Total RNA was extracted from cultured cells with TRIzol reagent (Invitrogen) according to the manufacturer's instructions and the cDNA was synthesized with PrimeScript RT reagent kit (Takara Bio). The expression of the genes encoding IL-10, TNF-α, MCP-1 and IL-6 was quantified by real-time PCR using a Lightcycler480 and SYBR Green system (Roche Diagnostic Systems, Somerville, NJ), following the manufacturer's protocol. The primer sequences used in this study are described previously [9].

Flow Cytometric Analysis

Peritoneal macrophages were treated with PBS, ALD-DNA (50 μg/ml) or ALD-DNA/MBL (50 μg/ml) for 48 h. To assess the expression of activation and other biological markers on macrophages, flow cytometric analysis was performed with FITC-labeled anti-MHC class II, PE-labeled anti-CD80 and PE-labeled anti-CD86 (BD Biosciences). For intracellular analysis of cytokine production, T cells were pre-stimulated with 10 ng/ml phorbol myristate acetate and 1 μg/ml ionomycin in the presence of 10 μg/ml brefeldin A for 5 to 6 hours. T cells were first stained for APC-labeled anti-CD4 (BD Biosciences), then fixed, permeabilized, and stained for FITC-labeled anti-IFN-γ and PE-labeled anti-IL-17 and analyzed by flow cytometry. All flow cytometry data were acquired on a FACSCalibur (BD Biosciences) in CellQuest (BD Biosciences) and analyzed by FlowJo software (Tree Star, Ashland, OR).

Cell Sorting

Murine renal tissues were surgical resected and dispersed in RPMI 1640 containing 5% FBS and 0.1% collagenase (Sigma-Aldrich) at 37°C for 30 min, followed by progressive sieving to obtain single-cell suspensions. To analyze gene expression in the renal macrophages, $CD11b^+/F4/80^{high}$ renal macrophages were sorted from nephritic single-cell suspensions using a FACSAria (BD Biosciences) with FITC-labeled anti-F4/80 and PE-labeled anti-CD11b (BD Biosciences). The purity of isolated cells was confirmed at 90%.

Western Blot Analysis

Western blot analysis was performed as described previously [35]. Abs used here were anti-mouse iNOS (Santa Cruz Biotechnology), anti-mouse MBL (Santa Cruz Biotechnology), anti-IκB (Cell Signaling Technology), anti–β-actin (Santa Cruz Biotechnology), anti-CREB (Cell Signaling Technology), anti–phospho-CREB (Cell Signaling Technology), anti-ERK1/2 (Cell Signaling Technology), anti-phospho-ERK1/2 (Cell Signaling Technology), anti-p38 (Cell Signaling Technology), anti-phospho-p38 (Cell Signaling Technology), anti-JNK (Cell Signaling Technology), anti-phospho-JNK (Cell Signaling Technology), anti-goat IgG-HRP (Santa Cruz Biotechnology), anti-mouse IgG-HRP (Santa Cruz Biotechnology), and goat anti-rabbit IgG-HRP (Santa Cruz Biotechnology).

Pathological Analysis

For histological analysis, murine kidney tissues were stained with H&E according to the manufacturer's instructions. Fluorescent staining of cryosections was used for IC deposition analysis in the glomeruli. Sections were fixed in acetone for 10 min and incubated with FITC-conjugated goat anti-mouse IgG (H+L chain-specific) Abs (Sigma-Aldrich) for 30 min. Pictures were acquired with Nikon SCLIPSS TE2000-S microscope (Nikon,

Melville, NY) equipped with ACT-1 software (Nikon; original magnification ×200).

Statistical Analysis

Statistical significance was assessed using Student's t-test or Mann–Whitney U-test unless otherwise noted, and data were given as mean $\pm$ SD unless otherwise noted. Statistical analyses of data were performed using the GraphPad Prism (version 4.0) statistical program. The statistical significance level was set as *$p<0.05$, **$p<0.01$, *** $p<0.001$.

Results

The Levels of MBL Decrease in Lupus Mice and are Negatively Correlated with SLE Disease

By means of immunization with ALD-DNA, we generated a murine model of SLE that developed high levels of anti-dsDNA antibodies (Figure S1A) and glomerulonephritis confirmed by urine protein quantification (Figure S1B), immune complex deposition assay (Figure S1C and S1D), and H&E staining of renal tissues (Figure S1E and S1F). To study whether MBL has a correlation to SLE disease, we first examined the levels of serum MBL in ALD-DNA–induced lupus mice and found that serum MBL levels increased slightly at week 2 but decreased sharply from week 4 (Figure 1A and 1B). From week 6, the levels of serum MBL in lupus mice were lower than those in controls. Enhanced circulating DNA levels were found in lupus mice (Figure 1C), which was consistent with our previous report [8], and the ratios of MBL to DNA were significantly lower in lupus mice than those in controls (Figure 1D). Furthermore, the levels of serum MBL were negatively correlated with the levels of anti-dsDNA antibodies and urine protein in SLE mice (Figure 1E and 1F). Taken together, these results indicate that MBL was insufficient in lupus mice.

MBL Blunts ALD-DNA–induced Macrophage M2b Polarization

Our previous studies revealed that ALD-DNA could induce macrophage M2b polarization, which exhibited significantly enhanced expression of IL-10, TNF-α, IL-6, MCP-1, and inducible NO synthase (iNOS) and played a pivotal role in the development of ALD-DNA–induced SLE disease [7,9]. To clarify whether MBL has any effect on the ALD-DNA–induced macrophage M2b polarization, we performed ELISA assay and real-time PCR to examine the expression of cytokines in mouse macrophage cell line RAW264.7 cells. We found that MBL could significantly suppress expression of the pro-inflammatory cytokines TNF-α, MCP-1 and IL-6 while greatly enhance expression of IL-10 at both mRNA and protein levels (Figure 2A and 2B). To examine whether the influence of MBL on the cytokine production of mouse primary macrophages is similar to its influence on those of RAW264.7 cells, ELISA assay and real-time PCR were performed to examine the expression of cytokines in peritoneal macrophages. Similar to what was observed in RAW264.7 cells, MBL treatment could suppress ALD-DNA–induced the expression of pro-inflammatory cytokines TNF-α, MCP-1 and IL-6 while significantly increase the expression of IL-10 in peritoneal macrophages (Figure 2C and 2D). Furthermore, we tested the protein expression of iNOS and found that MBL could suppress the level of iNOS induced by ALD-DNA (Figure 2E and 2F). Taken together, these results indicate that MBL treatment could modulate ALD-DNA–induced macrophage M2b polarization.

Regulation of Macrophage M2b Polarization by MBL is Associated with Repression of MAPK and NF-κB Signaling Pathway while Increase of CREB Activation

As MBL could blunt macrophage M2b polarization, we next investigated whether MBL has any effect on the signaling pathway induced by ALD-DNA. We performed western blot and found that MBL could significantly down-regulate the phosphorylation of ERK1/2, JNK and IκB (Figure 3B), which was consistent with our previous reports that ALD-DNA could induce macrophage M2b polarization by activating the MAPK and NF-κB signaling [9](Figure 3A). Previous data indicate that C1q could increase the phosphorylation of the transcription factors cAMP response element-binding protein (CREB) and induce CRE driven gene expression, which was able to stimulate IL-10 production and modulate M2 macrophage-specific gene expression [36,37]. Because MBL shared the similar structure and cell receptors with C1q [38], we investigated the phosphorylation of CREB and found that MBL could up-regulate the phosphorylation of CREB (Figure 3B). These results demonstrate that regulation of macrophage M2b polarization by MBL was associated with repression of MAPK and NF-κB signaling pathway while increase of CREB activation.

MBL Treatment Blunts Macrophage M2b Polarization and Ameliorates Lupus Nephritis in ALD-DNA–induced SLE Mice

To evaluate the effect of MBL treatment in mice, mice immunized with ALD-DNA were treated with pMBL or pcDNA3.1. The levels of serum MBL were significantly increased and the levels of serum circulating DNA were notably decreased in the mice treated with pMBL as compared with those in the mice treated with pcDNA3.1 (Figure S2 and S3). Our previous study has revealed that macrophage M2b polarization played a pivotal role in the development of SLE disease. Because MBL could blunt macrophage M2b polarization induced by ALD-DNA *in vitro*, we further investigated whether MBL treatment could modulate macrophage polarization and lupus nephritis in ALD-DNA–induced lupus mice. Consistent with above results *in vitro*, MBL treatment could suppress the pro-inflammatory cytokine TNF-α, MCP-1 and IL-6 while increase the expression of IL-10 in the renal macrophages (Figure 4A) and in serum of lupus mice (Figure 4B). More importantly, notably reduced the levels of anti-dsDNA autoantibodies (Figure 4C), urine protein (Figure 4D), IC deposition (Figure 4E and 4F), renal pathology (Figure 4G), and kidney score (Figure 4H) were found in the pMBL-treated lupus mice as compared with those of pcDNA3.1-treated lupus mice. These results suggest that MBL treatment could ameliorate ALD-DNA–induced lupus nephritis.

The Alleviation of SLE Disease by MBL Treatment might be Associated with Repression of the Ability of Macrophages to Polarize T Cells Toward Th1 and Th17 Cells

T cell differentiation plays an important role in the development of SLE disease. Activated macrophages with elevated expression of activation markers have the acquisition of antigen-presenting features, which lead to efficient Th1 and Th17 responses [39,40]. MBL could regulate ALD-DNA–induced macrophage activation and polarization, so we next investigated whether the regulation of T cell differentiation will occur in the development of modulation of ALD-DNA–induced immune responses by MBL. We applied flow cytometry and found that MBL could decrease the expression of MHC II, CD80 and CD86 (Figure 5A). So we suggested that

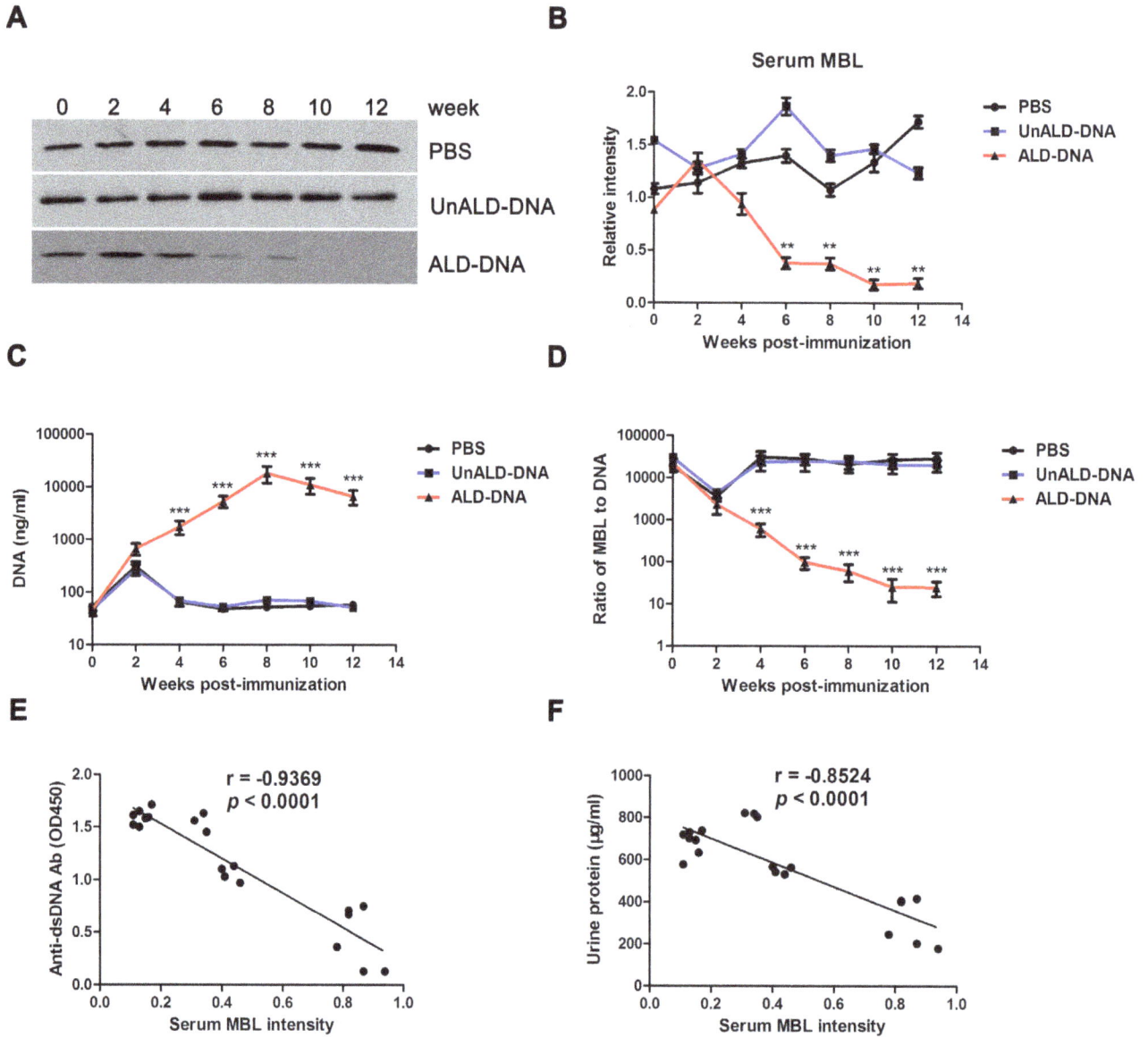

Figure 1. Serum MBL levels decrease in lupus mice and are negatively correlated with SLE disease. 6-week-old female BALB/c mice were immunized subcutaneously with ALD-DNA, UnALD-DNA, or PBS for 3 times in 4 weeks. n = 10. (A and B) Serum MBL levels in mice immunized with ALD-DNA, UnALD-DNA, or PBS were determined by western blot every 2 weeks and quantitative analysis of western blot of serum MBL levels was reflected as mean intensity. **$p<0.01$. n = 10. Data are representative of results obtained from 10 mice in each group. (C and D) The levels of serum circulating DNA were determined using a PicoGreen DNA detection kit and the ratios of MBL to DNA in SLE murine model and controls were presented. Data are means ± SD from 10 mice in each group. ***$p<0.001$. (E) The correlation between serum MBL and anti-dsDNA IgG level in SLE murine model (n = 20) was presented. Pearson correlation analysis was used to carry out the correlation study. r = −0.9369; $p<0.001$. (F) The correlation between serum MBL and urine protein level in SLE murine model (n = 20) was presented. Pearson correlation analysis was used to carry out the correlation study. r = −0.8524; $p<0.001$.

MBL could modulate the differentiation of T cells. To determine whether MBL influences the ability of macrophages to modulate the differentiation of T cells, we cultured peritoneal macrophages with PBS, ALD-DNA or ALD-DNA plus MBL for 48 h and then used them as APCs to stimulate the allogeneic naïve T cells for 6 days. It was found that there were significantly less IL-17 and IFN-γ production by CD4$^+$ T cells incubated with ALD-DNA/MBL–stimulated peritoneal macrophages than those incubated with ALD-DNA–stimulated peritoneal macrophages (Figure 5B and 5C). Further study showed that IL-17$^+$CD4$^+$ and IFN-γ^+CD4$^+$ T cells in lupus mice injected with ALD-DNA/MBL–treated

macrophages were decreased significantly as compared with those in lupus mice injected with ALD-DNA–treated macrophages (Figure S4A and S4B). These results suggest that MBL suppressed the ability of ALD-DNA–stimulated macrophages to promote the differentiation of CD4$^+$ T cells into the Th1 and Th17 phenotypes, which might be involved in the alleviation of ALD-DNA–induced SLE disease by MBL.

Discussion

It has been reported that MBL deficiency or low serum MBL levels caused by polymorphisms in the structural portion or

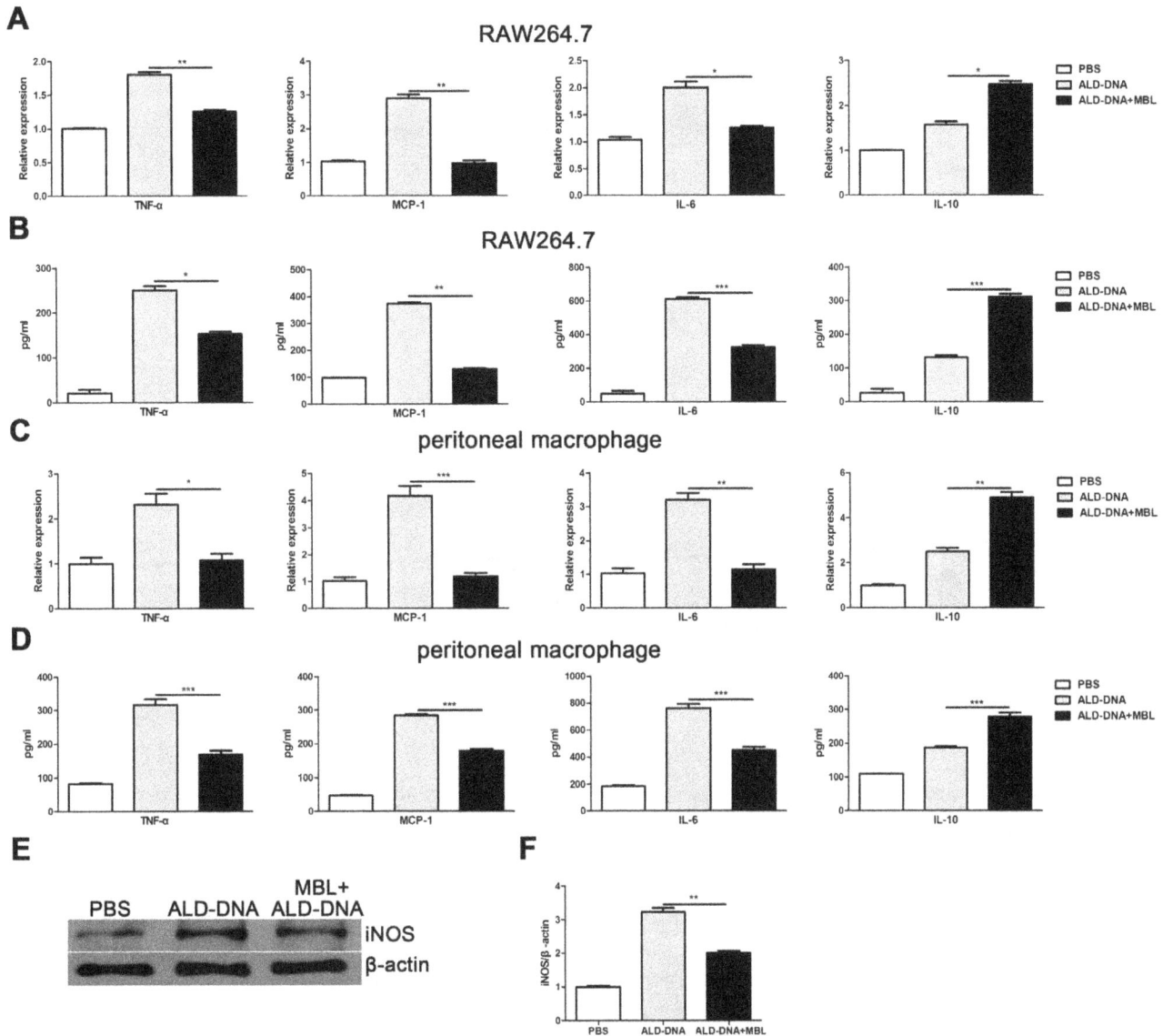

Figure 2. MBL modulates ALD-DNA–induced macrophage M2b polarization. ALD-DNA was pre-incubated with indicated mouse MBL for 2 h. RAW264.7 cells or peritoneal macrophages were cultured with PBS, ALD-DNA or ALD-DNA/MBL complexes for 24 h. (A and C) mRNA levels of TNF-α, MCP-1, IL-6 and IL-10 in RAW264.7 cells or peritoneal macrophages were analyzed by real-time PCR. (B and D) Protein levels of TNF-α, MCP-1, IL-6 and IL-10 in the supernatants of RAW264.7 cells or peritoneal macrophages were measured by ELISA. (E and F) RAW264.7 cells were cultured with PBS, ALD-DNA or ALD-DNA/MBL complexes for 24 h. Then cell lysates were prepared to measure the protein levels of iNOS by western blot analysis. All values are given relative to the expression level of the β-actin. Data are means ± SD of three independent experiments. *$p < 0.05$; **$p < 0.01$; ***$p < 0.001$.

promoter region of the MBL gene were observed in SLE patients [15,27,28]. However it remains unclear whether it contributes to the initiation and progression of SLE, especially the innate and adaptive immunity that occur in the development of autoimmune responses. Data presented in this study showed that the levels of MBL decreased in lupus mice and were negatively correlated with SLE disease. MBL blunted macrophage M2b polarization and suppressed the ability of macrophages to promote the differentiation of T cells. Furthermore, MBL treatment ameliorated ALD-DNA–induced lupus nephritis by reducing anti-dsDNA antibodies production and IC deposition.

It is now well established that exorbitant cell apoptosis has been found to occur frequently in SLE patients and lupus mice, which is caused by various factors including genetic susceptibility and

environmental factors [41,42]. Impaired clearance ability for apoptotic cells and cellular debris, including defects of macrophages and deficiency of serum factors such as complement, DNase I, pentraxins and IgM, may explain accumulation of self nuclear antigens released from noningested apoptotic cells [43–45]. Nuclear antigens including self-dsDNA released from these excessive apoptotic cells have been reported to contribute to the activation of pathological immune responses and the production of autoantibody, which lead to IC deposition and organ damage [46].

MBL is one member of complement components. In addition to the removal of microorganisms by activating the complement system, MBL could mediate the recognition and the clearance of modified self cells, such as apoptotic cells and cellular debris,

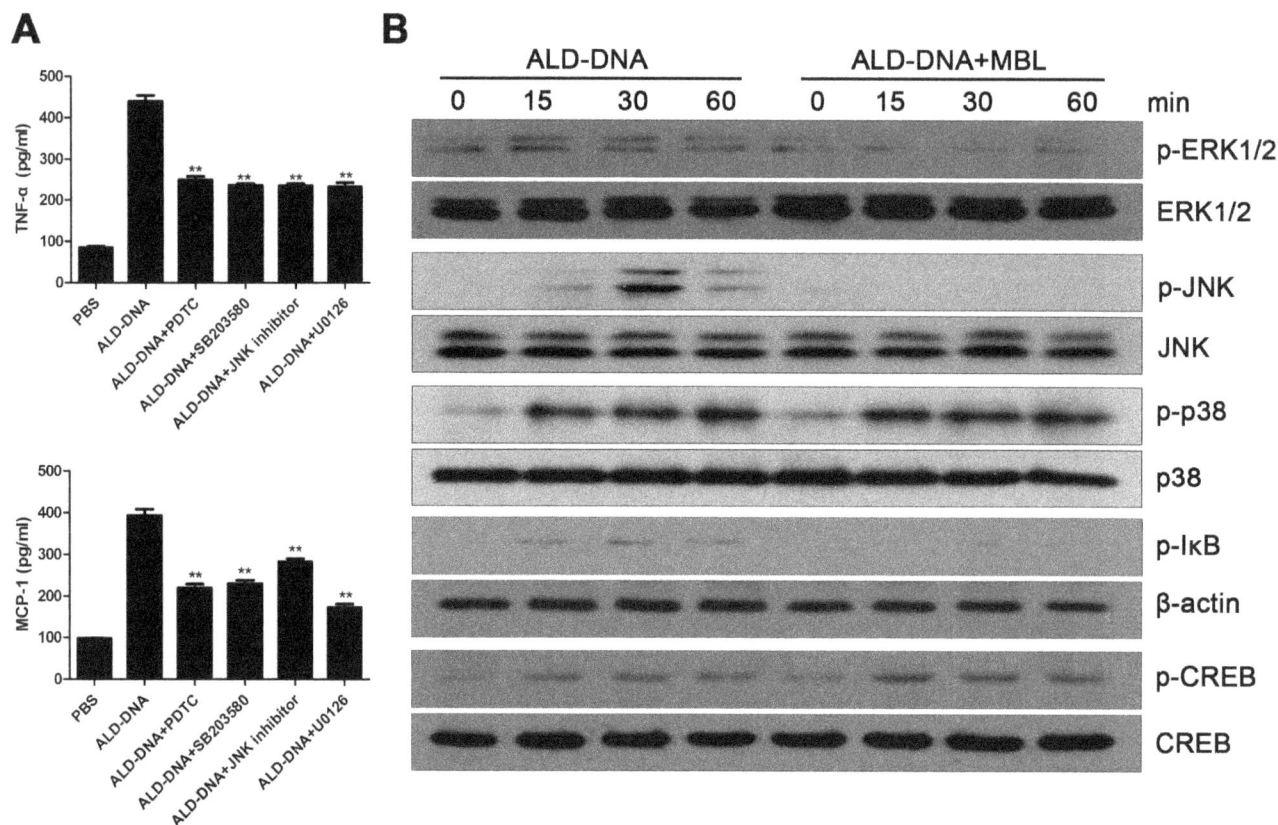

Figure 3. The signaling pathway of regulation of macrophage M2b polarization by MBL. (A) RAW264.7 cells were treated with a given inhibitor for 1 h before PBS or ALD-DNA stimulation and 24 h later the supernatants were collected for ELISA. (B) RAW264.7 cells were treated with ALD-DNA (50 µg/ml) or ALD-DNA (50 µg/ml) plus MBL (10 µg/ml) for the indicated times. The cells were harvested and β-actin, phosphorylated IκB, and the total and phosphorylated p38, ERK1/2, JNK and CREB were detected by western blot. Data are representative of results obtained in three independent experiments. **$p < 0.01$.

which is important for maintaining tissue homeostasis and avoiding autoimmune diseases such as SLE [22–25]. Previous studies have demonstrated that MBL deficiency or low serum MBL levels were observed in SLE patients [15,27,28], but whether MBL is involved in the development of SLE remains unclear. In our previous studies, we generated a novel murine model of SLE by immunizing the syngeneic female BALB/c mice with ALD-DNA, which developed high titers of anti-dsDNA antibodies, proteinuria, and glomerular nephritis that closely resembled human SLE [6–8]. The levels of serum MBL in lupus mice induced by ALD-DNA decreased and were negatively correlated with SLE disease, indicating that serum MBL was insufficient in SLE disease, which was consistent with previous reports on the serum MBL levels in SLE patients and MRL-lpr lupus mice [15,27,28,47]. Our results revealed that MBL treatment could enhance the clearance of DNA (Figure S3), indicating that MBL might play a protective role in the development of SLE. Previous studies indicated that MBL could enhance the clearance of modified cells and cells debris by the interaction with its receptors on the cell surface, such as C1q phagocytic receptor C1qRp (CD93), cC1qR (CRT) and CR1 (CD35) [19–25]. The involved receptor(s) of MBL in the process of DNA clearance remains to be further studied. In addition to the enhancement of DNA clearance, MBL was proved to bind to immunoglobulins and might facilitate the clearance of circulating immune complexes [48,49]. The clearance of DNA and immune complexes mediated by MBL might exhaust the serum MBL. Besides, it was observed

that there was a strong inverse correlation between anti-MBL autoantibodies and serum MBL levels [50]. The precise mechanism of decrease of serum MBL in ALD-DNA–induced lupus mice remains to be further studied. Furthermore, our study showed that MBL supplement *in vivo* could reduce the levels of anti-dsDNA autoantibodies, urine protein, IC deposition, renal pathology and kidney score. These data provide evidence to support the protective role of MBL in SLE disease.

Functional macrophage polarization represented different extremes of a continuum ranging from M1, M2a and M2b to M2c [9]. M1 polarization, driven by IFN-γ and LPS, typically acquires fortified cytotoxic and antitumoral properties; M2a polarization, induced by IL-4 and IL-13, and M2b polarization, induced by combined immune complexes with TLR or IL-1R agonists, exert immunoregulatory functions and drive type II responses, whereas M2c polarization, induced by IL-10, gains immunosuppression and tissue-remodeling activities. Our previous studies revealed that ALD-DNA could induce macrophage M2b polarization, which exhibited enhanced IL-10, TNF-α, IL-6, MCP-1 and iNOS [9]. Recent studies suggest that MBL could modulate macrophage-mediated inflammatory responses [29,30]. To study whether MBL has any influence on the immune responses induced by ALD-DNA, we examined cytokine production and found that MBL treatment leaded to the suppression of ALD-DNA–induced pro-inflammatory cytokines TNF-α, MCP-1 and IL-6, and an increase of anti-inflammatory cytokine IL-10 in macrophages, indicating that ALD-DNA/MBL treatment could

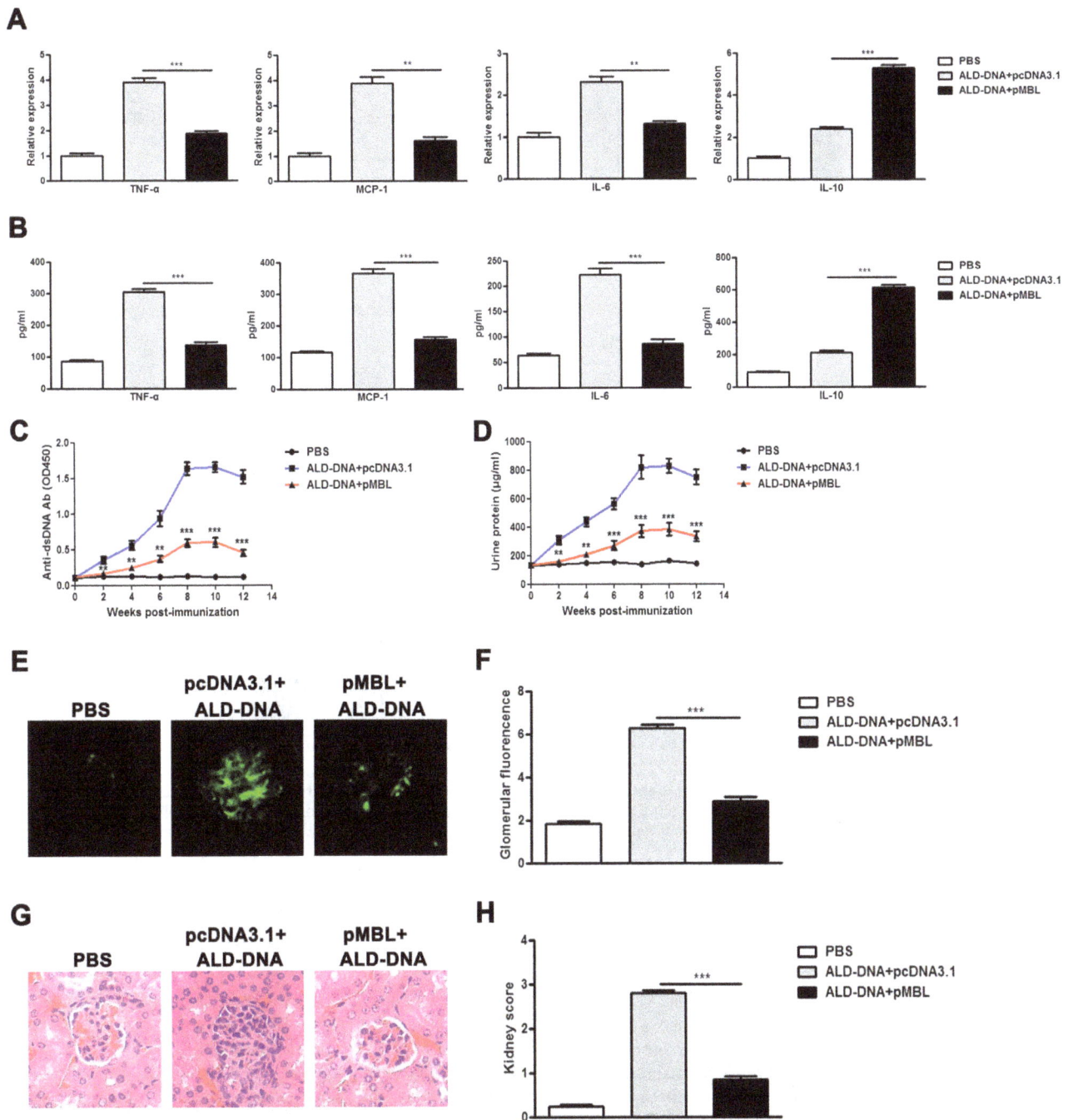

Figure 4. MBL treatment blunts macrophage M2b polarization and alleviates lupus nephritis. BALB/c mice were immunized subcutaneously with ALD-DNA (50 µg/mouse) or PBS for total 3 times in 4 weeks. Mice immunized with ALD-DNA were pre-treated intramuscularly with pMBL (100 µg/mice) or pcDNA3.1 (100 µg/mice), and injected every 2 weeks for total 5 times. (A) mRNA levels of TNF-α, MCP-1, IL-6 and IL-10 in renal macrophages purified from mice were evaluated by real-time PCR. Data are means ± SD of three independent experiments. **p<0.01; ***p<0.001. n=6. (B) Levels of TNF-α, MCP-1, IL-6 and IL-10 in serum were detected by ELISA assay. ***p<0.001. n=6. (C) Serum anti-dsDNA IgG levels of the mice were measured by ELISA assay every 2 weeks. **p<0.01; ***p<0.001. (D) Urine protein levels of the mice were assessed by BCA Protein Assay Kit every 2 weeks. **p<0.01; ***p<0.001. (E) The deposition of IgG-containing IC in glomeruli at week 12 after initial immunization. Imagines (×200) are representative of 10 mice in each group. (F) Mean glomerular fluorescence intensity (arbitrary units) was determined for IgG in ALD-DNA immunized lupus mice and control mice at week 12 after initial immunization. n=10. ***p<0.001. (G) 12 weeks after initial immunization, nephritic pathological changes were shown by H&E staining of renal tissues surgical resected from the mice. Imagines (×200) are representative of 10 mice in each group. (H) The kidney score was assessed using paraffin sections stained with H&E. n=10. ***p<0.001.

turn M2b macrophages to an anti-inflammatory phenotype. Further studies are needed to investigate the definitive anti-inflammatory phenotype induced by ALD-DNA/MBL. Impor-

tantly, we found that MBL could significantly down-regulate the phosphorylation of ERK1/2, JNK and IκB induced by ALD-DNA, which was consistent with our previous reports that MAPK

A

B

C

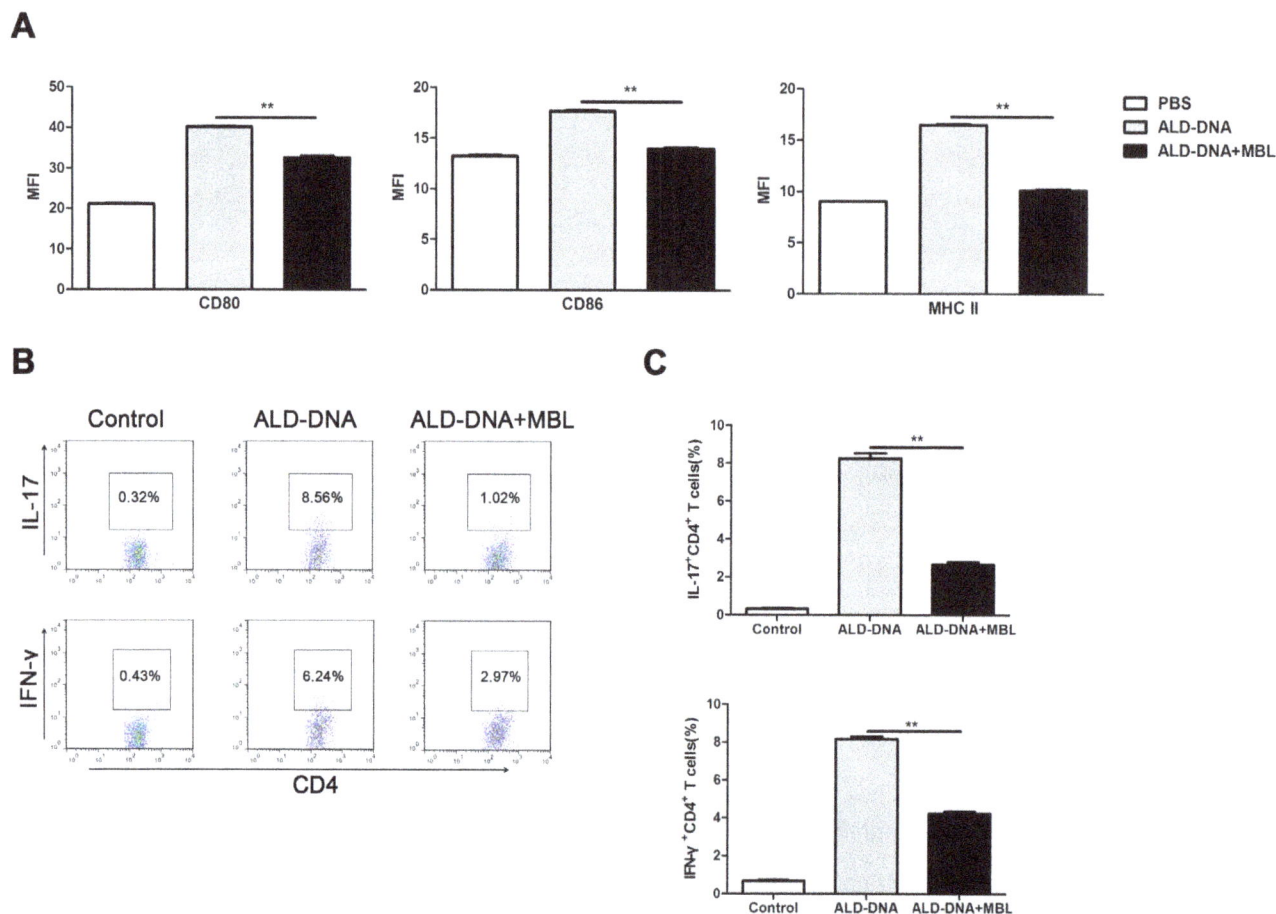

Figure 5. MBL alters the ability of ALD-DNA–stimulated macrophages to promote T cell differentiation. Peritoneal macrophages were incubated with PBS, ALD-DNA (50 μg/ml) or ALD-DNA (50 μg/ml) plus MBL (10 μg/ml) for 48 h. (A) The expression of MHC II, CD80 and CD86 was examined by flow cytometry and the levels of them were represented as mean fluorescent intensity (MFI). (B and C) These peritoneal macrophages and allogeneic T cells isolated from female BALB/c mice were cultured at a 1:5 ratio in the presence of ALD-DNA (50 μg/ml) for 6 days. For intracellular analysis of cytokine production, T cells were pre-stimulated with 10 ng/ml phorbol myristate acetate and 1 μg/ml ionomycin in the presence of 10 μg/ml brefeldin A for 5 to 6 hours. Cells were then fixed, permeabilized, and stained for IFN-γ and IL-17 and analyzed by flow cytometry. Average of percentage of IFN-γ$^+$ CD4$^+$ or IL-17$^+$CD4$^+$ T cells was presented in the bar charts. Data are means ± SD of three independent experiments. **$p < 0.01$.

and NF-κB signaling played an important role in ALD-DNA–induced macrophage M2b polarization [9]. A previous study has reported that C1q could increase the phosphorylation of CREB, which could induce CRE driven IL-10 production and modulate M2 macrophage-specific gene expression [36,37]. Because of the similar structure and cell receptors that MBL and C1q shared [38], we examined the phosphorylation of CREB and found MBL could up-regulate the phosphorylation of CREB, which might provide an interpretation of an increase of IL-10 in macrophages cultured with ALD-DNA/MBL. Apart from these signaling pathways, whether ALD-DNA/MBL modulates other signaling pathways remains to be investigated.

As antigen-presenting cells, activated macrophages can differentiate naïve T cells into Th1 cells and Th17 cells, which play a pivotal role in the development of SLE disease [51–53]. In this study, we found that MBL treatment decreased the expression of MHC II, CD80 and CD86, and leaded to the suppression of the ability of ALD-DNA–stimulated macrophages to promote the differentiation of CD4$^+$ T cells into the Th1 and Th17 phenotypes *in vitro* and *in vivo*, which might be involved in the alleviation of SLE disease by MBL. These data indicate that MBL played an

important role in the regulation of ALD-DNA–induced immune responses and would further our understanding of the regulatory function of MBL in the development of SLE.

In conclusion, our results presented in this study showed that the levels of serum MBL significantly decreased in lupus mice and were negatively correlated with SLE disease. MBL could blunt macrophage M2b polarization induced by ALD-DNA and suppress the ability of macrophages to promote T cell differentiation. MBL supplement *in vivo* could ameliorate ALD-DNA–induced lupus nephritis. Our findings provide a novel mechanism to understand the role of MBL in the pathogenesis of SLE and indicate that MBL might be a new candidate for modulating immune responses induced by DNA. So these results would open a new avenue for developing novel therapeutic approaches for DNA-induced autoimmune diseases such as SLE.

Supporting Information

Figure S1   ALD-DNA immunization induces high levels of anti-dsDNA antibody and lupus nephritis. 6-week-old female BALB/c mice were immunized subcutaneously with ALD-DNA, UnALD-DNA, or PBS for total 3 times in 4 weeks. n = 10.

(A) Serum anti-dsDNA IgG levels were measured by ELISA assay every 2 weeks after initial immunization. Data are means ± SD from 10 mice in each group. ***$p<0.001$. (B) Urine protein levels of the mice were assessed by BCA Protein Assay Kit every 2 weeks. Data are means ± SD from 10 mice in each group. ***$p<0.001$. (C) Glomerular immune complex deposition was detected by direct immunofluorescence for IgG in frozen kidney section from ALD-DNA-immunized lupus mice or control mice. Representative images (magnification×200) of 10 mice are shown for each group. (D) Mean glomerular fluorescence intensity (arbitrary units) was determined for IgG in ALD-DNA-immunized lupus mice and control mice. ***$p<0.001$. n = 10. (E) 12 weeks after initial immunization, nephritic pathology was evaluated by H&E staining of renal tissues. Imagines (magnification×200) are representative of at least 10 mice in each group. (F) The kidney score was assessed using paraffin sections stained with H&E. ***$p<0.001$.

Figure S2 pMBL treatment significantly increases the serum MBL levels. Mice immunized with ALD-DNA were treated intramuscularly with pMBL (100 μg/mice) or pcDNA3.1 (100 μg/mice), and injected every 2 weeks for total 5 times. The levels of serum MBL were detected by western blot every 2 weeks. Data are means ± SD from 10 mice in each group.

Figure S3 MBL treatment enhances the clearance of DNA *in vitro* and *in vivo*. ALD-DNA labeled with Alexa Fluor 488 (AF488-ALD-DNA) was incubated with MBL at 37°C for 2 h. And then RAW264.7 cells were cultured with PBS, AF488-ALD-DNA or AF488-ALD-DNA/MBL complexes for 30 minutes. (A and B) The intracellular AF488-ALD-DNA was determined by flow cytometry. ***$p<0.001$. (C) Mice immunized with ALD-DNA were treated intramuscularly with pMBL (100 μg/mice) or pcDNA3.1 (100 μg/mice), and injected every 2 weeks for total 5 times. 12 weeks after initial immunization, the levels of serum DNA in lupus mice treated with pMBL or pcDNA3.1 and control mice were detected using a PicoGreen DNA detection kit. Data are means ± SD from 10 mice in each group. *$p<0.05$.

Figure S4 MBL suppresses the ability of macrophages to promote T cell differentiation *in vivo*. For adoptive transfer of macrophages, we first treated peritoneal macrophages with ALD-DNA/MBL or ALD-DNA alone for 48 h. And then ALD-DNA–immunized mice were injected i.v with these macrophages (2.5×10^6 cells/mouse) at weeks 0, 2 and 4 after the initial immunization for a total of three times. (A and B) 8 weeks after initial immunization, splenocytes were collected and the levels of Th1 and Th17 cells were analyzed by flow cytometry. Data are means ± SD from 10 mice in each group. **$p<0.01$.

Acknowledgments

We thank Zhenke Wen for valuable discussions. And we also thank Xi Chen, Mudan Luo, and Furong Li for technical assistance.

Author Contributions

Conceived and designed the experiments: YC WZ SX. Performed the experiments: YC WZ. Analyzed the data: YC WZ SX. Contributed reagents/materials/analysis tools: YC WZ. Wrote the paper: YC WZ SX.

References

1. Buckner JH (2010) Mechanisms of impaired regulation by CD4(+)CD25(+)FOXP3(+) regulatory T cells in human autoimmune diseases. Nature Reviews Immunology 10: 849–859.
2. Charles N, Hardwick D, Daugas E, Illei GG, Rivera J (2010) Basophils and the T helper 2 environment can promote the development of lupus nephritis. Nature Medicine 16: 701–U107.
3. Hutcheson J, Scatizzi JC, Siddiqui AM, Haines GK, III, Wu T, et al. (2008) Combined deficiency of proapoptotic regulators Bim and Fas results in the early onset of systemic autoimmunity. Immunity 28: 206–217.
4. Nagata S, Hanayama R, Kawane K (2010) Autoimmunity and the Clearance of Dead Cells. Cell 140: 619–630.
5. Munoz LE, Janko C, Schulze C, Schorn C, Sarter K, et al. (2010) Autoimmunity and chronic inflammation - Two clearance-related steps in the etiopathogenesis of SLE. Autoimmunity Reviews 10: 38–42.
6. Qiao B, Wu J, Chu YW, Wang Y, Wang DP, et al. (2005) Induction of systemic lupus erythematosus-like syndrome in syngeneic mice by immunization with activated lymphocyte-derived DNA. Rheumatology 44: 1108–1114.
7. Zhang W, Xu W, Xiong S (2011) Macrophage Differentiation and Polarization via Phosphatidylinositol 3-Kinase/Akt-ERK Signaling Pathway Conferred by Serum Amyloid P Component. Journal of Immunology 187: 1764–1777.
8. Zhang W, Wu J, Qiao B, Xu W, Xiong S (2011) Amelioration of Lupus Nephritis by Serum Amyloid P Component Gene Therapy with Distinct Mechanisms Varied from Different Stage of the Disease. Plos One 6.
9. Zhang W, Xu W, Xiong S (2010) Blockade of Notch1 Signaling Alleviates Murine Lupus via Blunting Macrophage Activation and M2b Polarization. Journal of Immunology 184: 6465–6478.
10. Schiffer L, Bethunaickan R, Ramanujam M, Huang W, Schiffer M, et al. (2008) Activated renal macrophages are markers of disease onset and disease remission in lupus nephritis. Journal of Immunology 180: 1938–1947.
11. Walport MJ (2000) Lupus, DNase and defective disposal of cellular debris. Nature Genetics 25: 135–136.
12. Zipfel PF, Skerka C (2009) Complement regulators and inhibitory proteins. Nature Reviews Immunology 9: 729–740.
13. Ricklin D, Hajishengallis G, Yang K, Lambris JD (2010) Complement: a key system for immune surveillance and homeostasis. Nature Immunology 11: 785–797.
14. Dunkelberger JR, Song W-C (2010) Complement and its role in innate and adaptive immune responses. Cell Research 20: 34–50.
15. Nath SK, Kilpatrick J, Harley JB (2004) Genetics of human systemic lupus erythematosus: the emerging picture. Current Opinion in Immunology 16: 794–800.
16. Jeannin P, Jaillon S, Delneste Y (2008) Pattern recognition receptors in the immune response against dying cells. Current Opinion in Immunology 20: 530–537.
17. Netea MG, van der Meer JWM (2011) MECHANISMS OF DISEASE Immunodeficiency and Genetic Defects of Pattern-Recognition Receptors. New England Journal of Medicine 364: 60–70.
18. Ip WKE, Takahashi K, Ezekowitz RA, Stuart LM (2009) Mannose-binding lectin and innate immunity. Immunological Reviews 230: 9–21.
19. Csipo I, Kiss E, Bako E, Szegedi G, Kavai M (2005) Soluble complement receptor 1 (CD35) bound to immune complexes in sera of patients with systemic lupus erythematosus. Arthritis and Rheumatism 52: 2950–2951.
20. Marzocchi-Machado CM, Alves C, Azzolini A, Polizello ACM, Carvalho IF, et al. (2002) CR1 on erythrocytes of Brazilian systemic lupus erythematosus patients: The influence of disease activity on expression and ability of this receptor to bind immune complexes opsonized with complement from normal human serum. Journal of Autoimmunity 25: 289–297.
21. Takahashi K, Kozono Y, Waldschmidt TJ, Berthiaume D, Quigg RJ, et al. (1997) Mouse complement receptors type 1 (CR1; CD35) and type 2 (CR2; CD21) - Expression on normal B cell subpopulations and decreased levels during the development of autoimmunity in MRL/lpr mice. Journal of Immunology 159: 1557–1569.
22. Prodeus AP, Goerg S, Shen LM, Pozdnyakova OO, Chu L, et al. (1998) A critical role for complement in maintenance of self-tolerance. Immunity 9: 721–731.
23. Ghiran I, Barbashov SF, Klickstein LB, Tas S, Jensenius JC, et al. (2000) Complement receptor 1/CD35 is a receptor for mannan-binding lectin. Journal of Experimental Medicine 192: 1797–1807.
24. Ogden CA, deCathenneau A, Hoffmann PR, Bratton D, Ghebrehiwet B, et al. (2001) C1q and mannose binding lectin engagement of cell surface calreticulin and CD91 initiates macropinocytosis and uptake of apoptotic cells. Journal of Experimental Medicine 194: 781–795.
25. Takahashi K, Ip WKE, Michelow IC, Ezekowitz RAB (2006) The mannose-binding lectin: a prototypic pattern recognition molecule. Current Opinion in Immunology 18: 16–23.
26. Lee YH, Witte T, Momot T, Schmidt RE, Kaufman KM, et al. (2005) The Mannose-binding lectin gene polymorphisms and systemic lupus erythematosus -

Two case-control studies and a meta-analysis. Arthritis and Rheumatism 52: 3966–3974.

27. Kristjansdottir H, Saevarsdottir S, Grondal G, Alarcon-Riquelme ME, Erlendsson K, et al. (2008) Association of Three Systemic Lupus Erythematosus Susceptibility Factors, PD-1.3A, C4AQ0, and Low Levels of Mannan-Binding Lectin, With Autoimmune Manifestations in Icelandic Multicase Systemic Lupus Erythematosus Families. Arthritis and Rheumatism 58: 3865–3872.

28. Ip WK, Chan SY, Lau CS, Lau YL (1998) Association of systemic lupus erythematosus with promoter polymorphisms of the mannose-binding lectin gene. Arthritis and Rheumatism 41: 1663–1668.

29. Nadesalingam J, Dodds AW, Reid KBM, Palaniyar N (2005) Mannose-binding lectin recognizes peptidoglycan via the N-acetyl glucosamine moiety, and inhibits ligand-induced proinflammatory effect and promotes chemokine production by macrophages. Journal of Immunology 175: 1785–1794.

30. Jack DL, Read RC, Tenner AJ, Frosch M, Turner MW, et al. (2001) Mannose-binding lectin regulates the inflammatory response of human professional phagocytes to Neisseria meningitidis serogroup B. Journal of Infectious Diseases 184: 1152–1162.

31. Palaniyar N, Nadesalingam J, Clark H, Shih MJ, Dodds AW, et al. (2004) Nucleic acid is a novel ligand for innate, immune pattern recognition collectins surfactant proteins A and D and mannose-binding lectin. Journal of Biological Chemistry 279: 32728–32736.

32. Nakamura N, Nonaka M, Ma BY, Matsumoto S, Kawasaki N, et al. (2009) Characterization of the interaction between serum mannan-binding protein and nucleic acid ligands. Journal of Leukocyte Biology 86: 737–748.

33. Bidaud P, Hebert L, Barbey C, Appourchaux A-C, Torelli R, et al. (2012) Rhodococcus equi's Extreme Resistance to Hydrogen Peroxide Is Mainly Conferred by One of Its Four Catalase Genes. Plos One 7.

34. Tan SM, Chung MCM, Kon OL, Thiel S, Lee SH, et al. (1996) Improvements on the purification of mannan-binding lectin and demonstration of its Ca2+-independent association with a C1s-like serine protease. Biochemical Journal 319: 329–332.

35. Gao B, Duan Z, Xu W, Xiong S (2009) Tripartite Motif-Containing 22 Inhibits the Activity of Hepatitis B Virus Core Promoter, Which Is Dependent on Nuclear-Located RING Domain. Hepatology 50: 424–433.

36. Ruffell D, Mourkioti F, Gambardella A, Kirstetter P, Lopez RG, et al. (2009) A CREB-C/EBP beta cascade induces M2 macrophage-specific gene expression and promotes muscle injury repair. Proceedings of the National Academy of Sciences of the United States of America 106: 17475–17480.

37. Fraser DA, Arora M, Bohlson SS, Lozano E, Tenner AJ (2007) Generation of inhibitory NF kappa B complexes and phosphorylated cAMP response element-binding protein correlates with the anti-inflammatory activity of complement protein C1q in human monocytes. Journal of Biological Chemistry 282: 7360–7367.

38. Bottazzi B, Doni A, Garlanda C, Mantovani A (2010) An Integrated View of Humoral Innate Immunity: Pentraxins as a Paradigm. In: Paul WE, Littman DR, Yokoyama WM, editors. Annual Review of Immunology, Vol 28. 157–183.

39. Krausgruber T, Blazek K, Smallie T, Alzabin S, Lockstone H, et al. (2011) IRF5 promotes inflammatory macrophage polarization and T(H)1-T(H)17 responses. Nature Immunology 12: 231–U266.

40. Qin H, Yeh W-I, De Sarno P, Holdbrooks AT, Liu Y, et al. (2012) Signal transducer and activator of transcription-3/suppressor of cytokine signaling-3 (STAT3/SOCS3) axis in myeloid cells regulates neuroinflammation. Proceedings of the National Academy of Sciences of the United States of America 109: 5004–5009.

41. Rahman A, Isenberg DA (2008) Mechanisms of disease: Systemic lupus erythematosus. New England Journal of Medicine 358: 929–939.

42. Roszer T, Menendez-Gutierrez MP, Lefterova MI, Alameda D, Nunez V, et al. (2011) Autoimmune Kidney Disease and Impaired Engulfment of Apoptotic Cells in Mice with Macrophage Peroxisome Proliferator-Activated Receptor gamma or Retinoid X Receptor alpha Deficiency. Journal of Immunology 186: 621–631.

43. Gaipl US, Kuhn A, Sheriff A, Munoz LE, Franz S, et al. (2006) Clearance of apoptotic cells in human SLE. Apoptosis and Its Relevance to Autoimmunity 9: 173–187.

44. Savill J, Dransfield I, Gregory C, Haslett C (2002) A blast from the past: Clearance of apoptotic cells regulates immune responses. Nature Reviews Immunology 2: 965–975.

45. Hoffmann MH, Trembleau S, Muller S, Steiner G (2010) Nucleic acid-associated autoantigens: Pathogenic involvement and therapeutic potential. Journal of Autoimmunity 34: J178–J206.

46. Vinuesa CG, Goodnow CC (2002) Immunology - DNA drives autoimmunity. Nature 416: 595-+.

47. Trouw LA, Seelen MA, Duijs J, Wagner S, Loos M, et al. (2005) Activation of the lectin pathway in murine lupus nephritis. Molecular Immunology 42: 731–740.

48. Arnold JN, Dwek RA, Rudd PM, Sim RB (2006) Mannan binding lectin and its interaction with immunoglobulins in health and in disease. Immunology Letters 106: 103–110.

49. Saevarsdottir S, Steinsson K, Ludviksson BR, Grondal G, Valdimarsson H (2007) Mannan-binding lectin may facilitate the clearance of circulating immune complexes - implications from a study on C2-deficient individuals. Clinical and Experimental Immunology 148: 248–253.

50. Gupta B, Raghav SK, Agrawal C, Chaturvedi VP, Das RH, et al. (2006) Anti-MBL autoantibodies in patients with rheumatoid arthritis: prevalence and clinical significance. Journal of Autoimmunity 27: 125–133.

51. Garrett-Sinha LA, John S, Gaffen SL (2008) IL-17 and the Th17 lineage in systemic lupus erythematosus. Current Opinion in Rheumatology 20: 519–525.

52. Espinosa A, Dardalhon V, Brauner S, Ambrosi A, Higgs R, et al. (2009) Loss of the lupus autoantigen Ro52/Trim21 induces tissue inflammation and systemic autoimmunity by disregulating the IL-23-Th17 pathway. Journal of Experimental Medicine 206: 1661–1671.

53. Steinmetz OM, Turner J-E, Paust H-J, Lindner M, Peters A, et al. (2009) CXCR3 Mediates Renal Th1 and Th17 Immune Response in Murine Lupus Nephritis. Journal of Immunology 183: 4693–4704.

18

Safety of Hormonal Replacement Therapy and Oral Contraceptives in Systemic Lupus Erythematosus

Adriana Rojas-Villarraga[1]*, July-Vianneth Torres-Gonzalez[2], Ángela-María Ruiz-Sternberg[3]

1 Center for Autoimmune Diseases Research (CREA), School of medicine and health sciences, Universidad del Rosario, Bogotá, Colombia, 2 Medical social service provision mandatory, research assistant in partnership with the School of Medicine and Health Sciences, Universidad del Rosario, Bogotá, Colombia, 3 Departamento de investigación Grupo Investigación Clínica, School of Medicine and Health Sciences, Universidad del Rosario, Bogotá, Colombia

Abstract

Background: There is conflicting data regarding exogenous sex hormones [oral contraceptives (OC) and hormonal replacement therapy (HRT)] exposure and different outcomes on Systemic Lupus Erythematosus (SLE). The aim of this work is to determine, through a systematic review and meta-analysis the risks associated with estrogen use for women with SLE as well as the association of estrogen with developing SLE.

Methods and Findings: MEDLINE, EMBASE, SciElo, BIREME and the Cochrane library (1982 to July 2012), were databases from which were selected and reviewed (PRISMA guidelines) randomized controlled trials, cross-sectional, case-control and prospective or retrospective nonrandomized, comparative studies without language restrictions. Those were evaluated by two investigators who extracted information on study characteristics, outcomes of interest, risk of bias and summarized strength of evidence. A total of 6,879 articles were identified; 20 full-text articles were included. Thirty-two meta-analyses were developed. A significant association between HRT exposure (Random model) and an increased risk of developing SLE was found (Rate Ratio: 1.96; 95%-CI: 1.51–2.56; *P*-value<0.001). One of eleven meta-analyses evaluating the risk for SLE associated with OC exposure had a marginally significant result. There were no associations between HRT or OC exposure and specific outcomes of SLE. It was not always possible to Meta-analyze all the available data. There was a wide heterogeneity of SLE outcome measurements and estrogen therapy administration.

Conclusion: An association between HRT exposure and SLE causality was observed. No association was found when analyzing the risk for SLE among OC users, however since women with high disease activity/Thromboses or antiphospholipid-antibodies were excluded from most of the studies, caution should be exercised in interpreting the present results. To identify risk factors that predispose healthy individuals to the development of SLE who are planning to start HRT or OC is suggested.

Editor: Amr H. Sawalha, University of Michigan, United States of America

Funding: The authors have no support or funding to report.

Competing Interests: The authors have declared that no competing interests exist.

* Email: adrirojas@gmail.com

Introduction

Almost all autoimmune diseases (ADs) disproportionately affect middle-aged women and are among the leading causes of death for this group of patients. The female-to-male ratio for ADs becomes more prominent as patients age [1]. Systemic Lupus Erythematosus (SLE) is a complex and multifactorial disease. Although hormone differences may have a strong influence on the predisposition of women to SLE, genetic and environmental factors are also important [2].

Exogenous administration of estrogen has been clinically used in women for the treatment of symptoms associated with menopause, as hormone replacement therapy (HRT), in hormone contraception, and in inducing ovulation to manage infertility [3–7]. There is a widely held view that sexual steroid hormones, particularly

estrogens, may increase SLE activity, which is based on clinical and empirical observations that SLE is predominantly a female disease [8–10]. The female to male ratio of incidence rates, has been reported as high as 15:1, especially during reproductive years. In addition, altered estrone metabolism has been demonstrated in males and females affected with the disease and there are reports of disease flare-ups in SLE women treated with oral contraceptives (OC) and HRT, but the results have been conflicting [11–15].

Experiments with animal models of SLE have shown that prepuberal orchidectomy in males leads to disease activity that is comparable to that in females. In animals already affected with the disease, estrogen administration increases autoimmunity and mortality, while androgen administration reduces production of anti-DNA antibodies and ameliorates disease activity [16–18]. The effects of estrogen on murine models of SLE may be either harmful or beneficial depending on how they affect immune responses. Some estrogens can stimulate B cell activity, worsening complex-mediated glomerulonephritis, but they can also suppress some T cell-mediated responses, improving sialadenitis, renal vasculitis, and periarticular inflammation [19–21]. In fact, an imbalance between hormones can result in lower immune-suppressive androgens and higher immune-enhancing estrogens. Women with SLE tend to have lower androgen levels than healthy women [2].

There are reasonable concerns regarding estrogen usage in SLE women, primarily due to fear that the disease may be activated and the increased risk of venous and arterial thrombosis. On the other hand, Besides preventing accidental and unwanted pregnancies in women with SLE, OC have other potential benefits including control of cyclic disease activity, reduction of the risk of osteoporosis, and preservation of fertility in women treated with cyclophosphamide [7,22–26]. Yet, there are also circumstances that favor the use of estrogen. In the last few decades, SLE patients reached menopause more frequently due to improvements in prognosis and survival and a higher incidence of premature ovarian failure. They have an increased risk of osteoporosis and cardiovascular morbidity and mortality, and HRT is likely to be especially beneficial to them. Recent studies and meta-analyses have suggested that the effects of HRT on coronary heart disease (CHD) differ based on age and timing of initiation after menopause, and it may be beneficial for women under 60 who initiated HRT within ten years of menopause. [27] [28][29]. However, the benefits and risks of HRT on cardiovascular outcomes remain controversial. Since 2002 when The Women's Health Initiative (WHI) [30] and the Heart and Estrogen/ progestin Replacement Study (HERS) [31] questioned the cardiovascular protective effects of HRT, different authors have revisited the subject and have gotten contradictory results. A subsequent analysis of the WHI study showed that in women that initiated the therapy closer to menopause, there was no increased risk of CHD but rather a tendency to decreased risk [32]. This finding is consistent with the "timing hypothesis" [33]. The meta-analysis done by Yang et al. [34] found that HRT does not affect the incidence of CHD. Despite the above, results in women with SLE must be interpreted cautiously since their condition can coexist with pre-existing cardiovascular disease. The present study aimed to determine, through a systematic review and meta-analysis of published reports, the risks associated with estrogen use for women with SLE as well as the association of estrogen with developing SLE.

Methods

Study Design

A systematic literature review, focused on estrogen-based hormonal therapy in women with SLE, was carried out using the following databases: PubMed, EMBASE, COCHRANE, Virtual Health Library (VHL), and SciELO. It included articles published between January 1985 and July 2012. Two reviewers completed the search independently (JTG and ARV), applying the same selection criteria. The search results were compared and disagreements resolved by consensus. The Preferred Reporting Items for Systematic Reviews and Meta-analyses (PRISMA) guidelines were followed [35]. There were no limits regarding language or publication type. PubMed, COCHRANE and EMBASE databases were searched using MeSH terms and

Keywords while Scielo and VHL were searched using DeCS terms (**Appendix S1**).

Articles Selection

Abstracts and articles titles were reviewed by two authors (JTG and AMR) to find eligible studies. Once the articles were chosen, inclusion was discussed by all authors to resolve differences of opinion. For articles in languages other than English or Spanish, the abstracts were reviewed to determine eligibility. A study was included if (a) the abstract was available, (b) it contained original data, (c) it used accepted classification criteria for SLE according to American College of Rheumatology criteria (ACR) [36], (d) it contained information about exposure to HRT and/or OC, (e) it reported the impact of the use of estrogens (HRT or OC) in healthy women, and (f) it reported changes in the disease activity in women with SLE after exposure to estrogens (HRT or OC). Publications that provided epidemiologic data regarding risk factors such as relative risks (RR), odds ratios (OR) with confidence intervals (CI), and information necessary for calculating objective data were included in the meta-analysis.

Articles were excluded from the analysis if they: dealt with ADs other than SLE, analyzed gonadal hormones in plasma rather than clinical outcomes, were reviews, case reports or duplicated papers, discussed topics not related to disease activity, included the same data published in another study, or they reported on HRT or OC not containing estrogens.

Outcome Measures and Risk of Bias

The full text of each eligible study was read and classified based on the quality score of the studies using the levels established by the Oxford Centre for Evidence-based Medicine 2011 [37]. The Cochrane Collaboration's tool for assessing risk of bias in randomized trials was also implemented [38]. All authors independently extracted data (name of the author, country where the study took place, study design, outcomes evaluated, measurement of association, and groups compared). Articles were organized in two categories, according to the measured outcomes: (a) development of SLE in healthy women exposed to HRT or OC (any use, currently use, past use, time and dose) or (b) disease activity (flares, change in activity score measured by SLEDAI, SLAM, etc.) and different outcomes (i.e. hospitalization, death, thrombotic events, etc.) in women with SLE exposed to HRT or OC.

The sample size and proportion of subjects was specified when possible. For measurements of association, the adjusted effect size of the outcomes was extracted. If studies were not available on databases, they were requested and purchased or the author was contacted to obtain the original publication. If studies had a cohort design, the requirements included the number of subjects exposed, the number unexposed, and the number of subjects who developed the disease in both cases. Case-control studies required the number of subjects with SLE and controls that were exposed and not exposed. When the study did not report the number of subjects in each group, either the RR or the OR with the respective CI was necessary for inclusion in the meta-analysis calculations.

Statistical Analysis

Data were analyzed using the Comprehensive Meta-Analysis program, v.2 (Biostat, Englewood, NJ, 2004). Calculations were carried out for the whole group of articles depending on the binary data available for any exposure (HRT or OC independently), the number of subjects, and risk data (OR and RR with the corresponding 95% CI). The effect size was calculated based on

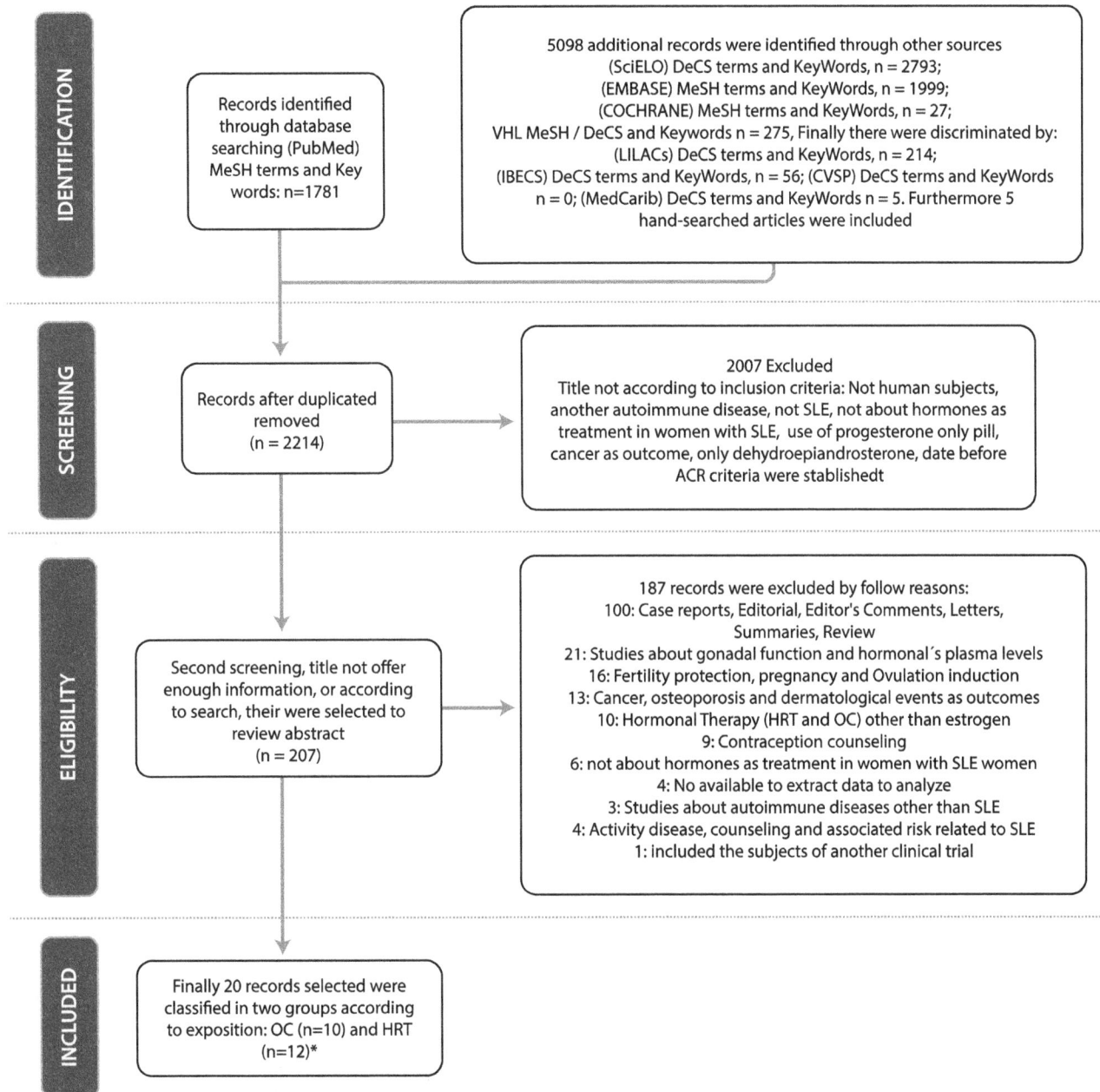

Figure 1. Flow Chart of the Systematic Literature Review. Footnote: VHL Virtual Health Library; MeSH Medical Medical Subject Headings; DeCS Health Sciences Descriptors; SLE Systemic Lupus Erythematosus; OC Oral contraceptives, HRT Hormonal Replacement Therapy *Two articles included exposition to both HRT and OC.

studies that only showed the OR (95% CI) and raw data from case-controlled, randomized clinical trials and cohort studies. A second effect size was calculated independently for studies that only showed the RR (95% CI) and raw data from randomized clinical trials and cohort studies. Different study designs were used to compute the same effect sizes, which had the same meaning in all studies and were comparable in relevant aspects. The association measures were transformed to log values, which were used in the pooled analysis, and then the results were converted back to ratio values for presentation. This approach prevented the omission of studies that used an alternative measure. When the studies reported means and standard deviations from a meaningful scale (i.e. SLEDAI), the preferred effect size was the raw mean

difference. The standardized mean difference (d or g) was implemented to transform all effect sizes to common metric values when different scales were applied.

A sensitivity analysis compared the meta-analysis results of the studies as a whole to the same meta-analysis with one study excluded in each round to determine how robust the findings were. It also evaluated the impact of decisions that lead to different data being used in the analysis and whether the conclusions reached might differ substantially if a single study or a number of studies were omitted. Additional meta-analyses were completed for studies with complex data structures and non-cumulative results since the information for the different effects was not totally independent (i.e. any-current exposure; different time points in the study; different SLE criteria applied in the same study, etc.). Supplementary analyses evaluated the association between each outcome and the exposure.

For each analysis, the final effect (RR and OR-95%CI) were obtained using both random and fixed effect models. The computational model was selected based on the expectation that studies shared a common effect size. The random effect model was preferred because it accepted that there is a distribution of true effect sizes rather than one true effect and assigned a more balanced weight to each study. It was also used because the studies were considered unequal in terms of specific exposures. Therefore, each study was weighted by the inverse of its variance including the within-studies variance plus the estimate of the between-studies variance [tau-squared (T^2)]. The method for estimating T^2 was the method of moments (or the DerSimonian and Laird).

Heterogeneity was calculated by means of Cochran's (Q) and Higgins's (I^2) tests. The I^2 test showed the proportion of observed dispersion that was real rather than spurious and was expressed as a ratio (0% to 100%). I^2 values of 25%, 50%, and 75% were qualitatively classified as low, moderate, and high, respectively. A significant Q-statistic ($P<0.10$) indicated heterogeneity across studies. Publication bias was determined using Funnel plots and Egger's regression asymmetry tests, and additional tests were applied if bias was found.

Results

Search strategy and data extraction

The PubMed search identified 1,781 articles and 5,098 additional records were identified through other sources (2,793 from SciELO, 1,999 from EMBASE, 27 from COCHRANE, and 275 from VHL, 5 hand-searched). Thus, a total of 6,879 articles were found. After screening, 207 full-text articles were assessed for eligibility. A previous meta-analysis was detected but it regarded hormone levels in plasma, rather than clinical outcomes and was not taken into account [39]. In addition, 3 systematic reviews were found and looked over to extract references according to inclusion criteria [40–42]. One included an article eligible for analysis [43]. Finally, after discarding 187 items for different reasons, 20 articles had adequate data for analysis [43–62] (**Appendix S2**). Two articles evaluated both OC and HRT exposure [49,51] and there were no missing items (**Figure 1 and Appendix S3**).

Meta-analysis

Overall results. Thirty-two meta-analyses were developed for all exposures; 13 evaluated HRT and 19 OC exposures.

Taking into account the fact that in the 20 articles included there were different outcomes which were evaluated (i.e. SLE development, different types of flares, death, hospitalization, and thrombosis) as well as different evaluation time points , different exposures (i.e. OC or HRT) or different SLE criteria for inclusion, we developed 32 meta-analyses in order to make the study as highly accurate as possible and avoid any bias. That is the reason data was grouped into independent subgroups based on the factors mentioned above. This approach was followed when it was not possible to synthesize diverse results based on biological plausibility or there were no statistical techniques to combine the results.

Meta-analyses of hormonal replacement therapy exposure. We found a significant association between HRT exposure and an increased risk of developing SLE (**Table 1**). **Figure 2** shows the forest plot for the meta-analysis including the most relevant outcome per author. The final common effect size, based on a random model, was statistically significant (Rate Ratio:1.96; 95%CI: 1.51–2.56; P-value<0.001). The results of

different measures of heterogeneity calculated for the analysis are shown in **Figure 2** as follows: Q-value: 3.37; degree of freedom (Q):5; P-value: 0.643; I^2: 0%; T^2: 0. Significant publication bias was not identified using the Egger test (P-value 2-tailed: 0.48; intercept:1.61). This meta-analysis included results taking into account two different criteria for SLE (i.e. ACR criteria and ACR plus physician diagnosis) in the study of Sanchez-Guerrero et al [48,54] corresponding to four outcomes (i.e. current and past use) in addition to two outcomes from the study of Costenbader et al [49] (i.e. current and past use). When the meta-analysis included results concerning only ACR criteria, the result remained significant (**Figure 3**) (Rate Ratio: 1.87; 95%CI: 1.38–2.54; P-value<0.001). When the analysis was run searching for associations between HRT exposure and SLE development, including case control studies [51,61], the results were not significant (OR: 0.84; 95%CI: 0.51–1.39; P-value: 0.51).

There were no associations between HRT exposure and specific outcomes of SLE (OR or RR calculations). Six meta-analyses (**Appendix S4**) were run evaluating different outcomes: death, all flares, multiple flares, major flares, thrombosis (arterial or venous compiled), and coronary disease. None were significant. When the change in SLE activity was analyzed, measured through different scales (SLEDAI, SLAM, SDI), the final standardized mean difference or the mean change SLEDAI (g Hedges) was not significant. The mean change in SLEDAI was not significant by three different meta-analyses, including studies with 12 or more months of follow-up.

Meta-analyses of oral contraceptives exposure. One of eleven meta-analyses evaluating the risk for SLE associated with OC exposure had a marginally significant result. This meta-analysis included the SLE outcome from patients with any use and included two population-based nested cases-control studies [51,56] and two case-control [60,62] studies. The final common effect size (**Figure 4**) based on a random model, was statistically significant (OR: 1.44; 95%CI: 1.00–2.08; P-value: 0.047). One of the four studies included [60] in this meta-analysis grouped the patients by age, and in this case, the group exposed was 36–45 years old. However, if all the groups were included, the results were not significant (**Table 1 and Appendix S5**). In a sub-analysis taking into account the studies that followed the patients for the first year (any exposure) the result was near significant (**Figure 5**) (OR: 1.44; 95%CI: 0.99–2.10; P-value: 0.053). This trend of association was lost (**Table 1**) when studies following the patients during the second year were analyzed (OR: 2; 95%CI: 0.29–13.6; P-value: 0.47). When the results were limited to patients currently exposed, the analysis was not significant (OR: 1.33; 95%CI: 0.75–2.36; P-value: 0.32). It was also not significant when limited to past use (OR: 1.14; 95%CI: 0.95–1.36; P-value: 0.13). Analyses searching for associations between OC exposure and different outcomes of SLE (death, hospitalization, all flares, major flares, and thrombosis) were not significant (**Table 1** and **Appendix S5**). After developing a sensitivity analysis that excluded one study at a time for all the meta-analyses, the results were similar to the cumulative analysis (**Appendix S5**).

Discussion

The present study included a rigorous systematic search that let us identify the majority of studies published on HRT and OC in SLE.

We were able to perform calculations through a meta-analysis and make conclusions based on the outcomes analyzed. After performing several analyses, including different studies on patients exposed to HRT, we demonstrated this exposure increased the risk

Study name	Time point	Rate ratio	Lower limit	Upper limit	Z-Value	p-Value	Rate ratio and 95% CI	Relative weight
Costenbader K, et al. 2007-2	Past Use	1,800	1,032	3,139	2,071	0,038		22,69
Costenbader K, et al. 2007-3	Current Use	1,634	0,973	2,742	1,858	0,063		26,18
Sanchez-Guerrero J, et al. 1995-2	Current Use	2,879	1,451	5,712	3,025	0,002		14,95
Sanchez-Guerrero J, et al. 1995-3	Past Use	1,604	0,751	3,426	1,220	0,223		12,18
Sanchez-Guerrero J, et al. 1995-5	Current Use	2,953	1,420	6,138	2,900	0,004		13,11
Sanchez-Guerrero J, et al. 1995-6	Past Use	1,696	0,760	3,786	1,290	0,197		10,89
		1,968	1,510	2,565	5,008	0,000		

0,01   0,1   1   10   100

Non Exposed   Exposed

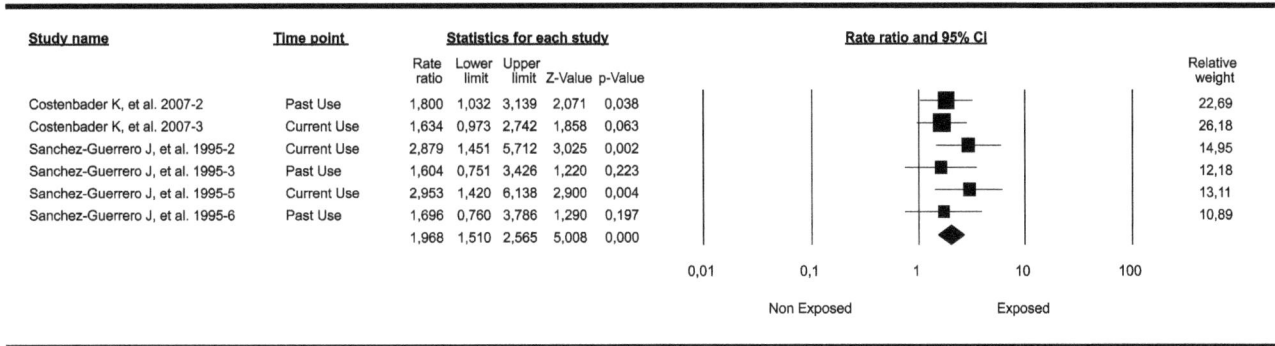

Figure 2. Forest plot of studies meta-analyzed: association between HRT exposure and risk of developing SLE. Footnote: Final common effect size based on a random model. CI: confidence intervals; SLE: Systemic Lupus Erythematosus; HRT: hormonal replacement therapy.

of SLE development in healthy women (RR: 1.96; 95%CI: 1.51–2.56; *P*-value<0.001). Therefore, we can conclude that there is a moderately increased risk of developing SLE for women using HRT. A limitation of the analysis was the overlapping information retrieved from two studies. Sanchez-Guerrero et al. [54] and Costenbader et al. [49] followed the same population from the Nurses'Health Study (NHS) cohort, the first between 1976 and 1990 and the second between 1976 and 2002. Results should also interpreted with caution since these two studies have limitations inherent to self-reported data and since women with HRT that regularly attend medical check-ups may more often be diagnosed with SLE.

When evaluating the data included from Costenbader K et al. [49], it is striking that the mean age at onset of menopause in women who later developed SLE was 51.6 (3.9) years [mean (SD)]; whereas, it was 52.7 (4.3) years in the rest of the NHS cohort (*P*< 0.01 by t-test). The mean age at diagnosis was 52.4 (8.3), which is consistent with estimates of mean age and the incidence in the US. In both NHS cohorts, rates of SLE diagnosis were highest in the youngest women and declined with age. It is important to note that the relationship between hormones and SLE development is clearly complex and there may be genetic, immunological, or biological mechanisms related to SLE development and early menopause, which may represent confounding factors since women with early menopause are more likely to be treated with HRT.

The present meta-analysis did not find a significant association when analyzing the risk for SLE among OC users. Studies with different designs have found conflicting results. Some studies found a significantly increased risk of developing SLE [49,56]; while, others studies did not [51,58].

In the studies included in the present meta-analysis, OC and HRT generally did not affect the course of lupus activity at a clinically significant level. Two randomized clinical trials [48,50] of HRT vs. placebo failed to find differences in disease activity or the incidence of severe flares in the two groups; however, one found the incidence of mild to moderate disease and the probability of suffering flares of any type were higher in the group that received HRT [50]. The results of this clinical trial are in contrast with other cohort and case control studies in which there were no differences in the rate of flares nor in the disease activity scores in postmenopausal women with SLE treated with HRT compared with postmenopausal SLE women not treated with HRT [52,53,55]. Interestingly, Kreidstein [53] found that although there was not a difference in the incidence of total flares, pure serological flares were more common in HRT users and clinical flares more common in non-users.

Oral contraceptive use has been associated with lupus exacerbation in anecdotal reports and descriptive studies. To date, two well-designed randomized clinical trials [44,57] have addressed this and found no differences in disease activity or incidences of flares or severe flares. It is noteworthy that subjects in both trials had clinically stable disease; therefore, results cannot be extrapolated to all SLE patients and should be interpreted with caution. One previous systematic review has addressed the topic of sex hormones in SLE. The review included only contraceptive

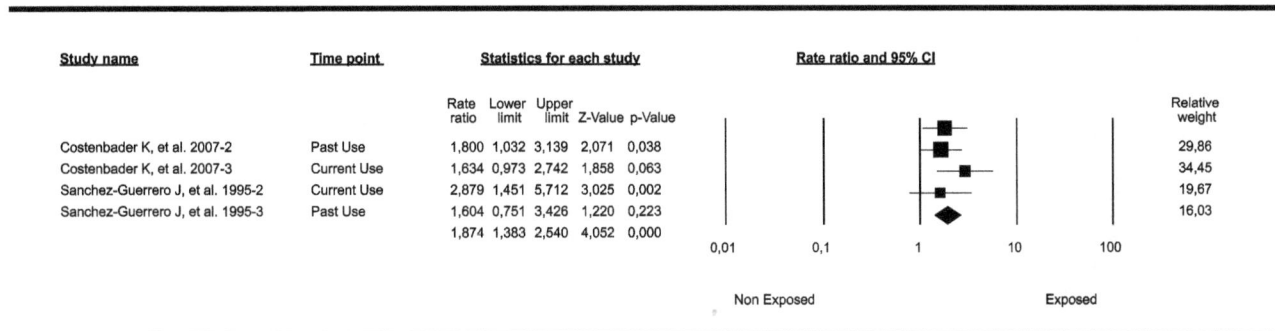

Study name	Time point	Rate ratio	Lower limit	Upper limit	Z-Value	p-Value	Rate ratio and 95% CI	Relative weight
Costenbader K, et al. 2007-2	Past Use	1,800	1,032	3,139	2,071	0,038		29,86
Costenbader K, et al. 2007-3	Current Use	1,634	0,973	2,742	1,858	0,063		34,45
Sanchez-Guerrero J, et al. 1995-2	Current Use	2,879	1,451	5,712	3,025	0,002		19,67
Sanchez-Guerrero J, et al. 1995-3	Past Use	1,604	0,751	3,426	1,220	0,223		16,03
		1,874	1,383	2,540	4,052	0,000		

0,01   0,1   1   10   100

Non Exposed   Exposed

Figure 3. Forest plot of studies meta-analyzed: association between HRT exposure and risk of developing SLE (ACR criteria only). Footnote: Final common effect size based on a random model. CI: confidence intervals; SLE: Systemic Lupus Erythematosus; ACR: American College of Rheumatology criteria; HRT: hormonal replacement therapy.

Table 1. Meta analyses results.

HRT

Outcome	Number of studies (Subgroups) [Ref]	Time Point of exposure	Measure of association	Study Design	Effect size (Random model)	CI 95%	P value	I^2	P value	Egger
SLE	2 (6)[a,b] [49,54]	Current and Past	RaR	Cohort	1,96	1,51–2,56	<0,001	0,00	0,64	0,48
SLE	2 (4)[b,c] [49,54]	Current and Past	RaR	Cohort	1,87	1,38–2,54	<0,001	0,00	0,58	0,61
SLE	2 (4) [51,61]	Current, ever and Past	OR	Population based CC and Database nested CC	0,93	0,64–1,37	0,74	0,00	0,42	0,70
SLE	2 (4) [51,61]	Current and Past	OR	Population based CC and Database nested CC	0,84	0,51–1,39	0,51	14,1	0,32	0,66
Multiple Flares	2 [48,50]	12 and 24 months	DIM (SE)	RCT	0,17 (0,16)[†]	–0,14–0,49	0,29	46,9	0,17	NA
Major Flares	2 [48,50]	12 and 24 months	RR	RCT	1,48	0,65–3,39	0,34	0,00	0,352	NA
Flares	3 [48,53,55]	12 months and more	OR	CC, RCT and RCS	1,01	0,35–2,9	0,98	52,6	0,123	0,006[¶]
All Thrombosis	4 [47,48,50,55]	12 months and more	OR	RCT, RCS and Cohort nested CS	0,92	0,23–3,66	0,91	51,1	0,10	0,31
Coronary Disease	2 [45,46]	Ever use	OR	CS and Mixed Cohort nested CC study	2,72	0,20–35,9	0,44	87,8	0,004	NA
SLEDAI[d]	2 [48,50]	12 months	DIM (SE)	RCT	0,21 (0,33)[‡]	–0,43–0,86	0,52	0,00	0,42	NA
SLEDAI[e]	2 [48,50]	12 and 24 months	DIM (SE)	RCT	0,22 (0,33)[‡]	–0,42–0,87	0,5	0,00	0,62	NA
SLEDAI	2 [48,50,52]	12 and 24 months	g Hedges	RCT	–0,66(0,46)	–1,58––0,25	0,15	93,1	0,000	0,24
Death	2 [48,50]	12 and 24 months	OR	RCT	1,69	0,20–13,6	0,63	0,00	0,61	NA

OC

Outcome	Number of studies (Subgroups) [Ref]	Time Point of exposure	Measure of association	Study Design	Effect size (Random model)	CI 95%	P value	I^2	P value	Egger
SLE	2 (2)[c] [51,56]	Current	OR	CC	1,33	0,75–2,36	0,32	79,2	0,02	NA
SLE	4 (8)[f] [51,56,60,62]	Ever Use	OR	CC	1,20	0,94–1,54	0,13	53,9	0,03	0,56
SLE	4 (4)[g] [51,56,60,62]	Ever Use	OR	CC	1,34	0,88–2,03	0,16	76,3	0,00	0,97
SLE	4 (4)[h] [51,56,60,62]	Ever Use	OR	CC	1,37	0,93–2,01	0,10	73,9	0,00	0,89
SLE	4 (4)[c,i] [51,56,60,62]	Ever Use	OR	CC	1,44	1,00–2,08	0,04	69,4	0,02	0,73
SLE	4 (4)[j] [51,56,60,62]	Ever Use	OR	CC	1,41	0,95–2,11	0,08	71,0	0,01	0,85
SLE	4 (4)[k] [51,56,60,62]	Ever Use	OR	CC	1,41	0,94–2,11	0,09	71,4	0,01	0,87
SLE	2 (2)[c] [51,62]	Ever Use*	OR	CC	1,44	0,99–2,10	0,05	0,00	0,77	NA
SLE	2 (2)[c] [51,62]	Ever Use**	OR	CC	2,00	0,29–13,61	0,47	92,4	0,00	NA
SLE	2 (2)[c] [51,56]	Past Use	OR	CC	1,14	0,95–1,36	0,13	0,00	0,44	NA
SLE	3 (3) [51,56,60]	Past Use and 3 years before Diagnosis	OR	CC	1,07	0,86–1,33	0,52	24,3	0,26	0,01[¶]

Table 1. Cont.

oc

Outcome	Number of studies (Subgroups) [Ref]	Time Point of exposure	Measure of association	Study Design	Effect size (Random model)	CI 95%	P value	I²	P value	Egger
Thrombosis	2 [43,44]	During study	OR	Mixed RCT and Cohort nested CS	4,29	0,65–28,27	0,12	0,00	0,33	NA
Any Thrombosis	3 (4) [43,44,57]	Any time about study	OR	Mixed RCT and Cohort nested CS	1,47	0,34–6,37	0,60	24,4	0,26	0,86
Thrombosis after therapy	2 [44,57]	During study	RR	RCT	0,63	0,12–3,19	0,57	0,00	0,38	NA
Flares^c	2 (3) [44,57]	12 months	RR	RCT	1,01	0,83–1,25	0,85	25,2	0,26	0,67
Major Flares^§	2 [44,57]	12 months	RR	RCT	0,78	0,29–2,04	0,61	0,00	0,77	NA
SLEDAI	2 [44,57]	12 months	DIM (SE)	RCT	6,28 (5,85)	−5,19–17,7	0,28	99,1	0,00	NA
Hospitalized	2 [44,57]	12 months and more	RR	RCT	1,19	0,70–1,99	0,51	0,00	0,93	NA
Death	2 [44,57]	12 months and more	RR	RCT	1,008	0,10–9,57	0,99	0,00	0,34	NA

RaR: Rate Ratio. CI: Confidence interval. CC: Case-control design. CS: cross-sectional. RCT: Randomized Clinical Trial. RCS: Retrospective Cross sectional. DIM: Difference in means.
[a]ACR criteria and ACR plus physician diagnosis included.
[b]the cohorts between 1976 and 1990 and between1976 and 2002 were overlapped between the two studies.
[c]Only ACR criteria included.
[d]means change in SLEDAI.
[e]the means change in SLEDAI on max time of follow-up from both studies.
[f]There were included all subgroups from a study which is clustered by age (67).
[g]There were selected ever use in 25 years old and lower, data from one study (67).
[h]There were selected ever use in 26–35 years old data from one study (67).
[i]There were selected ever use in 36–45 years old data from one study (67).
[j]There were selected ever use in 46–55 years old data from one study (67).
[k]there were selected ever use in older 56 years old data from one study (67).
[‡]Variance = 0.11.
[†]Variance = 0.02.
[*]1–11 months,
[**]12 months or more.
[§]Severe flares and major flares.
[e]Flares combined by subtypes.
[¶]Begg and Mazumdar p = 0.29. Trim and fill procedures showed a similar effect size. 25 articles with an effect size of zero would be needed to nullify the observed effect.

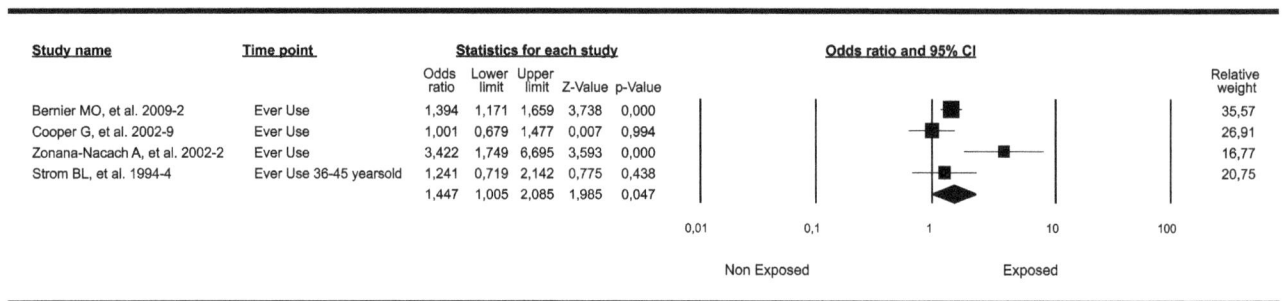

Study name	Time point	Odds ratio	Lower limit	Upper limit	Z-Value	p-Value	Odds ratio and 95% CI	Relative weight
Bernier MO, et al. 2009-2	Ever Use	1,394	1,171	1,659	3,738	0,000		35,57
Cooper G, et al. 2002-9	Ever Use	1,001	0,679	1,477	0,007	0,994		26,91
Zonana-Nacach A, et al. 2002-2	Ever Use	3,422	1,749	6,695	3,593	0,000		16,77
Strom BL, et al. 1994-4	Ever Use 36-45 yearsold	1,241	0,719	2,142	0,775	0,438		20,75
		1,447	1,005	2,085	1,985	0,047		

Figure 4. Forest plot of studies meta-analyzed: association between OC exposure and risk of developing SLE (limited to patients with OC ever use). Footnote: Final common effect size based on a random model. CI: confidence intervals; SLE: Systemic Lupus Erythematosus; OC: oral contraceptives.

methods and was limited to women already diagnosed with SLE ([40]). The authors included case series that lack statistical validity since they use no control group to compare outcomes and did not include some important studies that provided valuable information for our study. Nor did they do a meta-analysis due to the heterogeneity found across the studies. However, the conclusions they reached were similar to ours. Oral Contraceptives did not alter the activity of SLE in patients with inactive or stable disease and even though the risk of thromboembolic events increases in SLE, the evidence from their study suggests that this is only true for patients who are positive for antiphospholipid antibodies (APLA).

The use of HRT and OC in SLE patients potentially increases the risk for arterial or venous thrombosis especially in women with APS. Different mechanisms have been implicated including endothelial cell proliferation as well as changes in coagulation factors, platelets, and the fibrinolytic system. The findings of the present study did not support this hypothesis. Most of the studies included in the analysis did not find an association between HRT use and thrombotic events [48,53,55]. Furthermore, in a longitudinal study of outcomes in SLE, HRT was significantly and negatively associated with vascular arterial events, although this association was no longer significant after adjusting for propensity score; in addition, the study did not find an association between HRT and venous thrombosis [47]. However, Chooji-tarom K et al. [43] showed that thrombotic events appear to be associated with OC use in SLE women who test positive for APLA. Generally, the studies included in the present meta-analysis involved SLE patients with low disease activity and the majority excluded patients with APLA or previous thrombotic events.

The relation between SLE and hormonal exposure, especially from HRT, appears to be significant. It is well known that SLE is a complex and clinically heterogeneous AD. Genetic predisposition has been implicated in the pathogenesis of SLE, which has a relatively strong genetic component (sibling risk ratio~30), compared with many other ADs [63]. There is substantial information supporting that some of the pathways involved in the causality of SLE are under the control of environmental and hormonal factors, such as estrogen exposure [2,64,65]. In different ADs, estrogen has demonstrated anti-inflammatory activity by inhibiting many proinflammatory pathways of innate immunity, adaptive immunity, and inflammatory tissue responses; in addition, proinflammatory responses have also been shown, including anti-apoptotic effects on immune cells, promotion of neoangiogenesis, and stimulation of B cells (unfavorable in B cell-driven diseases such as SLE) [66].

There are reports of beneficial effects of estrogens in other ADs such as rheumatoid arthritis [67], multiple sclerosis [68], systemic sclerosis [69], and Sjögren's syndrome [70], as well as evidence supporting an activating or impairment role [65,66,71–75]. Understanding the pathways of ADs etiology will become more important for understanding the causality of them and their associations with external factors such estrogens.

Limitations

We found wide heterogeneity of SLE activity indexes; characteristics of women included in the studies in terms of severity of disease, lupus activity, and the presence of APLA; HRT and OC doses; combinations of estrogen and progesterone formulations;

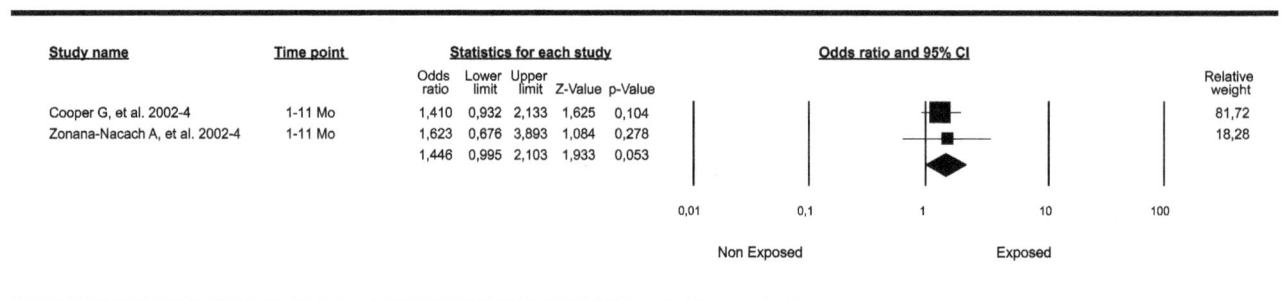

Study name	Time point	Odds ratio	Lower limit	Upper limit	Z-Value	p-Value	Odds ratio and 95% CI	Relative weight
Cooper G, et al. 2002-4	1-11 Mo	1,410	0,932	2,133	1,625	0,104		81,72
Zonana-Nacach A, et al. 2002-4	1-11 Mo	1,623	0,676	3,893	1,084	0,278		18,28
		1,446	0,995	2,103	1,933	0,053		

Figure 5. Forest plot of studies meta-analyzed: association between OC exposure and risk of developing SLE (limited to patients followed for the first year). Footnote: Final common effect size based on a random model. CI: confidence intervals; SLE: Systemic Lupus Erythematosus; OC: oral contraceptives.

and routes of administrations, which limits comparisons and generalizations. If all studies in a meta-analysis are based on the same kind of data (means, binary, or correlational), the researcher should select an effect size based on that kind of data. When some studies use means and others use binary data or correlational data, we can apply formulas to convert among effect sizes [76]. In the present research, it was not always possible to meta-analyze all the available data. It is clear that studies that used different measures may differ from each other in substantive ways, and this needs to be considered when deciding to include the various studies in the same analysis. Integrating all of them in a meta-analysis requires an effect-size index that can be applied to both types of outcomes [76].

In addition, some studies report data with a rate-ratio effect size (i.e. the ratio of the rate in the experimental intervention group to the rate in the control group). Analyzing count data as rates is not always appropriate and is uncommon because the assumption of a constant underlying risk may not be suitable and statistical methods for this data are not well developed [77]. Therefore, it was not possible to disclose the type of association by computing additional data.

An additional limitation of the study was the presence of high heterogeneity in most of the studies (i.e. I^2, the proportion of observed dispersions that are real, rather than spurious). The heterogeneity in effect sizes revealed the variation in the true effect sizes; in addition, the variation observed was partly spurious, incorporating both (true) heterogeneity and also random error.

Conclusions

It has been suggested that estrogens should not be used in SLE women with active disease, severe organ involvement, history of deep vein thrombosis or who are positive for APLA. HRT and OC are clearly underutilized in SLE patients [11,78]. The mean age for menopause in SLE patients is approximately 10 years earlier than in healthy women [79] and osteoporosis is frequently more severe due not only to the effects of early menopause but also to the effects of inflammatory mediators on bone turnover. Despite the clear beneficial effects that HRT has shown, even in women with SLE [55,80], fears that sexual steroid hormones, particularly estrogens, may increase SLE activity prevented its use by rheumatologists and gynecologists. HRT or OC use should be recommended in certain women with SLE after careful consideration of possible risks, benefits, and personal preferences. Taking

into account the selection bias of the studies included in the meta-analysis, which in general, excluded women with high disease activity or with APLA or history of thrombosis which limited the generalizability of results of the present study, the recommendations for using these agents on women with known SLE, must be followed cautiously.

In conclusion, an association between HRT exposure and SLE causality was observed. The present meta-analysis did not find a significant association when analyzing the risk for SLE among OC users. The relationship between hormones and SLE development is clearly complex and there may be genetic, immunological, or biological mechanisms related to SLE development. Future research on environmental and hormonal exposure will enhance our knowledge of the common mechanisms associated with ADs.

Supporting Information

Appendix S1   Data sources and searches (complementary information).

Appendix S2   Articles included in the Systematic Literature Review and meta-analysis.

Appendix S3   Cochrane Collaboration's tool for assessing risk of bias in randomized trials.

Appendix S4   Supplementary meta-analysis, sensitivity analyses and risk of bias analyses (HRT exposure).

Appendix S5   Supplementary meta-analysis, sensitivity analyses and risk of bias analyses (OC exposure).

Checklist S1   PRISMA checklist.

Author Contributions

Conceived and designed the experiments: ARV AMRS. Performed the experiments: ARV AMRS JVTG. Analyzed the data: ARV JVTG. Contributed reagents/materials/analysis tools: AMRS JVTG. Contributed to the writing of the manuscript: ARV AMRS JVTG. Interpreted the statistical data: ARV AMRS JVTG.

References

1. Anaya J-M (2010) The autoimmune tautology. Arthritis Res Ther 12: 147.
2. Quintero OL, Amador-Patarroyo MJ, Montoya-Ortiz G, Rojas-Villarraga A, Anaya J-M (2012) Autoimmune disease and gender: plausible mechanisms for the female predominance of autoimmunity. J Autoimmun 38: J109–19.
3. Panay N (2012) Treatment of premenstrual syndrome: a decision-making algorithm. Menopause Int 18: 90–92.
4. Santen RJ, Allred DC, Ardoin SP, Archer DF, Boyd N, et al. (2010) Postmenopausal hormone therapy: an Endocrine Society scientific statement. J Clin Endocrinol Metab 95: s1–s66.
5. Darroch JE (2013) Trends in contraceptive use. Contraception 87: 259–263.
6. Blockeel C, Engels S, De Vos M, Haentjens P, Polyzos NP, et al. (2012) Oestradiol valerate pretreatment in GnRH-antagonist cycles: a randomized controlled trial. Reprod Biomed Online 24: 272–280.
7. Tartagni M, Damiani GR, Di Naro E, Persiani P, Crescini C, et al. (2011) Pregnancy in a woman with premature ovarian insufficiency undergoing intracytoplasmic sperm injection after pretreatment with estrogens followed by therapy with estrogens associated with ovarian stimulation with gonadotropins: remarks about oocyte and emb. Menopause 18: 932–934.
8. Ackerman LS (2006) Sex hormones and the genesis of autoimmunity. Arch Dermatol 142: 371–376.
9. Masi AT, Kaslow RA (1978) Sex effects in systemic lupus erythematosus: a clue to pathogenesis. Arthritis Rheum 21: 480–484.
10. Alekberova ZS, Folomeev MI, Polyntsev I V (1990) [The role of estrogen-androgen imbalance in rheumatic diseases]. Ter Arkh 62: 17–21.
11. Buyon JP, Kalunian KC, Skovron ML, Petri M, Lahita R, et al. (1995) Can Women with Systemic Lupus Erythematosus Safely Use Exogenous Estrogens? J Clin Rheumatol 1: 205–212.
12. Gompel A, Piette JC (2007) Systemic lupus erythematosus and hormone replacement therapy. Menopause Int 13: 65–70.
13. Julkunen H (2000) Hormone replacement therapy in women with rheumatic diseases. Scand J Rheumatol 29: 146–153.
14. Schwarz EB, Lohr PA (2006) Oral contraceptives in women with systemic lupus erythematosus. N Engl J Med 354: 1203–4; author reply 1203–4.
15. Lakasing L, Khamashta M (2001) Contraceptive practices in women with systemic lupus erythematosus and/or antiphospholipid syndrome: what advice should we be giving? J Fam Plann Reprod Health Care 27: 7–12.
16. Roubinian JR, Talal N, Greenspan JS, Goodman JR, Siiteri PK (1978) Effect of castration and sex hormone treatment on survival, anti-nucleic acid antibodies, and glomerulonephritis in NZB/NZW F1 mice. J Exp Med 147: 1568–1583.
17. Carlsten H, Nilsson N, Jonsson R, Tarkowski A (1991) Differential effects of oestrogen in murine lupus: acceleration of glomerulonephritis and amelioration of T cell-mediated lesions. J Autoimmun 4: 845–856.
18. Steinberg AD, Klassen LW, Raveche ES, Gerber NL, Reinertsen JL, et al. (1978) Study of the multiple factors in the pathogenesis of autoimmunity in New Zealand mice. Arthritis Rheum 21: S190–201.

19. Jiang B, Sun L, Hao S, Li X, Xu Y, et al. (2008) Estrogen modulates bone marrow-derived DCs in SLE murine model-(NZB x NZW) F1 female mice. Immunol Invest 37: 227–243.

20. Talal N, Dang H, Ahmed SA, Kraig E, Fischbach M (1987) Interleukin 2, T cell receptor and sex hormone studies in autoimmune mice. J Rheumatol Suppl 14 Suppl 1: 21–25.

21. Nagy G, Koncz A, Perl A (2005) T- and B-cell abnormalities in systemic lupus erythematosus. Crit Rev Immunol 25: 123–140.

22. Shabanova SS, Ananieva LP, Alekberova ZS, Guzov II (2008) Ovarian function and disease activity in patients with systemic lupus erythematosus. Clin Exp Rheumatol 26: 436–441.

23. Mok CC, Wong RW, Lau CS (1999) Ovarian failure and flares of systemic lupus erythematosus. Arthritis Rheum 42: 1274–1280.

24. Somers EC, Marder W, Christman GM, Ognenovski V, McCune WJ (2005) Use of a gonadotropin-releasing hormone analog for protection against premature ovarian failure during cyclophosphamide therapy in women with severe lupus. Arthritis Rheum 52: 2761–2767.

25. Silva CAA, Hilário MO, Febrônio M V, Oliveira SK, Terreri MT, et al. (2007) Risk factors for amenorrhea in juvenile systemic lupus erythematosus (JSLE): a Brazilian multicentre cohort study. Lupus 16: 531–536.

26. Medeiros PB, Febrônio M V, Bonfá E, Borba EF, Takiuti AD, et al. (2009) Menstrual and hormonal alterations in juvenile systemic lupus erythematosus. Lupus 18: 38–43.

27. Schierbeck LL, Rejnmark L, Tofteng CL, Stilgren L, Eiken P, et al. (2012) Effect of hormone replacement therapy on cardiovascular events in recently postmenopausal women: randomised trial. BMJ 345: e6409.

28. Salpeter SR, Walsh JM, Ormiston TM, Greyber E, Buckley NS, et al. (2006) Meta-analysis: effect of hormone-replacement therapy on components of the metabolic syndrome in postmenopausal women. Diabetes Obes Metab 8: 538–554.

29. Salpeter SR, Cheng J, Thabane L, Buckley NS, Salpeter EE (2009) Bayesian meta-analysis of hormone therapy and mortality in younger postmenopausal women. Am J Med 122: 1016–1022.e1.

30. Rossouw JE, Anderson GL, Prentice RL, LaCroix AZ, Kooperberg C, et al. (2002) Risks and benefits of estrogen plus progestin in healthy postmenopausal women: principal results From the Women's Health Initiative randomized controlled trial. JAMA 288: 321–333.

31. Herrington DM, Vittinghoff E, Lin F, Fong J, Harris F, et al. (2002) Statin therapy, cardiovascular events, and total mortality in the Heart and Estrogen/Progestin Replacement Study (HERS). Circulation 105: 2962–2967.

32. Rossouw JE, Prentice RL, Manson JE, Wu L, Barad D, et al. (2007) Postmenopausal hormone therapy and risk of cardiovascular disease by age and years since menopause. JAMA 297: 1465–1477.

33. Hodis HN, Collins P, Mack WJ, Schierbeck LL (2012) The timing hypothesis for coronary heart disease prevention with hormone therapy: past, present and future in perspective. Climacteric 15: 217–228.

34. Yang D, Li J, Yuan Z, Liu X (2013) Effect of hormone replacement therapy on cardiovascular outcomes: a meta-analysis of randomized controlled trials. PLoS One 8: e62329.

35. Liberati A, Altman DG, Tetzlaff J, Mulrow C, Gøtzsche PC, et al. (2009) The PRISMA statement for reporting systematic reviews and meta-analyses of studies that evaluate health care interventions: explanation and elaboration. J Clin Epidemiol 62: e1–34.

36. Tan EM, Cohen AS, Fries JF, Masi AT, McShane DJ, et al. (1982) The 1982 revised criteria for the classification of systemic lupus erythematosus. Arthritis Rheum 25: 1271–1277.

37. Howick J, Chalmers I, Glasziou P, Greenhalgh T, Heneghan C, et al. (2011) Oxford Centre for Evidence-Based Medicine 2011 Levels of Evidence. OCEBM Levels Evid Work Gr. Available: http://www.cebm.net/index.aspx?o = 5653.

38. Higgins JP, Altman DG, Gøtzsche PC, Jüni P, Moher D, et al. (2011) The Cochrane Collaboration's tool for assessing risk of bias in randomised trials. BMJ 343: d5928.

39. McMurray RW, May W (2003) Sex hormones and systemic lupus erythematosus: review and meta-analysis. Arthritis Rheum 48: 2100–2110.

40. Culwell KR, Curtis KM, del Carmen Cravioto M (2009) Safety of contraceptive method use among women with systemic lupus erythematosus: a systematic review. Obstet Gynecol 114: 341–353.

41. Li RH, Gebbie AE, Wong RW, Ng EH, Glasier AF, et al. (2011) The use of sex hormones in women with rheumatological diseases. Hong Kong Med J 17: 487–491.

42. Vinet E, Lee J, Pineau C, Clarke AE, Bernatsky S (2010) Oral contraceptives and risk of systemic lupus erythematosus. Int J Clin Rheumtol 5: 169–175.

43. Choojitarom K, Verasertniyom O, Totemchokchyakarn K, Nantiruj K, Sumethkul V, et al. (2008) Lupus nephritis and Raynaud's phenomenon are significant risk factors for vascular thrombosis in SLE patients with positive antiphospholipid antibodies. Clin Rheumatol 27: 345–351.

44. Petri M, Kim MY, Kalunian KC, Grossman J, Hahn BH, et al. (2005) Combined oral contraceptives in women with systemic lupus erythematosus. N Engl J Med 353: 2550–2558.

45. Kiani AN, Vogel-Claussen J, Magder LS, Petri M (2010) Noncalcified coronary plaque in systemic lupus erythematosus. J Rheumatol 37: 579–584.

46. Hochman J, Urowitz MB, Ibañez D, Gladman DD (2009) Hormone replacement therapy in women with systemic lupus erythematosus and risk of cardiovascular disease. Lupus 18: 313–317.

47. Fernández M, Calvo-Alén J, Bertoli AM, Bastian HM, Fessler BJ, et al. (2007) Systemic lupus erythematosus in a multiethnic US cohort (LUMINA L II): relationship between vascular events and the use of hormone replacement therapy in postmenopausal women. J Clin Rheumatol 13: 261–265.

48. Sánchez-Guerrero J, González-Pérez M, Durand-Carbajal M, Lara-Reyes P, Jiménez-Santana L, et al. (2007) Menopause hormonal therapy in women with systemic lupus erythematosus. Arthritis Rheum 56: 3070–3079.

49. Costenbader KH, Feskanich D, Stampfer MJ, Karlson EW (2007) Reproductive and menopausal factors and risk of systemic lupus erythematosus in women. Arthritis Rheum 56: 1251–1262.

50. Buyon JP, Petri MA, Kim MY, Kalunian KC, Grossman J, et al. (2005) The effect of combined estrogen and progesterone hormone replacement therapy on disease activity in systemic lupus erythematosus: a randomized trial. Ann Intern Med 142: 953–962.

51. Cooper GS, Dooley MA, Treadwell EL, St Clair EW, Gilkeson GS (2002) Hormonal and reproductive risk factors for development of systemic lupus erythematosus: results of a population-based, case-control study. Arthritis Rheum 46: 1830–1839.

52. Mok CC, Lau CS, Ho CT, Lee KW, Mok MY, et al. (1998) Safety of hormonal replacement therapy in postmenopausal patients with systemic lupus erythematosus. Scand J Rheumatol 27: 342–346.

53. Kreidstein S, Urowitz MB, Gladman DD, Gough J (1997) Hormone replacement therapy in systemic lupus erythematosus. J Rheumatol 24: 2149–2152.

54. Sánchez-Guerrero J, Liang MH, Karlson EW, Hunter DJ, Colditz GA (1995) Postmenopausal estrogen therapy and the risk for developing systemic lupus erythematosus. Ann Intern Med 122: 430–433.

55. Arden NK, Lloyd ME, Spector TD, Hughes GR (1994) Safety of hormone replacement therapy (HRT) in systemic lupus erythematosus (SLE). Lupus 3: 11–13.

56. Bernier M-O, Mikaeloff Y, Hudson M, Suissa S (2009) Combined oral contraceptive use and the risk of systemic lupus erythematosus. Arthritis Rheum 61: 476–481.

57. Sánchez-Guerrero J, Uribe AG, Jiménez-Santana L, Mestanza-Peralta M, Lara-Reyes P, et al. (2005) A trial of contraceptive methods in women with systemic lupus erythematosus. N Engl J Med 353: 2539–2549.

58. Sanchez-Guerrero J, Karlson EW, Liang MH, Hunter DJ, Speizer FE, et al. (1997) Past use of oral contraceptives and the risk of developing systemic lupus erythematosus. Arthritis Rheum 40: 804–808.

59. Grimes D, LeBolt S, Grimes K, Wingo P (1985) Systemic lupus Erythematosus and reproductive function: A case control study. Am J Obstet Gynecol 153: 179–186.

60. Strom BL, Reidenberg MM, West S, Snyder ES, Freundlich B, et al. (1994) Shingles, allergies, family medical history, oral contraceptives, and other potential risk factors for systemic lupus erythematosus. Am J Epidemiol 140: 632–642.

61. Meier CR, Sturkenboom MC, Cohen AS, Jick H (1998) Postmenopausal estrogen replacement therapy and the risk of developing systemic lupus erythematosus or discoid lupus. J Rheumatol 25: 1515–1519.

62. Zonana-Nacach A, Rodríguez-Guzmán LM, Jiménez-Balderas FJ, Camargo-Coronel A, Escobedo-de la Peña J, et al. (2002) [Risk factors associated with systemic lupus erythematosis in a Mexican population]. Salud Publica Mex 44: 213–218.

63. Han S, Kim-Howard X, Deshmukh H, Kamatani Y, Viswanathan P, et al. (2009) Evaluation of imputation-based association in and around the integrin-alpha-M (ITGAM) gene and replication of robust association between a non-synonymous functional variant within ITGAM and systemic lupus erythematosus (SLE). Hum Mol Genet 18: 1171–1180.

64. Schwartzman-Morris J, Putterman C (2012) Gender differences in the pathogenesis and outcome of lupus and of lupus nephritis. Clin Dev Immunol 2012: 604892.

65. Cutolo M, Capellino S, Straub RH (2008) Oestrogens in rheumatic diseases: friend or foe? Rheumatology (Oxford) 47 Suppl 3: iii2–5.

66. Straub RH (2007) The complex role of estrogens in inflammation. Endocr Rev 28: 521–574.

67. Bhatia SS, Majka DS, Kittelson JM, Parrish LA, Ferucci ED, et al. (2007) Rheumatoid factor seropositivity is inversely associated with oral contraceptive use in women without rheumatoid arthritis. Ann Rheum Dis 66: 267–269.

68. Kipp M, Amor S, Krauth R, Beyer C (2012) Multiple sclerosis: neuroprotective alliance of estrogen-progesterone and gender. Front Neuroendocrinol 33: 1–16.

69. Beretta L, Caronni M, Origgi L, Ponti A, Santaniello A, et al. (2006) Hormone replacement therapy may prevent the development of isolated pulmonary hypertension in patients with systemic sclerosis and limited cutaneous involvement. Scand J Rheumatol 35: 468–471.

70. Mostafa S, Seamon V, Azzarolo AM (2012) Influence of sex hormones and genetic predisposition in Sjögren's syndrome: a new clue to the immunopathogenesis of dry eye disease. Exp Eye Res 96: 88–97.

71. Somogyi A, Müzes G, Molnár J, Tulassay Z (1998) Drug-related Churg-Strauss syndrome? Adverse Drug React Toxicol Rev 17: 63–74.

72. D'Onofrio F, Miele L, Diaco M, Santoro L, De Socio G, et al. (2006) Sjogren's syndrome in a celiac patient: searching for environmental triggers. Int J Immunopathol Pharmacol 19: 445–448.

73. Onel K, Bussel JB (2004) Adverse effects of estrogen therapy in a subset of women with ITP. J Thromb Haemost 2: 670–671.

74. Li Y, Xiao B, Xiao L, Zhang N, Yang H (2010) Myasthenia gravis accompanied by premature ovarian failure and aggravation by estrogen. Intern Med 49: 611–613.

75. Capellino S, Montagna P, Villaggio B, Soldano S, Straub RH, et al. (2008) Hydroxylated estrogen metabolites influence the proliferation of cultured human monocytes: possible role in synovial tissue hyperplasia. Clin Exp Rheumatol 26: 903–909.

76. Borenstein M, Higgins J, Rothstein H (2009) Introduction to Meta-Analysis. Statistics in Practice [Hardcover]. Wiley.

77. Higgins J, Green S (2011) Cochrane Handbook for Systematic Reviews of Interventions Version 5.1.0 [updated March 2011]. Higgins JPT GS, editor The Cochrane Collaboration. Available: www.cochrane-handbook.org.

78. Julkunen HA, Kaaja R, Friman C (1993) Contraceptive practice in women with systemic lupus erythematosus. Br J Rheumatol 32: 227–230.

79. Sánchez-Guerrero J (1999) Age at menopause and clinical characteristics. Arthritis Rheum 42: S71–S407. doi:10.1002/art.1780422107.

80. Cravioto M-D-C, Durand-Carbajal M, Jiménez-Santana L, Lara-Reyes P, Seuc AH, et al. (2011) Efficacy of estrogen plus progestin on menopausal symptoms in women with systemic lupus erythematosus: a randomized, double-blind, controlled trial. Arthritis Care Res (Hoboken) 63: 1654–1663.

Increased Risk of Chronic Obstructive Pulmonary Disease in Patients with Systemic Lupus Erythematosus

Te-Chun Shen[1,2], Cheng-Li Lin[3,4], Chia-Hung Chen[1], Chih-Yen Tu[1], Te-Chun Hsia[1]*, Chuen-Ming Shih[1], Wu-Huei Hsu[1], Yen-Jung Chang[5]*

1 Division of Pulmonary and Critical Care Medicine, Department of Internal Medicine, China Medical University Hospital and China Medical University, Taichung, Taiwan, 2 Division of Pulmonary and Critical Care Medicine, Department of Internal Medicine, Chu Shang Show Chwan Hospital, Nantou, Taiwan, 3 Department of Public Health, China Medical University, Taichung, Taiwan, 4 Management Office for Health Data, China Medical University Hospital, Taichung, Taiwan, 5 Department of Health Promotion and Health Education, National Taiwan Normal University, Taipei, Taiwan

Abstract

Background: There is increasing evidence that autoimmune disease is associated with development of chronic obstructive pulmonary disease (COPD). We aim to assess the relationship between systemic lupus erythematosus (SLE) and COPD risk in a nationwide population.

Methods: We conducted a retrospective cohort study using the catastrophic illness registry of the Taiwan National Health Insurance Research Database (NHIRD). We identified 10,623 patients with SLE newly diagnosed between 2000 and 2010. Each patient was randomly frequency-matched with four people without SLE on age, sex, and index year from the general population. Both cohorts were followed up until the end of 2010 to measure the incidence of COPD. The risk of COPD was analyzed using Cox proportional hazards regression models including age, sex, index year and comorbidities.

Results: The overall incidence rate of COPD was 1.73-fold higher in the SLE cohort than in the control cohort (17.4 vs. 10.1 per 10,000 person-years, 95% CI = 1.62–1.84). Age related analysis showed increased incidence of COPD with age in both SLE and control cohorts. However, adjusted HR maximum was observed in the youngest age group (adjusted HR: 4.33, 95% CI, 2.39–7.85) while adjusted HR minimum was witnessed in the oldest age group (adjusted HR: 1.19, 95% CI, 0.85–1.22).

Conclusion: Patients with SLE have a significant risk of developing COPD than the control population. Based on the findings from this study, it can be hypothesized that in addition to cigarette smoke SLE may be a determining factor for COPD incidence. However, further investigation is needed to corroborate this hypothesis.

Editor: Antony Bayer, Cardiff University, United Kingdom

Funding: This work was supported by Taiwan Department of Health Clinical Trial and Research Center and for Excellence (DOH102-TD-B-111-004) and Taiwan Department of Health Cancer Research Center for Excellence (DOH102-TD-C-111-005). The funders had no role in study design, data collection and analysis, decision to publish, or preparation of the manuscript. No additional external funding was received for this study.

Competing Interests: The authors have declared that no competing interests exist.

* E-mail: yjchang2012@gmail.com (YC); derrick.hsia@msa.hinet.net (TH)

Introduction

Systemic lupus erythematosus (SLE), an autoimmune disease that affects multiple organ systems, is more prevalent in women, particularly of child-bearing age. Although the exact mechanism of SLE initiation and progression is unknown, several risk factors, such as heredity, hormonal abnormalities, environmental pollutants, and viral infections, have been recognized as important contributors toward SLE development. An important clinical evidence of this disease is the presence of anti-double-stranded DNA (anti-ds DNA) autoantibodies, which are highly specific and can be used as diagnostic markers for disease activity and progression [1]. The annual incidence of SLE in adults ranges from 2.0 to 7.6 cases per 100,000 person-years in developed countries [2]. A recent population-based study from Taiwan found

that the average incidence of SLE cases was 4.87 per 100,000 person-years between 2003 and 2008 [3].

Chronic obstructive pulmonary disease (COPD) is a slow progressive disease characterized by obstruction of airflow in the lungs due to chronic inflammation on the lining of airways. It is the 4th leading cause of death worldwide, with reported prevalence rates between 5% and 13% [4,5]. Although exposure to cigarette smoke plays a pivotal role in COPD development, a substantial group of patients with COPD has been identified as nonsmokers [6,7]. Therefore, in addition to tobacco smoke, relevance of other contributing factors in COPD development cannot be ignored; thus, other contributing factors exist and one of them may be autoimmunity. The role of autoimmune pathology in the development and progression of COPD is becoming increasingly appreciated [8].

Smoking is a common environmental risk factor for COPD, but COPD development in patients with SLE may not be attributed to cigarette smoke alone. SLE may play an independent role in COPD incidence. Even smokers with SLE may display a different time course in COPD development compared with non-SLE individuals who were addicted to smoking. A recent epidemiological study from Israel has reported that rheumatoid arthritis, also an autoimmune disease, is significantly associated with COPD; the study was adjusted by controlling confounders including smoking [9]. Other study sources have revealed that the majority of patients with COPD contain increased levels of serum antibodies capable of interacting with self-antigens [10–16], and occurrence of antibodies to specific autoantigens correlates with disease severity [12–14,16]. The mechanism of interactions between autoimmunity and COPD is still inconclusive.

The primary aim of our study is to determine whether a differential risk of developing COPD for adults exists with and without SLE by examining a relatively large population cohort in Taiwan. The results in this study were generated from a population-based retrospective cohort obtained from the National Health Insurance (NHI) system's database. To the best of our knowledge, this is the first nationwide population-based study evaluating the relationship between SLE and the risk of developing COPD.

Methods

Data Source

The National Health Insurance (NHI) program in Taiwan was first established in 1995, since then it has covered approximately 99% of Taiwan's population (23.74 million) [17]. The National Health Research Institute (NHRI) of Taiwan, in co-operation with the National Health Insurance Bureau (NHIB), has established a National Health Insurance Research Database (NHIRD), from which data were pooled for our study [18,19]. The International Classification of Disease, 9th Revision, Clinical Modification (ICD-9-CM) was used for SLE diagnosis. Following regulations implemented by the Department of Health, the identity of each patient was encrypted for privacy and data security. This study was exempted from full ethical review by the International Review Board, China Medical University and Hospital Research Ethics Committee (IRB permit number: CMU-REC-101-012).

Study Population

Patients certified with catastrophic illnesses including SLE were exempted from paying a copayment and therefore could be easily identified from the Registry of Catastrophic Illness Patient Database (RCIPD). A catastrophic illness is defined as a severe illness requiring advanced health care. Catastrophic illnesses usually involve high health care costs and may incapacitate the person from working, creating a financial hardship. All patients with SLE are categorized to have a catastrophic illness in the NHI system of Taiwan [3]. Patients certified with SLE catastrophic illness certification (ICD-9-CM code 710.0) as identified from the RCIPD covering a period of 10 years (2000–2010) were selected for this study. The index date for patients with SLE was assigned to be the date on which symptoms of SLE were first revealed. For comparison study, a non-SLE cohort control was randomly selected (4 for every patient in the SLE cohort) from the list of insured persons without a history of SLE and was matched for age, sex, and index year of SLE diagnosis. Patients in both cohorts with prior incidence of COPD (ICD-9 code 491, 492, and 496) or with missing information related to age and/or sex were excluded from this study.

Outcome and Comorbidities

All study patients were followed until they were diagnosed with COPD as evident from the medical records. To measure the incidence of COPD, the SLE and non-SLE cohort were followed until COPD was diagnosed or death of the subject occurred or patients failed to follow-up or 31 December 2010, whichever came first. Comorbidities including hypertension (ICD-9-CM codes 401–405), diabetes (ICD-9-CM code 250), hyperlipidemia (ICD-9-CM code 272), coronary artery disease (CAD) (ICD-9-codes 410-414), cerebrovascular accident (CVA) (ICD-9-codes 430-438), and end-stage renal disease (ESRD) (ICD-9-CM code 585) were defined as diseases diagnosed before the index date.

Statistical analysis

All statistical analyses were performed using SAS software, version 9.1.3 (SAS Institute, Cary, NC, USA). A two-sided statistical test with $p<0.05$ was considered statistically significant. The SLE cohort and non-SLE cohort data were compared using the Chi-square test for categorical variables and unpaired Student t-test for continuous variables. For comparisons between the SLE cohort and the non-SLE cohort, the incidence rate ratio (IRR) of COPD and 95% confidence interval (CI) were measured using the Poisson regression model. The univariable and multivariable Cox proportional hazard regression models were applied to measure the hazard ratio (HR) and 95% confidence interval (CI) of COPD incidence for the SLE cohort compared with that of the non-SLE cohort. Variables in the multivariable model included age, sex, hypertension, diabetes, hyperlipidemia, CAD, CVA, and ESRD. The Cox model was also used to estimate age, sex, and comorbidity specific HR. The Kaplan–Meier method was used to estimate cumulative incidence and the differences between the curves were tested with two-tailed log-rank test.

Results

The demographics and medical comorbidities of patients enrolled in the study program are depicted in (Table 1). A total of 53,115 patients were enrolled in this study. The mean age ($\pm$SD) was 37.3$\pm$11.5 years for the SLE cohort and 37.1$\pm$11.9 years for the non-SLE control cohort.

The majority of the subjects selected for this study were female (88.3%) and nearly (73.8%) of the subjects were aged 20–49 years (43.8%). When compared with the non-SLE control cohort, patients with SLE displayed higher proportion of comorbidities including hypertension (19.0% vs. 6.71%), diabetes (5.08% vs. 3.97%), hyperlipidemia (6.08% vs. 1.80%), CAD (4.84% vs. 2.41%), CVA (5.98% vs. 2.52%), and ESRD (3.29% vs. 0.46%). The mean follow up duration was 5.13$\pm$3.29 years for the SLE cohort and 5.32$\pm$3.24 years for the non-SLE cohort. The SLE cohort group reported higher rate of COPD incidence compared with the control cohort (17.4 vs. 10.1 per 10,000 person-years, 95% CI, 1.62–1.84, adjusted HR: 1.92, 95% CI, 1.50–2.44) (Table 2). The cumulative incidence of COPD by the end of follow-up period was approximately 0.55% higher in the SLE cohort than the non-SLE cohort (1.53% vs. 0.98%; $P<0.001$) (Figure 1). The sex specific risk analysis for both the cohorts revealed that both genders were equally susceptible in developing COPD (adjusted HR for women: 2.10, 95% CI, 1.55–2.83 vs. adjusted HR for men: 1.88, 95% CI, 1.24–2.86). Age related analysis showed increased incidence of COPD with age in both SLE and non-SLE cohorts. However, adjusted HR maximum was witnessed in the age range 20–49 years (adjusted HR: 4.33, 95% CI, 2.39–7.85) while adjusted HR minimum was observed in the oldest age group (>65 years) (Table 2). The multivariable Cox

Table 1. Demographic characteristics and comorbidities in patients with and without systemic lupus erythematosus.

Variable	SLE, n(%)		p value
	No	Yes	
	N = 42492	N = 10623	
Sex			
Female	37508(88.3)	9377(88.3)	0.99
Male	4984(11.7)	1246(11.7)	
Age, mean(SD)	37.1(11.9)	37.3(11.5)	0.07[#]
Age			
20–34 years	18596(43.8)	4649(43.8)	0.99
35–49 years	14012(33.0)	3503(33.0)	
50–64 years	6480(15.3)	1620(15.3)	
65+ years	3404(8.01)	851(8.01)	
Comorbidities			
Hypertension	2853(6.71)	2017(19.0)	<0.0001
Diabetes	1687(3.97)	540(5.08)	<0.0001
Hyperlipidemia	765(1.80)	646(6.08)	<0.0001
CAD	1023(2.41)	514(4.84)	<0.0001
CVA	1071(2.52)	635(5.98)	<0.0001
ESRD	197(0.46)	350(3.29)	<0.0001

Chi-square test, [#]: Two sample t-test.

proportional hazard regression model showed an increased risk of COPD in patients with SLE with one of following characteristics: men (adjusted HR: 2.33, 95% CI, 1.84–2.94), older age (adjusted HR: 61.9, 95% CI, 34.7–110.7), diabetes (adjusted HR: 1.52, 95% CI, 1.16–1.99), CAD (adjusted HR: 1.86, 95% CI, 1.41–2.45), and CVA (adjusted HR: 1.99, 95% CI, 1.51–1.36) (Table 3).

Discussion

To the best of our knowledge, this is the first nationwide population-based study evaluating the relationship between SLE and COPD risk. In this study, there was a significantly higher incidence of COPD among patients with COPD than that in the general population. Further age related risk analysis indicated higher COPD incidence in aged patients although adjusted HR progressively decreased with age. This apparent contradictory finding could be explained by assuming aged patients may be exposed to cigarette smoke for a prolonged period of time or they could present with a large number of comorbid diseases. Therefore, the adjusted HR of oldest age group was not statistically relevant.

Another remarkable finding from this study revealed that the HR of developing COPD was comparatively higher (adjusted HR: 9.45, 95% CI, 2.81–31.9) in men aged 21–49 years with SLE than in men with similar age range in the control cohort. The differences in smoking rate might account for this observation. The smoking rate in men of the SLE cohort may be higher than that of the non-SLE cohort. Alternatively, SLE could be considered as an independent risk factor for COPD or smokers with SLE developed COPD within a short time frame. A recent public health report released from the Ministry of Health and Welfare of Taiwan, has reported that about 42.8% of males with age ranging from 20 to 50 years are smokers [20]. Although the

NHI database does not contain information about personal smoking habits, we reasoned this value could be attributed to male smokers aged 20–50-years old in the non-SLE cohort. Therefore, to explain the occurrence of such a high HR, we hypothesized that either SLE directly causes COPD incidence or facilitates shortening of the disease course. However, further investigation is needed to corroborate this hypothesis.

For our study purpose, exposure to tobacco smoke is still considered as the most important confounding factor for COPD. Unfortunately, the NHI database does not provide any information on personal smoking habits. Freemer *et al* note that exposure to tobacco smoke has been associated with several autoimmune diseases [21]. Majka *et al* report the relationship between the development of SLE and cigarette smoking is less affirmative [22]. We have searched for previous publications which involved smoking rate among SLE patients and general population. We found that some studies with no significant difference between the two groups [23–26]. It is inconclusive that patients with SLE have a significant high smoking rate in all races. We roughly estimated the current smoking rate of non-SLE cohorts by considering data from public health reports obtained from the Ministry of Health and Welfare of Taiwan (Table 2). The overall smoking rate in the general population is 19.8% (males, 35.0%, females, 4.1%). Therefore, we considered combined effects of SLE and smoking for evaluation of increased incidence of COPD in this study.

Based on disease definition in the registry system as established by NHIRD of Taiwan, SLE is categorized as a "catastrophic illness" and patients diagnosed with SLE are entitled to receive the "catastrophic illness certification" issued by the government. The catastrophic illness certified patient is eligible for a great deal of discount benefits with regard to medical expenses. The certification process requires critical evaluation of medical records, serological, and/or pathological reports by experts specialized in the disease field [27]. The diagnosis of COPD is based on target history and requires comprehensive pulmonary function assessment. The criteria set forth by the GOLD guideline are usually followed in concluding the diagnosis of COPD [28]. A spot check is also performed regularly. Therefore, NHIRD provides a reliable data source for SLE and COPD occurrences. Moreover, any pre-existing condition of COPD would be detected by rheumatologists during comprehensive evaluation of patient's medical history while confirming SLE diagnosis. Therefore, patients diagnosed with COPD afterwards could be considered as new cases.

The exact link between inflammation and autoimmune disorders is not known. However, smoking serves as an important bridging link between the two diseases. Smoking is a well-known risk factor associated with several autoimmune diseases. Chronic exposure to cigarette smoke may be detrimental to the regular functioning of the body at the intracellular level. For example, smoking induces production of intracellular antigens [29–31], augments B cell autoreactivity and stimulates the proliferation of peripheral T-lymphocytes, and actively promotes generation of endogenous oxidative free radicals [29,32–33]. Harmful toxins present in cigarette smoke may interact with DNA and cause genetic mutations, which ultimately lead to altered gene expressions resulting in autoimmune diseases [9]. COPD is a representative example of inflammatory disease. Although the exact underlying mechanism causing COPD has not been established, several mechanisms have been implicated in the pathogenesis of smoking induced COPD. Sirtuin 1 (SIRT1) is a deacetylase anti-inflammatory protein, the important functions of which are mediated by several different transcription factors (e.g., NF-kappaB). Decreased levels of SIRT1 and NF-kappaB activity have been reported in smokers exhibiting COPD conditions [34].

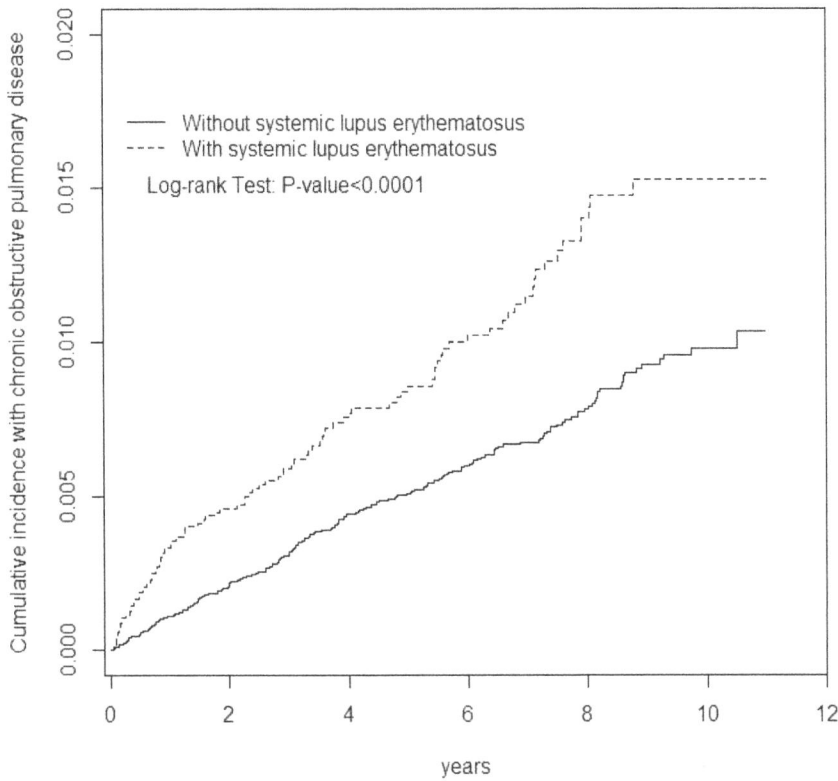

Figure 1. Cummulative incidence of COPD for subjects with and without systemic lupus erythematosus using the Kaplan–Meir method.

Table 2. Sex- and age-specific incidence rates of COPD in subjects with and without systemic lupus erythematosus (SLE) and Cox model estimated hazard ratios for patients with SLE.

Variables (smoking rate %)‡	SLE						IRR*(95% CI)	Adjusted HR† (95% CI)
	No			Yes				
	Event	PY	Rate#	Event	PY	Rate#		
All	228	226007	10.1	95	54533	17.4	1.73(1.62, 1.84)***	1.92(1.50, 2.44)***
20–49 (25.0%)	21	176590	1.19	30	43844	6.84	5.75(5.34, 6.20)***	4.33(2.39, 7.85)***
50–64 (14.9%)	33	34499	9.57	21	7763	27.1	2.83(2.43, 3.29)***	2.38(1.37, 4.13)***
65+ (11.0%)	174	14918	116.6	44	2926	150.4	1.29(1.05, 1.58)*	1.19(0.85, 1.66)
Women	146	200870	7.27	63	48708	12.9	1.78(1.66, 1.91)***	2.10(1.55, 2.83)***
20–49 (5.6%)	17	159543	1.07	20	39726	5.03	4.72(4.37, 5.11)***	3.30(1.66, 6.58)***
50–64 (2.2%)	21	29555	7.11	13	6698	19.4	2.73(2.30, 3.24)***	2.20(1.09, 4.45)*
65+ (1.0%)	108	11773	91.7	30	2283	131.4	1.43(1.14, 1.81)**	1.45(0.96, 2.17)
Men	82	25137	32.6	32	5825	54.9	1.68(1.42, 2.00)***	1.88(1.24, 2.86)**
20–49 (42.8%)	4	17047	2.35	10	4117	24.3	10.4(8.17, 13.1)***	9.45(2.81, 31.9)***
50–64 (30.1%)	12	4944	24.3	8	1065	75.1	3.09(2.19, 4.38)***	2.81(1.14, 6.95)*
65+ (19.4%)	66	3145	209.9	14	643	217.7	1.04(0.68, 1.58)	1.01(0.56, 1.82)

Rate#, incidence rate per 10,000 person-years.
IRR*, incidence rate ratio.
†Model was adjusted for age, sex, and comorbidities.
‡Current smoking rate of general population in Taiwan (%).
* p<0.05, ** p<0.01, *** p<0.001.

Table 3. Cox model with hazard ratios and 95% confidence intervals of COPD associated with systemic lupus erythematosus and covariates.

Variable	Crude		Adjusted[†]	
	HR	(95% CI)	HR	(95% CI)
Age				
20–34 years	1	(Reference)	1	(Reference)
35–49 years	3.74	(1.99, 7.03)***	3.62	(1.93, 6.79)***
50–64 years	12.1	(6.63, 22.2)***	9.03	(4.90, 16.6)***
65+ years	115.6	(66.0, 202.3)***	61.9	(34.7, 110.7)***
Sex				
Male	4.38	(3.48, 5.50)***	2.33	(1.84, 2.94)***
Female	1	(Reference)	1	(Reference)
Baseline comorbidities (yes vs no)				
SLE	1.72	(1.36, 2.19)***	1.82	(1.43, 2.31)***
Hypertension	9.53	(7.66, 11.8)***	1.28	(0.97, 1.68)
Diabetes	9.17	(7.20, 11.7)***	1.52	(1.16, 1.99)**
Hyperlipidemia	4.34	(3.06, 6.17)***	0.87	(0.60, 1.26)
CAD	13.1	(10.3, 16.7)***	1.86	(1.41, 2.45)***
CVA	12.2	(9.56, 15.6)***	1.99	(1.51, 2.620***
ESRD	2.20	(1.09, 4.43)*	0.67	(0.33, 1.36)

[†]Adjusted HR: multivariable analysis including for age, sex, hypertension, diabetes, hyperlipidemia, CAD, CVA, and ESRD.
*p<0.05, ** p<0.01, *** p<0.001.

Vascular endothelial growth factor (VEGF) signaling is a crucial event associated with lung structure maintenance. Bronchiolar expressions of VEGF and VEGF2 receptors are significantly lower in smokers with COPD [35]. The toll-like receptors in the lung epithelium plays a pivotal role in host defense mechanism. Tobacco smoke has been identified as a potential modulator of expression of toll-like receptor 4 (TLR4) in respiratory epithelium [36].

The strength of our study lies in the use of population-based data that are highly representative of the general population. However, our study has several limitations. First, the National Health Insurance Research Database (NHIRD) does not contain detailed information regarding smoking habits, body weight index (BMI), diet preference, drug use, and family history of systemic diseases, all of which may be associated risk factors for COPD development. Second, the evidence derived from a retrospective cohort study is statistically less relevant than information obtained from randomized trials because of potential biases related to adjustments made for confounding variables. Despite our meticulous study design, biases resulting from unknown confounding factors may have affected our results. Third, all data in the NHIRD are anonymous. Thus, relevant clinical variables, such as serum laboratory data, pulmonary function tests, imaging results, and pathology findings were unavailable for patients in our study.

Conclusion

To the best of our knowledge, our study is the first nationwide population-based study evaluating the risk of developing COPD in patients with SLE. Patients with SLE have a significant risk of developing COPD than the control population. Based on the findings from this study, it can be hypothesized that in addition to cigarette smoke SLE may be a determining factor for COPD incidence. However, further investigation is needed to corroborate this hypothesis.

Author Contributions

Conceived and designed the experiments: TS CC CT. Performed the experiments: TS TH CS WH. Analyzed the data: CL YC. Contributed reagents/materials/analysis tools: CL YC. Wrote the paper: TS CL YC.

References

1. Pons-Estel GJ, Alarco'n GS, Scofield L, Reinlib L, Cooper GS (2010) Understanding the epidemiology and progression of systemic lupus erythematosus. Semin Arthr Rheum 39: 257–68.
2. Fessel WJ (1988) Epidemiology of systemic lupus erythematosus. Rheum Dis Clin N Am 14: 15–23.
3. Yeh KW, Yu CH, Chan PC, Horng JT, Huang JL (2013) Burden of systemic lupus erythematosus in Taiwan: a population-based survey. Rheumatol Int DOI: 10.1007/s00296-012-2643-6.
4. Vestbo J, Hurd SS, Agusti AG, Jones PW, Vogelmeier C, et al. (2013) Global strategy for the diagnosis, management, and prevention of chronic obstructive pulmonary disease: GOLD executive summary. Am J Respir Crit Care Med 187: 347–65.
5. Mannino DM, Buist AS (2007) Global burden of COPD: risk factors, prevalence, and future trends. Lancet 370: 765–73.
6. Birring SS, Brightling CE, Bradding P, Entwisle JJ, Vara DD, et al. (2002) Clinical, radiologic, and induced sputum features of chronic obstructive pulmonary disease in nonsmokers: a descriptive study. Am J Respir Crit Care Med 166: 1078–83.
7. Hagstad S, Ekerljung L, Lindberg A, Backman H, Rönmark E, et al. (2012) COPD among non-smokers—Report from the Obstructive Lung Disease in Northern Sweden (OLIN) studies. Respir Med 106: 980–8.
8. Packard TA, Li QZ, Cosgrove GP, Bowler RP, Cambier JC (2013) COPD is associated with production of autoantibodies to a broad spectrum of self-antigens, correlative with disease phenotype. Immunol Res 55: 48–57.
9. Bieber V, Cohen AD, Freud T, Agmon-Levin N, Gertel S, et al. (2013) Autoimmune smoke and fire—coexisting rheumatoid arthritis and chronic obstructive pulmonary disease: a cross-sectional analysis. Immunol Res 56: 261–6.
10. Feghali-Bostwick CA, Gadgil AS, Otterbein LE, Pilewski JM, Stoner MW, et al. (2008) Autoantibodies in patients with chronic obstructive pulmonary disease. Am J Respir Crit Care Med 177: 156–63.
11. Karayama M, Inui N, Suda T, Nakamura Y, Nakamura H, et al. (2010) Antiendothelial Cell Antibodies in Patients With COPD. Chest 138: 1303–8.
12. Kirkham PA, Caramori G, Casolari P, Papi AA, Edwards M, et al. (2011) Oxidative stress-induced antibodies to carbonyl-modified protein correlate with severity of chronic obstructive pulmonary disease. Am J Respir Crit Care Med 184: 796–802.
13. Kuo YB, Chang CA, Wu YK, Hsieh MJ, Tsai CH, et al. (2010) Identification and clinical association of anti-cytokeratin 18 autoantibody in COPD. Immunol Lett 128: 131–6.
14. Lee SH, Goswami S, Grudo A, Song LZ, Bandi V, et al. (2007) Antielastin autoimmunity in tobacco smoking-induced emphysema. Nat Med 13: 567–9.
15. Leidinger P, Keller A, Heisel S, Ludwig N, Rheinheimer S, et al. (2009) Novel autoantigens immunogenic in COPD patients. Respir Res 10: 20.
16. Núñez B, Sauleda J, Antó JM, Julià MR, Orozco M, et al. (2011) Anti-tissue antibodies are related to lung function in chronic obstructive pulmonary disease. Am J Respir Crit Care Med 183: 1025–31.
17. Cheng TM (2009) Taiwan's national health insurance system: high value for the dollar. Six Countries, Six Reform Models: Their Healthcare Reform: Experience of Israel, the Netherlands, New Zealand, Singapore, Switzerland and Taiwan. Hackensack, NJ: World Scientific 171–204.
18. Shen TC, Tu CY, Lin CL, Wei CC, Li YF (2014) Increased risk of asthma in patients with systemic lupus erythematosus. Am J Respir Crit Care Med 189: 496–9.
19. Shen TC, Lin CL, Wei CC, Tu CY, Li YF (2014) The risk of asthma in rheumatoid arthritis: a population-based cohort study. QJM Jan 20.
20. Health Promotion Administration, Ministry of Health and Welfare of Taiwan website. Available: http://www.hpa.gov.tw/BHPNet/Web/HealthTopic/Topic.aspx?id=200712250024. Accessed 2014 Feb 18.
21. Freemer MM, King TE Jr, Criswell LA (2006) Association of smoking with dsDNA autoantibody production in systemic lupus erythematosus. Ann Rheum Dis 65: 581–4.
22. Majka DS, Holers VM (2006) Cigarette smoking and the risk of systemic lupus erythematosus and rheumatoid arthritis. Ann Rheum Dis 65: 561–3.

23. Drenkard C, Rask KJ, Easley KA, Bao G, Lim SS (2013) Primary preventive services in patients with systemic lupus erythematosus: study from a population-based sample in Southeast U.S. Semin Arthritis Rheum 43: 209–16.
24. Petri M, Thompson E, Abusuwwa R, Huang J, Garrctt E (2001) BALES: the Baltimore Lupus Environmental Study. Arthritis Rheum 44 Suppl 9: S331.
25. Cooper GS, Dooley MA, Treadwell EL, St Clair EW, Gilkeson GS (2001) Smoking and use of hair treatments in relation to risk of developing systemic lupus erythematosus. J Rheumatol 28: 2653–6.
26. Reidenberg MM, Drayer DE, Lorenzo B, Strom BL, West SL, et al. (1993) Acetylation phenotypes and environmental chemical exposure of people with idiopathic systemic lupus erythematosus. Arthritis Rheum 36: 971–3.
27. Tan EM, Cohen AS, Fries JF, Masi AT, McShane DJ, et al. (1982) Special article: the 1982 revised criteria for the classification of systemic lupus erythematosus. Arthritis Rheum 25: 1271–7.
28. The Global Initiative for Chronic Obstructive Lung Disease website. Available: http://www.goldcopd.org/. Accessed 2013 Nov 20.
29. Arnson Y, Shoenfeld Y, Amital H (2010) Effects of tobacco smoke on immunity, inflammation and autoimmunity. J Autoimmun 34: J258–65.
30. Zifman E, Amital H, Gilburd B, Shoenfeld Y (2008) Antioxidants and smoking in autoimmune disease–opposing sides of the seesaw? Autoimmun Rev 8: 165–9.
31. Carmi G, Amital H (2011) The geoepidemiology of autoimmunity: capsules from the 7th International Congress on Autoimmunity, Ljubljana, Slovenia, May 2010. Isr Med Assoc J 13: 121–7.
32. Bengtsson AA, Rylander L, Hagmar L, Nived O, Sturfelt G (2002) Risk factors for developing systemic lupus erythematosus: a casecontrol study in southern Sweden. Rheumatology [Oxford] 41: 563–71.
33. Vermeulen A (1993) Environment, human reproduction, menopause, and andropause. Environ Health Perspect 101 (Suppl2): 91–100.
34. Rajendrasozhan S, Yang SR, Edirisinghe I, Yao H, Adenuga D, et al. (2008) Deacetylases and NF-kappaB in redox regulation of cigarette smoke-induced lung inflammation: epigenetics in pathogenesis of COPD. Antioxid Redox Signal 10: 799–811.
35. Suzuki M, Betsuyaku T, Nagai K, Fuke S, Nasuhara Y, et al. (2008) Decreased airway expression of vascular endothelial growth factor in cigarette smoke-induced emphysema in mice and COPD patients. Inhal Toxicol 20: 349–59.
36. MacRedmond RE, Greene CM, Dorscheid DR, McElvaney NG, O'Neill SJ (2007) Epithelial expression of TLR4 is modulated in COPD and by steroids, salmeterol and cigarette smoke. Respir Res 8: 84.

Clinical and Serological Features of Patients Referred through a Rheumatology Triage System because of Positive Antinuclear Antibodies

Christie Fitch-Rogalsky[1], Whitney Steber[1], Michael Mahler[2], Terri Lupton[1], Liam Martin[1], Susan G. Barr[1], Dianne P. Mosher[1], James Wick[1], Marvin J. Fritzler[1]*

1 Faculty of Medicine, University of Calgary, Calgary, Alberta, Canada, **2** INOVA Diagnostics Inc., San Diego, California, United States of America

Abstract

Background: The referral of patients with positive anti-nuclear antibody (ANA) tests has been criticized as an inappropriate use of medical resources. The utility of a positive ANA test in a central triage (CT) system was studied by determining the autoantibody profiles and clinical diagnoses of patients referred to rheumatologists through a CT system because of a positive ANA test.

Methods: Patients that met three criteria were included: (1) referred to Rheumatology CT over a three year interval; (2) reason for referral was a "positive ANA"; (3) were evaluated by a certified rheumatologist. The CT clinical database was used to obtain demographic and clinical information and a serological database was used to retrieve specific ANA and/or extractable nuclear antigen (ENA) test results. Clinical information was extracted from the consulting rheumatologist's report.

Results: 15,357 patients were referred through the CT system; 643 (4.1%) of these because of a positive ANA and of these 263 (40.9%) were evaluated by a certified rheumatologist. In 63/263 (24%) of ANA positive patients, the specialist provided a diagnosis of an ANA associated rheumatic disease (AARD) while 69 (26.2%) had no evidence of any disease; 102 (38.8%) had other rheumatologic diagnoses and 29 (11%) had conditions that did not meet AARD classification criteria. Of ANA positive archived sera, 15.1% were anti-DFS70 positive and 91.2% of these did not have an AARD.

Conclusions: This is the first study to evaluate the serological and clinical features of patients referred through a CT system because of a positive ANA. The spectrum of autoantibody specificities was wide with anti-Ro52/TRIM21 being the most common autoantibody detected. Approximately 15% of referrals had only antibodies to DFS70, the vast majority of which did not have clinical evidence for an AARD. These findings provide insight into the utility of autoantibody testing in a CT system.

Editor: Masataka Kuwana, Keio University School of Medicine, Japan

Funding: This project was funded and supported by resources from Mitogen Advanced Diagnostics Laboratory and as well as funds allocated to the Arthritis Society Research Chair by the University of Calgary, Division of Rheumatology, at the University of Calgary. The funders had no role in the study design, data collection and analysis, decision to publish, or preparation of the manuscript.

Competing Interests: This study was partly supported by the Mitogen Advanced Diagnostics Laboratory. M. Mahler is an employee of INOVA Diagnostics Inc. (San Diego), a manufacturer of autoantibody diagnostic kits. The HEp-2 slides were a kind gift from ImmunoConcepts Inc. (Sacramento, CA), and the anti-DFS70 assay kits were a gift of INOVA Diagnostics (San Diego, CA). M. Fritzler is a paid consultant, has received honoraria or has received gifts in kind from ImmunoConcepts Inc. (Sacramento, CA), Bio-Rad (Hercules, CA) and INOVA Diagnostics (San Diego, CA), Mikrogen GmbH (Neuried, Germany), Euroimmun GmbH (Lubeck, Germany) and Dr. Fooke Laboratorien GmbH (Neuss, Germany). There are no further patents, products in development or marketed products to declare.

* E-mail: fritzler@ucalgary.ca

Introduction

The detection of anti-nuclear antibodies (ANA) has been established as an important adjunct to the diagnosis and classification of ANA-associated rheumatic diseases (AARD) such as systemic lupus erythematosus (SLE), systemic sclerosis (SSc), mixed connective tissue disease (MCTD), idiopathic inflammatory myopathies (IIM) and Sjögren's syndrome (SjS) [1]. Nevertheless, concerns have been raised about the ANA test as a screen for AARD [2,3] and that positive tests inappropriately prompt unwarranted referrals from primary and secondary care physicians to tertiary care specialists [4–6]. Some concerns about ANA tests as an approach to screening for AARD are based on studies of the frequency of ANA in the healthy individuals [7] and calculations of pre-test probabilities and the clinical challenge of interpreting a positive test when the patient has no apparent evidence for a definitive diagnosis of, nor meets the classification criteria for, an AARD [3–5,8].

The limitations of ANA and the related ENA tests have been offset by at least three key findings. First, for several decades it has been appreciated that some autoantibodies are highly specific for certain AARD [9,10]. Hence, when disease specific autoantibodies, such as anti-dsDNA antibodies in SLE, anti-centromere antibodies in SSc and anti-Jo-1 antibodies in IIM are detected in the absence of diagnostic or classification criteria for these conditions the clinician is often uncertain about the advice to give to the referring physician or the patient. This issue is linked to a second key finding wherein it now well established that ANA and disease-specific autoantibodies can pre-date the clinical diagnosis of AARD by as many as two decades [11–13]. Thus, in the context of a person with a positive ANA where the specific autoantibody is known, the physician should take care before advising the patient that they do not have an AARD. Third, there is growing evidence that autoantibodies directed against the dense fine speckled 70 (DFS70) antigen without accompanying disease specific antibodies are rare in AARD and may be useful biomarker to rule out these conditions [14–17]. All three of these issues are of particular importance when patients are referred to a rheumatology central triage system because of a positive ANA test. Key questions are: 1) are such referrals inappropriate and a waste of health care resources, and 2) can the specificities of ANA and related autoantibodies inform the triage process to define the urgency of a specific referral to a specialist? Accordingly, the goals of this study were firstly to examine the ANA/ENA profiles of patients referred through a rheumatology central triage system; secondly, to determine if ANA/ENA of a given specificity were attended by a specific diagnosis and, thirdly, to determine the frequency of autoantibodies directed to DFS70 in a ANA referral cohort and elucidate the possible association of these antibodies to a specific diagnosis.

Materials and Methods

Ethics Statement

This study was approved by the University of Calgary Conjoint Health Research Ethics Board (Ethics ID#: E-24353). Under the terms of this approval, all patient records and information was anonymized and de-identified prior to analysis, precluding the requirement of written informed consent. All clinical investigation was conducted according to the principles expressed in the Declaration of Helsinki.

Patients, Selection Criteria, Demographic and Clinical Information

We utilized an anonymous administrative database to evaluate the utility of autoantibody testing in the context of triage of referrals to the rheumatology service through a Central Referral and Triage (CReATe) service in the Calgary Health Region (Calgary, Alberta, Canada). This database includes the reason that the patient was referred for consultation, such as abnormal laboratory tests, signs or symptoms thought to suggest a rheumatic disease as well as baseline demographic data, working diagnoses and wait times. Of particular relevance to this study was the identification of patients referred to the rheumatology service because they had a positive ANA (ANA Referral Cohort: ARC). All individuals included in the ARC met the following criteria: (1) referred to Rheumatology Central Triage from in a sequential three year calendar time frame (n = 15,537); (2) reason for referral was a "positive ANA (n = 643); (3) were evaluated by certified rheumatology specialists at regional referral centres (n = 263) in Calgary, Alberta, Canada.

After the patient was seen by the consulting rheumatologist, a form was completed and information expressing the appropriateness of triage and final diagnosis was entered into the database. Final diagnoses were categorized as non-inflammatory disorders (e.g. fibromyalgia, osteoarthritis, tendonitis, and bursitis) or

inflammatory diseases, including AARDs, rheumatoid arthritis (RA) and other systemic inflammatory arthritis. Accordingly, patients were grouped into three diagnostic categories (AARD, non-AARD and unresolved AARD). The AARD group included patients with a diagnosis of SLE, SSc, MCTD, IIM and SjS. The non-AARD included patients who had a definitive diagnosis but AARD was excluded. The third group (unresolved) consisted of patients without a final diagnosis or patients in which AARD insufficient classification criteria were not met and AARD could not be ruled out.

A second anonymous database that contained the serological data (see below) was extracted from the Mitogen Advanced Diagnostics Laboratory (MADL), Calgary, Alberta, Canada) master database. The two anonymous databases (CReATe and MADL) devoid of unique patient identifiers were merged using an anchored scrambled unique alphanumeric lifetime identifier (ULI) in order to maintain confidentiality.

A descriptive analysis of the combined dataset was performed, including the origin and number of referrals and autoantibody tests and results, triage categories, wait times and any delays in patient care resulting from requests for autoantibody tests. The number of patients referred because of a positive ANA test and their final diagnoses was tabulated. The primary analysis was the ability of an individual autoantibody to predict the diagnosis recorded by the consulting rheumatologist. This was gauged by determining the sensitivity, specificity, positive predictive value, negative predictive value and likelihood ratios for each test in relation to the final diagnosis, as well as the diagnostic categories described above. Secondary outcomes included the ability of individual or combined autoantibody results to predict the working diagnosis and triage category in order to assess how these results influence the triage process as it is currently designed. Agreement between the working diagnosis and the final diagnosis was assessed as a marker of referral quality.

Autoantibody Testing

The MADL performs ANA and ENA tests for the Calgary Health Region and surrounding catchment areas. ANA testing (including pattern and titer assessment) utilized HEp-2 cell substrates (HEp-2000, ImmunoConcepts Inc., Sacramento, CA) to screen for autoantibodies by indirect immunofluorescence (IIF) at a dilution of 1/160 [7] on the sera stored at MADL. All available samples were also tested for ANA specificities included in the ENA screening panel (chromatin, ribosomal P, Sm, U1RNP (ribonucleoprotein), SS-A/Ro60, Ro52/TRIM21, SS-B/La, Scl-70 (topoisomerase I), Jo-1 (histidyl tRNA synthetase) by addressable laser bead immunoassay (FIDIS, TheraDiag: Paris, France), anti-centromere by IIF pattern on HEp-2 cells and dsDNA by the *Crithidia lucilliae* IIF test (ImmunoConcepts, Sacramento, CA) [18]. Last, antibodies to DFS70/LEDGF were detected by a chemiluminescent immunoassay (QUANTA Flash DFS70, INOVA Diagnostics, San Diego, CA)[16,17].

Statistics

The data were evaluated using the Analyse-it software (Version 1.62; Analyse-it Software, Ltd., Leeds, UK). Positive and negative likelihood ratios (LR) were calculated for the individual autoantibodies. For statistical analysis, patients were grouped into AARD (SLE, SSc, SjS, IIM and MCTD) and non-AARD patients. Individuals in which diagnosis was not fully established and verified or in which AARD could not be ruled out were excluded from respective analyses.

Results

The clinical spectrum and referral diagnosis of all 15,357 patients referred to the Rheumatology service is represented in Figure 1. The majority of referrals were for evaluation of an inflammatory arthropathy (23.9%), arthralgia (26.6%) or a previously diagnosed AARD (12.1%), while smaller proportions were referred for consultation with respect to management of spondyloarthropathy (7.3%), osteoarthritis (6.7%), soft tissue rheumatism (3.1%) or vasculitis (1.4%). The ARC cohort of 263 patients from this referral group had an average age of 48.7 years (range 18–86, SD 83.53) and 92% were female. Approximately 68% of patients were referred from an urban center and 83.7% were referred by a family physician while the remainder were referred by subspecialist physicians: (in order of decreasing frequency) general internal medicine, neurology, respirology, otolaryngology, ophthalmology, dermatology, cardiology, hematology, obstetrics, general surgery, psychiatry. The mean interval from date of referral to when the patient was seen by the consultant was 165.4 days (range 25–551 days; SD 83.53).

Clinical information of the 263 ARC is summarized in Table 1. In total, 24% (n = 63) had a diagnosis of an AARD: SLE (9.1%; n = 24), SjS (9.1%; n = 24), SSc (2.3%; n = 6) and MCTD (1.9%; n = 5) followed by a spectrum of other AARDs or closely related conditions. Twenty-nine patients (11%) had equivocal evidence for an AARD and either did not meet sufficient criteria for classification or the consulting physician was unable to provide a definitive diagnosis (i.e. unresolved diagnosis): 13 (4.9%) undifferentiated connective tissue disease, 8 (3%) Raynaud's phenomenon, 5 (1.9%) inflammatory polyarthropathy and 3 (1.1%) discoid or cutaneous lupus. By comparison, 102 (38.8%) had a rheumatologic diagnosis but did not have an AARD, with osteoarthritis (9.9%), fibromyalgia (8.7%), arthralgia/myalgia (7.9%) and rheumatoid arthritis (RA) (2.3%) being the most common. Of note, 69 (26.2%) patients had no evidence for either an autoimmune or rheumatic disease. One hundred and sixteen patients (44.1%) of the ARC had a positive ENA test with the most common specificity being autoantibodies directed to Ro52/TRIM21 (n = 53; 45.7%), SS-A/Ro60 (n = 40; 34.5%), chromatin (n = 21; 18.5%), and SS-B/La (n = 19; 16.4%) (Table 2). The

Table 1. Consultant's Opinion of 263 Patients in the ARC.

Consultant's Diagnosis	N	%
AARD	**63**	**24**
Systemic lupus erythematosus	24	9.1
Sjögren's syndrome	24	9.1
Systemic sclerosis	6	2.3
Mixed connective tissue disease	5	1.9
Drug-induced lupus	2	0.8
Dermatomyositis	2	0.8
Unresolved AARD	**29**	**11**
Undifferentiated connective tissue disease	13	4.9
Raynaud's phenomenon	8	3.0
Inflammatory polyarthropathy	5	1.9
Discoid and cutaneous lupus	3	1.1
Other rheumatologic diagnoses	**102**	**38.8**
Osteoarthritis	26	9.9
Fibromyalgia	23	8.7
Arthralgia/myalgia	21	7.9
Rheumatoid arthritis	6	2.3
Neuromuscular/neuropathy	6	2.3
Mechanical back pain	5	1.9
Vasculitis/polymyalgia rheumatica	2	0.8
Other*	13	4.9
No findings for rheumatic or autoimmune disease	**69**	**26.2**

*Other includes gout, tendonitis, bursitis, patellofemoral syndrome, palindromic rheumatism, spondyloarthropathy, psoriatic arthritis, unspecified polyarthropathy.

consultant's diagnosis linked to these anti-ENA autoantibodies is shown in Table S1 in File S1.

The IIF results of the ARC showed that the three most common primary ANA IIF patterns were speckled (n = 158; 60.1%),

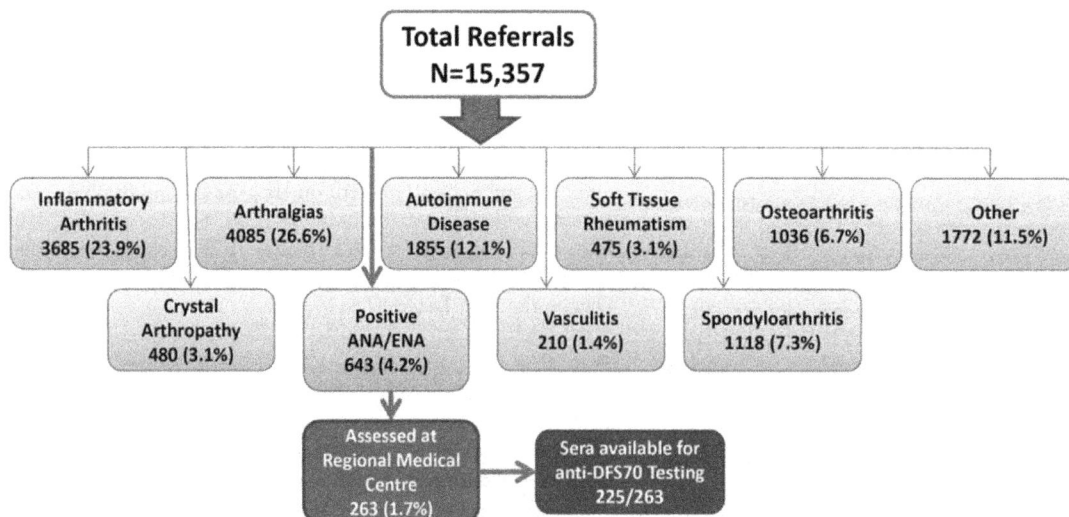

Figure 1. Derivation of the ARC via the diagnostic profile of 15,537 patients referred to rheumatology central triage over a three year audit period.

Table 2. Autoantibody Specificities of the 116 patients in the ARC with a positive anti-ENA*.

ENA Autoantibody**	N	%
Ro52/TRIM21	53	45.7
SS-A/Ro60	40	34.5
Chromatin	21	18.1
SS-B/La	19	16.4
Topoisomerase I (Scl-70)	17	14.7
U1 Ribonucleoprotein	17	14.7
Sm	14	12.1
Ribosomal P*	10	13.2
dsDNA*	10	13.2
Centromere	3	2.6
Jo-1	3	2.6
Unidentified	1	0.8

Note: 116/263 patients referred with a positive ANA had a detectable ENA autoantibody. Some patients had more than 1 autoantibody, hence % totals will not = 100.
*results available for 76 samples.
**Clinical diagnoses associated with specific autoantibodies see Table S1 in File S1.

nucleolar (n = 66; 25.1%), and homogeneous speckled (n = 55; 20.9%), with titers ranging from 1/160-1/5120 (Table S2 in File S1). Other IIF staining patterns included cytoplasmic (27.4%), multiple nuclear dots (26%), nuclear matrix and centromere (7.6%) and other less common patterns (Table S2 in File S1).

Anti-DFS70 antibodies

Thirty-four of the 225 (15.1%) archived sera tested positive for anti-DFS70 antibodies (Figure 2) and was the sole autoantibody detected in 24/34 (70.6%) of the sera. Among the anti-DFS70 antibody positive cohort, 33 had a definite diagnosis (one was unresolved) and of those 31/33 (93.9%) had no evidence of or fulfilled classification criteria for an AARD (Figure 3). The two patients with an AARD had SjS (one with coexistent anti-Ro52/TRIM21 antibodies). Sixteen (47.1%) anti-DFS70 positive patients had no evidence for any disease although three of these had autoantibodies typically associated with an AARD: one with anti-Scl-70/topo I and two with anti-chromatin antibodies. Other diagnoses in the anti-DFS70 antibody positive patients included Raynaud's phenomenon, osteoarthritis, RA, fibromyalgia and individual patients with polymyalgia rheumatica and psoriatic arthritis (Figure 2).

To analyze if autoantibodies might provide value in determining the urgency of referral we calculated the LRs for all anti-ENAs and for anti-DFS70 antibodies (Figure 3). The LR+ for AARD showed significant variations ranging from 0.0 (anti-Jo-1 antibodies) to 8.6 (anti-Ribo-P antibodies). The LR+ for non-AARD for anti-DFS70 antibodies was 5.4 and when considered in conjunction with other autoantibodies (no coexisting antibody/monospecific for anti-DFS70 antibodies) the LR+ increase to 10.9. Clarity on the usefulness of ANA, anti-ENA and anti-DFS70 antibody testing was illustrated by a supervised cluster analysis (Figure 4).

Discussion

Diagnosis of Patients with Positive ANA/anti-ENA antibodies

One of the time honored adjuncts to diagnosis of AARD or the broader spectrum of systemic autoimmune rheumatic diseases is autoantibody testing. In most of these conditions, autoantibodies are included as part of validated disease classification criteria [19–22]. Accordingly, on the backdrop of a wide range of protean clinical signs and symptoms, autoantibody tests, and the ANA test in particular, are often used as a screening tool for AARD by referring physicians [3,5,23–25]. The referral of patients with positive ANA and/or ENA to tertiary care specialists is a common practice that has met with some criticism [3,5,23,26,27], with one claim being that because pre-test probabilities of AARD is low, such referrals are unnecessary and a burden on the health care system resulting increased wait times for rheumatology consultations. This can be complicated when the referring physician has told the patient that they do or do not have an AARD. Such misdiagnoses (over-diagnosis or under-diagnosis) can have emotional and insurability consequences for the patient and a serious negative impact on health care resources, including inappropriate or delays in appropriate therapy culminating in poor clinical outcomes, such as irreversible organ damage or failure [5,28–30]. These issues also have ethical implications [31] and algorithms for how cost-effective and rational autoantibody testing could be harmonized and developed into a standardized schema is gaining international attention [23,24,32,32–37].

In 1989 Shiel and Jason [38] reported that patients referred to a community rheumatologist because of a positive ANA with a titer of 1/40 or greater (comprising 8.8% of all referrals compared to 4.1% in our study) received a specific diagnosis in 86.6% and of those, 51.4% had a connective tissue disease [38]. An interesting study by Narain et al [5] reported that of 263 patients referred with a presumptive diagnosis of SLE, 48% received a diagnosis of other conditions and 29% were seropositive for ANA but did not have autoimmune disease. Disconcertingly, 39 patients who were seropositive for ANA but had no autoimmune disease had been treated with corticosteroids at dosages as high as 60 mg/d. By comparison, a more recent study by Abeles and Ables [27] found that none of the patients referred to a specialist clinic with an ANA titer of <1/160 had an AARD, and like previous studies [39], the majority had soft tissue rheumatism and other pain syndromes. In our study, where the screening ANA test was performed at a serum dilution of 1/160, approximately 27% of patients referred because of a positive ANA/ant-ENA antibody test had an AARD, approximately 10% had equivocal evidence for AARD, and the remainder had a wide variety of rheumatic (i.e. rheumatoid arthritis) and non-rheumatic conditions. In another study of 50 ANA positive patients that did not fulfill sufficient criteria for classification of SLE, anti-Ro60/SS-A and anti- La/SS-B antibodies were the most common detectable anti-ENA antibodies (6%) using a limited diagnostic profile and while none of the patients with leukopenia, thrombocytopenia, fatigue and arthralgia did not evolve to a full diagnosis of SLE, the authors concluded that ANA positivity connoted a form of systemic autoimmunity [40]. By comparison, patients with arthritis, rash, Raynaud's phenomenon and anti- Ro60/SS-A autoantibodies did evolve to SLE. These observations are interesting in the context of our study since we have initiated a longitudinal study to determine which ACR patients with a positive ANA or anti-ENA antibody test that did not meet criteria for an AARD evolve into an AARD such as SLE.

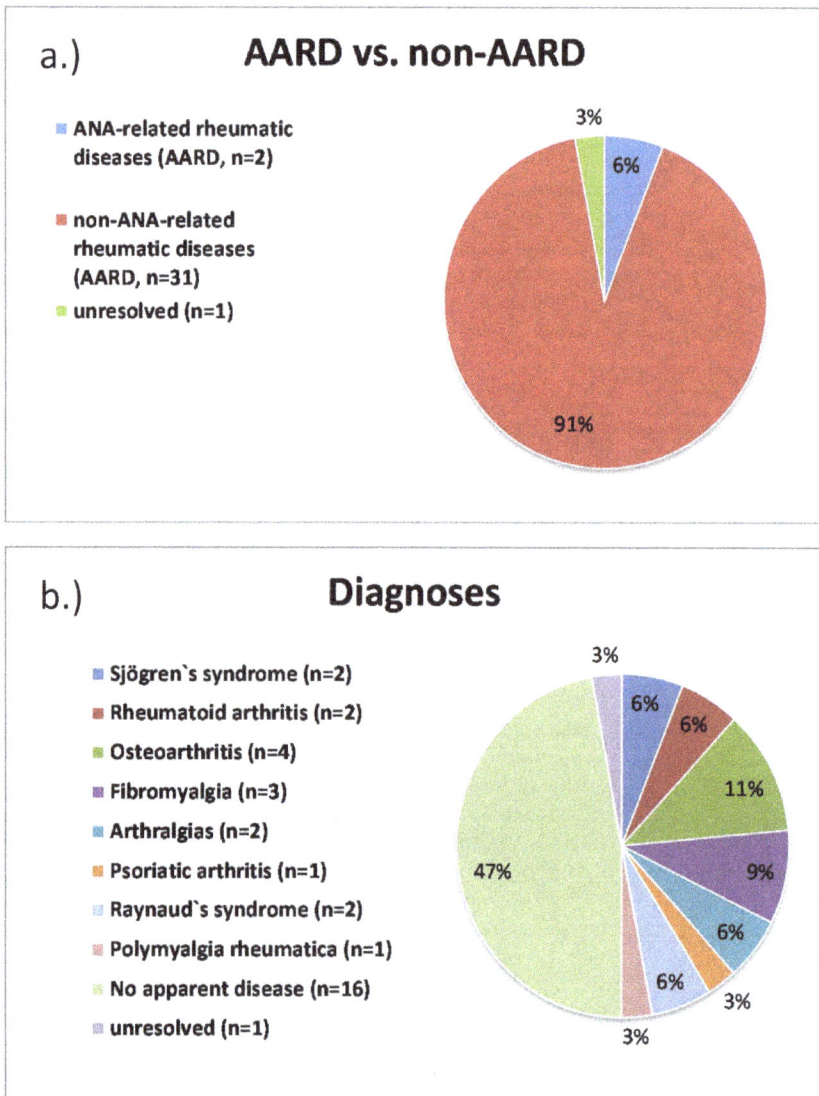

Figure 2. Clinical diagnoses of 34 patients with anti-DFS70 antibodies. Panel a.) frequency (%) of ANA-associated rheumatic diseases (AARD) and non-AARD. One patient with undifferentiated connective tissue disease did not match AARD or non-AARD and was classified as "unresolved". Panel b.) frequency of diagnoses of the patients with anti-DFS70 antibodies is shown.

The serum dilution at which screening ANA tests are performed lacks uniformity from laboratory to laboratory. A study by an international advisory committee comprised of representatives from fifteen participating laboratories concluded that the ANA screening dilution should be set at 1/160 to increase the specificity of the ANA test [7]. Nevertheless, as exemplified by the report of Abeles and Abeles [27] and others [38], many laboratories continue to test sera at lower screening dilutions. Based on our study it appears that even if the screening serum dilution is set at 1/160, more than one-half of patients do not have sufficient clinical evidence or classification criteria to make a diagnosis of an AARD at the time of evaluation by the consulting rheumatologist.

There is hope that a more thorough understanding of ANA and anti-ENA antibody specificities can help address some of the inherent shortcomings of ANA and anti-ENA antibody specificity and sensitivity. For example, mounting evidence indicates that the presence of anti-DFS70 antibodies is a useful biomarker found in ANA positive individuals the vast majority of whom did not have an AARD [14–17]. In the present study, approximately 15% of

the ARC had antibodies directed to DFS70 and in the majority (73.5%) it was the only detectable autoantibody. Of these anti-DFS70 positive patients, only 2/33 (6.1%) had an AARD while approximately one-third had either no evidence for a disease or a variety of other non-AARD diagnoses such as osteoarthritis and fibromyalgia. In summation, our findings support previous studies indicating that anti-DFS70 antibodies tend to exclude the diagnosis of AARD [16,17,41] and the observation that the majority are "monospecific" for anti-DFS70 antibodies add further evidence to the potential value of routinely testing for these autoantibodies.

Use of Autoantibody Profiles to inform Patient Triage and Referral Systems

This is the first published study to evaluate the clinical diagnoses and serological parameters of patients referred to rheumatologists through a central triage system because of a positive ANA test. Access to rheumatologists is often inadequate to meet patient

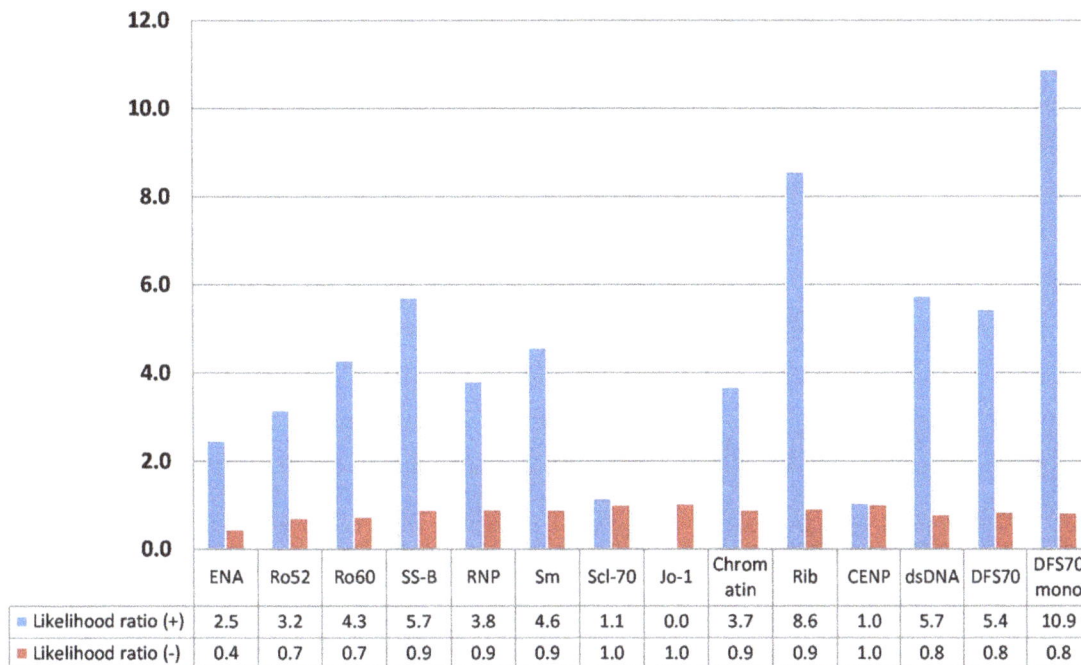

	ENA	Ro52	Ro60	SS-B	RNP	Sm	Scl-70	Jo-1	Chrom atin	Rib	CENP	dsDNA	DFS70	DFS70 mono
Likelihood ratio (+)	2.5	3.2	4.3	5.7	3.8	4.6	1.1	0.0	3.7	8.6	1.0	5.7	5.4	10.9
Likelihood ratio (-)	0.4	0.7	0.7	0.9	0.9	0.9	1.0	1.0	0.9	0.9	1.0	0.8	0.8	0.8

Figure 3. Likelihood ratios differentiate AARD from non-AARD in ANA positive patients (n = 208, 55 excluded due to missing results; dsDNA based on 76 samples). NOTE: Anti-DFS70 positivity was indicative for non-AARD. 'DFS70 mono' represents patients that have anti-DFS70, but no other detectable autoantibody.

needs due to population growth, aging of the population, and a declining supply of specialists [42]. In our study, the average waiting time from referral to when the patient was seen by the consulting rheumatologist was 165 days (> five months). Although it is intuitive, there is evidence that an early and accurate diagnosis of patients with rheumatic diseases improves health outcomes while reducing health care costs [35,43–48]. In our study, the vast majority (~80%) of referrals for a positive ANA was from general practitioners (GPs) and at least one study has shown that the threshold used by GPs for referral to rheumatologists is low leading to lengthy wait times [49]. It was suggested that more frequent use of telephone consultations and improved diagnostic skills of GPs may alleviate the wait times. Another suggested approach was to use registered nurses and GPs themselves to do the triage [50], an approach that had a degree of diagnostic accuracy rivaling that of experienced rheumatologists. The limitation to this approach is

that it seems an assumption that GPs are available for such activity because they are not as busy as rheumatologists. Using appropriately trained registered nurses and/or other allied health care personnel is the approach that we have taken to screen and adjudicate referrals as a "team" approach as recommended by others [51].

A key component to improving timely, efficient and appropriate access to specialist consultation and care is the ability of the triage team to assign a level of urgency to the referral. An effective and efficient triage system requires the formulation of a working diagnosis based on the information included in the referral letter [52]. This may be particularly difficult in rheumatology, as there are few diagnostic tests that can firmly establish a diagnosis. The diagnosis of AARD relies on a complete history, physical examination and investigations [34], and depends on the expertise of the care provider. In the context of rheumatology referrals

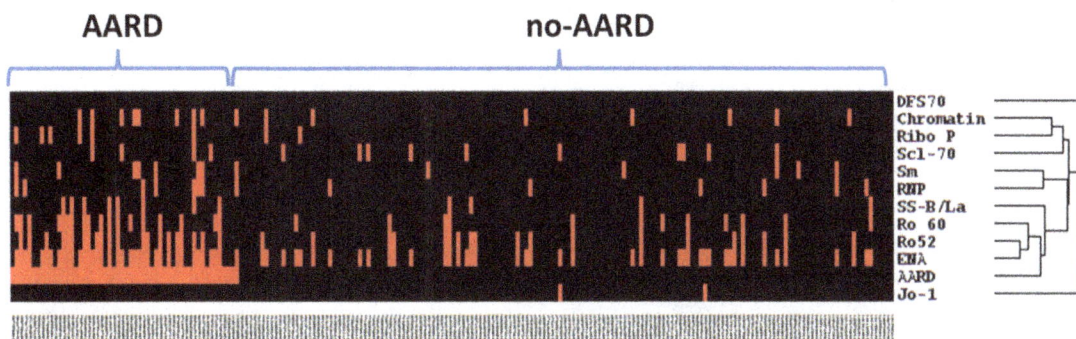

Figure 4. Supervised cluster analysis with patients sorted according to the presence or absence of ANA associated rheumatic disease (AARD) was performed with antibodies to extractable nuclear antigens (ENA), chromatin, ribosomal P and to DFS70. ENA, Ro52/TRIM21, SS-A/Ro60 and SS-B/La cluster most closely with AARD whereas DFS70 antibodies and Jo-1 demonstrate high distance clustering.

because of a positive ANA, our data suggest that patients with isolated anti-DFS70 autoantibodies do not require urgent referral to a specialist, whereas patients with anti-ENA antibodies and other AARD-specific autoantibodies, where early and accurate diagnosis is a goal, require rapid assessment for an AARD.

Limitations

This study was a cross-sectional study without patient follow-up to determine the longer term outcome of patients. The utility of ANA testing in a triage or referral setting or in diagnostic algorithms is complicated by a number of factors, most notably that autoantibodies often precede symptoms and overt evidence of disease by as much as two decades [53,54]. While this phenomenon is well established in medical literature, many physicians have yet to embrace the concept in their clinical evaluation of patients. To help understand the use of autoantibodies as predictors of diseases, the ARC in this study is being followed for long term clinical outcomes.

In addition, this study did not assess the economic impacts of the referral system. The cost effectiveness of autoantibody testing and its effective application to the clinical setting is clearly required [35], and if there were more effective ways to triage patients that will never develop an AARD, cost savings could be significant. To date, rather than a holistic cost-benefit analysis, cost analyses have tended to focus on the cost of the ANA test itself and related algorithms [3,23,36,37]. Of note, it has already been suggested that the detection of anti-DFS70 autoantibodies may result in meaningful cost savings [14,55] by the potential of reducing the additional testing in search of establishing the diagnosis of a systemic autoimmune rheumatic disease and in some cases the initiation of inappropriate therapy [5].

Future Considerations and Conclusions

With the emergence of novel biomarkers for AARD, it is thought that disease prevention and morbidity amelioration by establishing an early and accurate diagnosis will likely not rely on a single or any one class of biomarkers (i.e. autoantibody, genetic, metabolomic). Rather than a single autoantibody marker (i.e. anti-Scl-70/topo I, anti-dsDNA, anti-DFS70) it is likely that multiplexed autoantibody profiles will provide more important clinical information in the future. Our study suggests that the fine specificities of ANA and other autoantibodies are important to decide whether or not an urgent referral is needed. For example, based on other corroborating studies [15–17], our present study indicates that if the patient has isolated anti-DFS70 antibodies, then urgent referral is likely not required. However, if patients have certain anti-ENA, such as anti-dsDNA or anti-ribosomal P, then more urgent assessment is indicated.

Supporting Information

File S1 File contains Table S1 and Table S2. Table S1: Consultant Diagnosis of anti-ENA Antibody Positive Individuals. Table S2: Indirect Immunofluorescence Patterns of Sera from Patients in the Referral Cohort.

Acknowledgments

The authors acknowledge the technical support of Ms. Haiyan Hou, Jane Yang, Meifeng Zhang and the clinical input of the members of the Division of Rheumatology at the University of Calgary. The HEp-2 slides were a kind gift from ImmunoConcepts Inc. (Sacramento, CA) and the anti-DFS70 assay kits were a gift of INOVA Diagnostics (San Diego, CA).

Author Contributions

Conceived and designed the experiments: SB LM MJF. Performed the experiments: CR WS TL JW MJF. Analyzed the data: CR WS TL SB LM MM DM JW MJF. Contributed reagents/materials/analysis tools: MM MJF. Wrote the paper: CR WS MM MJF.

References

1. Mahler M, Fritzler MJ (2010) Epitope specificity and significance in systemic autoimmune diseases. Ann N Y Acad Sci 1183: 267–287.
2. Juby A, Johnston C, Davis P (1991) Specificity, sensitivity and diagnostic predictive value of selected laboratory generated autoantibody profiles in patients with connective tissue diseases. J Rheumatol 18: 354–358.
3. Man A, Shojania K, Phoon C, Pal J, de Badyn MH, et al. (2013) An evaluation of autoimmune antibody testing patterns in a Canadian health region and an evaluation of a laboratory algorithm aimed at reducing unnecessary testing. Clin Rheumatol 32: 601–608.
4. Esdaile JM, Joseph L, Abrahamowicz M, Li Y, Danoff D, et al. (1996) Routine immunologic tests in systemic lupus erythematosus: Is there a need for more studies? J Rheumatol 23: 1891–1896.
5. Narain S, Richards HB, Satoh M, Sarmiento M, Davidson R, et al. (2004) Diagnostic accuracy for lupus and other systemic autoimmune diseases in the community setting. Arch Intern Med 164: 2435–2441.
6. Yazdany J, Schmajuk G, Robbins M, Daikh D, Beall A, et al. (2013) Choosing wisely: the American College of Rheumatology's Top 5 list of things physicians and patients should question. Arthritis Care Res (Hoboken) 65: 329–339.
7. Tan EM, Feltkamp TEW, Smolen JS, Butcher B, Dawkins R, et al. (1997) Range of antinuclear antibodies in "healthy" individuals. Arthritis Rheum 40: 1601–1611.
8. Suarez-Almazor ME, Gonzalez-Lopez L, Gamez-Nava JI, Belseck E, Kendall CJ, et al. (1998) Utilization and predictive value of laboratory tests in patients referred to rheumatologists by primary care physicians. J Rheumatol 25: 1980–1985.
9. von Muhlen CA, Tan EM (1995) Autoantibodies in the diagnosis of systemic rheumatic disease. Semin Arthritis Rheum 24: 323–358.
10. Wiik AS (2005) Anti-nuclear autoantibodies: clinical utility for diagnosis, prognosis, monitoring, and planning of treatment strategy in systemic immunoinflammatory diseases. Scand J Rheumatol 34: 260–268.
11. Arbuckle MR, McClain MT, Rubertone MV, Scofield RH, Dennis GJ, et al. (2003) Development of autoantibodies before the clinical onset of systemic lupus erythematosus. N Engl J Med 349: 1526–1533.
12. Heinlen LD, McClain MT, Merrill J, Akbarali YW, Edgerton CC, et al. (2007) Clinical criteria for systemic lupus erythematosus precede diagnosis, and associated autoantibodies are present before clinical symptoms. Arthritis Rheum 56: 2344–2351.
13. Conrad K, Schlösser W, Fritzler MJ (2007) The predictive relevance of autoantibodies. In: Conrad K, Chan EKL, Fritzler MJ, Sack U, Shoenfeld Y, et al. editors. From Etiopathogenesis to the Prediction of Autoimmune Diseases: Relevance of Autoantibodies. Langerich, Germany: Pabst Scientific Publishers. pp. 16–31.
14. Muro Y, Sugiura K, Morita Y, Tomita Y (2008) High concomitance of disease marker autoantibodies in anti-DFS70/LEDGF autoantibody-positive patients with autoimmune rheumatic disease. Lupus 17: 171–176.
15. Mahler M, Hanly JG, Fritzler MJ (2012) Importance of the dense fine speckled pattern on HEp-2 cells and anti-DFS70 antibodies for the diagnosis of systemic autoimmune diseases. Autoimmun Rev 11: 642–645.
16. Mahler M, Parker T, Peebles CL, Andrade LE, Swart A, et al. (2012) Anti-DFS70/LEDGF Antibodies Are More Prevalent in Healthy Individuals Compared to Patients with Systemic Autoimmune Rheumatic Diseases. J Rheumatol 39: 2104–2110.
17. Miyara M, Albesa R, Charuel JL, El Amri M, Fritzler MJ, et al. (2013) Clinical phenotypes of patients with anti-DFS70/LEDGF antibodies in a routine ANA referral cohort. Clin Dev Immunol 2013: 703759.
18. Stinton LM, Barr SG, Tibbles LA, Yilmaz S, Sar A, et al. (2007) Autoantibodies in lupus nephritis patients requiring renal transplantation. Lupus 16: 394–400.
19. Petri M, Orbai AM, Alarcon GS, Gordon C, Merrill JT, et al. (2012) Derivation and validation of systemic lupus international collaborating clinics classification criteria for systemic lupus erythematosus. Arthritis Rheum 64: 2677–2686.
20. Funovits J, Aletaha D, Bykerk V, Combe B, Dougados M, et al. (2010) The 2010 American College of Rheumatology/European League Against Rheumatism classification criteria for rheumatoid arthritis: Methodological Report Phase I. Ann Rheum Dis 69: 1589–1595.
21. Johnson SR, Fransen J, Khanna D, Baron M, van den Hoogen F, et al. (2012) Validation of potential classification criteria for systemic sclerosis. Arthritis Care Res (Hoboken) 64: 358–367.

22. van den Hoogen F, Khanna D, Fransen J, Johnson S, Baron M, et al. (2013) Classification Criteria for Systemic Sclerosis: An ACR-EULAR Collaborative Initiative. Arthritis & Rheumatism 65: 2737–2747.

23. Tampoia M, Fontana A, Di Serio F, Maggiolini P, Pansini N (2003) Application of a diagnostic algorithm in autoantibody testing: assessment of clinical effectiveness and economic efficiency. Clin Chim Acta 333: 181–183.

24. Stinton LM, Fritzler MJ (2007) A clinical approach to autoantibody testing in systemic autoimmune rheumatic disorders. Autoimmun Rev 7: 77–84.

25. Lyons R, Narain S, Nichols C, Satoh M, Reeves WH (2005) Effective use of autoantibody tests in the diagnosis of systemic autoimmune disease. Ann N Y Acad Sci 1050: 217–228.

26. Fritzler MJ (2011) The antinuclear antibody (ANA) test: Last or lasting gasp? Arthritis Rheum 16: 19–22.

27. Abeles AM, Abeles M (2013) The clinical utility of a positive antinuclear antibody test result. Am J Med 126: 342–348.

28. Wiik AS, Gordon TP, Kavanaugh AF, Lahita RG, Reeves W, et al. (2004) Cutting edge diagnostics in rheumatology: on the role of patients, clinicians, and laboratory scientists in optimizing the use of autoimmune serology. Arthritis Care Res 51: 291–298.

29. Lateef A, Petri M (2012) Unmet medical needs in systemic lupus erythematosus. Arthritis Res Ther 14 Suppl: S4.

30. Bellando-Randone S, Guiducci S, Matucci-Cerinic M (2012) Very early diagnosis of systemic sclerosis. Pol Arch Med Wewn 122 Suppl 1:18–23: 18–23.

31. Bossuyt X, Louche C, Wiik A (2008) Standardisation in clinical laboratory medicine: an ethical reflection. Ann Rheum Dis 67: 1061–1063.

32. Kavanaugh AF, Solomon DH (2002) Guidelines for immunologic laboratory testing in the rheumatic diseases: Anti-DNA antibody tests. Arthritis Rheum 47: 546–555.

33. Solomon DH, Kavanaugh AJ, Schur PH (2002) Evidence-based guidelines for the use of immunologic tests: antinuclear antibody testing. Arthritis Rheum 47: 434–444.

34. Shojania K (2001) Rheumatology: 2. What laboratory tests are needed? Can Med Assoc J 162: 1157–1163.

35. Shoenfeld Y, Cervera R, Haass M, Kallenberg C, Khamashta M, et al. (2007) EASI - The European Autoimmunity Standardisation Initiative: a new initiative that can contribute to agreed diagnostic models of diagnosing autoimmune disorders throughout Europe. Ann N Y Acad Sci 1109: 138–144.

36. Bonaguri C, Melegari A, Dall'Aglio P, Ballabio A, Terenziani P, et al. (2009) An italian multicenter study for application of a diagnostic algorithm in autoantibody testing. Ann N Y Acad Sci 1173: 124–129.

37. Bonaguri C, Melegari A, Ballabio A, Parmeggiani M, Russo A, et al. (2011) Italian multicentre study for application of a diagnostic algorithm in autoantibody testing for autoimmune rheumatic disease: conclusive results. Autoimmun Rev 11: 1–5.

38. Shiel WC, Jason M (1989) The diagnostic associations of patients with antinuclear antibodies referred to a community rheumatologist. J Rheumatol 16: 782–785.

39. Gamez-Nava JI, Gonzalez-Lopez L, Davis P, Suarez-Almazor ME (1998) Referral and diagnosis of common rheumatic diseases by primary care physicians. Br J Rheumatol 37: 1215–1219.

40. Vlachoyiannopoulos PG, Tzavara V, Dafni U, Spanos E, Moutsopoulos HM (1998) Clinical features and evolution of antinuclear antibody positive individuals in a rheumatology outpatient clinic. J Rheumatol 25: 886–891.

41. Mariz HA, Sato EI, Barbosa SH, Rodrigues SH, Dellavance A, et al. (2011) ANA HEp-2 pattern is a critical parameter for discriminating ANA-positive healthy individuals and patietns with autoimmune rheumatic diseases. Arthritis Rheum 63: 191–200.

42. Qian J, Ehrmann FD, Bissonauth A, Menard HA, Panopalis P, et al. (2010) A retrospective review of rheumatology referral wait times within a health centre in Quebec, Canada. Rheumatol Int 30: 705–707.

43. Wiles NJ, Lunt M, Barrett EM, Bukhari M, Silman AJ, et al. (2001) Reduced disability at five years with early treatment of inflammatory polyarthritis: results from a large observational cohort, using propensity models to adjust for disease severity. Arthritis Rheum 44: 1033–1042.

44. Lard LR, Visser H, Speyer I, vander Horst-Bruinsma IE, Zwinderman AH, et al. (2001) Early versus delayed treatment in patients with recent-onset rheumatoid arthritis: comparison of two cohorts who received different treatment strategies. Am J Med 111: 446–451.

45. Emery P, Breedveld FC, Dougados M, Kalden JR, Schiff MH, et al. (2002) Early referral recommendation for newly diagnosed rheumatoid arthritis: evidence based development of a clinical guide. Ann Rheum Dis 61: 290–297.

46. Trouw LA, Mahler M (2012) Closing the serological gap: promising novel biomarkers for the early diagnosis of rheumatoid arthritis. Autoimmun Rev 12: 318–322.

47. Meacock R, Dale N, Harrison MJ (2013) The humanistic and economic burden of systemic lupus erythematosus: a systematic review. Pharmacoeconomics 31: 49–61.

48. Yang P, Kruh JN, Foster CS (2012) Antiphospholipid antibody syndrome. Curr Opin Ophthalmol 23: 528–532.

49. Lyons PA, Rayner TF, Trivedi S, Holle JU, Watts RA, et al. (2012) Genetically distinct subsets within ANCA-Associated Vasculitis. N Engl J Med 367: 214–223.

50. Gormley GJ, Steele WK, Gilliland A, Leggett P, Wright GD, et al. (2003) Can diagnostic triage by general practitioners or rheumatology nurses improve the positive predictive value of referrals to early arthritis clinics? Rheumatology (Oxford) 42: 763–768.

51. Wiik AS, Bizzaro N (2012) Missing links in high quality diagnostics of inflammatory systemicrheumatic diseases. It is all about the patient! Autoimmunity Highlights 3: 35–49.

52. Gran JT, Nordvag BY (2000) Referrals from general practice to an outpatient rheumatology clinic: disease spectrum and analysis of referral letters. Clin Rheumatol 19: 450–454.

53. Fritzler MJ (2011) Autoantibody Testing: Current Challenges and Future Opportunities. In: Conrad K, Chan EKL, Fritzler MJ, Humbel RL, Meroni PL, et al. editors. From Prediction to Prevention of Autoimmune Diseases. Berlin: Pabst Science Publishers.pp. 584–596.

54. Fritzler MJ (2012) Toward a new autoantibody diagnostic orthodoxy: understanding the bad, good and indifferent. Autoimmunity Highlights 3: 51–58.

55. Watanabe A, Kodera M, Sugiura K, Usuda T, Tan EA, et al. (2004) Anti-DFS70 antibodies in 597 healthy hospital workers. Arthritis Rheum 50: 892–900.

TRIpartite Motif 21 (TRIM21) Differentially Regulates the Stability of Interferon Regulatory Factor 5 (IRF5) Isoforms

Elisa Lazzari[1], Justyna Korczeniewska[2], Joan Ní Gabhann[1], Siobhán Smith[1], Betsy J. Barnes[2], Caroline A. Jefferies[1]*

1 Molecular and Cellular Therapeutics, Research Institute, Royal College of Surgeons in Ireland, Dublin, Ireland, 2 Department of Biochemistry and Molecular Biology, Rutgers Biomedical and Health Sciences, Newark, New Jersey, United States of America, Rutgers Biomedical and Health Sciences, New Jersey Medical School- Cancer Center, Newark, New Jersey, United States of America

Abstract

IRF5 is a member of the Interferon Regulatory Factor (IRF) family of transcription factors activated downstream of the Toll-Like receptors (TLRs). Polymorphisms in *IRF5* have been shown to be associated with the autoimmune disease Systemic Lupus Erythematosus (SLE) and other autoimmune conditions, suggesting a central role for IRF5 in the regulation of the immune response. Four different IRF5 isoforms originate due to alternative splicing and to the presence or absence of a 30 nucleotide insertion in *IRF5* exon 6. Since the polymorphic region disturbs a PEST domain, a region associated with protein degradation, we hypothesized that the isoforms bearing the insertion might have increased stability, thus explaining the association of individual IRF5 isoforms with SLE. As the E3 ubiquitin ligase TRIpartite Motif 21 (TRIM21) has been shown to regulate the stability and hence activity of members of the IRF family, we investigated whether IRF5 is subjected to regulation by TRIM21 and whether dysregulation of this mechanism could explain the association of IRF5 with SLE. Our results show that IRF5 is degraded following TLR7 activation and that TRIM21 is involved in this process. Comparison of the individual IRF5 variants demonstrates that isoforms generated by alternative splicing are resistant to TRIM21-mediated degradation following TLR7 stimulation, thus providing a functional link between isoforms expression and stability/activity which contributes to explain the association of IRF5 with SLE.

Editor: Luwen Zhang, University of Nebraska-Lincoln, United States of America

Funding: This work was supported by Health Research Board grant number HRB/RP/2008/234 (www.hrb.ie), the Arthritis Foundation (www.arthritis.org), and the Alliance for Lupus Research (www.lupusresearch.org). The funders had no role in study design, data collection and analysis, decision to publish, or preparation of the manuscript.

Competing Interests: The authors have declared that no competing interests exist.

* Email: cjefferies@rcsi.ie

Introduction

Systemic lupus erythematosus (SLE) is a chronic autoimmune disease characterised by a complex interplay between innate and adaptive immune systems. Nucleic acid sensing receptors such as TLR7 and TLR9, which recognise RNA and DNA, respectively, have been shown to contribute to autoantibody and type I interferon (IFN) production in SLE [1–4]. In this context the transcription factor IRF5, which promotes pro-inflammatory cytokines and type I IFN production in response to both TLR7 and -9 activation, has been genetically and functionally associated with SLE [5–7].

Polymorphisms in the *IRF5* gene define haplotypes that can have a protective or exacerbating (risk) effect on lupus susceptibility, with the risk haplotype being characterized by the presence of Single Nucleotide Polymorphisms (SNPs) in the promoter region and 3′ untranslated region (UTR) which result in enhanced levels of IRF5 mRNA. In addition, different isoforms of the IRF5 protein are expressed due to the presence or absence of a 30 nucleotide insertion in exon 6, which has also been included in the risk haplotype. Furthermore, *IRF5* exon 6 contains an alternative splice site 48 nucleotides downstream of the 5′ end, and different

combinations of insertion/deletion and alternative/conventional splicing lead to the expression of four IRF5 isoforms (IRF5-V1, -V2, -V3 and -V5) presenting different deletion patterns in their central region. Since *IRF5* exon 6 encodes for part of a PEST domain normally present in proteins characterised by rapid turnover, one hypothesis is that the presence or absence of the insertion and the mechanism of splicing may influence the stability of the different IRF5 isoforms [8–11]. Indeed, enhanced levels of IRF5 mRNA and proteins were observed in Peripheral Blood Mononuclear Cells (PBMCs) from SLE patients and importantly, the increased levels of IRF5 correlates with elevated levels of circulating IFNα, thus highlighting the link between *IRF5* genotype and dysregulation of IRF5 function and consequentially of type I IFN expression [9,10,12–15].

The E3 ubiquitin ligase TRIM21 plays an important role in regulating the stability and hence activity of the IRF family of transcription factors. TRIM21 is in fact able to interact with IRF3, IRF7 and IRF8 upon TLR stimulation, resulting in TRIM21-mediated ubiquitination, subsequent degradation and hence termination of signaling [16–18]. Although the role of TRIM21 as a negative regulator of IRF-mediated responses is well established, recent studies demonstrate that in resting cells and in the early phase of the immune response TRIM21 may act to enhance IRF3 and IRF8 transcriptional activity, while other factors may cooperate with TRIM21 for IRF degradation in the late phase of signaling [17,19,20]. Regardless of the specific molecular mechanisms involved, the importance of TRIM21 as a regulator if IFN responses is nonetheless demonstrated by the severe "lupus-like" disease developed by *Trim21* knock out mice, characterized by enhanced production of pro-inflammatory cytokines such as type I interferons, IL-12 and IL-23, all of which are known to be regulated by IRF family members [16,18,20–22].

In this context, investigating the interplay between IRF5 and TRIM21 and the stability of individual IRF5 isoforms is of particular relevance for understanding the *IRF5* risk haplotype and the contribution of IRF5 to the disease. Given that exon 6 encodes for a Proline-, Glutamic acid-, Serine-, Threonine-rich (PEST) domain potentially important for IRF5 stability, we hypothesized that the various IRF5 isoforms generated from insertion/deletion and/or alternative splicing may have altered stability, potentially as a result of altered ability to interact with TRIM21, and hence downstream effects on IRF5-mediated gene transcription. We demonstrated that IRF5 can directly interact with TRIM21 and interestingly the interaction is inducible upon TLR7 stimulation, thus suggesting that TRIM21 may target IRF5 in this pathway. Contrary to our initial hypothesis, mapping of IRF5 domains involved in the interaction revealed that the IRF5 polymorphic region is dispensable for the association between IRF5 and TRIM21, and in fact we demonstrate that all of the IRF5 isoforms investigated in this study interact with TRIM21 to a similar extent. In determining the functional consequences of this interaction we observed that IRF5 isoforms originating from alternative splicing (IRF5-V2 and IRF5-V3) are resistant to TRIM21-mediated degradation whereas IRF5-V1 and IRF5-V5 are targeted for TRIM21-mediated degradation in TLR7-stimulated cells. The inability of TRIM21 to degrade IRF5-V2 and IRF5-V3 results in abrogation of TRIM21-mediated inhibition of IRF5-driven reporter activity, and corresponds with previously reported enhanced expression and activity in SLE [23]. Altogether, these results demonstrate that dysregulation of the IRF5-TRIM21 regulatory loop or expression of more stable isoforms in SLE patients could represent a novel mechanism of pathogenesis in SLE and possibly other autoimmune diseases.

Materials and Methods

Cell culture

Human embryonic kidney (HEK)-293T (ECACC, United Kingdom) and HEK-TLR7 (InvivoGen) cells were cultured in Dulbecco's Modified Essential Medium (DMEM) supplemented with 10% (v/v) heat inactivated fetal calf serum (FCS), 100 units/ml Penicillin and 100 µg/ml Streptomycin. Blasticidin (Invivo-Gen) was added to a final concentration of 10 µg/ml for culture of HEK-TLR7. THP-1 cells (ECACC, United Kingdom) were cultured in RPMI-1640 supplemented with 10% (v/v) fetal calf serum and 100 units/ml Penicillin and 100 µg/ml Streptomycin. All cells were maintained at 37°C in 5% CO_2. Primary human peripheral blood mononuclear cells (PBMCs) were isolated from whole blood from healthy donors, under ethical approval from Royal College of Surgeons in Ireland research ethics committee REC269, using a Ficoll gradient and cultured in RPMI-1640 media supplemented with 10% (v/v) heat inactivated fetal calf serum and 100 units/ml Penicillin and 100 µg/ml Streptomycin. Informed consent from all participants involved in this study was obtained in a written manner. Participants involved in this study

were only recruited from, and experimentation conducted at, Royal College of Surgeons in Ireland.

Plasmids and reagents

Plasmids encoding Myc-tagged IRF5 isoforms were a kind gift of Dr. Frank Neipel (Virologisches Institut - Klinische und Molekulare Virologie, Erlangen, Germany). Plasmids encoding Xpress-TRIM21 and GST-TRIM21 PRY/SPRY domain were a gift from Dr. David Rhodes (Cambridge Institute for Medical Research, Cambridge, UK). HA-ubiquitin wild type and mutants were a gift from Dr. James Burrows (Centre for Cancer Research and Cell Biology, Belfast, UK). Plasmids encoding FLAG-tagged IRF5 full length and deletion mutants were described previously [24]. Myc-MyD88 construct was a kind gift from Dr. Alberto Mantovani (Istituto Clinico Humanitas, Milan, Italy). pGL3-IFNA4 luciferase and pGL4-TK-Renilla were a kind gift from Dr. John Hiscott (Lady Davis Institute, Montreal, Canada) and Dr. Kate Fitzgerald (UMASS, Massachusetts, USA), respectively. Plasmids encoding shRNA targeting TRIM21 and scrambled negative control were described previously [16]. TLR ligands were purchased from InvivoGen (California, USA). Primary antibodies used were anti-FLAG (Sigma), anti-c-Myc and anti-β-Actin (Abcam), anti-GST (GE Healthcare), anti-Xpress (Invitrogen), anti-IRF5 (Cell Signaling) and anti-α-actinin, anti-HA and anti-TRIM21 (Santa Cruz).

Immunoprecipitation and western blot analysis

Immunoblots were performed as previously described [16]. For immunoprecipitations, cells were transfected as indicated and lysed in RIPA buffer (PBS containing 0.5% (w/v) sodium deoxycholate, 0.1% (w/v) SDS and 1% (v/v) Nonidet P40) supplemented with protease inhibitors (PMSF 1 mM, Na_3VO_4 1 mM, KF 1 mM, Pepstatin A 1 µg/ml and Leupeptin HCl 1 µg/ml). Cleared cell lysates were incubated with HA-agarose (Sigma) or with 1 µg of anti-Xpress antibody followed by incubation with protein G sepharose (GE Healthcare). For recombinant pull-downs, cells were lysed in Tris-HCl lysis buffer (50 mM Tris-HCl pH 7.4, 1% (v/v) Nonidet P40, 0.25% (w/v) sodium deoxycholate, 150 mM NaCl, 1 mM EDTA) supplemented with protease inhibitors and incubated with 1 µg of Glutathione S-Transferase (GST) or GST-PRY/SPRY TRIM21 bound to glutathione agarose (Qiagen). Isolated proteins were separated by 10% SDS-PAGE.

Real-time polymerase chain reaction (PCR)

RNA was extracted from cell cultures using TRIzol reagent (Sigma) and reverse transcribed to complementary DNA using Tetro cDNA synthesis kit (Bioline) according to the manufacturer's recommendations. Real-time quantitative PCR was performed with SYBR Green Taq ReadyMix (Sigma), using the following primer pairs for human IL-6: sense 5′-AGTTCCTGCA-GAAAAAGGCA-3′ and antisense 5′-AAAGCTGCGCAGAAT-GAGAT-3′ and human 18sRNA: sense 5′-GGGAGGTAGT-GACGAAAAAT-3′ and antisense 5′-ACCAACAAAATAGAACCGCG-3′. Data were analyzed using an ABI Prism 7900 system (Applied Biosystems) and were normalized to a GAPDH reference. Real-time PCR data were analyzed using the $2^{-\Delta\Delta Ct}$ method [25].

Pulse-chase experiments to determine IRF5 stability

HEK-TLR7 cells transfected with individual isoforms were pre-treated for 30 minutes with cycloheximide (100 µg/ml, Sigma) followed by stimulation with CL097 (5 µg/ml). Samples were

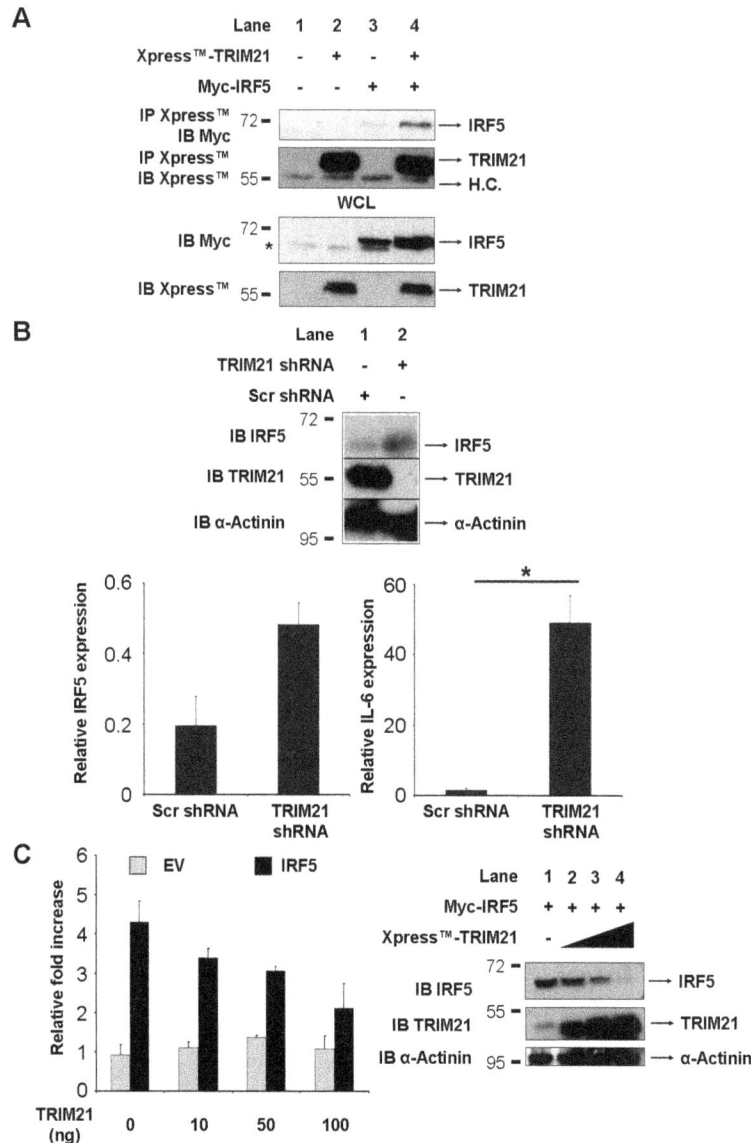

Figure 1. TRIM21 interacts with IRF5 and regulates its stability and activity. A, Myc-IRF5 and Xpress-TRIM21 were overexpressed in HEK-293T cells. 24 hours post-transfection cells were lysed, Xpress-TRIM21 was immunoprecipitated from cell lysates and association of TRIM21 with IRF5 was assessed by anti-Myc immunoblot. WCL, whole cell lysate; H.C., Heavy Chain; *indicates non-specific signal. B, HEK-293T cells were transfected with 2 μg of plasmids encoding shRNA targeting TRIM21 or scrambled shRNA as a negative control. 48 hours after transfection cells were lysed and levels of IRF5, TRIM21 and α-actinin were determined by western blot. Bottom graphs show densitometric analysis of relative IRF5 levels (left) and expression of IL-6 as determined by RT-PCR of RNA extracted from the same samples (right). C, HEK293T were transfected with plasmids encoding the luciferase reporter gene under the control of the IFNA4 promoter and Myc-tagged IRF5 in presence of increasing amounts of Xpress-TRIM21. The TK-Renilla plasmid was used as internal control. Luciferase activity was measured 48 hours after transfection and normalized to renilla activity. Results are shown as fold activation over Empty Vector control. Expression of IRF5, TRIM21 and α-actinin was determined by western blot with anti-Myc, anti-Xpress and anti-α-actinin, respectively. *$p<0.05$ as determined by Student's t-test.

harvested after 4 and 8 hours of treatment and proteins resolved by 10% SDS-PAGE. Densitometric analysis was performed using GeneTools software (Syngene) in order to calculate the ratio between IRF5 and α-actinin levels in each sample.

Confocal microscopy

HeLa cells were transfected with 500 ng of GFP-IRF5 and 500 ng of mRFP-TRIM21 for 18–24 hr and were then treated with Imiquimod (20 μg/ml) for 3 hr. Cells were fixed with 4% paraformaldehyde (Sigma) and mounted in DAPI containing

mounting media (Dako). Cells were imaged by confocal microscopy on a Zeiss LSM 510 META (Oberkochen, Germany).

Reporter gene assay

HEK-293T (1×10^4 per well) were seeded in a 96-well plate 24 hours prior to transfection with 50 ng of reporter gene (firefly luciferase controlled by the IFNA4 promoter) and 50 ng IRF5 in presence of increasing amounts (10–100 ng) of Xpress-TRIM21, or 50 ng MyD88 and 100 ng Xpress-TRIM21. Renilla luciferase (5 ng) was used as internal control. All transfections were carried out using Metafectene (Biontex) according to the manufacturer's

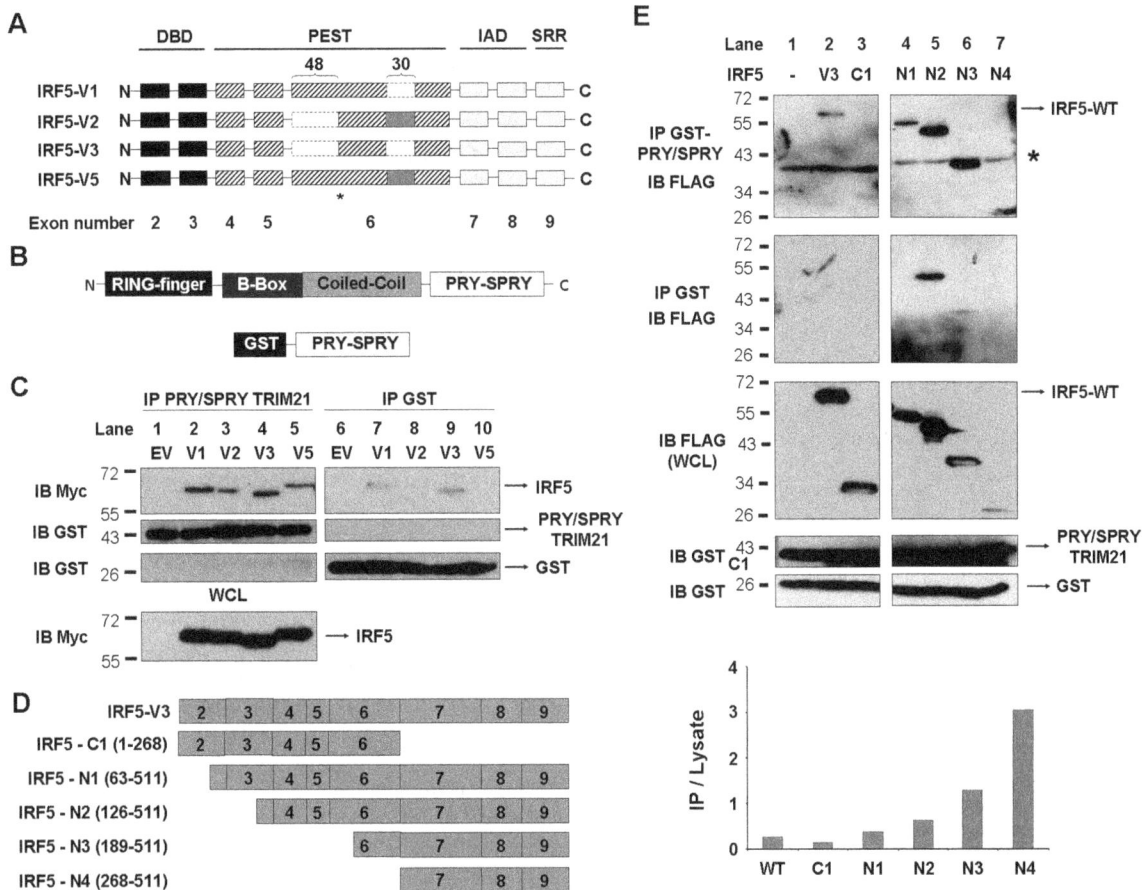

Figure 2. Analysis of interaction domains of IRF5 and TRIM21. A, Exon schematic of IRF5 isoforms structure. DBD, DNA binding domain; PEST, region rich in proline (P), glutamic acid (E), serine (S) and threonine (T) residues; IAD, IRF association domain; SRR, Serine-Rich Region. Dotted lines represent deleted regions. The dark grey box in exon 6 represents the polymorphic 30 nucleotide insertion while *indicates the position of the alternative splicing site 48 nucleotides from exon 6 5′ end. B, Domain structure of TRIM21 (top) and GST-tagged PRY/SPRY domain (bottom). C, Myc-IRF5 isoforms were overexpressed in HEK-293T and lysates were incubated with GST-PRY/SPRY TRIM21 (left panel) or GST alone (right panel) bound to glutathione agarose. Interaction of IRF5 isoforms was assessed by immunoblot (top panels) and total IRF5 expression in the whole cell lysate (WCL) is shown in the bottom panel. D, Schematic diagram of exons encoding full length IRF5-V3 (top) and exons deletions originating C-terminal (C1) or N-terminal (N1–N4) truncated proteins. E, Full length FLAG-IRF5 or deletion mutants were overexpressed in HEK-293T and lysates were incubated with GST-PRY/SPRY TRIM21 (top panel) or GST alone bound to glutathione agarose. Interaction of IRF5 was assessed by anti-FLAG immunoblot and total IRF5 expression in the whole cell lysate (WCL) is shown. Anti-GST immunoblots (bottom panels) show amount of GST-PRY/SPRY TRIM21 or GST incubated with cell lysates. *indicates non-specific signal. Band intensity was calculated and ratio between pulled-down signal and total expression in the whole cell lysate is shown (bottom graph).

instructions. Luciferase activity was analyzed 48 hours post-transfection and standardized to Renilla luciferase activity to normalize for transfection efficiency.

Results

TRIM21 interacts with IRF5 and regulates its stability and activity

Regulation of transcription factor turnover is an important mechanism to control gene expression. The E3 ubiquitin ligase TRIM21 plays a major role in regulating the immune response by controlling stability and activity of various members of the interferon regulatory factor family. Interestingly, the ability of TRIM21 to ubiquitinate IRF5 has previously been demonstrated, but the effects of this post-translational modification on IRF5 stability and activity have yet to be elucidated [18]. We first investigated whether IRF5 and TRIM21 could interact directly *in vivo* by overexpressing plasmids encoding Myc-tagged IRF5

and Xpress-tagged TRIM21 in HEK-293T cells followed by immunoprecipitation of TRIM21 from cell lysates. As figure 1A shows, blotting of immunocomplexes with anti-Myc revealed a direct interaction between the two proteins (figure 1A, upper panel, lane 4).

We next assessed the effect of TRIM21 depletion on IRF5 stability and activity. HEK-293T cells were transfected with shRNA targeting TRIM21 or scrambled shRNA as control for off-target effects. Western blot analysis of IRF5 levels shows a marked increase in IRF5 expression in cells depleted of TRIM21, thus indicating that TRIM21 has a negative effect on IRF5 stability (figure 1B, upper panel, compare lane 2 with lane 1), as confirmed by densitometric analysis (figure 1B, bottom panel, left). Accordingly, the expression of an IRF5-controlled gene, IL-6 [6], was found to be dramatically enhanced in absence of TRIM21, in keeping with the elevated levels of IRF5 observed in these samples (figure 1B, bottom panel, right). To confirm that TRIM21 can negatively regulate IRF5 transcriptional activity, we examined the effect of TRIM21 on the ability of one of the IRF5 isoforms examined in this study, IRF5-V1 (described below), to activate an IFNA4-dependent promoter. As figure 1C shows, the activity of IRF5 is dose-dependently inhibited by TRIM21 (figure 1C, left), and the reduction in activity results from TRIM21-mediated degradation of IRF5 as shown by western blot performed on lysates from the corresponding samples (figure 1C, right).

The IRF association domain of IRF5 interacts with TRIM21 via its PRY/SPRY domain

Having shown that TRIM21 can interact with IRF5 and has an effect on its stability and activity, we next sought to investigate which domains in IRF5 and TRIM21 were important to mediate this interaction. We first assessed the ability of IRF5 variants arising from the combination of insertion/deletion and alternative use of the 5' splice site in exon 6 (shown in figure 2A and hereafter referred to as IRF5-V1, -V2, -V3 and -V5) to interact *in vitro* with recombinant GST-tagged TRIM21 PRY/SPRY domain (figure 2B), previously shown to be necessary for interaction with its identified substrates such as IRF3, IRF8 and DDX41 [16,17,19,26,27]. Lysates from HEK-293T cells overexpressing Myc-tagged IRF5 isoforms were incubated with GST-tagged TRIM21 PRY/SPRY domain or GST alone as a negative control and proteins were resolved by SDS-PAGE. Figure 2C (upper panel, lanes 2–5) shows that all the isoforms interact with TRIM21 PRY/SPRY domain in a similar manner, suggesting that polymorphisms in the region encoded by exon 6 in IRF5 do not affect IRF5-TRIM21 interaction and confirming that the C-terminal PRY/SPRY domain in TRIM21 can mediate the interaction between the two proteins.

In order to determine which domain in IRF5 was necessary for the interaction and to further investigate the possible involvement of IRF5 polymorphic region in mediating the association with TRIM21, we next assessed the interaction properties of TRIM21 with full length IRF5 or various IRF5 deletion mutants (as outlined in figure 2D). Like other IRF family members, IRF5 is composed of a conserved N-terminal DNA binding domain, a central linker region/PEST domain and a C-terminal IRF Association Domain (IAD) known to mediate interaction of IRF5 with transcriptional activators such as CBP/p300 [28]. We therefore incubated lysates from HEK-293T overexpressing full length or truncated variants of IRF5 with recombinant GST-tagged TRIM21 PRY/SPRY domain or GST alone as a negative control. As figure 2E shows, interaction between recombinant TRIM21 PRY/SPRY and an IRF5 mutant lacking the C-terminal IAD (IRF5-C1) was nearly completely abolished as compared to the full length IRF5 protein, thus demonstrating that the IAD domain is critically important for mediating protein-protein interactions in IRF5 (figure 2E, upper panel, lane 3). Indeed, we observed that the IAD domain of IRF5 alone, encoded by exons 7 through 9, could interact with recombinant TRIM21 PRY/SPRY (figure 2E, upper panel, lane 7), thus indicating that the IAD is sufficient to mediate IRF5-TRIM21 interaction. Interestingly we observed that, as compared to IRF5 full length, mutants bearing N-terminal truncations (IRF5-N1-N3) showed enhanced interaction with TRIM21, thus suggesting that IRF5 N-terminal domains may have an inhibitory effect on this interaction (figure 2E, upper panel, lanes 4–6 and corresponding densitometry graph, bottom panel). Taken together, these results indicate that an intact C-terminal IAD domain of IRF5 is required and sufficient to mediate the interaction with the PRY/SPRY domain of TRIM21 (figure 2E, upper panel, lane 7), indicating therefore that the polymorphic region encoded by exon 6 is not directly involved in binding TRIM21. Furthermore, these experiments confirm that the C-terminal PRY/SPRY domain in

TRIM21 can mediate the association with IRF5, in keeping with an increasing body of evidence indicating that the C-terminal region represents the substrate interaction domain in TRIM21 [29].

Different IRF5 isoforms interact with TRIM21 equally upon TLR7 stimulation and act as substrates for TRIM21-mediated ubiquitination

The effect of TRIM21 on IRF stability relies on its E3 ubiquitin ligase activity: by adding poly-ubiquitin chains on specific lysine residue(s) on the IRFs, TRIM21, like other E3 ubiquitin ligases, creates a signal that targets the activated transcription factor for proteasomal- or lysosomal-mediated degradation, thus achieving termination of signaling [16,21,30]. Having shown that all the isoforms interact with TRIM21 uniformly, we next assessed the ability of TRIM21 to ubiquitinate the single IRF5 isoforms. Myc-tagged IRF5 isoforms along with HA-ubiquitin were over-expressed in HEK-293T cells in presence or absence of Xpress-TRIM21. Following isolation of HA-ubiquitin-bound proteins from the cell lysates, the extent of ubiquitination for each isoform was determined by immunoblotting with anti-Myc antibody. As figure 3A shows, all IRF5 isoforms appear to be moderately ubiquitinated when co-transfected with ubiquitin alone (figure 3A, upper panel, lanes 3–6); however, ubiquitination dramatically increases in presence of TRIM21 for all isoforms, confirming that IRF5 is a substrate for TRIM21 ubiquitin-ligase activity (figure 3A, lanes 7–10). In order to investigate the mechanism by which ubiquitination may affect either IRF5 stability or activity, the extent of TRIM21-mediated IRF5 ubiquitination was assessed using ubiquitin mutants lacking lysines at position 48 or 63 and thus unable to form K48- or K63-linked poly-ubiquitin chains (figure S1), respectively, or mutants carrying only lysines at position 48 or 63 (figure S2). In all cases TRIM21 retained the ability to ubiquitinate IRF5 isoforms in presence of the various ubiquitin mutants, albeit with slightly different banding patterns, thus indicating that TRIM21 may target IRF5 with different types of ubiquitin chains and may thus have multiple roles in regulating IRF5 activity.

We next investigated whether the interaction between IRF5 and TRIM21 could be affected by TLR stimulation, previously shown to enhance TRIM21 affinity for its substrates, focusing in particular on the TLR7 pathway known to activate IRF5 and of primary importance in SLE [5,16,21,31,32]. THP-1 cells were stimulated with the TLR7 ligand Imiquimod and cell lysates were incubated with recombinant GST-PRY/SPRY TRIM21. Results shown in figure 3B (upper panels, lane 3) show that in the late phase of TLR7 stimulation the affinity of IRF5 for TRIM21 is slightly increased, suggesting therefore that TRIM21 can target IRF5 in this pathway. In keeping with the ability of Imiquimod to induce an interaction between TRIM21 and IRF5, TLR7 stimulation of PBMCs resulted in a time dependent degradation of IRF5 (figure 3B, lower panels, lanes 5 and 6), confirming that degradation can be induced following TLR-mediated activation.

In order to investigate how TLR7 stimulation would modulate the affinity of individual IRF5 isoforms for TRIM21, we overexpressed plasmids encoding TRIM21 and IRF5 isoforms in HEK-TLR7 cells. Following treatment with the TLR7 ligand CL097, preferred to Imiquimod given the enhanced ability of CL097 to activate IRF5 in this cell line (data not shown), TRIM21 was immunoprecipitated from cell lysates and association with IRF5 isoforms was assessed by anti-Myc immunoblot. As shown in figure 3C, TRIM21 interacted with each of the isoforms to a similar extent in resting cells (figure 3C, upper panel, lanes 1, 3, 5

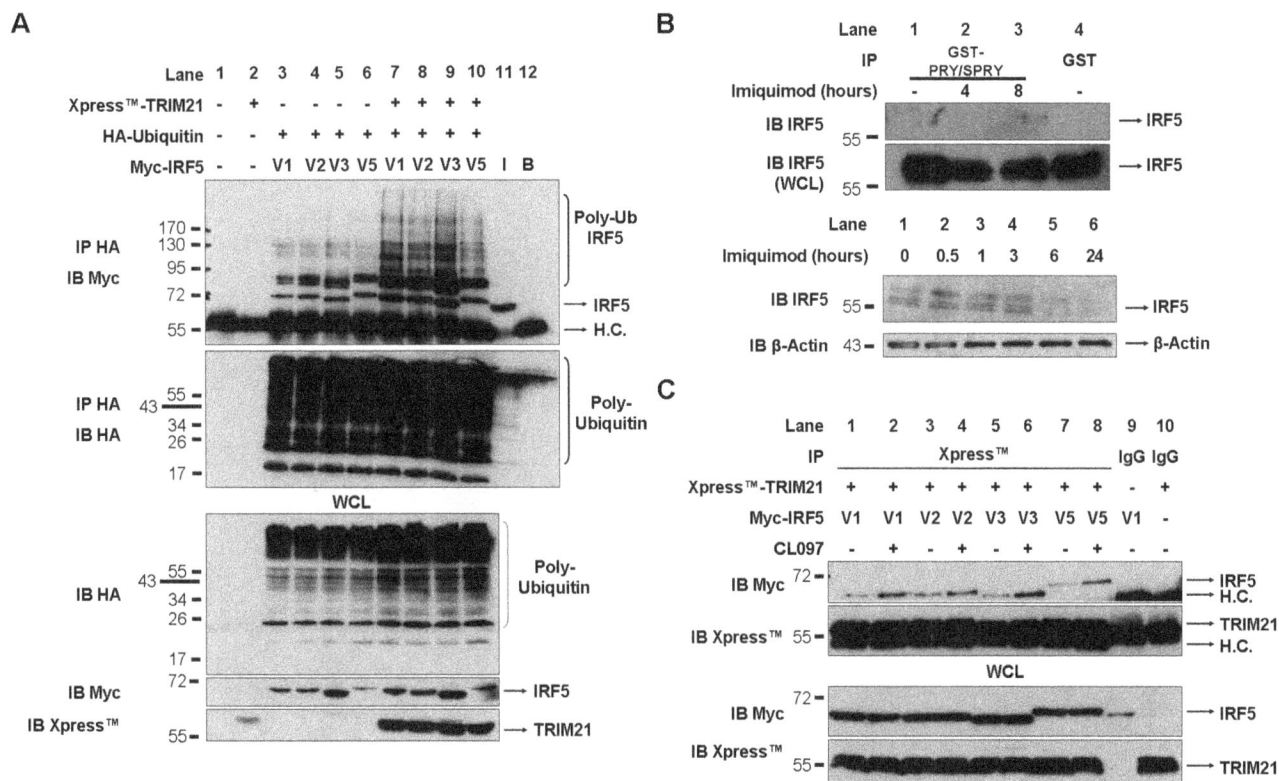

Figure 3. TRIM21 ubiquitinates IRF5 and interacts with IRF5 isoforms upon TLR7 stimulation. A, Myc-tagged IRF5 isoforms and HA-Ubiquitin were overexpressed in HEK-293T in presence or absence of Xpress-TRIM21. Lysates were incubated with HA agarose and the extent of IRF5 ubiquitination was assessed by anti-Myc immunoblot (top panel). Expression of IRF5 and TRIM21 in the Whole Cell Lysate (WCL) is shown in the bottom panels. I (lane 11), Myc-IRF5-V1 Input; B (lane 12), HA-agarose beads alone; H.C., Heavy Chain. B, Top panel: THP-1 were stimulated with Imiquimod (10 µg/ml) for 4 and 8 hours and lysates were incubated with GST-PRY/SPRY TRIM21 (lanes 1–3) or GST alone (lane 4) bound to glutathione agarose. Interaction of IRF5 and total IRF5 expression in the whole cell lysate (WCL) was assessed by immunoblot. Bottom panel: PBMCs were treated with 10 µg/ml Imiquimod for the indicated times. Proteins were resolved by SDS PAGE and immunoblotting performed with anti-IRF5 and anti-β-Actin antibodies. C, Myc-IRF5 isoforms and Xpress-TRIM21 were overexpressed in HEK-TLR7 cells. Following 8 hours treatment with CL097 (5 µg/ml) Xpress-TRIM21 was immunoprecipitated from cell lysates and association of TRIM21 with IRF5 isoforms was assessed by anti-Myc immunoblot. Normal mouse IgG (lanes 9 and 10) was used as negative control. WCL, whole cell lysate; H.C., Heavy Chain.

and 7), with the interaction increasing in each case following TLR7 stimulation (figure 3C, upper panel, lanes 2, 4, 6 and 8).

TRIM21 regulates IRF5 stability and activity in an isoform-specific manner

Having shown that TLR7 stimulation promotes IRF5 degradation and interaction of IRF5 isoforms with TRIM21, we next investigated how TRIM21 affected the stability of the individual isoforms by performing a series of pulse-chase experiments in HEK-TLR7 cells. IRF5 isoforms were over-expressed in HEK-TLR7 cells in presence or absence of TRIM21 and, following treatment with the protein synthesis inhibitor cycloheximide, cells were stimulated with the TLR7 ligand CL097 and relative IRF5 protein levels were assessed by western blot (figure S3) and normalized to α-actinin levels. As figure 4A–D shows, TRIM21 overexpression in HEK-TLR7 cells treated with cycloheximide and CL097 promoted the degradation of IRF5-V1 at the early time point (figure 4A, top panel, left) and IRF5-V5 in the late phase of treatment (figure 4D, top panel, left), whilst no appreciable effect of TRIM21 on the stability of IRF5-V2 and IRF5-V3 was observed (figure 4B and C, top panels, left). Taken together these results therefore indicate that isoforms originating from alternative splicing (IRF5-V2 and IRF5-V3), lacking the first 48 nucleotides encoding the PEST domain, are resistant to

TRIM21-mediated degradation following TLR7 stimulation, whilst the presence or absence of the 30 nucleotide insertion within the PEST domain encoding region has no effect on the stability of IRF5 isoforms. In keeping with the stability data, confocal analysis of GFP-IRF5 and RFP-TRIM21 subcellular localization in HeLa cells treated with Imiquimod reveals that IRF5 isoforms targeted for degradation (V1 and V5) co-localize with TRIM21 in vesicular structures which may represent sites of degradation of poly-ubiquitinated proteins such as autophagosomes/lysosomes (figure 4A and D, bottom panels), whilst no co-localization in such structures can be observed for the stable isoforms V2 and V3 (figure 4B and C, bottom panels).

TRIM21 was previously shown to inhibit IRF7- and IRF3-mediated activation of IFNα and IFNβ promoters [16,21], and we thus next investigated whether the same regulatory mechanism could apply to IRF5 and whether differences could be observed between the different isoforms, given the differential ability of TRIM21 to selectively degrade only IRF5 isoforms originated by conventional splicing (IRF5-V1 and IRF5-V5). We therefore used reporter gene assays to measure IRF5 isoforms activity in presence or absence of TRIM21. HEK-293T cells were transfected with a reporter gene controlled by the IFNA4 promoter together with plasmids encoding IRF5 isoforms and MyD88 to mimic TLR-mediated IRF5 activation (figure 4A–D, upper panels, right). In

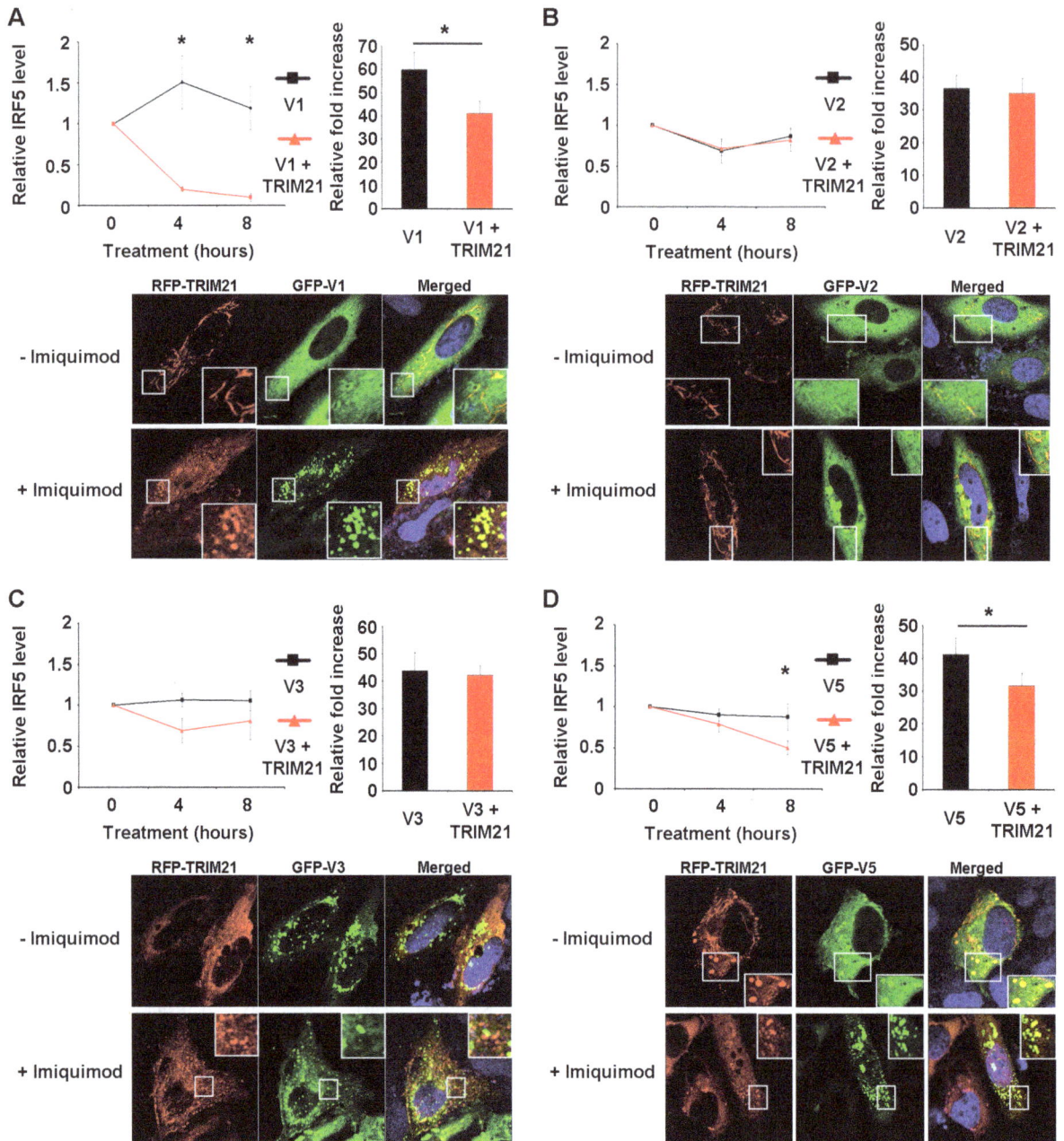

Figure 4. TRIM21 differentially regulates the stability of IRF5 isoforms. A–D, top left, HEK-TLR7 cells were transfected with Myc-tagged IRF5 isoforms (A, V1; B, V2; C, V3; D, V5) in presence or absence of Xpress-TRIM21. The day after transfection cells were treated with cycloheximide (100 μg/ml) in combination with CL097 (5 μg/ml) for the indicated times. Levels of IRF5, TRIM21 and α-Actinin were determined by immunoblot and levels of IRF5 normalized to α-Actinin were calculated and plotted, *$p<0.05$. A–D, top right, HEK293T were transfected with plasmids encoding the luciferase reporter gene under the control of the IFNA4 promoter, Myc-tagged IRF5 isoforms and MyD88 in presence or absence of Xpress-TRIM21. The TK-Renilla plasmid was used as internal control. Luciferase activity was measured 48 hours after transfection and normalized to renilla activity. Results are shown as fold activation over Empty Vector control, *$p<0.05$. A–D, bottom, HeLa cells were transfected with 1 μg of plasmids encoding GFP-tagged IRF5 (green) and mRFP-TRIM21 (red) and left untreated or stimulated with Imiquimod for 3 hours. Cells were fixed mounted in DAPI in order to visualize nuclei (blue) and images were taken under oil immersion at 63× magnification. Images shown are from a single experiment and are representative of three independent experiments.

keeping with the stability data, we observed significant TRIM21-mediated inhibition of IRF5-V1 and IRF5-V5 activity, whilst IRF5-V2 and IRF5-V3 activity was not affected by TRIM21 co-transfection. Taken together our results indicate that TRIM21 interacts with all isoforms of IRF5 thus far studied and that it contributes to TLR7-mediated destabilisation of IRF5 in an isoform-specific manner. Most importantly, the ability of TRIM21

to promote destabilisation of IRF5-V1 and -V5 translates to inhibitory effects on TLR7-mediated activation of the IFNA4 promoter. Thus TRIM21 can affect IRF5-mediated signal transduction and gene expression in an isoform specific manner.

Discussion

Despite an increasing body of evidence suggesting that genetic variants in *IRF5* are linked to enhanced susceptibility to the autoimmune disease SLE, a comprehensive functional characterization of these variants is still missing. As one such polymorphism is a 30 nucleotide insertion in the PEST domain-encoding exon 6 of the *IRF5* gene, we investigated the stability of four IRF5 isoforms bearing different combinations of insertion/deletions in the PEST domain due to the presence or absence of the insertion and/or generated via alternative splicing. By investigating the molecular mechanism of IRF5 degradation following TLR stimulation we have identified IRF5 as a substrate of the E3 ubiquitin ligase TRIM21, previously shown to target other IRFs for degradation post-pathogen recognition [16,20,21]. Interestingly, analysis of the single isoforms revealed that IRF5 variants originating from alternative splicing (V2 and V3) and missing the first 48 nucleotides of the PEST domain-encoding region are resistant to TRIM21-mediated degradation and inhibition, thus suggesting that the enhanced expression of these isoforms in SLE patient monocytes may be as a result of decreased ability of TRIM21 to degrade them [23].

Previous studies have shown that TRIM21 interacts with its substrates via its C-terminal PRY/SPRY domain [16,17,19,26,27]. Whilst all TRIM proteins share a common structure composed of an N-terminal RING domain followed by one or two B-Box domains and a Coiled-Coil region, the C-terminal domain is more variable and considered to be important in mediating substrate specificity [33]. The PRY/SPRY domain in particular has evolved in parallel with adaptive immune mechanisms and is present in many TRIM members involved in regulation of the immune response (TRIM16, -20, -21, -22, -25, -27) or restriction of viral replication (TRIM5α) [34–36]. Several disease-associated mutations of *TRIM* genes have been identified in regions encoding this C-terminal domain, thus highlighting the importance of this protein region for substrate recognition and ultimately TRIM function [29]. As already observed for other IRF family members, our results demonstrate that the interaction between TRIM21 and IRF5 requires the PRY/SPRY domain, thus indicating a common mechanism for TRIM21 to target this family of transcription factors. Importantly, TLR-mediated phosphorylation of tyrosine residues in this domain was shown to be necessary to enhance affinity of TRIM21 for IRF3 [27]. The recombinant PRY/SPRY TRIM21 we used in this study, although an invaluable tool to examine the interaction properties of various overexpressed IRF5 isoforms or deletion mutants, likely does not mimic TLR-activated TRIM21. As such, the weakness of the interaction we observed between recombinant PRY/SPRY TRIM21 and endogenous IRF5 may suggest that TLR-induced post-translational modification of both IRF5 and TRIM21 is necessary to mediate a strong association between the two proteins.

When we analyzed the interaction properties of individual IRF5 isoforms we observed comparable levels of association between TRIM21 and all IRF5 isoforms investigated, suggesting that the IRF5 polymorphic region was not involved in mediating the interaction with TRIM21. Indeed, analysis of the interaction properties of various IRF5 deletion mutants indicated the C-terminal IAD domain (encoded by exons 7 to 9) to be necessary and sufficient to mediate the interaction with TRIM21, thus confirming that polymorphisms in the region encoded by *IRF5* exon 6 do not alter the affinity of IRF5 for TRIM21. Interestingly the interaction was enhanced following TLR7 stimulation for all isoforms suggesting, as mentioned previously, that TLR-mediated

activation of IRF5 triggers post-translational modifications that increase IRF5 affinity for TRIM21. The C-terminal IAD domain in IRF5, which we show to mediate the interaction between IRF5 and TRIM21, has indeed been shown to undergo structural changes following TLR-mediated phosphorylation of conserved serine residues in this region. Phosphorylation-dependent dislocation of an autoinhibitory helix is necessary to expose IRF5 dimerization domain and to allow the formation of homo- and heterodimers which can then associate with other transcriptional co-activators such as CBP/p300 [12,37]. Furthermore, analysis of the crystal structure of the closely related IRF3 and other IRF family members suggests the possibility that, in an inactive state, the N-terminal DNA binding domain of IRFs may be folded upon the C-terminal interaction domain [38–40]. Thus, virus-induced IRF phosphorylation could induce dislocation of C-terminal autoinhibitory structures and repositioning of the N-terminal DNA binding domain, resulting in unmasking of the DNA binding residues and the IAD interaction domain. In keeping with this hypothesis, we observed enhanced interaction with TRIM21 PRY/SPRY domain of IRF5 mutants lacking N-terminal domains (N1–N4) as compared to IRF5 full length, thus indicating an inhibitory effect of IRF5 N-terminal on IRF5-TRIM21 interaction. Interestingly, the phosphorylation-dependent switch from an autoinhibited form to the active one observed for IRF5 is shared by other members of the IRF family, such as IRF3 and IRF7, all of which are targeted by TRIM21 for degradation post-pathogen recognition [37,39,41]. Thus, regulatory mechanisms common to different IRFs suggest that phosphorylation, which allows for dimerization and activation of this family of transcription factors, also represents a signal for degradation, as already shown for IRF3, with TRIM21 emerging as the key E3 ubiquitin ligase targeting the IRF family [42]. It has recently been shown that an intact IAD is necessary to mediate IRF3 and IRF7 degradation by the rotavirus non-structural protein NSP1, suggesting that this conserved common region may be similarly targeted by cellular and viral E3 ligases in order to achieve termination of IRF-mediated signaling [43]. In this context, it is possible therefore that the IAD domain of IRF proteins, conserved in all members from IRF3 to IRF9, may be a common target for TRIM21-mediated degradation of this family of transcription factors.

With respect to a role for TRIM21 in regulating IRF5 stability, we observed enhanced IRF5 expression in cells depleted of TRIM21 by targeted shRNA silencing. Interestingly, expression of one of the genes controlled by IRF5, IL-6, was also enhanced in these samples, thus indicating that TRIM21 can regulate IRF5 turnover and consequently IRF5-mediated gene expression. In keeping with this, we observed that TRIM21 can dose-dependently inhibit IRF5-mediated activation of the IFNA4 promoter as analyzed by reporter gene assay. Collectively, our results therefore indicates that IRF5 is a novel target for TRIM21 and that dysregulation of TRIM21 activity in SLE may thus contribute to enhanced IRF5 levels and consequently to the enhanced levels of type I IFN and pro-inflammatory cytokines, in part regulated by IRF5, observed in SLE patients [44,45]. Analysis of the single IRF5 isoforms examined revealed that, whilst all isoforms interacted with and were ubiquitinated by TRIM21 to a similar degree, their turnover rate presented differences, thus suggesting that ubiquitination may not be the sole determinant of IRF5 isoforms stability. In particular, we observed TRIM21-dependent degradation of IRF5 variants originating by conventional splicing (V1 and V5) following TLR7 stimulation, whilst IRF5 isoforms originating from alternative splicing (V2 and V3) were resistant to TRIM21-mediated degradation. Confocal analysis of IRF5 and TRIM21 subcellular localization in TLR7-

stimulated cells provided a useful insight into the probable mechanism of TRIM21-mediated degradation of IRF5 and potentially explains the differences observed between the various IRF5 isoforms. We observed in fact co-localization of the conventionally spliced and unstable isoforms V1 and V5 with TRIM21 in vesicular cytoplasmic structures resembling autophagosomes/lysosomes, previously shown to mediate degradation of intracellular ubiquitinated proteins [46,47], whilst no co-localization of TRIM21 with the stable isoforms V2 and V3 in such structures was observed. The ubiquitin-binding protein p62 was previously shown to be necessary for formation and degradation of polyubiquitin-containing bodies by autophagy [48], and interestingly, p62 cooperates with TRIM21 in orchestrating IRF8 degradation. Thus, while TRIM21-mediated ubiquitination of IRF8 was shown to initially enhance its activity, p62 binding to ubiquitinated IRF8 in the late phase of the response was shown to be necessary to promote its degradation [17,20]. Our results suggest that a similar mechanism may be in place in regulating IRF5 stability, and the differences observed between the various IRF5 isoforms may therefore reflect differences in their affinity for p62, since we did not observe differences in the affinity of IRF5 isoforms for TRIM21. Further studies in the role of p62 in regulating the stability of IRF5 isoforms will help to precisely define the mechanism of IRF5 degradation.

Regardless of the specific mechanism involved, the finding that alternatively spliced isoforms have increased stability in TLR7-stimulated cells is of particular relevance in the context of SLE, since elevated levels and activity of spliceosome components have been observed in PBMCs from SLE patients indicating therefore that the more stable alternatively spliced IRF5 isoforms (IRF5-V2 and -V3) may be over-represented in SLE patients' immune cells [12]. Indeed, Stone et al recently reported that the stable isoform IRF5-V2 mRNA is significantly overexpressed in monocytes from SLE patients as compared to controls [23]. Furthermore, the same study identified a large number of novel IRF5 variants, many of which, like the stable isoforms V2 and V3 investigated here, are generated by alternative splicing of the 5' region of exon 6 and are therefore likely to escape TRIM21-mediated negative regulation possibly due to alterations in their PEST domain structure. In keeping with the stability data, analysis of the effect of TRIM21 on the ability of IRF5 isoforms to activate the IFNA4 promoter indicated that the activity of IRF5 isoforms V1 and V5, targeted by TRIM21 for degradation in TLR7-activated cells, is inhibited in presence of TRIM21, whilst the stable isoforms V2 and V3 are resistant to TRIM21-mediated degradation and can not be inhibited by TRIM21.

Taken together, our results indicate that interaction of IRF5 with TRIM21 and its subsequent ubiquitination occurs regardless of the isoforms examined here. However, the effects of TRIM21 are indeed isoform specific, with V1 and V5 being destabilised by TRIM21 whilst V2 and V3, which arise from alternative splicing of exon 6 and have therefore altered PEST domain structure, are stable in presence of TRIM21. Our finding that alternative splicing of the IRF5 transcript results in expression of isoforms, like

V2 and V3 examined in this study, able to escape TRIM21-mediated degradation and therefore not inhibited by TRIM21 upon TLR activation, suggests that the presence of SLE-specific, degradation-resistant IRF5 isoforms may mediate the enhanced production of type I IFN and proinflammatory cytokines known to play a critical role in SLE development and pathogenesis.

Supporting Information

Figure S1 TRIM21 ubiquitinates IRF5 isoforms with both K48- and K63-linked polyubiquitin chains. Myc-tagged IRF5 isoforms and HA-Ubiquitin wild type, K48R or K63R mutants were overexpressed in HEK-293T in presence or absence of Xpress-TRIM21. Lysates were incubated with HA agarose and the extent of IRF5 ubiquitination was assessed by anti-Myc immunoblot (top panels). Expression of IRF5 and TRIM21 in the Whole Cell Lysate (WCL) is shown in the bottom panels. A, IRF5-V1 (IRF5 lysates membrane was reblotted with anti-Xpress and *indicates the residual Myc signal detected in the Xpress immunoblot); B, IRF5-V2; C, IRF5-V3; D, IRF5-V5.

Figure S2 TRIM21 ubiquitinates IRF5 isoforms with both K48- and K63-linked polyubiquitin chains. Myc-tagged IRF5 isoforms and HA-Ubiquitin R48K (panel A) or R63K (panel B) mutants were overexpressed in HEK-293T in presence (lanes 7–10) or absence (lanes 3–6) of Xpress-TRIM21. Lysates were incubated with HA agarose and the extent of IRF5 ubiquitination was assessed by anti-Myc immunoblot (top panels). Expression of TRIM21 in the whole cell lysates (WCL) is shown on the bottom panels. *indicates the residual Myc signal detected in the Xpress immunoblot.

Figure S3 TRIM21 differentially regulates the stability of IRF5 isoforms - Western blot analysis. A–D, HEK-TLR7 cells were transfected with Myc-tagged IRF5 isoforms (A, V1; B, V2; C, V3; D, V5) in presence or absence of Xpress-TRIM21. The day after transfection cells were treated with cycloheximide (100 µg/ml) in combination with CL097 (5 µg/ml) for the indicated times. Levels of IRF5, TRIM21 and α-Actinin were determined by immunoblot.

Acknowledgments

We thank F. Neipel, D. Rhodes, J. Burrows, A. Mantovani, J. Hiscott and K. Fitzgerald for reagents.

Author Contributions

Conceived and designed the experiments: EL JK JNG SS BJB CAJ. Performed the experiments: EL JK JNG SS BJB CAJ. Analyzed the data: EL JK JNG SS BJB CAJ. Contributed reagents/materials/analysis tools: EL JK JNG SS BJB CAJ. Contributed to the writing of the manuscript: EL JK JNG SS BJB CAJ.

References

1. Christensen SR, Kashgarian M, Alexopoulou L, Flavell RA, Akira S, et al. (2005) Toll-like receptor 9 controls anti-DNA autoantibody production in murine lupus. The Journal of Experimental Medicine 202: 321–331.
2. Christensen SR, Shupe J, Nickerson K, Kashgarian M, Flavell RA, et al. (2006) Toll-like receptor 7 and TLR9 dictate autoantibody specificity and have opposing inflammatory and regulatory roles in a murine model of lupus. Immunity 25: 417–428.
3. Kono DH, Haraldsson MK, Lawson BR, Pollard KM, Koh YT, et al. (2009) Endosomal TLR signaling is required for anti-nucleic acid and rheumatoid

factor autoantibodies in lupus. Proceedings of the National Academy of Sciences 106: 12061–12066.
4. Lee PY, Kumagai Y, Li Y, Takeuchi O, Yoshida H, et al. (2008) TLR7-dependent and FcγR-independent production of type I interferon in experimental mouse lupus. The Journal of Experimental Medicine 205: 2995–3006.
5. Schoenemeyer A, Barnes BJ, Mancl ME, Latz E, Goutagny N, et al. (2005) The interferon regulatory factor, IRF5, is a central mediator of toll-like receptor 7 signaling. J Biol Chem 280: 17005–17012.

6. Takaoka A, Yanai H, Kondo S, Duncan G, Negishi H, et al. (2005) Integral role of IRF-5 in the gene induction programme activated by Toll-like receptors. Nature 434: 243–249.

7. Hellquist A, Järvinen TM, Koskenmies S, Zucchelli M, Orsmark-Pietras C, et al. (2009) Evidence for Genetic Association and Interaction Between the TYK2 and IRF5 Genes in Systemic Lupus Erythematosus. The Journal of Rheumatology 36: 1631–1638.

8. Rogers S, Wells R, Rechsteiner M (1986) Amino acid sequences common to rapidly degraded proteins: the PEST hypothesis. Science 234: 364–368.

9. Graham RR, Kyogoku C, Sigurdsson S, Vlasova IA, Davies LR, et al. (2007) Three functional variants of IFN regulatory factor 5 (IRF5) define risk and protective haplotypes for human lupus. Proc Natl Acad Sci USA 104: 6758–6763.

10. Kozyrev SV, Lewen S, Reddy PM, Pons-Estel B, Witte T, et al. (2007) Structural insertion/deletion variation in IRF5 is associated with a risk haplotype and defines the precise IRF5 isoforms expressed in systemic lupus erythematosus. Arthritis Rheum 56: 1234–1241.

11. Niewold TB, Kelly JA, Kariuki SN, Franek BS, Kumar AA, et al. (2012) IRF5 haplotypes demonstrate diverse serological associations which predict serum interferon alpha activity and explain the majority of the genetic association with systemic lupus erythematosus. Annals of the Rheumatic Diseases.

12. Feng D, Stone RC, Eloranta M-L, Sangster-Guity N, Nordmark G, et al. (2010) Genetic variants and disease-associated factors contribute to enhanced interferon regulatory factor 5 expression in blood cells of patients with systemic lupus erythematosus. Arthritis & Rheumatism 62: 562–573.

13. Graham RR, Kozyrev SV, Baechler EC, Reddy MV, Plenge RM, et al. (2006) A common haplotype of interferon regulatory factor 5 (IRF5) regulates splicing and expression and is associated with increased risk of systemic lupus erythematosus. Nat Genet 38: 550–555.

14. Sigurdsson S, Goring HH, Kristjansdottir G, Milani L, Nordmark G, et al. (2008) Comprehensive evaluation of the genetic variants of interferon regulatory factor 5 (IRF5) reveals a novel 5 bp length polymorphism as strong risk factor for systemic lupus erythematosus. Hum Mol Genet 17: 872–881.

15. Niewold TB, Kelly JA, Flesch MH, Espinoza LR, Harley JB, et al. (2008) Association of the IRF5 risk haplotype with high serum interferon-alpha activity in systemic lupus erythematosus patients. Arthritis Rheum 58: 2481–2487.

16. Higgs R, Ni Gabhann J, Ben Larbi N, Breen EP, Fitzgerald KA, et al. (2008) The E3 ubiquitin ligase Ro52 negatively regulates IFN-β production post-pathogen recognition by polyubiquitin-mediated degradation of IRF3. J Immunol 181: 1780–1786.

17. Kong HJ, Anderson DE, Lee CH, Jang MK, Tamura T, et al. (2007) Cutting Edge: Autoantigen Ro52 Is an Interferon Inducible E3 Ligase That Ubiquitinates IRF-8 and Enhances Cytokine Expression in Macrophages. The Journal of Immunology 179: 26–30.

18. Espinosa A, Dardalhon V, Brauner S, Ambrosi A, Higgs R, et al. (2009) Loss of the lupus autoantigen Ro52/Trim21 induces tissue inflammation and systemic autoimmunity by disregulating the IL-23-Th17 pathway. J Exp Med 206: 1661–1671.

19. Yang K, Shi HX, Liu XY, Shan YF, Wei B, et al. (2009) TRIM21 is essential to sustain IFN regulatory factor 3 activation during antiviral response. J Immunol 182: 3782–3792.

20. Kim JY, Ozato K (2009) The sequestosome 1/p62 attenuates cytokine gene expression in activated macrophages by inhibiting IFN regulatory factor 8 and TNF receptor-associated factor 6/NF-κB activity. J Immunol 182: 2131–2140.

21. Higgs R, Lazzari E, Wynne C, Ni Gabhann J, Espinosa A, et al. (2010) Self protection from anti-viral responses–Ro52 promotes degradation of the transcription factor IRF7 downstream of the viral Toll-Like receptors. PLoS One 5: e11776.

22. Smith S, Gabhann JN, Higgs R, Stacey K, Wahren-Herlenius M, et al. (2012) Enhanced interferon regulatory factor 3 binding to the interleukin-23p19 promoter correlates with enhanced interleukin-23 expression in systemic lupus erythematosus. Arthritis & Rheumatism 64: 1601–1609.

23. Stone RC, Du P, Feng D, Dhawan K, Rönnblom L, et al. (2013) RNA-Seq for Enrichment and Analysis of IRF5 Transcript Expression in SLE. PLoS One 8: e54487.

24. Korczeniewska J, Barnes BJ (2012) The COP9 Signalosome Interacts with and Regulates Interferon Regulatory Factor 5 Protein Stability. Molecular and Cellular Biology 33: 1124–1138.

25. Livak KJ, Schmittgen TD (2001) Analysis of Relative Gene Expression Data Using Real-Time Quantitative PCR and the 2−ΔΔCT Method. Methods 25: 402–408.

26. Zhang Z, Bao M, Lu N, Weng L, Yuan B, et al. (2013) The E3 ubiquitin ligase TRIM21 negatively regulates the innate immune response to intracellular double-stranded DNA. Nat Immunol 14: 172–178.

27. Stacey KB, Breen E, Jefferies CA (2012) Tyrosine Phosphorylation of the E3 Ubiquitin Ligase TRIM21 Positively Regulates Interaction with IRF3 and Hence TRIM21 Activity. PLoS One 7: e34041.

28. Feng D, Sangster-Guity N, Stone R, Korczeniewska J, Mancl ME, et al. (2010) Differential Requirement of Histone Acetylase and Deacetylase Activities for IRF5-Mediated Proinflammatory Cytokine Expression. The Journal of Immunology 185: 6003–6012.

29. James LC, Keeble AH, Khan Z, Rhodes DA, Trowsdale J (2007) Structural basis for PRYSPRY-mediated tripartite motif (TRIM) protein function. Proceedings of the National Academy of Sciences 104: 6200–6205.

30. Niida M, Tanaka M, Kamitani T (2010) Downregulation of active IKK-β by Ro52-mediated autophagy. Molecular Immunology 47: 2378–2387.

31. Savarese E, Chae O-w, Trowitzsch S, Weber G, Kastner B, et al. (2006) U1 small nuclear ribonucleoprotein immune complexes induce type I interferon in plasmacytoid dendritic cells through TLR7. Blood 107: 3229–3234.

32. Santiago-Raber M-L, Baudino L, Izui S (2009) Emerging roles of TLR7 and TLR9 in murine SLE. Journal of Autoimmunity 33: 231–238.

33. Meroni G, Diez-Roux G (2005) TRIM/RBCC, a novel class of 'single protein RING finger' E3 ubiquitin ligases. Bioessays 27: 1147–1157.

34. Ozato K, Shin DM, Chang TH, Morse HC 3rd (2008) TRIM family proteins and their emerging roles in innate immunity. Nat Rev Immunol 8: 849–860.

35. Jefferies C, Wynne C, Higgs R (2011) Antiviral TRIMs: friend or foe in autoimmune and autoinflammatory disease? Nat Rev Immunol 11: 617–625.

36. Nisole S, Stoye JP, Saib A (2005) TRIM family proteins: retroviral restriction and antiviral defence. Nat Rev Micro 3: 799–808.

37. Chen W, Lam SS, Srinath H, Jiang Z, Correia JJ, et al. (2008) Insights into interferon regulatory factor activation from the crystal structure of dimeric IRF5. Nat Struct Mol Biol 15: 1213–1220.

38. Lin R, Mamane Y, Hiscott J (1999) Structural and Functional Analysis of Interferon Regulatory Factor 3: Localization of the Transactivation and Autoinhibitory Domains. Molecular and Cellular Biology 19: 2465–2474.

39. Qin BY, Liu C, Lam SS, Srinath H, Delston R, et al. (2003) Crystal structure of IRF-3 reveals mechanism of autoinhibition and virus-induced phosphoactivation. Nat Struct Biol 10: 913–921.

40. Brass AL, Kehrli E, Eisenbeis CF, Storb U, Singh H (1996) Pip, a lymphoid-restricted IRF, contains a regulatory domain that is important for autoinhibition and ternary complex formation with the Ets factor PU.1. Genes & Development 10: 2335–2347.

41. Marié I, Smith E, Prakash A, Levy DE (2000) Phosphorylation-Induced Dimerization of Interferon Regulatory Factor 7 Unmasks DNA Binding and a Bipartite Transactivation Domain. Molecular and Cellular Biology 20: 8803–8814.

42. Lin R, Heylbroeck C, Pitha PM, Hiscott J (1998) Virus-Dependent Phosphorylation of the IRF-3 Transcription Factor Regulates Nuclear Translocation, Transactivation Potential, and Proteasome-Mediated Degradation. Molecular and Cellular Biology 18: 2986–2996.

43. Arnold MM, Barro M, Patton JT (2013) Rotavirus NSP1-Mediates Degradation of Interferon Regulatory Factors Through Targeting of the Dimerization Domain. Journal of Virology.

44. Gröndal G, Gunnarsson I, Rönnelid J, Rogberg S, Klareskog L, et al. (2000) Cytokine production, serum levels and disease activity in systemic lupus erythematosus. Clinical and experimental rheumatology 18: 565–570.

45. Baechler EC, Batliwalla FM, Karypis G, Gaffney PM, Ortmann WA, et al. (2003) Interferon-inducible gene expression signature in peripheral blood cells of patients with severe lupus. Proc Natl Acad Sci USA 100: 2610–2615.

46. Kim PK, Hailey DW, Mullen RT, Lippincott-Schwartz J (2008) Ubiquitin signals autophagic degradation of cytosolic proteins and peroxisomes. Proceedings of the National Academy of Sciences 105: 20567–20574.

47. Kirkin V, McEwan DG, Novak I, Dikic I (2009) A Role for Ubiquitin in Selective Autophagy. Molecular Cell 34: 259–269.

48. Pankiv S, Clausen TH, Lamark T, Brech A, Bruun J-A, et al. (2007) p62/SQSTM1 Binds Directly to Atg8/LC3 to Facilitate Degradation of Ubiquitinated Protein Aggregates by Autophagy. Journal of Biological Chemistry 282: 24131–24145.

Rapid Resolution Liquid Chromatography Coupled with Quadrupole Time-of-Flight Mass Spectrometry-Based Metabolomics Approach to Study the Effects of Jieduquyuziyin Prescription on Systemic Lupus Erythematosus

Xinghong Ding[1⑨], Jinbo Hu[2⑨], Chengping Wen[3], Zhishan Ding[4], Li Yao[2], Yongsheng Fan[3]*

1 Analysis and Testing Center, Zhejiang Chinese Medical University, Hangzhou, China, 2 College of Pharmaceutical Science, Zhejiang Chinese Medical University, Hangzhou, China, 3 College of Basic Medicine, Zhejiang Chinese Medical University, Hangzhou, China, 4 College of Life Science, Zhejiang Chinese Medical University, Hangzhou, China

Abstract

Jieduquyuziyin prescription (JP), a traditional Chinese medicine (TCM) prescription, has been widely used for the clinical treatment of systemic lupus erythematosus (SLE). However, the complex chemical constituents of JP and the multifactorial pathogenesis of SLE make research on the therapeutic mechanism of JP in SLE challenging. In this paper, a serum metabolomics approach based on rapid resolution liquid chromatography coupled with quadrupole time-of-flight mass spectrometry (RRLC-Q-TOF/MS) was employed to acquire the metabolic characteristics of serum samples obtained from mice in the SLE model group, JP-treated group, prednisone acetate (PA)-treated group and control group. The orthogonal partial least squares (OPLS) was applied to recognize metabolic patterns, and an obvious separation of groups was obtained. Thirteen metabolites, namely, phosphatidylethanolamine (PE 20:3), hepoxilin B3, lyso- phosphatidylethanolamine (lyso-PE 22:6), 12S-hydroxypentaenoic acid (12S-HEPE), traumatic acid, serotonin, platelet-activating factor (PAF), phosphatidylcholine (PC 20:5),eicosapentaenoic acid (EPA), 12(S)-hydroxyei- cosatetraenoic acid (12S-HETE), 14-hydroxy docosahexaenoic acid (14-HDOHE), lyso-phosphatidylcholine (lyso-PC 20:4), and indole acetaldehyde, were identified and characterized as differential metabolites involved in the pathogenesis of SLE. After treatment with JP, the relative content of 12(S)-HETE, PAF, 12(S)-HEPE, EPA, PE (20:3), Lyso-PE(22:6), and 14-HDOHE were effectively regulated, which suggested that the therapeutic effects of JP on SLE may involve regulating disturbances to the metabolism of unsaturated fatty acid, tryptophan and phospholipid. This research also demonstrated that metabolomics is a powerful tool for researching complex disease mechanisms and evaluating the mechanism of action of TCM.

Editor: Shervin Assassi, University of Texas Health Science Center at Houston, United States of America

Funding: This study was supported by grants from the National Natural Science Foundation of China (No. 81001515), the Research Fund for the Doctoral Program of Higher Education of China (No. 20093322120001). The funders had no role in study design, data collection and analysis, decision to publish, or preparation of the manuscript.

Competing Interests: The authors have declared that no competing interests exist.

* E-mail: applezjtcm@126.com

⑨ These authors contributed equally to this work.

Introduction

Systemic lupus erythematosus (SLE), a complex systemic autoimmune disease, is a multifactorial process characterized by multi-system and multi-organ impairment. A commonly accepted viewpoint holds that uncontrolled lymphocyte autoreactivity and dysregulated production of auto-antibodies by B cells lead to formation of immune complexes that can precipitate in the organs and cause tissue damage [1]. The multifactorial process of SLE makes research on its pathogenesis and therapeutic approach challenging [2]. Glucocorticoids and immunosuppressors are effective in the clinical treatment of SLE but are accompanied by serious side effects, such as femoral head necrosis and hypertension [3].

As a refractory disease, SLE involves multiple mechanisms, which suggests that traditional Chinese medicine (TCM), being based on holistic concepts and systems thinking, may have a good therapeutic effect. TCM is a treasure of Chinese civilization and has experienced a history of thousands of years of clinical practice. Jieduquyuziyin prescription (JP), which contains *Radix Paeoniae Rubra*, *Radix Rehmanniae*, *Carapax Trionycis*, *Radix Glycyrrhizae*, et al, is widely used for SLE treatment in China and has a good therapeutic effect on SLE [4]. More importantly, JP has fewer side effects than glucocorticoids and immunosuppressors, even after long-term use [5]. However, the complexity of the chemical constituents of JP makes study of its efficacy challenging.

Metabolomics is considered "the quantitative measurement of the dynamic multi-parametric metabolic response of living systems to pathophysiological stimuli or genetic modification" [6], and is also an important part of systems biology. Metabolomics studies the body from a holistic perspective, which coincides with the theory of TCM [7]. This specialty of metabolomics not only helps to reveal the scientific basis of TCM, but is also beneficial to understanding the pathogenesis and diagnosis of disease, as well as toxicological research [8]. Serum is commonly and effectively used as an object of metabolomic analysis because the serum metabolome is rich, comprising various classes of important biomolecules [9,10]. Mass spectrometry (MS)-based metabolomics is well suited for reliably coping with high-throughput samples with respect to both technical accuracy and the identification and quantitation of low-molecular-weight metabolites which is primary concern of metabolomics [11]. Rapid resolution liquid chromatography coupled with quadrupole time-of-flight mass spectrometry (RRLC-Q-TOF/MS) is widely used for metabolomics studies because of its outstanding dynamic range and high sensitivity, which means that even low-response metabolites can be collected and identified [12]. In addition, MS and MS/MS information on metabolites acquired from RRLC-Q-TOF/MS are helpful for metabolite identification.

Mice treated with a single intraperitoneal injection of the pristane develop a lupus-like disease characterized by the production of autoantibodies directed against many lupus autoantigens [13,14]; and with in-depth understanding of the mechanisms of pristane-induced SLE model, which are associated with IFN-I dysregulation, the mice model has been thought to highly relevant to human SLE [15]. In this paper, a RRLC-Q-TOF/MS-based metabolomics method was established to study the metabolic profiles and differential metabolites associated with SLE by analyzing serum specimens collected from the SLE model group, prednisone acetate (PA)-treated group, JP-treated group, and control group. Furthermore, some active compounds of JP were quantified by a rapid resolution liquid chromatography system coupled with triple quadrupole mass spectrometry (RRLC-QQQ/MS). This study may facilitate understanding of the pathological changes in SLE and the therapeutic mechanism of JP.

Experimental Methods

Chemicals and reagents

An HPLC grade of formic acid and acetonitrile were purchased from Tedia (Fairfield, OH, USA). Prednisone acetate tablets were purchased from Lisheng (Tianjin, China). Water was purified by a Milli-Q water purification system (Millipore, Bedford, MA, USA). Reference and calibration solutions were purchased from Agilent (Agilent, Santa Clara, CA, USA). Standards of catalpol, paeoniflorin, ferulic acid, liquiritin, rutin, hesperidin, quercetin, asiaticoside and glycyrrhizic acid were purchased from the National Institutes for Food and Drug Control, China.

Raw herbal medicines and JP extract

The following raw herbal medicines were purchased from the Chinese Herbal Medicine Co. Ltd. of Zhejiang Chinese Medical University (Hangzhou, China). JP was a combination of dried root of *Radix Rehmanniae, Carapax Trionycis, Herba Artemisiae Annuae, Rhizoma Cimicifugae foetidae, Herba Hedyotidis, Radix Paeoniae Rubra, Herba Centellae Asiaticae, Semen Coicis, Fructus Citri Sarcodactylis* and *Radix Glycyrrhizae* (at ratios of 5:4:4:9:5:4:5:5:3:2). Next, 120 g JP was cut into small pieces and soaked in water (1/10 w/v) for 1 h, then boiled for 2 h. The filtrate was collected and the residue was extracted again with the same volume of water for another 2 h. The filtrates were combined and concentrated under vacuum to make a 1200 mL volume of JP.

Quantitative analysis of active compounds of JP

Some active compounds of JP, including catalpol, paeoniflorin, hesperidin, asiaticoside, glycyrrhetinic acid, quercetin, rutin and ferulic acid were quantified. The standards were precisely weighed and dissolved in methanol to plot the calibration curve of the standards. The extracted 100 mL JP was freeze-dried. Ultrasonic waves were used to help dissolve the residue in 20 mL methanol, and then the solution was filtered through 0.22 μm nylon filters.

JP was analyzed on an Agilent 1290 RRLC coupled to a 6460 QQQ/MS system with an ESI (Electron spray ionization) source (Agilent Technologies, Santa Clara, CA, USA). Samples were separated on an Agilent Eclipse Plus C18 column (2.1×50 mm, 1.8 μm) using 0.1% formic acid in water (A) and 0.1% formic acid in acetonitrile (B). The sample glass vials and column temperature were maintained at 4°C and 35°C, respectively. The gradient elution program was 5% B at 0 to 3 min, 5% to 15% B at 3 to 12 min, maintenance at 15% B for 6 min, 15% to 65% B at 18 to 35 min, 65% to 95% B at 35 to 39 min, and maintenance at 95% B for 2 min. The flow rate was kept constant at 0.3 mL min^{-1}, and the post time was set at 4 min.

The parameters of the ESI source were optimized. The negative ion mode was applied; nebulizer gas was set at 35 psig, capillary voltage at 3,500 V, drying gas (N$_2$) flow rate and temperature at 9 L min^{-1} and 350°C, respectively. The specific optimized MS and MS/MS parameters of the standards are shown in Table 1.

Ethics statement

All procedures were conducted in accordance to Animal Care and Use Committee guidelines of the Zhejiang Chinese Medical University. All methods were approved by the Institutional Animal Care and Use Committee of Zhejiang Chinese Medical University (Permission number: SYXK-ZHE-2008-0115).

Animals and treatments

40 female C57BL/6J mice, 8 weeks old and weighing 22 to 26 g, were purchased from the Experimental Animal Center of Zhejiang Chinese Medical University and were housed in four cages. The mice were housed in a specific-pathogen-free (SPF) environment and had free access to a standard diet and tap water. All animals were kept in an animal room with suitable conditions: temperature at 20 ± 2°C, relative humidity at 55% ± 10%, and 12 h dark-to-light cycle. All animals were allowed to acclimate for 1 week before the experiment. The mice were randomly divided into four groups (n = 10): JP-treated group, PA-treated group, SLE model group, and control group; and JP-treated group, PA-treated group, SLE model group were given a single 0.5 mL intraperitoneal injection of pristane (Sigma-Aldrich, Louis, MO, USA). JP and PA were given orally (daily) to JP-treated group and PA-treated group, respectively, from 1 month after pristane injection and continued till 5 months [16]. PA was dissolved in physiological saline as a concentration of 0.69 mg mL^{-1}, and the dosage was 18 mL kg^{-1} per day. The dosage of JP was also 18 mL kg^{-1} per day, and the SLE model group and control group were administered orally with an equivalent volume of physiological saline.

RRLC-Q-TOF/MS analysis of metabolic profiling

After 10 weeks of treatment, blood samples were collected from the abdominal aorta to centrifuge tubes. Then 30 min later, the samples were centrifuged at 3,000 rpm for 10 min. Serum was transferred into other tubes and stored at −80°C until analysis.

Serum samples were thawed at room temperature, and then 450 μL acetonitrile was added to 150 μL serum and vortex-mixed

Table 1. The MS and MS/MS parameters of the standards and their quantitative results.

Name	No.	Retention time (min)	Fragmentor voltages (V)	Productor ion (m/z)	Collision energy (eV)	Product ion(m/z)	Content (µg/mL)	CV (%) (n = 5)	Accuracy%
Catalpol	1	0.66	120	(M+COOH)-:407.1	7	199.0, 361.0	4.07± 0.12	2.9%	97.4%
Paeoniflorin	2	10.91	120	(M+COOH)-:525.0	8	449.0, 121.0	230.15± 6.54	2.8%	102.4%
Ferulic acid	3	12.87	135	(M-H)-:193.0	12	133.8, 177.7	14.72± 0.45	3.0%	101.5%
Liquiritin	4	13.97	150	(M-H)-:417.1	15	254.9	6.58± 0.12	1.8%	98.2%
Rutin	5	14.96	150	(M-H)-:609.0	32	299.9	13.73± 0.51	3.7%	99.1%
Hesperidin	6	18.72	150	(M-H)-:609.1	20	300.9	10.13± 0.18	1.7%	103.4%
Quercetin	7	24.384	150	(M-H)-:301.0	20	150.9, 120.9	15.86± 0.64	4.0%	98.5%
Asiaticoside	8	25.67	150	(M+COOH)-:1003.4	18	957.3, 469.0	26.12± 1.04	3.9%	104.2%
Glycyrrhizic acid	9	28.98	160	(M-H)-:821.3	46	351.2, 193.1	120.66±3.63	3.0%	97.8%

for 1 min. The mixture was placed at 4°C for 10 min, and then centrifuged at 13,000 rpm for 10 min at 4°C. The supernatant was filtered through 0.22 µm nylon filter film and transferred to an autosampler vial, after which 4 µL of the sample was injected into the column.

Serum samples were analyzed on an Agilent 1260 RRLC coupled to a 6520 Q-TOF/MS system with a dual ESI source (Agilent Technologies, Santa Clara, CA, USA). Serum samples were separated on an Agilent Eclipse Plus C18 column (2.1×50 mm, 1.8 µm). The column temperature was set at 35°C and the flow rate was 0.3 mL min^{-1}. The optimal mobile phase consisted of water with 0.1% formic acid (A) and acetonitrile with 0.1% formic acid (B). From 0 to 2 min, mobile phase B was maintained at 20%, from 2 to 12 min increased linearly from 20% to 65%, then increased to 95% in the next 13 min and kept at 95% for 3 min. The post time was set at 4 min. The sample glass vials were maintained at 4°C. The drying gas (N$_2$) had a flow rate of 9 L min^{-1} and a temperature of 350°C. The positive and negative ionization modes were applied to acquire MS data, and the capillary voltages were at 4,000 V and 3,500 V, respectively. The skimmer voltage was set at 65 V and the fragmentor voltage at 135 V. MS data was acquired in full-scan mode from m/z 50 to 1,000 at the rate of 2 spectra s^{-1}, and the collision energy of MS/MS data acquisition was set at 20 eV. The reference solution was continuously introduced into the MS system during analysis as an internal calibration of the Q-TOF system.

Data analysis

The raw data were analyzed by an Agilent Mass Hunter (version 4.0 Qualitative Analysis, Agilent). The molecular feature extraction (MFE) algorithm was applied to extract metabolic features including m/z, retention time, and ion intensities from the total ion current (TIC) chromatograms. The main parameters of MFE were optimized as follows: the range of m/z values was 50 to 1000, and the thresholds of peak filters and compound filters set at 300 counts and 1000 counts, respectively. The abundance of each compound was defined as the summation of the isotopic peaks, adduct ion peaks and base peak of the compound. The results of MFE were imported into Mass Profiler Professional (MPP) software (version B 12.00, Agilent) for further data filtering, which included alignment, normalization, median-centering, and filtering by frequency. Firstly, the compounds with abundance greater than 3000 were aligned by accurate mass and retention time; the tolerance windows of mass and retention time were 10 ppm and 0.3 min, respectively. Secondly, the abundance of compounds was normalized and media-centered. Thirdly, missing peaks were filtered according to their frequency, and compounds that appeared in more than 80% of samples in at least one group were retained. The final compounds were exported to an Excel table (Microsoft, Redmond, USA). OPLS of SIMCA-P (Umetrics AB, Umea, Sweden) was applied to give a comprehensive view of clustering trends for the multidimensional data [17].

Results and Discussion

Quantitative analysis of active compounds in JP

Base peak chromatogram (BPC) of the standards (Fig. 1A) and JP (Fig. 1B) were acquired. Calibration curves for the standards were plotted as the abundance of product ions versus concentration, and all r^2 values were more than 0.994. The coefficient of variation (CV) and accuracy of the calibration curves, combined with the quantitative results are represented in Table 1.

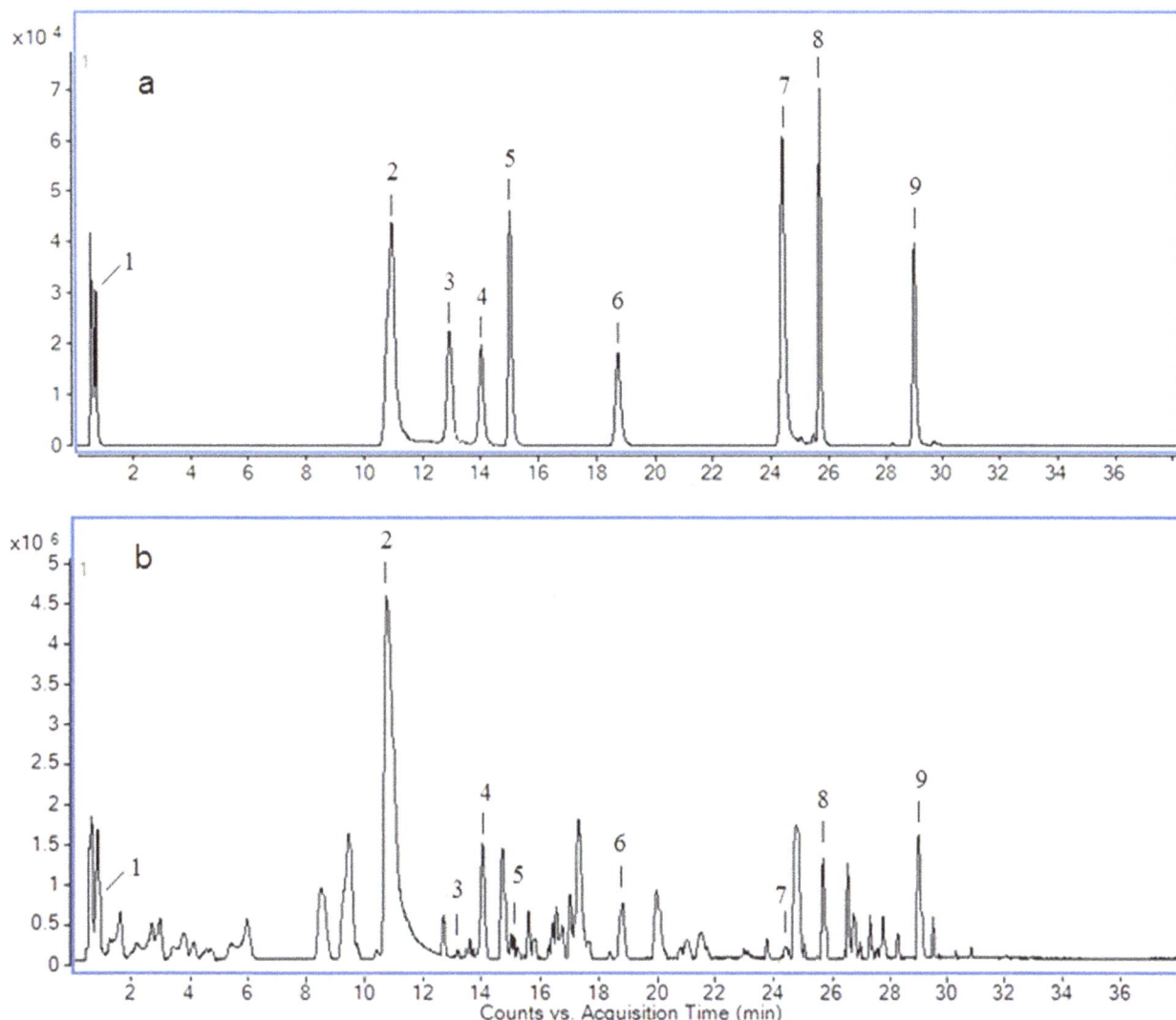

Figure 1. BPC of standards (a) and JP (b).

Method development and validation

The total protein concentration of blood serum is 60 to 80 g L^{-1} [18]; the high protein content of serum necessitates protein removal, for which the most commonly used method is protein precipitation with an organic solvent [19]. The optimal volume ratio of sample to acetonitrile was tested and used for protein precipitation [20]; a ratio of 1:3 was employed, according to our usual practice. For the method validation study, 50 μL of serum the samples from each of the four groups were pooled to get a quality control (QC)specimen, and preparation of the QC specimen was the same as the samples. A number of consecutive injections of the QC sample were made to obtain a stable Q-TOF/MS system before experimental data acquisition, and then acquisition of data for the serum samples was started. QC specimens were analyzed every ten specimens throughout the whole analysis procedure.

For the QC sample, five characteristic ions (252.1336, 308.2324, 184.1462, 445.1456, 514.3085) were picked out to examine the drift of retention times, m/z and peak areas. The results showed that variations in the retention times were less than 0.17 min, drift values of m/z were less than 6 ppm and the relative standard deviation (RSD) of each peak area was below 8%, demonstrating that the system had excellent stability and repeatability during the analysis procedure.

Metabolic profile of SLE

The typical TIC chromatograms of serum were acquired in positive ionization mode (Fig. 2A) and negative ionization mode (Fig. 2B). Alignment, normalization, median-centering, and filtering by frequency of MPP were applied to process the data, and finally 948 compounds of the positive and negative ion modes were obtained. Multivariate statistical analysis can give a comprehensive view of the clustering trend for complex metabolomics data [21]. The OPLS of SIMCA-P was used for multivariate analysis, and the CV-ANOVA (Analysis of variance testing of cross-validated residuals) was performed to validate the OPLS model. The p-value of CV-ANOVA was far lower than 0.01, and those results interpreted that the OPLS model was a significant model. A OPLS score plot base on all 948 compounds using 3 components ($R^2X = 0.536$, $R^2Y = 0.931$ and $Q^2 = 0.917$) showed a obvious separation of the control group and the SLE model group(Fig. 3A). SLE model mice deviated from control

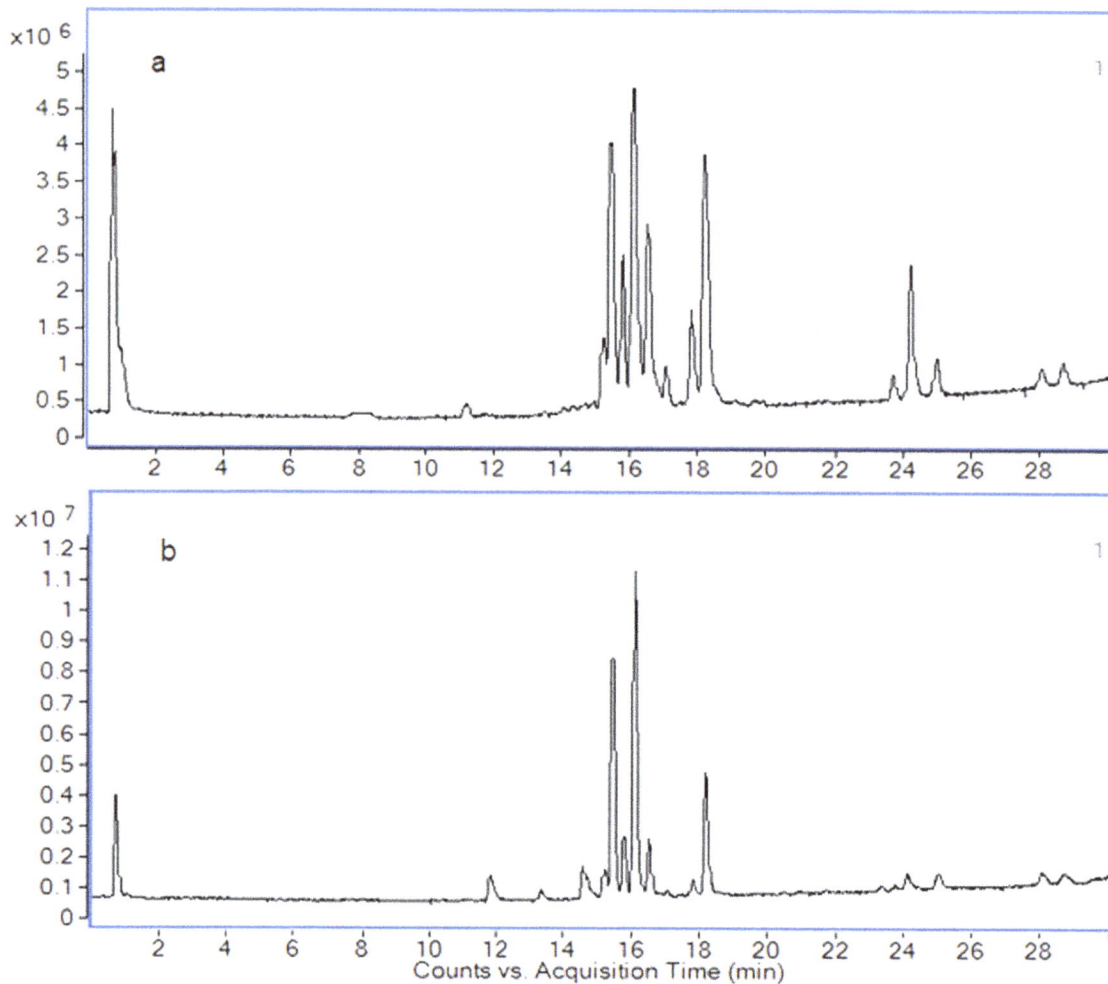

Figure 2. Typical TIC chromatograms for serum obtained in the positive ion mode (a) and negative ion mode (b).

mice in their metabolic profile, indicating that the metabolic networks of SLE mice were disordered. The differential metabolites associated with SLE were found according to the loading plot of OPLS (Fig. 3B) and the p-value of student's t-test.

Differential metabolites were identified according to their MS and MS/MS information. The m/z 343.2275 was taken to illustrate the process of differential metabolite identification. Firstly, according to data analysis results of differential metabolites, the relative content of m/z 343.2275 was significantly different, and was determined as an [M-H]- ion by its MFE and MS information. Secondly, the extracted ion chromatograms (EIC) of m/z 343.2275 of all samples were obtained, and these chromatograms were merged (Fig. 4). The merged EIC visual reflects the relative content change of metabolites among groups and confirms that a suitable statistical method was used for data analysis. Thirdly, the MS/MS information about the fragmentation pattern of m/z 343.2275 was acquired from the Q-TOF system with 20 eV of collision energy. The following main fragment ions were acquired: 59.0141, 107.0868, 161.1324, 121.0645, 133.1018 (Fig. 5). The METLIN database was searched for the MS/MS information [22], and m/z 343.2275 was identified as 14-hydroxy docosahexaenoic acid (14-HDOHE). The identification process of other differential metabolites was similar to that of 14-HDOHE;

the identification results and their trends of change among groups are shown in table 2.

Therapeutic effect of JP on SLE

The results of differential metabolite identification suggest that the development of SLE involves serious disorders of the metabolism of unsaturated fatty acids (UFAs), phospholipid and tryptamine. The dysfunction of the immune system in SLE mice may be caused by metabolic disorders. Disorders of UFA metabolism, especially of arachidonic acid (AA), eicosapentaenoic acid (EPA), and docosahexaenoic acid (DHA), probably aggravate the multi-organ and multi-system inflammatory response, thus promoting the development of SLE. After treatment with JP or PA, the score plot ($R^2X = 0.489$, $R^2Y = 0.894$ and $Q^2 = 0.786$) of OPLS (Fig. 6) showed that there was a significant difference in the metabolic profile of the SLE model group, PA-treated group, JP-treated group and control group. This difference confirmed that JP and PA can play a role in regulating the abnormal metabolic network of SLE mice. PA could effectively regulate the relative content of differential metabolites such as traumatic acid, due to its anti-inflammatory and immunosuppressive function. JP, which exerts a multi-pathway and multi-target role in the body, effectively regulated the metabolic disorders of mice with SLE. The relative content of EPA, 12S-hydroxyeicosatetraenoic acid

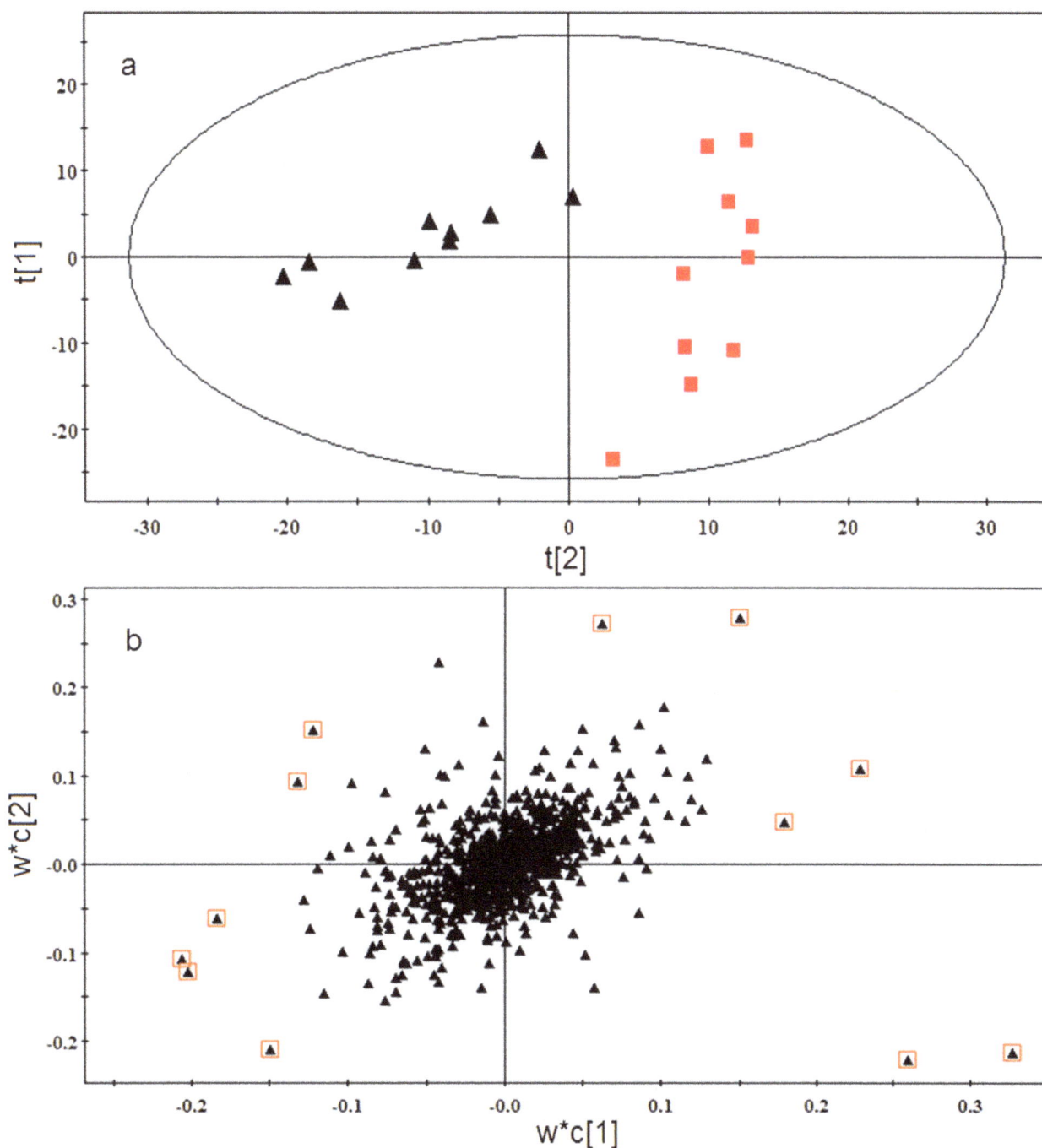

Figure 3. (a) OPLS score plot of the SLE model group (▲) and control group (■). (b) OPLS loading plot of the SLE model group and control group. The 12 metabolites far from the origin that contributed significantly to differentiating the clustering of the SLE model group from the control group were defined as differential metabolites.

(12S-HETE), 14-HDOHE, 12(S)-HEPE, and Platelet-activating factor (PAF) in the JP-treated group were prominently regulated, and the content of these differential metabolites trended to the level of the control group (Table 2). JP effectively repaired the UFA metabolic network, thus alleviating the adverse effects of differential metabolites on immune response and inflammation, ameliorating the dysfunction of the immune system and the multi-organ inflammatory response during the development of SLE, thereby inhibiting the progression of SLE.

Biochemical interpretation of differential metabolites

Fig. 7 shows the perturbed metabolic network associated with SLE. The metabolic pathways of UFAs, tryptophan and phospholipid were involved in the pathogenesis of SLE. UFAs perform an important role in maintaining normal physiological function, including regulation of the immune response. Deficiency of UFA can accentuate or improve the symptoms of certain autoimmune diseases in animals [23]. In this experiment, multiple metabolites of UFA metabolic pathways were involved in the

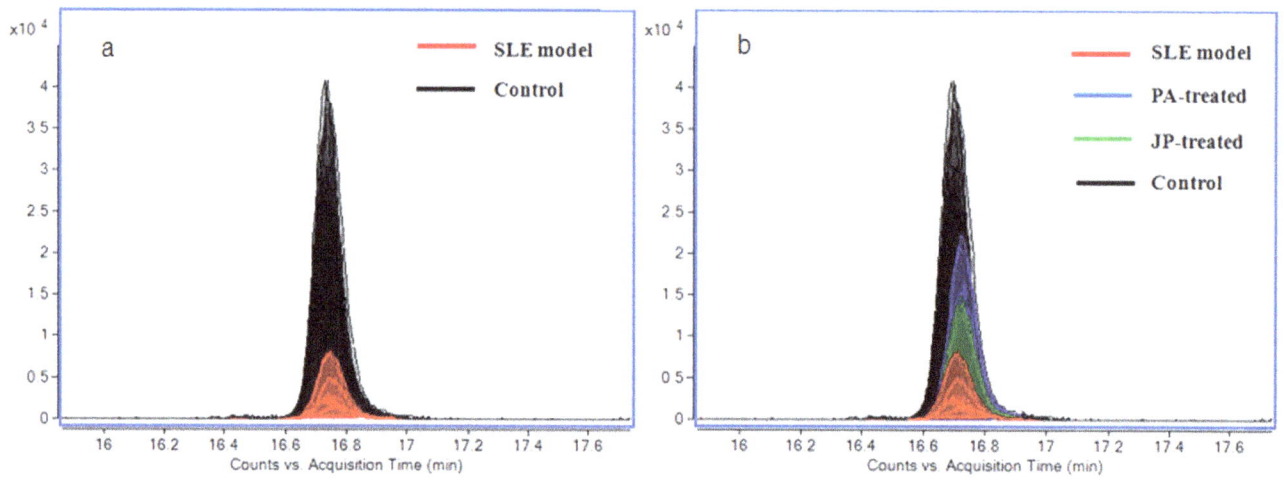

Figure 4. (a) Merged EIC of 14-HDOHE based on the SLE model group and control group. The relative content of 14-HDOHE significantly increased in SLE model mice. (b) Merged EIC of 14-HDOHE based on SLE model group, control group, JP-treated group, and PA-treated group.

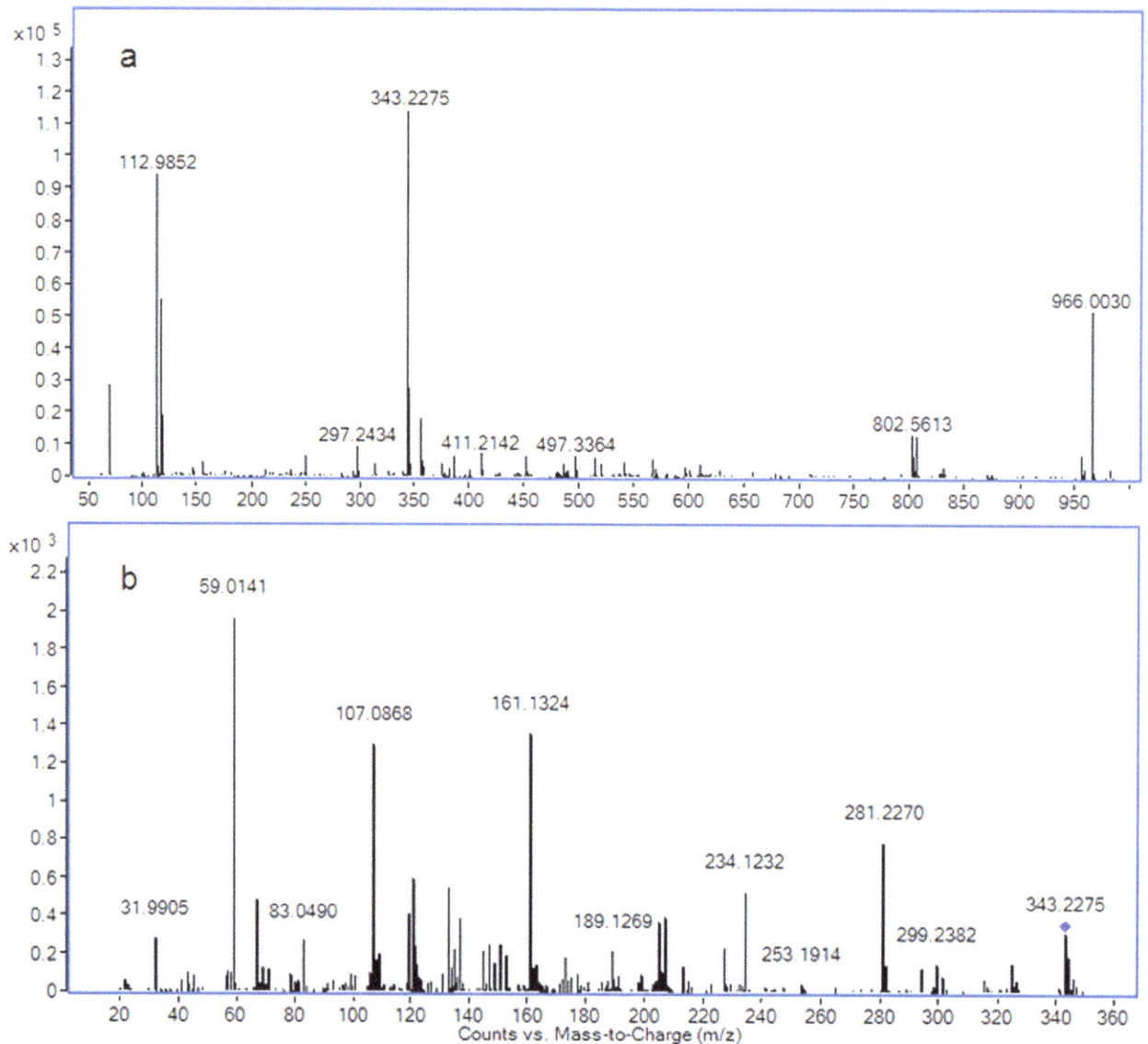

Figure 5. MS (a) and MS/MS (b) information of 14-HDOHE.

Table 2. Identification and trends of change for differential metabolites.

Mass	Retention time (min)	Acquisition Mode	Name	Formula	Metabolic pathway	Trend in SLE model group [a]	Trend in JP-treated group [b]	Trend in PA-treated group [b]
159.0682	0.77	ESI+	Indole acetaldehyde	$C_{10}H_9NO$	Tryptophan metabolism	↓**	←	←
176.0948	0.78	ESI+	Serotonin	$C_{10}H_{12}N_2O$	Tryptophan metabolism	↓**	→	←
228.1361	12.21	ESI+	Traumatic acid	$C_{12}H_{20}O4$	α- Linolenic acid metabolism	↑**	→	↑*
302.2245	16.18	ESI+	EPA	$C_{20}H_{30}O_2$	Fatty acid biosynthesis	↓**	↑**	↑**
523.3637	17.45	ESI+	PAF	$C_{26}H_{54}NO_7P$	Phosphatidic metabolism	↑**	↓*	↑**
543.3331	15.45	ESI+	Lyso-PC(20:4)	$C_{28}H_{50}NO_7P$	Phospholipid metabolism	↓**	—	—
541.3162	14.66	ESI+	PC (20:5)	$C_{28}H_{48}NO_7P$	Phospholipid metabolism	↓**	—	—
503.2992	18.05	ESI+	PE (20:3)	$C_{25}H_{46}NO_7P$	Phospholipid metabolism	↑*	→*	↑*
320.2354	17.85	ESI-	12(S)-HETE	$C_{20}H_{32}O_3$	Arachidonic acid metabolism	↑**	→**	→*
318.2195	16.19	ESI-	12(S)-HEPE	$C_{20}H_{30}O_3$	EPA metabolism	↑**	←**	←*
344.2353	17.53	ESI-	14-HDOHE	$C_{22}H_{32}O_3$	DHA metabolism	↓**	↑*	↑**
336.2304	16.43	ESI-	Hepoxilin B3	$C_{20}H_{32}O_4$	Arachidonic acid metabolism	↓**	←	←
525.2857	15.38	ESI-	Lyso-PE(22:6)	$C_{27}H_{44}NO_7P$	Phospholipid metabolism	↑*	→*	→*

[a]Change trend compared with control group.
[b]Change trend compared with SLE model group.
The levels of differential metabolites were marked with (↓) down-regulated, (↑) up-regulated and (—) no significant change (*P<0.05; **P<0.01).

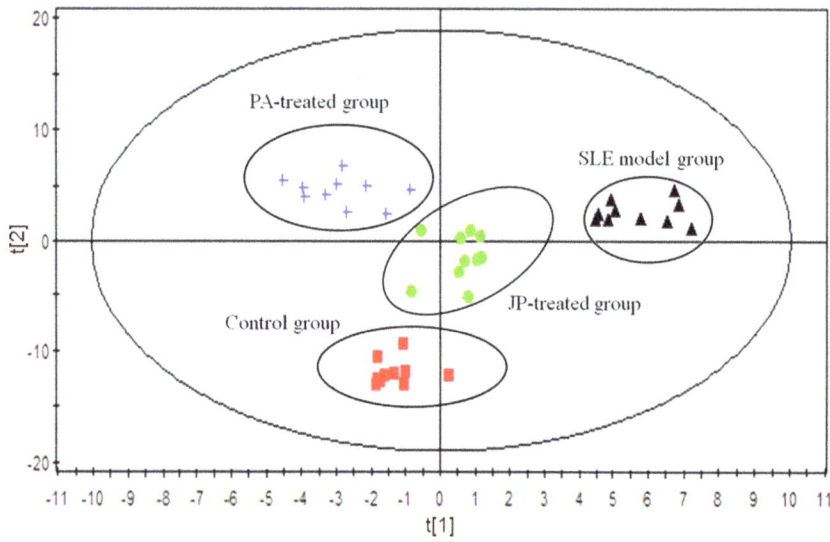

Figure 6. OPLS score plot of the SLE model group, PA-treated group, JP-treated group and control group by SIMCA-P11.0 (n = 10 in each group).

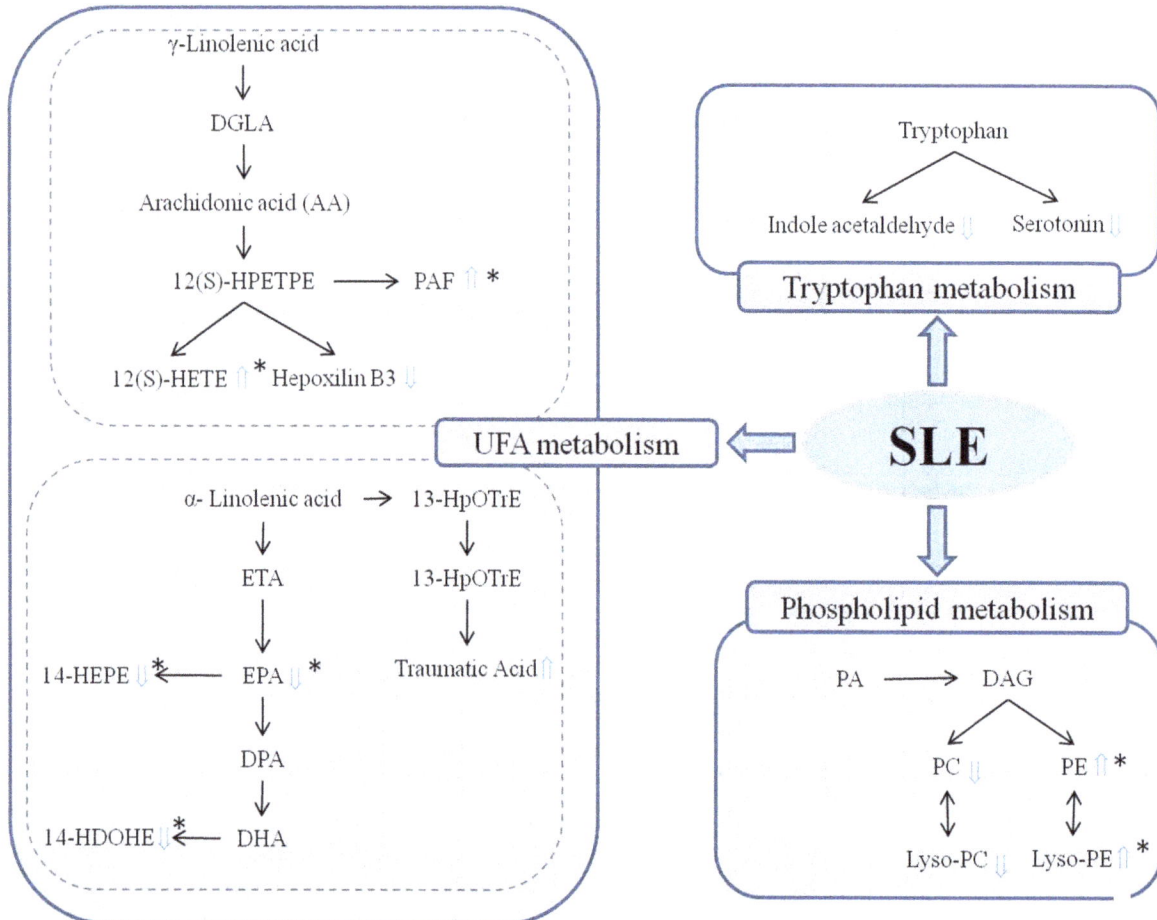

Figure 7. The perturbed metabolic network associated with SLE. The differential metabolite levels of the SLE model group compared to the control group were marked with (⇑) upregulated and (⇓) downregulated. (*Differential metabolites which could be effectively regulated by JP).

pathogenesis of SLE. The relative content of 14-HDOHE, EPA and its active metabolite 12S-hydroxypentaenoic acid (12S-HEPE) were decreased in the serum of the SLE model group, while the content of 12(S)-HETE, and traumatic acid were elevated. These results indicate that UFA metabolism is involved in the development of SLE. 12(S)-HEPE originating from 12-lipoxygenase (12-LOX) oxidation of EPA is thought to elicit an inhibitory effect on platelet aggregation. DHA and EPA metabolism produce a variety of metabolites; these weaker physiologically active metabolites competitively inhibit the biosynthesis of inflammatory mediators such as leukotrienes B_4 (LTB$_4$) and prostaglandin E_2 (PGE$_2$), and have an anti-inflammatory efficacy [24]. Metabolic disturbances to EPA and DHA may affect their ability to regulate the immune response, thereby increasing the symptoms of SLE. 12(S)-HETE is an active metabolite of arachidonic acid produced through the 12-lipoxygenase pathway. It has a powerful role in promoting inflammation and causes the accumulation of extracellular matrix and induces mesangial cell hypertrophy via p38 MAPK [25]. The role of 12(S)-HETE in the pathogenesis of diabetic nephropathy has been confirmed [26]. Increased 12(S)-HETE may promote kidney inflammation and cell hypertrophy when SLE occurs, thereby aggravating the symptoms of kidney disease. UFA metabolic disorders would result in a low serum level of anti-inflammatory metabolites and a high serum level of pro-inflammatory metabolites; these abnormal alterations may be one factor to explain why the pathogenesis of SLE is accompanied by a systemic inflammatory response.

Moreover, there is evidence indicating that perturbations of intestinal microbiota composition or function may play an important role in the development of diseases associated with altered metabolism [27], and that the intestinal microbiota can regulate the absorption, metabolism and storage of host lipid and UFAs via numerous microbial activities [28,29]. Therefore, the immune system disorder associated with SLE may be related to the intestinal microbiota dysfunction that adversely affects UFA metabolism. On the other hand, the dysbiosis of intestinal microbiota also can directly perturb the immune regulatory networks [30]. The close links between the intestinal microbiota, the immune system and lipid metabolism inspires an idea that incorporates intestinal microbial function into an in-depth study of the prominent disorders of UFA metabolism and the immune system in SLE model mice, as well as the possibility of treating SLE by regulating the intestinal microbiota.

Phospholipid metabolites, including phosphatidylcholine (PC 20:5), Lyso-PC (20:4), phosphatidylethanolamine (PE 20:3), Lyso-PE(22:6) and PAF were identified as the differential metabolites of SLE. The phospholipids are important precursors for many biologically active mediators of metabolism including eicosanoids, diacylglycerol and PAF. PEs also play important roles in biological processes such as apoptosis and cell signaling [31]. The abnormal phospholipid metabolic pathway may not only result in the abnormal of physiology and metabolism via a variety of pathways, but also promote the systemic inflammatory state [32]. PAF, a highly bioactive inflammatory phospholipid mediator, plays an important role in the pathogenesis of allergic reactions, acute and chronic inflammatory reactions, and arthritis [33]. PAF is also believed to play a role in various syndromes or diseases, including renal diseases, by favoring immune complex formation and modulating the subsequent inflammatory reaction [34]. PAF-induced proteinuria could be prevented by a PAF receptor antagonist, which further illustrates the physiological role of PAF in glomerular permeability [35]. In this study, SLE model mice showed obviously elevated serum levels of PAF, which is probably related to the serious lupus nephritis. PAF can promote platelet aggregation and can also stimulate the generation of auto-antibodies by activating platelets. In brief, activated platelets aggregated with circulating antigen-presenting cells, including monocytes and plasmacytoid dendritic cells, thus stimulating significant auto-antibody [36]. Therefore, PAF may become a new target for the treatment of SLE: PAF enzymes or PAF receptor antagonists may restrain the effects of PAF action, thereby inhibiting the proinflammatory and platelet activation it causes [37].

Indole acetaldehyde and serotonin are tryptophan metabolites, whose content declined in the SLE model group. Tryptophan has a very sensitive regulation function for the T cell cycle and can promote the conversion of T cells in the spleen [38]. However, tryptophan is susceptible to the influence of kidney disease and immune system disorders leading to metabolic disorders [39]. The tryptophan metabolic pathway was significantly affected by SLE, and disorder of tryptophan metabolism is also been reported in MRL/lpr mice, a spontaneous SLE model, in our previous study [40]. Therefore, the tryptophan metabolism is susceptible in process of SLE, and the abnormal tryptophan metabolism can influence the apoptosis of T cell [41], and impact the development of SLE.

Conclusion

RRLC-Q-TOF/MS-based serum metabolomics analysis combined with multivariate statistical analysis was applied to evaluate the pathogenesis of SLE and the mechanism of action of JP in SLE model mice. There was a prominent metabolic profile difference between SLE model mice and control mice according to OPLS. Thirteen differential metabolites in the SLE model were identified by the MS and MS/MS information. These differential metabolites confirm that SLE is associated with specific abnormalities in the metabolism of UFAs, tryptophan and phospholipid. JP can effectively regulate the UFA and phospholipid metabolic pathway and exert a good therapeutic effect on SLE. These results provide a better understanding of the pathogenesis of SLE and the mechanism of action of JP in SLE. Our results also prove that metabolomics is a powerful technology platform for studying the mechanism of action of TCM and investigating disease pathogenesis.

Author Contributions

Conceived and designed the experiments: XD JH YF. Performed the experiments: XD JH ZD LY. Analyzed the data: XD JH. Contributed reagents/materials/analysis tools: XD CW ZD LY. Wrote the paper: XD JH.

References

1. Tsokos GC (2011) Systemic lupus erythematosus. N Engl J Med 365: 2110–2121.
2. Gurevitz SL, Snyder JA, Wessel EK, Frey J, Williamson BA (2013) Systemic lupus erythematosus: A review of disease and treatment options. Consult Pharm 28: 110–121.
3. Irastorza l GR, Danza A, Khamashta M (2012) Glucocorticoid use and abuse in SLE. Rheumatology 51: 1145–1153.
4. Fan YS, Wen CP, Wu GL, Li MX (2005) Investigation into preventive an therapeutic effects of jiduquyuziyin methods in treating corticosteroid osteoporosis in systemic lupus erythematosus. Chin J Traditi Chin Med Pharm 20: 667–669.
5. Wen CP, Fan YS, Li XY, Lu KD, Wang XC (2007) Investigation on the effect of traditional Chinese medical jieduquyuziyin methods on the quality of life with systemic lupus erythematosus. Chin Arch Traditi Chin Med 25: 1599–1602.

6. Nicholson JK, Lindon JC, Holmes E (1999) 'Metabolomics': understanding the metabolic responses of living systems to pathophysiological stimuli via multivariate statistical analysis of biological NMR spectroscopic data. Xenobiotica 29: 1181–1189.

7. Xu GW, Kong HW, Wang JS, Lu X (2009) Investigation of traditional Chinese medicine based on systems thinking: a summary of recent research work in the authors' group. World Sci Technol Modernization Traditi Chin Med 11:107–119.

8. Vuckovic D (2012) Current trends and challenges in sample preparation for global metabolomics using liquid chromatography–mass spectrometry. Anal Bioanal Chem 403: 1523–1548.

9. Psychogios N, Hau DD, Peng J, Guo AC, Mandal R, et al. (2011) The human serum metabolome. PLoS One 6: e16957.

10. Gika H, Theodoridis G (2011) Sample preparation prior to the LC–MS-based metabolomics/metabonomics of blood-derived samples. Bioanalysis 3: 1647–1661.

11. Weckwerth W (2003) Metabolomics in systems biology. Annu Rev Plant Biol 54: 669–689.

12. An Z, Chen Y, Zhang R, Song Y, Sun JH, et al. (2010) Integrated ionization approach for RRLC-MS/MS-based metabonomics: finding potential biomarkers for lung cancer. J Proteome Res 9:4071–4081.

13. Satoh M, Reeves WH (1994) Induction of lupus-associated autoantibodies in BALB/c mice by intraperitoneal injection of pristane. J Exp Med 180: 2341–2346.

14. Thibault DL, Graham KL, Lee LY, Balboni I, Hertzog PJ, et al (2009) Type I interferon receptor controls B-cell expression of nucleic acid-sensing Toll-like receptors and autoantibody production in a murine model of lupus. Arthritis Res Ther 11: R112.

15. Reeves WH, Lee PL, Weinstein JS, Satoh M, Lu L (2009) Induction of autoimmunity by pristine and other naturally occurring hydrocarbons. Trends Immunol 30: 455–464.

16. Minhas U, Minz R,Das P, Bhatnagar A (2012) Therapeutic effect of Withania somnifera on pristane-induced model of SLE. Inflammopharmacol 20: 195–205.

17. Gabrielsson J, Jonsson H, Airiau C, Schmidt B, Escott R, et al. (2006) OPLS methodology for analysis of pre-processing effects on spectroscopic data. Chemometr Intell Lab 84: 153–158.

18. Gika HG, Macpherson E, Theodoridis GA, Wilson ID (2008) Evaluation of the repeatability of ultra-performance liquid chromatography-TOF-MS for global metabolic profiling of human urine samples. J Chromatogr B 871: 299–305.

19. Theodoridis G, Gika HG, Wilson ID (2008) LC-MS-based methodology for global metabolite profiling in metabonomics/metabolomics. TrAC-Trends Anal Chem 27: 251–260.

20. Vuckovic D (2012) Current trends and challenges in sample preparation for global metabolomics using liquid chromatography-mass spectrometry. Anal Bioanal Chem 403: 1523–1548.

21. Goodpaster AM, Kennedy MA (2011) Quantification and statistical significance analysis of group separation in NMR-based metabonomics studies. Chemometr Intell Lab 109: 162–170.

22. Theodore RS, Joseph CR, Li XD, Waddell K, Fischer SM (2008) Molecular Formula and METLIN Personal Metabolite Database Matching Applied to the Identification of Compounds Generated by LC/TOF-MS. J Biomol Tech 19: 258–266.

23. Hwang D (1989) Essential fatty acids and immune response. FASEB J 3: 2052–2061.

24. Mori TA, Beilin LJ (2004) Omega-3 fatty acids and inflammation. Curr Atheroscler Rep 6: 461–467.

25. Reddy MA, Adler SG, Kim YS, Lanting L, Rossi J, et al. (2002) Interaction of MAPK and 12-lipoxygenase pathways in growth and matrix protein expression in mesangial cells. Am J Physiol Renal Physiol 283: F985–F994.

26. Kang SW, Adler SG, Nast CC, Lapage J, Gu JL, et al. (2001) 12-Lipoxygenase is increased in glucose-stimulated mesangial cells and in experimental diabetic nephropathy. Kidney Int 59: 1354–1362.

27. Velagapudi VR, Hezaveh R, Reigstad CS, Gopalacharyulu P, Yetukuri L, et al. (2010) The gut microbiota modulates host energy and lipid metabolism in mice. J Lipid Res 51: 1101–1112.

28. Lahti L, Salonen A, Kekkonen RA, Salojarvi J, Jalamka-tuovinen J, et al. (2013) Associations between the human intestinal microbiota, *Lactobacillus rhamnosus* GG and serum lipids indicated by integrated analysis of high-throughput profiling data. Peer J 1:e32.

29. Laparra JM, Sanz Y (2010) Interactions of gut microbiota with functional food components and nutraceuticals. Pharmacol Res 61: 219–225.

30. Maynard CL, Elson CO, Hatton RD, Weaver CT (2012) Reciprocal interactions of the intestinal microbiota and immune system. Nature 489: 231–241.

31. Vance JE (2008) Phosphatidylserine and phosphatidylethanolamine in mammalian cells: two metabolically related aminophospholipids. J Lipid Res 49: 1377–1387.

32. Manzi S, Wasko MC (2000) Inflammation-mediated rheumatic diseases and atherosclerosis. Ann Rheum Dis 59: 321–325.

33. Yost CC, Weyrich AS, Zimmerman GA (2010) The platelet activating factor (PAF) signaling cascade systemic inflammatory responses. Biochimie 92: 692–697.

34. Papavasiliou EC, Gouva C, Siamopoulos KC, Tselepis AD (2005) Erythrocyte PAF-acetylhydrolase activity in various stages of chronic kidney disease: Effect of long-term therapy with erythropoietin. Kidney Int 68: 246–255.

35. Perico N, Delaini F, Tagliaferri M, Remuzzi G (1988) Effect of platelet-activating factor and its specific receptor antagonist on glomerular permeability to proteins in isolated perfused rat kidney. Lab Invest 58: 163–171.

36. Duffau P, Seneschal J, Nicco C, Nicco C, Richez C, et al. (2010) Platelet CD154 potentiates interferon-α secretion by plasmacytoid dendritic cells in systemic lupus erythematosus. Sci Transl Med 2 :47ra63.

37. Price S (2010) Connective tissue diseases: Activated platelets as a target for SLE therapy. Nat Rev Rheumatol 6: 613.

38. Mellor AL, Munn DH (2004) IDO expression by dendritic cells: Tolerance and tryptophan catabolism. Nat Rev Immunol 4: 762–774.

39. Alegre E, López AS, Diaz-Lagares A, González A (2008) Study of the plasmatic levels of tryptophan and kynurenine throughout pregnancy. Clinica Chimica Acta 393, 132–134.

40. Hu JB, Jiang FS, Gu HC, Ding ZS, Yao L, et al. (2013) Metabolomics Study on the Effects of Jieduquyuziyin Prescription on Systemic Lupus Erythematosus Mice by LC-Q-TOF/MS. Chromatographia 76: 791–800.

41. Rand LeS, Gonzale A, Gonzale AS, Carosell ED, Rouas-Freiss N (2005) Indoleamine 2,3 dioxygenase and human leucocyte antigen-G inhibit the T-cell alloproliferative response through two independent pathways. Immunology 116:297–307.

Meta-Analysis of Associations of IL1 Receptor Antagonist and Estrogen Receptor Gene Polymorphisms with Systemic Lupus Erythematosus Susceptibility

Li Cai[1,9], Jin-wei Zhang[2,9], Xing-xin Xue[1], Zhi-gang Wang[3], Jia-jia Wang[1], Shai-di Tang[1], Shao-wen Tang[1], Jie Wang[4,5], Yun Zhang[1,6]*, Xian Xia[3]*

1 Department of Epidemiology and Biostatistics, School of Public Health, Nanjing Medical University, Jiangning District, Nanjing, Jiangsu, China, 2 Department of Anesthesiology, Affiliated Drum Tower Hospital of Medical College of Nanjing University, Gulou District, Nanjing, Jiangsu, China, 3 Department of Nosocomial Infection Control, General Hospital of Beijing Military Region, Dongcheng District, Beijing, China, 4 State Key Laboratory of Reproductive Medicine, Nanjing Medical University, Jiangning District, Nanjing, Jiangsu, China, 5 Department of General Practice, Kangda College, Nanjing Medical University, Jiangning District, Nanjing, Jiangsu, China, 6 Institute of Epidemiology and Microbiology, Huadong Research Institute for Medicine and Biotechnics, Nanjing, Jiangsu, China

Abstract

Systemic lupus erythematosus (SLE) is an autoimmune disease that affects a number of different organs and tissues. Interleukin-1 (IL1) and estrogen are considered potential elements in the pathology of SLE. Recently, the variable number of tandem repeats (VNTR) polymorphism in the IL1 receptor antagonist gene (IL1-RN) and PvuII (rs2234693) and XbaI (rs9340799) polymorphisms in the estrogen receptor 1 gene (ESR1) have been associated with a predisposition to SLE. However, the evidence for these associations is inconclusive. We therefore conducted a meta-analysis to validate the roles of these polymorphisms in SLE susceptibility. We searched four databases and identified a total of 17 eligible articles comprising 24 studies. The Newcastle-Ottawa quality assessment scale was used to assess the qualities of the selected studies. We assessed the strengths of the associations using odds ratios (ORs) with 95% confidence intervals (95% CIs). Regarding the IL-1RN VNTR, the 2 allele significantly increased SLE susceptibility (2 vs. L: OR = 1.34, 95% CI = 1.03–1.73, $P = 0.03$). The ESR1 PvuII CC/CT genotype was also associated with SLE susceptibility (CC/CT vs. TT: OR = 1.25, 95% CI = 1.06–1.47, $P = 0.01$), and the difference was especially pronounced among Asians (CC/CT vs. TT: OR = 1.33, 95% CI = 1.04–1.69, $P = 0.02$). No significant association between the ESR1 XbaI polymorphism and SLE susceptibility was observed in the overall analysis. However, a marginally significant association between the GG/GA genotype was found in individuals of Asian descent (GG/GA vs. AA: OR = 1.30, 95% CI = 1.01–1.67, $P = 0.04$). These results indicate that the IL1-RN VNTR 2 allele, ESR1 PvuII CC/CT genotype and ESR1 XbaI GG/GA genotype may increase SLE susceptibility, especially in Asian individuals.

Editor: Shervin Assassi, University of Texas Health Science Center at Houston, United States of America

Funding: This study was supported by grants from the National Natural Science Foundation of China (Grant No. 81273146, 81102165). (http://www.nsfc.gov.cn) The funders had no role in study design, data collection and analysis, decision to publish, or preparation of the manuscript.

Competing Interests: The authors have declared that no competing interests exist.

* Email: zhangyunvip@126.com (YZ); r_summer@163.com (Xian Xia)

9 These authors contributed equally to this work.

Introduction

Systemic lupus erythematosus (SLE) is an autoimmune disease that affects various organs and tissues, involving the production of a range of autoantibodies against serological, intracellular, nucleic acid and cell surface antigens [1]. Although the mechanisms underlying SLE are not fully understood, genetic, environmental and hormonal factors are all thought to impact on the development of the disease [2].

Cytokines are considered to be potential elements in the pathology of SLE. These include interleukin-1 (IL1), which plays a key regulatory role in initiating and modulating immunologic and inflammatory events [3,4]. Animals with experimental SLE produced increased levels of IL1 throughout the disease course [5]. The IL1 family consists of IL1α, IL1β and IL1 receptor

antagonist (IL1-RA) [6]. IL1-RA is an important anti-inflammatory molecule that binds to IL1 receptors in competition with IL1α and IL1β, thus inhibiting their activities and modulating a variety of IL1-related immune and inflammatory activities [7]. The IL1-RA gene (IL1-RN) has a variable number of tandem repeats (VNTR) polymorphism of 86 base pairs (bp) in intron 2. Five alleles correspond to allele 1 (four repeats), allele 2 (two repeats), allele 3 (five repeats), allele 4 (three repeats) and allele 5 (six repeats), which can be further categorized into a long allele (L: 3–6 repeats) and a short allele (2:2 repeats). The genotypes are therefore classified as LL, 2L and 22 [8]. Blakemore et al. [9] first revealed that the frequency of the IL1-RN VNTR 2 allele was increased in SLE patients, since when mounting studies have explored the relationship between the IL1-RN VNTR polymorphism and SLE susceptibility in different populations; however, the findings have been controversial [10–12].

Estrogen is another underlying element in the pathology of SLE. SLE typically presents in women of childbearing age [13] and its morbidity falls remarkably after the menopause, in line with the decline in endogenous estrogen [14]. In an SLE mouse model, female mice had poorer outcomes than male mice, and estrogens exacerbated, while androgens ameliorated, the disease [15]. One possible mechanism is that physiological concentrations of estrogen could affect the secretion of cytokines such as IL1 [16–18]. However, the roles of estrogen and IL1 in SLE remain unclear. Estrogen acts on target cells through binding to estrogen receptors (ERs). ERα, encoded by the ER 1 gene (*ESR1*), is the main form of ER. Two polymorphisms, *ESR1 PvuII* T/C (rs2234693) and *ESR1 XbaI* A/G (rs9340799), located in the first intron of the *ESR1* gene, have been extensively studied, but the associations between these polymorphisms and SLE susceptibility remain controversial [19,20].

Limited sample sizes and inadequate statistical power mean that the results of studies of the relationships between the *IL1-RN* VNTR, *ESR1 PvuII*, and *ESR1 XbaI* polymorphisms and SLE susceptibility remain conflicting, rather than conclusive [9–12,19–31]. Given the potentially important roles of these three polymorphisms in the pathological process and the increasing numbers of studies in different populations, we performed a meta-analysis to derive a more precise estimation of the associations between the *IL1-RN* VNTR, *ESR1 PvuII*, and *ESR1 XbaI* polymorphisms and SLE susceptibility.

Materials and Methods

Search strategy

We searched the PubMed, Embase, Wanfang and Chinese National Knowledge Infrastructure databases using the search terms: 'systemic lupus erythematosus' or 'SLE', 'polymorphism' or 'allele' or 'genotype', 'interleukin-1 receptor antagonist' or '*IL1-RN*' or 'estrogen receptor' or '*ER*'. The literature search was updated on December 2013 and there was no date limit. The results were also supplemented with manual searches of references from the final published articles.

Study selection

The inclusion criteria were: (1) case-control design; (2) studies investigating the relationship between the *IL1-RN* VNTR, *ESR1 PvuII* or *ESR1 XbaI* polymorphisms and SLE susceptibility; (3) studies with sufficient data to provide odds ratios (ORs) and 95% confidence intervals (CIs); and (4) diagnosis of SLE patients performed according to the American College of Rheumatology criteria [32,33]. The exclusion criteria were: (1) studies with overlapping populations; and (2) studies with insufficient data.

Data extraction

The following information was sought from each publication: first author's surname, year of publication, participants' country, ethnicity, sex distribution, genotyping methods, the source of control groups (population-based or hospital-based controls) and matching numbers of genotyped cases and controls. The literature search, eligible study selection and data extraction were carefully conducted independently by two reviewers (Cai and Zhang) and consensuses were reached on all items.

Quality appraisal

Two reviewers (Cai and Zhang) independently rated the methodological quality of every included study according to the

Newcastle-Ottawa quality assessment scale [34]. This scale contains nine items (1 point for each) in three parts: selection (four items), comparability (two items) and exposure (three items).

Statistical analysis

Statistical manipulations were conducted using Stata 10.0 (Stata Corporation, College Station, TX, USA). A χ^2 test for goodness of fit was used to test for Hardy-Weinberg equilibrium (HWE) in the control group, with $P<0.05$ indicating a deviation from HWE. Crude ORs and 95% CIs were used to assess the strengths of the associations between the *IL1-RN* and *ESR1* polymorphisms and SLE susceptibility. The statistical significance of the pooled ORs was determined by the Z test, with $P<0.05$ considered significant. Statistical heterogeneity among studies was assessed by the Q-test and the I^2 statistic was used to estimate heterogeneity quantitatively [35]. In the absence of heterogeneity ($P>0.10$ or $I^2<50\%$), pooled ORs and 95% CIs were calculated by the fixed-effects model (Mantel-Haenszel method), otherwise the random-effects model (DerSimonian-Laird method) was used. Sensitivity analysis was used to evaluate the stability of the results of the meta-analysis by removing one study at a time to determine the influence of the individual data set on the pooled OR. Potential publication bias was examined by a funnel plot of log OR against its standard error using Begg's test, and the degree of asymmetry was assessed by Egger's unweighted regression asymmetry test. Publication bias may be present if $P<0.05$ [36].

Results

Study characteristics

A detailed flow chart of the inclusion and exclusion processes is presented in Figure 1. Overall, 86 studies (44 in English and 42 in Chinese) were retrieved based on the search terms. Of these, 69 studies were excluded according to the inclusion and exclusion criteria and 17 eligible articles representing 24 studies were identified (one article was considered as several separate studies if it involved different populations or different target single nucleotide polymorphisms). Eleven studies including 1171 SLE patients and 1834 controls described *IL-1RN* VNTR genotypes, seven studies including 1012 SLE patients and 2442 controls described *ESR1 PvuII* genotypes and six studies including 816 SLE patients and 1478 controls described *ESR1 XbaI* genotypes. The first author's surname, publication year, ethnicity, quality score, sex distribution, frequencies of various genotypes in SLE patients and controls and HWE in controls for each study are listed in Tables 1, 2 and 3. The mean score of the quality appraisal was 6.54. In addition, most of the eligible studies were population-based and polymerase chain reaction was performed in all studies. Genotype distributions in the control populations agreed with HWE in all except seven studies [12,19,22,23,25,29,30].

Quantitative synthesis

Eleven studies including 1171 SLE patients and 1834 controls assessed the relationship between *IL1-RN* VNTR polymorphisms and SLE susceptibility. *IL1-RN* VNTR polymorphism showed no significant association with SLE susceptibility in a dominant model (22/2L vs. LL: OR = 1.11, 95% CI = 0.87−1.40, $P=0.40$), recessive model (22 vs. LL/2L: OR = 1.32, 95% CI = 0.88−1.97, $P=0.17$) or additive model (22 vs. LL: OR = 1.32, 95% CI = 0.88−1.98, $P=0.19$, Table 4). However, a significant association was observed in an allelic contrast model (2 vs. L: OR = 1.34, 95% CI = 1.03−1.73, $P=0.03$, Figure 2). After excluding the studies in which the genotype distributions in the control groups deviated from HWE, the *IL1-RN* VNTR

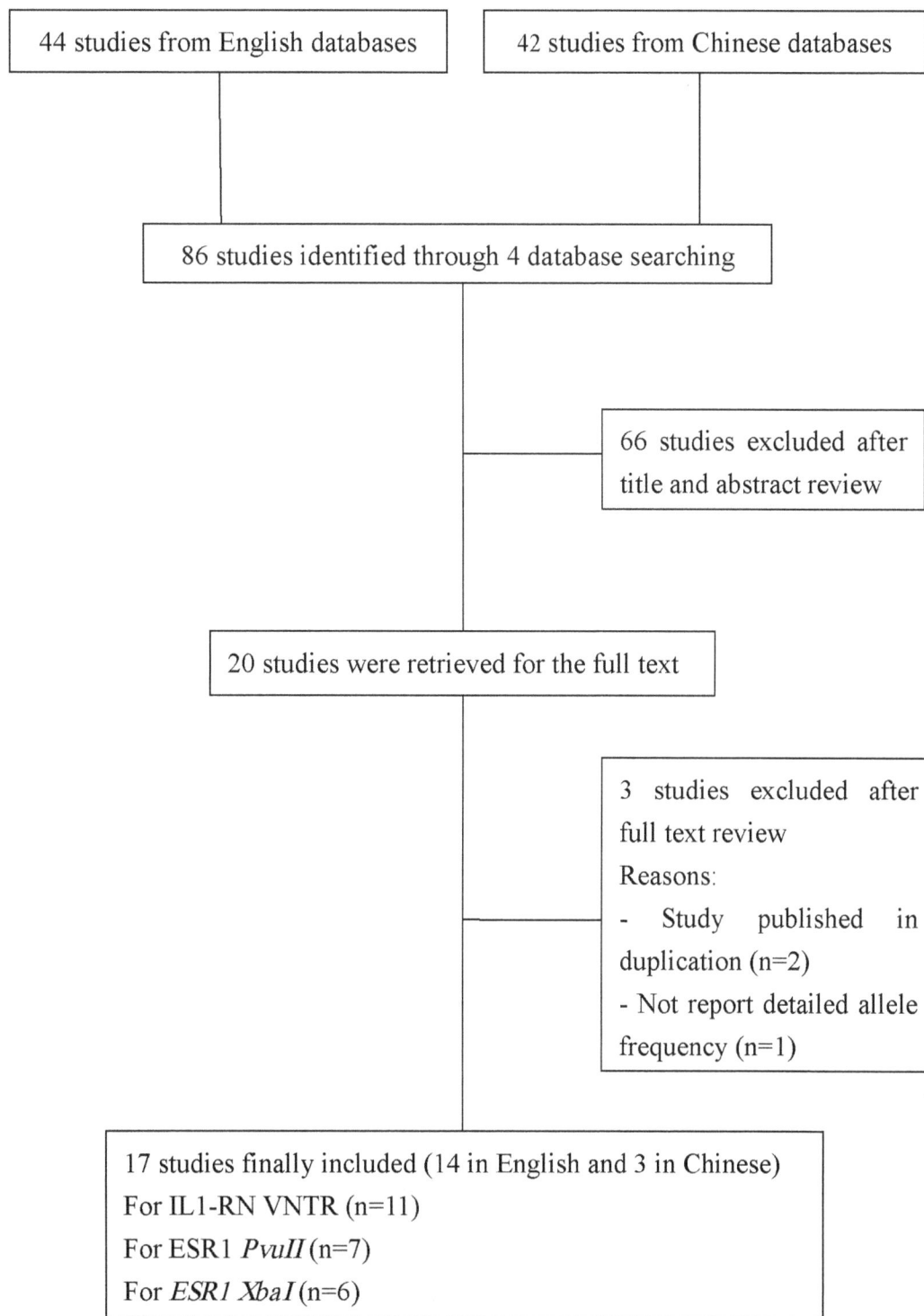

Figure 1. Flow diagram of studies included in the meta-analysis.

polymorphism showed no significant association with SLE susceptibility in all genetic models (Table S1). We performed subgroup analyses in Asian and Caucasian populations and found no significant differences in either ethnic subgroup (Table S1).

Seven studies compared the *ESR1 Pvu*II polymorphism in SLE patients and controls. Individuals carrying variant genotypes had an increased risk of SLE in the dominant model (CC/CT vs. TT:

OR = 1.25, 95% CI = 1.06–1.47, P = 0.01, Figure 3) but not in other genetic models (CC vs. TT/CT: OR = 0.96, 95% CI = 0.79–1.17, P = 0.71; CC vs. TT: OR = 1.10, 95% CI = 0.88–1.38, P = 0.41; C vs. T: OR = 1.28, 95% CI = 0.95–1.74, P = 0.11, Table 4). After excluding the study in which the genotype distribution in the control group deviated from the HWE, *ESR1 Pvu*II polymorphism was significantly associated

Table 1. Characteristics and IL1-RN VNTR polymorphism genotype distributions in studies included in the meta-analysis.

Author, year	Ethnicity	Quality score[a]	Control					Case					P_{HWE}
			LL	2L	22	L	2	LL	2L	22	L	2	
Tsai 2006 [10]	Taiwan(Asian)	6	-	-	-	142	6	-	-	-	198	10	-
Lee 2004 [11]	Korean(Asian)	7	109	18	0	236	18	83	10	0	176	10	0.39
Parks 2004 [12]	United States(Caucasian)	7	169	18	15	356	48	66	12	8	144	28	**<0.01**
Parks 2004 [12]	United States(African-American)	7	69	3	0	141	3	137	6	1	280	8	0.86
Jonsen2004 [21]	Sweden(Caucasian)	6	111	75	14	297	103	86	38	14	210	66	0.78
Huang 2002 [22]	Taiwan(Asian)	7	96	6	1	198	8	43	8	1	94	10	**0.03**
Zhu 2000 [23]	China(Asian)	5	15	31	4	61	39	26	52	2	104	56	**0.03**
Tjernstrom 1999 [24]	Sweden(Caucasian)	7	-	-	-	339	39	-	-	-	130	32	-
Heward 1999 [25]	Caucasian(Caucasian)	4	312	7	19	631	45	106	4	6	216	16	**<0.01**
Suzuki 1997 [26]	Japan(Asian)	4	-	-	-	418	18	-	-	-	354	38	-
Blakemore 1994 [9]	England(Caucasian)	7	152	92	17	396	126	39	31	11	109	53	0.54

aThe quality score was determinded by using the Newcastle-Ottawa quality assessment scale.
IL1-RN: Interleukin-1 receptor antagonist gene; VNTR: variable number of tandem repeats; HWE: Hardy-Weinberg equilibrium.

Table 2. Characteristics and ESR1 PvuII polymorphism genotype distributions in studies included in the meta-analysis.

Author, year	Ethnicity	Quality score[a]	Gender (M/F)		Control					Case					P_{HWE}
			Control	Case	TT	TC	CC	T	C	TT	TC	CC	T	C	
Kisiel 2011 [20]	Poland (Caucasian)	6	482/482	14/182	270	467	227	1007	921	44	101	51	189	203	0.36
Wang 2010 [23]	United States(Mixed)	8	0/102	0/46	38	48	15	124	78	9	26	11	44	48	0.98
Lu 2009 [28]	China(Asian)	7	0/157	0/221	83	56	18	222	92	95	92	34	282	160	0.08
Li 2008 [29]	China(Asian)	6	0/200	0/70	86	82	32	254	146	23	39	8	85	55	0.10
Chen 2008 [30]	China(Asian)	5	36/46	6/76	30	31	21	91	73	37	30	15	104	60	**0.03**
Johansson 2005 [31]	Sweden(Caucasian)	9	180/490	40/220	208	332	130	748	592	83	132	45	298	222	0.90
Lee 2004 [19]	Korean(Asian)	7	0/268	0/137	114	110	44	338	198	46	76	15	106	168	0.05

aThe quality score was determinded by using the Newcastle-Ottawa quality assessment scale.
ESR1: estrogen receptor 1 gene; M: Male; F: Female; HWE: Hardy-Weinberg equilibrium.

Table 3. Characteristics and *ESR1 XbaI* polymorphism genotype distributions in studies included in the meta-analysis.

Author, year	Ethnicity	Quality score[a]	Gender (M/F) Control	Gender (M/F) Case	Control AA	AG	GG	A	G	Case AA	AG	GG	A	G	P_{HWE}
Wang 2010 [23]	United States(Mixed)	8	0/102	0/46	48	44	9	140	62	14	24	8	52	40	0.81
Lu 2009 [28]	China(Asian)	7	0/157	0/221	112	38	7	262	52	138	73	10	349	93	0.12
Li 2008 [29]	China(Asian)	6	0/200	0/70	144	46	10	334	66	46	19	5	111	29	**0.02**
Chen 2008 [30]	China(Asian)	5	36/46	6/76	45	29	8	119	45	48	31	3	127	37	0.31
Johansson 2005 [31]	Sweden(Caucasian)	9	180/490	40/220	332	281	57	945	395	145	94	21	384	136	0.82
Lee 2004 [19]	Korean(Asian)	7	0/268	0/137	192	62	14	446	90	89	38	10	216	58	**<0.01**

[a]The quality score was determinded by using the Newcastle-Ottawa quality assessment scale.
ESR1: estrogen receptor 1 gene; M: Male; F: Female; HWE: Hardy-Weinberg equilibrium.

with SLE susceptibility in both dominant and allelic contrast models (Table S2). When grouped by ethnicity, a significant association was still observed in the dominant model in the Asian group (CC/CT vs. TT: OR = 1.33, 95% CI = 1.04–1.69, P = 0.02, Table S2) but not in the Caucasian group (CC/CT vs. TT: OR = 1.11, 95% CI = 0.88–1.40, P = 0.38, Table S2).

Six studies investigated the association between *ESR1 XbaI* polymorphism and SLE susceptibility. No significant relationships were identified for any of the genetic models in the whole study set (GG/GA vs. AA: OR = 1.19, 95% CI = 0.88–1.62, P = 0.27; GG vs. AA/GA: OR = 1.08, 95% CI = 0.77–1.51, P = 0.67; GG vs. AA: OR = 1.09, 95% CI = 0.77–1.54, P = 0.64; G vs. A: OR = 1.15, 95% CI = 0.89–1.49, P = 0.27, Table 4). Exclusion of the two studies in which the genotype distributions in the control groups deviated from the HWE had no significant effect on the results (Table S3). However, stratified analysis by ethnicity demonstrated a marginally significant association in the dominant model (GG/GA vs. AA: OR = 1.30, 95% CI = 1.01–1.67, P = 0.04, Figure 4, Table S3) in individuals of Asian descent.

Tests of heterogeneity

For *IL1-RN* VNTR, *ESR1 Pvu*II, and *ESR1 Xba*I, heterogeneity between studies was observed in the overall analysis of the allelic contrast model ($P_{heterogeneity}$ = 0.02, 0.00, 0.03, respectively, Table 4). In addition, heterogeneity was also found for *ESR1 Xba*I in the dominant model ($P_{heterogeneity}$ = 0.03). Ethnicity was assessed as a potential source of heterogeneity. Ethnicity (χ^2 = 11.49, df = 2, P = 0.003) contributed to the heterogeneity for *ESR1 Pvu*II. Ethnicity also contributed to the heterogeneity for the dominant model (χ^2 = 10.00, df = 2, P = 0.007) and the allelic contrast model (χ^2 = 8.83, df = 2, P = 0.010) for *ESR1 Xba*I.

Sensitivity analysis

Sensitivity analysis revealed that heterogeneity decreased after some studies were removed: Jonsen *et al.* 2004 [21] for *IL1-RN* VNTR (2 vs. L: $P_{heterogeneity}$ = 0.08, I^2 = 41.8%); Johansson *et al.* 2005 [31] for *ESR1 Xba*I (G vs. A: $P_{heterogeneity}$ = 0.25, I^2 = 26.4%); and Johansson *et al.* 2005 [31] for *ESR1 Xba*I (GG/GA vs. AA: $P_{heterogeneity}$ = 0.48, I^2 = 0.0%). The results of the association between *ESR1 Pvu*II and SLE susceptibility were not substantially altered.

Publication bias

No publication bias was detected among studies regarding the association between the *IL1-RN* VNTR polymorphism and SLE (P = 0.83 for 2 vs. L, Figure 5). Similarly, the results of Egger's and Begg's tests showed no publication bias for the *ESR1 Pvu*II or *ESR1 Xba*I polymorphisms in all models.

Discussion

Studies of gene polymorphisms potentially related to SLE have recently attracted growing attention. In the present study, we performed a meta-analysis of the associations between *IL1-RN* VNTR, *ESR1 Pvu*II, and *ESR1 Xba*I polymorphisms and SLE susceptibility. The analysis indicated an association between the 2 allele of the VNTR polymorphism in intron 2 of *IL1-RN* and increased SLE susceptibility (2 vs. L: OR = 1.34, 95% CI = 1.03–1.73, P = 0.03). There was also an association between *ESR1 Pvu*II and SLE in the dominant model (CC/CT vs. TT: OR = 1.25, 95% CI = 1.06–1.47, P = 0.01), which was pronounced among Asian individuals (CC/CT vs. TT: OR = 1.33, 95% CI = 1.04–1.69, P = 0.02). There was no significant association between the *ESR1 Xba*I polymorphism and SLE suscepti-

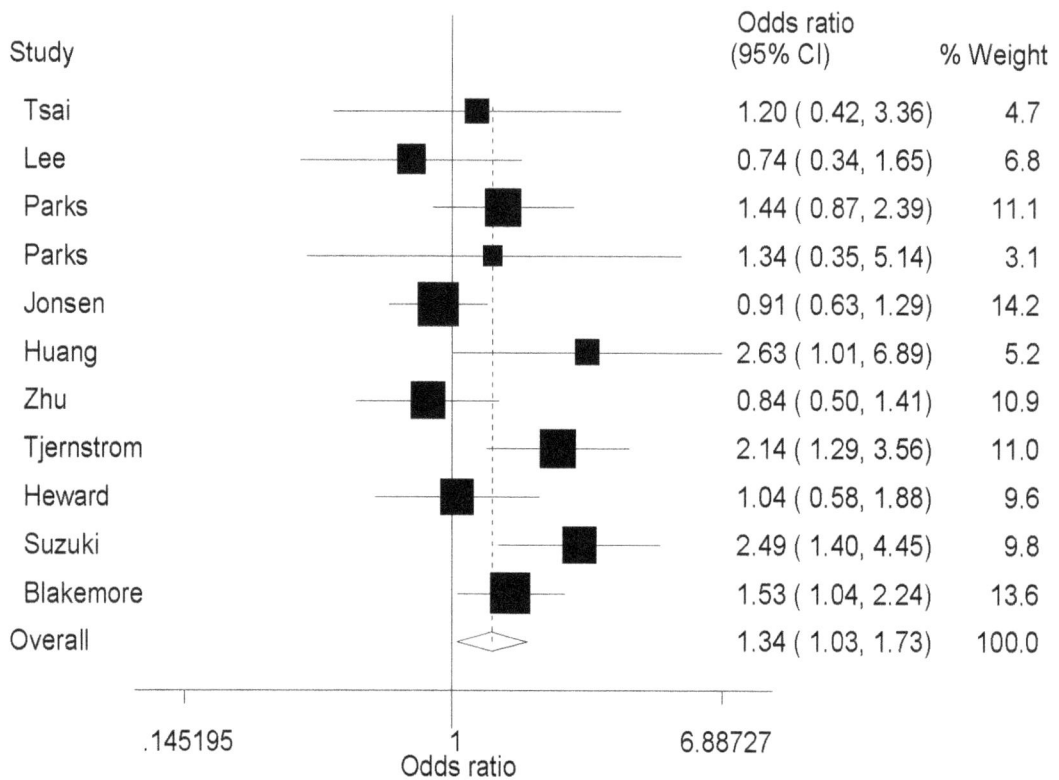

Figure 2. Forest plot of the association between SLE susceptibility and *IL1-RN* VNTR polymorphism (2 versus L).

bility in the overall analysis, but the GG/GA genotype was associated with SLE susceptibility in Asians (GG/GA vs. AA: OR = 1.30, 95% CI = 1.01–1.67, P = 0.04).

IL1 is a potent pro-inflammatory cytokine in acute and chronic inflammation in SLE [37]. IL1RA is a natural antagonist of IL1

and its anti-inflammatory activity is mediated through several different pathways [38] and investigations found decreased production of IL1RA in active SLE [39]. The *IL1-RN* VNTR 2 allele was associated with increased production of IL1β *in vitro* [40,41] and the concentration of IL1RA was shown to be

Table 4. Main results of meta-analysis of the association of *IL1-RN* VNTR, *ESR1 PvuII* and *ESR1 XbaI* polymorphisms with SLE susceptibility.

Gene and Genetic models	Number of study	$P_{heterogeneity}$	I^2(%)	Type of effect model	ORs (95% CI)	P
IL1-RN VNTR						
Dominant (22/2L vs. LL)	8	0.19	29.3	Fixed	1.11 (0.87–1.40)	0.40
Recessive (22 vs. LL/2L)	7	0.50	0	Fixed	1.32 (0.88–1.97)	0.17
Additive (22 vs. LL)	7	0.46	0	Fixed	1.32 (0.88–1.98)	0.19
Allelic contrast (2 vs. L)	11	**0.02**	51.4	Random	**1.34 (1.03–1.73)**	**0.03**
ESR1 PvuII						
Dominant (CC/CT vs. TT)	7	0.10	43.3	Fixed	**1.25 (1.06–1.47)**	**0.01**
Recessive (CC vs. TT/CT)	7	0.22	26.8	Fixed	0.96 (0.79–1.17)	0.71
Additive (CC vs. TT)	7	0.11	42.5	Fixed	1.10 (0.88–1.38)	0.41
Allelic contrast (C vs. T)	7	**0.00**	85.5	Random	1.28 (0.95–1.74)	0.11
ESR1 XbaI						
Dominant(GG/GA vs. AA)	6	**0.03**	58.8	Random	1.19 (0.88–1.62)	0.27
Recessive(GG vs. AA/AG)	6	0.39	6.1	Fixed	1.08 (0.77–1.51)	0.67
Additive(GG vs. AA)	6	0.17	35.1	Fixed	1.09 (0.77–1.54)	0.64
Allelic contrast(G vs. A)	6	**0.03**	60.4	Random	1.15 (0.89–1.49)	0.27

IL1-RN: Interleukin-1 receptor antagonist gene; VNTR: variable number of tandem repeats; *ESR1*: estrogen receptor 1 gene; OR: odds ratio; CI: confidence interval.

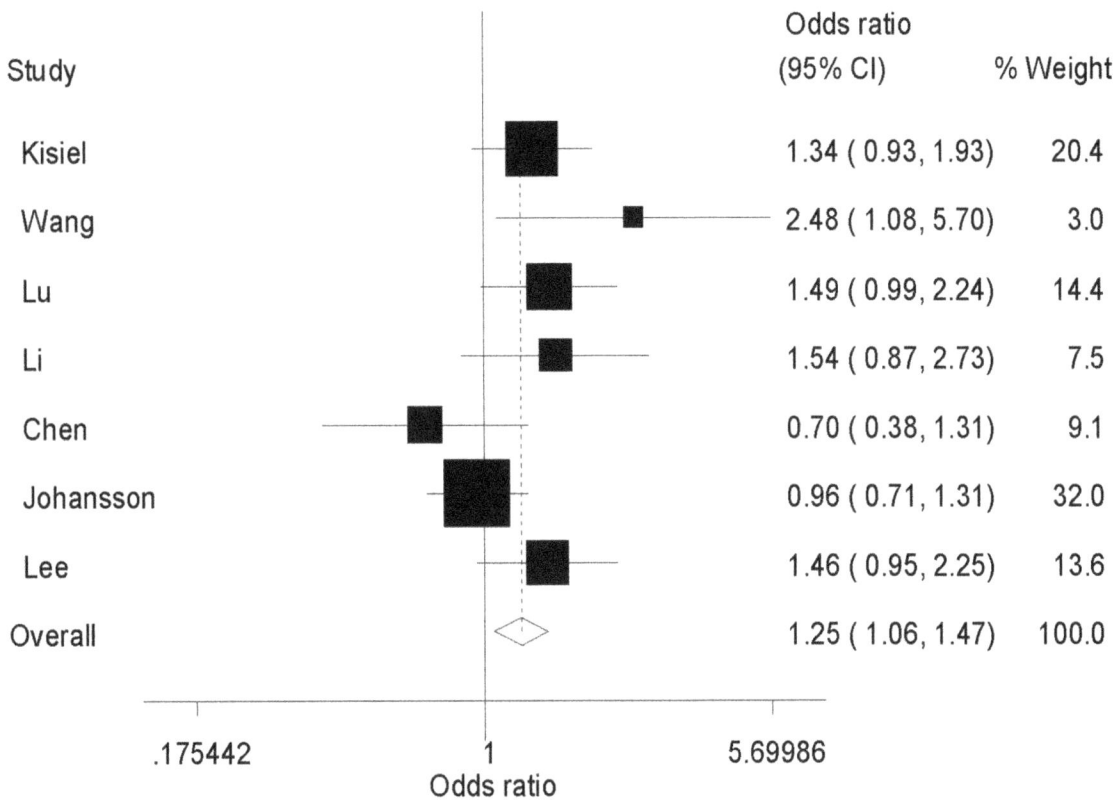

Figure 3. Forest plot of the association between SLE susceptibility and *ESR1 Pvu*II polymorphism (CC/CT versus TT).

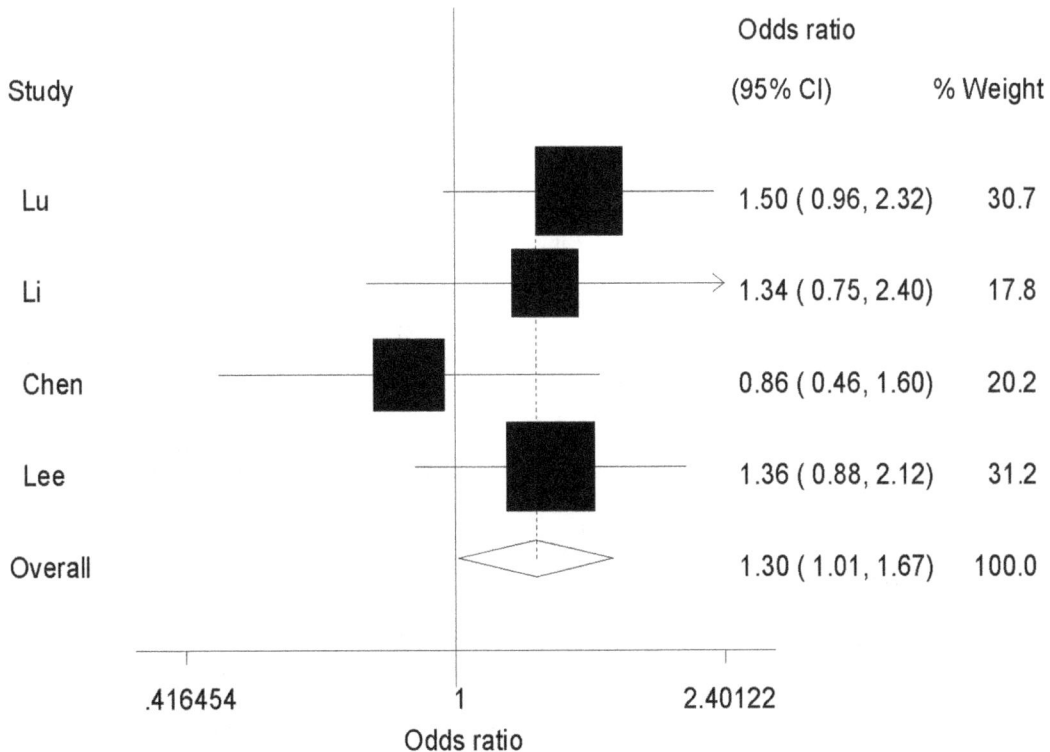

Figure 4. Forest plot of the association between SLE susceptibility and *ESR1 Xba*I polymorphism in Asian descent (GG/GA versus AA).

Begg's funnel plot with pseudo 95% confidence limits

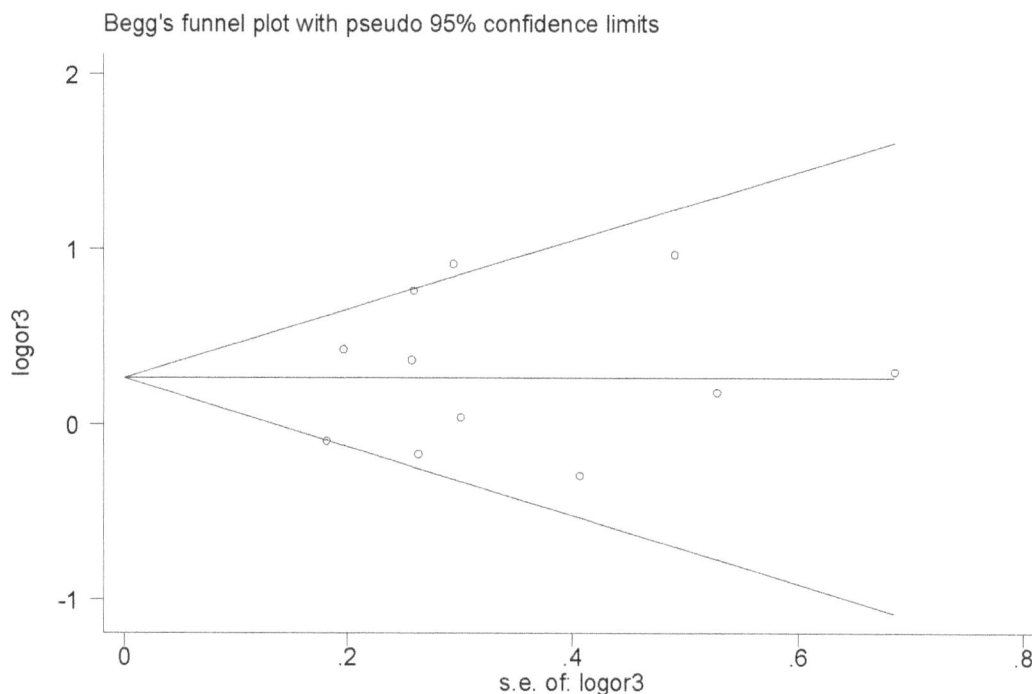

Figure 5. Begg's funnel plot for publication bias test. *IL1-RN* VNTR: 2 versus L.

correlated with IL1β [42]. Also, this meta-analysis identified carriage of the 2 allele as a risk factor for SLE susceptibility (2 vs. L: OR = 1.34, 95% CI = 1.03–1.73, $P = 0.03$). In support of this, the *IL1-RN* VNTR contains three potential protein-binding sites: an acute phase response element, an interferon α and an interferon β silencer B [43]. The 2 allele of *IL1-RN* VNTR only has 2 repeats. This could affect mRNA length and subsequent protein processing and stability [44], which could in turn affect the production of IL1RA.

Our study also showed that the *ESR1 Pvu*II CC/CT and *ESR1 Xba*I GG/GA genotypes could increase susceptibility to SLE. Estrogen can affect both innate and adaptive immune responses in mice [45] and SLE patients [46] through different pathways [47–49], and estrogen receptors are expressed in most immunocompetent cells [50]. Some researchers determined that IL1β levels were higher during the luteal period compared with the follicular period of the female reproductive cycle, which was consistent with the results of *in vivo* [51–53] and *in vitro* tests [18]. The polymorphisms *Pvu*II and *Xba*I are located in intron 1 of *ESR1* but are still able to affect the gene, and thus affect estrogen concentrations. The C allele of *Pvu*II can produce a binding site for the B-myb transcription factor, which could enhance the ability to up-regulate downstream receptor structures compared with the T allele [54]. In the present study, SLE susceptibility was associated with the *ESR1 Pvu*II C allele but not with *Xba*I in overall analysis. However, we could not rule out the possibility of an association between the *ESR1 Xba*I polymorphism and SLE susceptibility because *Pvu*II and *Xba*I are tightly linked [55] and it is difficult to identify which one has a role to play.

Given its multifactorial nature, it is likely that the pathogenesis of SLE may be modulated by age, gender, ethnicity, environmental factors and other variables. We therefore carried out subgroup analysis based on ethnicity. Associations between SLE

susceptibility and the *ESR1 Pvu*II C allele and the *ESR1 Xba*I G allele were found in individuals of Asian descent. This may be attributable to genetic heterogeneity among different populations. Consistent with this, ethnicity contributed to the heterogeneity for *ESR1 Pvu*II and *ESR1 Xba*I. Moreover, sensitivity analysis revealed that the heterogeneity was reduced by removing Johansson *et al.*'s [31] study, which was the only study in the meta-analysis of the association between *ESR1 Xba*I polymorphism and SLE susceptibility that was based on Caucasians. It is also possible that differences in lifestyle and environmental factors between different populations may interact with genes to affect the pathogenesis of SLE.

This meta-analysis had some inevitable limitations. First, three studies on the *IL1-RN* VNTR polymorphism did not provide genotype data, and the data used to analyze the various genetic models were thus not completely consistent. This may lead to misinterpretation of the association between the *IL1-RN* VNTR polymorphism and SLE susceptibility. Second, although all eligible studies were included in our study, the small sample size and low statistical power (Table S4, S5 and S6) associated with the low incidence of SLE means that there is a possibility of false negative results. We expect more participants being tested in the future to draw a more reliable conclusion. Third, deviation of genotype distributions from HWE in the control populations in some studies may reflect genotyping errors or control selection bias. The results relating to *IL1-RN* VNTR and *ESR1 Pvu*II changed when these studies were excluded, suggesting that these results should be interpreted with caution. Fourth, as mentioned above, various factors affect the pathology of SLE; the lack of individual data meant that we only pooled the data based on unadjusted information. Finally, the quality scores were not high for some studies and these studies may have distorted the results.

In conclusion, this meta-analysis indicated that the *IL1-RN* VNTR 2 allele and the *ESR1 Pvu*II CC/CT and *ESR1 Xba*I

GG/GA genotypes may increase the susceptibility to SLE, especially in individuals of Asian descent. However, this conclusion should be interpreted cautiously because of the low statistical power and considerable heterogeneity. Also, further functional studies are needed to investigate the functions of these alleles. Well-designed, large studies in different ethnic groups and with more detailed information on age, sex, and age of onset of the disease are needed to validate our results. Studies of gene-environment interactions in relation to *IL1-RN-ESR1* should also be performed to confirm our preliminary findings.

Supporting Information

Table S1 Meta analysis of the association of *IL1-RN VNTR* polymorphism with SLE susceptibility.

Table S2 Meta analysis of the association of *ESR1 Pvu*II polymorphism with SLE susceptibility.

Table S3 Meta analysis of the association of *ESR1 Xba*I polymorphism with SLE susceptibility.

Table S4 The statistical power of *IL1-RN VNTR* 2 allele in studied included in the meta-analysis.

Table S5 The statistical power of *ESR1 Pvu*II CC/CT genotypes in studied included in the meta-analysis.

Table S6 The statistical power of *ESR1 Xba*I GG/GA genotypes in studied included in the meta-analysis.

Author Contributions

Conceived and designed the experiments: X. Xia YZ. Performed the experiments: LC JWZ Jia-jia Wang. Analyzed the data: LC JWZ. Contributed reagents/materials/analysis tools: X. Xue ZGW Shao-wen Tang Jie Wang. Wrote the paper: LC JWZ Shai-di Tang.

References

1. Tsokos GC (2011) Systemic lupus erythematosus. N Engl J Med 365: 2110–2121.
2. D'Cruz DP, Khamashta MA, Hughes GR (2007) Systemic lupus erythematosus. Lancet 369: 587–596.
3. Yap DY, Lai KN (2013) The role of cytokines in the pathogenesis of systemic lupus erythematosus - from bench to bedside. Nephrology (Carlton) 18: 243–255.
4. Boswell JM, Yui MA, Burt DW, Kelley VE (1988) Increased tumor necrosis factor and IL-1 beta gene expression in the kidneys of mice with lupus nephritis. J Immunol 141: 3050–3054.
5. Segal R, Bermas BL, Dayan M, Kalush F, Shearer GM, et al. (1997) Kinetics of cytokine production in experimental systemic lupus erythematosus: involvement of T helper cell 1/T helper cell 2-type cytokines in disease. J Immunol 158: 3009–3016.
6. Smith DE, Renshaw BR, Ketchem RR, Kubin M, Garka KE, et al. (2000) Four new members expand the interleukin-1 superfamily. J Biol Chem 275: 1169–1175.
7. Dinarello CA (1998) Interleukin-1, interleukin-1 receptors and interleukin-1 receptor antagonist. Int Rev Immunol 16: 457–499.
8. Vamvakopoulos JE, Taylor CJ, Morris-Stiff GJ, Green C, Metcalfe S (2002) The interleukin-1 receptor antagonist gene: a single-copy variant of the intron 2 variable number tandem repeat (VNTR) polymorphism. Eur J Immunogenet 29: 337–340.
9. Blakemore AI, Tarlow JK, Cork MJ, Gordon C, Emery P, et al. (1994) Interleukin-1 receptor antagonist gene polymorphism as a disease severity factor in systemic lupus erythematosus. Arthritis Rheum 37: 1380–1385.
10. Tsai IJ, Lan JL, Lin CY, Hsiao SH, Tsai LM, et al. (2006) The different expression patterns of interleukin-1 receptor antagonist in systemic lupus erythematosus. Tissue Antigens 68: 493–501.
11. Lee YH, Kim HJ, Rho YH, Choi SJ, Ji JD, et al. (2004) Interleukin-1 receptor antagonist gene polymorphism and rheumatoid arthritis. Rheumatol Int 24: 133–136.
12. Parks CG, Cooper GS, Dooley MA, Treadwell EL, St Clair EW, et al. (2004) Systemic lupus erythematosus and genetic variation in the interleukin 1 gene cluster: a population based study in the southeastern United States. Ann Rheum Dis 63: 91–94.
13. Ansar Ahmed S, Penhale WJ, Talal N (1985) Sex hormones, immune responses, and autoimmune diseases. Mechanisms of sex hormone action. Am J Pathol 121: 531–551.
14. Tucker LB, Menon S, Schaller JG, Isenberg DA (1995) Adult- and childhood-onset systemic lupus erythematosus: a comparison of onset, clinical features, serology, and outcome. Br J Rheumatol 34: 866–872.
15. Roubinian JR, Talal N, Greenspan JS, Goodman JR, Siiteri PK (1978) Effect of castration and sex hormone treatment on survival, anti-nucleic acid antibodies, and glomerulonephritis in NZB/NZW F1 mice. J Exp Med 147: 1568–1583.
16. Yuan Y, Shimizu I, Shen M, Aoyagi E, Takenaka H, et al. (2008) Effects of estradiol and progesterone on the proinflammatory cytokine production by mononuclear cells from patients with chronic hepatitis C. World J Gastroenterol 14: 2200–2207.
17. Cunningham M, Gilkeson G (2011) Estrogen receptors in immunity and autoimmunity. Clin Rev Allergy Immunol 40: 66–73.
18. Kim C, Cadet P (2010) Environmental toxin 4-nonylphenol and autoimmune diseases: using DNA microarray to examine genetic markers of cytokine expression. Arch Med Sci 6: 321–327.
19. Lee YJ, Shin KS, Kang SW, Lee CK, Yoo B, et al. (2004) Association of the oestrogen receptor alpha gene polymorphisms with disease onset in systemic lupus erythematosus. Ann Rheum Dis 63: 1244–1249.
20. Kisiel BM, Kosinska J, Wierzbowska M, Rutkowska-Sak L, Musiej-Nowakowska E, et al. (2011) Differential association of juvenile and adult systemic lupus erythematosus with genetic variants of oestrogen receptors alpha and beta. Lupus 20: 85–89.
21. Jonsen A, Bengtsson AA, Sturfelt G, Truedsson L (2004) Analysis of HLA DR, HLA DQ, C4A, FcgammaRIIa, FcgammaRIIIa, MBL, and IL-1Ra allelic variants in Caucasian systemic lupus erythematosus patients suggests an effect of the combined FcgammaRIIa R/R and IL-1Ra 2/2 genotypes on disease susceptibility. Arthritis Res Ther 6: R557–562.
22. Huang CM, Wu MC, Wu JY, Tsai FJ (2002) Interleukin-1 receptor antagonist gene polymorphism in chinese patients with systemic lupus erythematosus. Clin Rheumatol 21: 255–257.
23. Zhu W, Xie HF, Shi W, Liu ZR (2000) Interleukin-1 receptor antagonist gene polymorphism in patients with systemic lupus erythematosus. Chin J Dermatol 33: 35.
24. Tjernstrom F, Hellmer G, Nived O, Truedsson L, Sturfelt G (1999) Synergetic effect between interleukin-1 receptor antagonist allele (IL1RN*2) and MHC class II (DR17,DQ2) in determining susceptibility to systemic lupus erythematosus. Lupus 8: 103–108.
25. Heward J, Allahabadia A, Gordon C, Sheppard MC, Barnett AH, et al. (1999) The interleukin-1 receptor antagonist gene shows no allelic association with three autoimmune diseases. Thyroid 9: 627–628.
26. Suzuki H, Matsui Y, Kashiwagi H (1997) Interleukin-1 receptor antagonist gene polymorphism in Japanese patients with systemic lupus erythematosus. Arthritis Rheum 40: 389–390.
27. Wang J, Nuite M, McAlindon TE (2010) Association of estrogen and aromatase gene polymorphisms with systemic lupus erythematosus. Lupus 19: 734–740.
28. Lu ZM, Wang ZE, Wu CX, Wang CY, Zhang BC, et al. (2009) Association of Estrogen Receptor α Gene Polymorphisms with Cytokine Genes Expression in Systemic Lupus Erythematosus. Croatian Medical Journal 50: 117–123.
29. Li F, Che ZX, Liu YQ, Fu HL, Wang ZE, et al. (2008) Association between estrogen receptor α gene polymorphisms and systemic lupus erythematosus in Chinese women. Chin J Clinical Laboratory Science 26: 112–114.
30. Chen H, Fan Y, Men JL (2008) Relationship between estrogen receptor gene polymorphisms and SLE. Chin J Dermatol 41: 46–48.
31. Johansson M, Arlestig L, Moller B, Smedby T, Rantapaa-Dahlqvist S (2005) Oestrogen receptor {alpha} gene polymorphisms in systemic lupus erythematosus. Ann Rheum Dis 64: 1611–1617.
32. Tan EM, Cohen AS, Fries JF, Masi AT, McShane DJ, et al. (1982) The 1982 revised criteria for the classification of systemic lupus erythematosus. Arthritis Rheum 25: 1271–1277.
33. Hochberg MC (1997) Updating the American College of Rheumatology revised criteria for the classification of systemic lupus erythematosus. Arthritis Rheum 40: 1725.
34. Wells GA, Shea B, O'Connell D, Peterson J, Welch V, et al. Home>Our Research>Research Programs>Clinical Epidemiology>The Newcastle-Ottawa Scale (NOS) for Assessing the Quality of Nonrandomised Studies in Meta-analyses [Web page]. Ottawa, ON: Ottawa Hospital Research Institute; n.d. [Available online at: http://www.ohri.ca/programs/clinical_epidemiology/oxford.asp; Accessed 2012 February 10.
35. Higgins JP, Thompson SG, Deeks JJ, Altman DG (2003) Measuring inconsistency in meta-analyses. BMJ 327: 557–560.

36. Egger M, Davey Smith G, Schneider M, Minder C (1997) Bias in meta-analysis detected by a simple, graphical test. BMJ 315: 629–634.

37. Rus V, Atamas SP, Shustova V, Luzina IG, Selaru F, et al. (2002) Expression of cytokine- and chemokine-related genes in peripheral blood mononuclear cells from lupus patients by cDNA array. Clin Immunol 102: 283–290.

38. Garat C, Arend WP (2003) Intracellular IL-1Ra type 1 inhibits IL-1-induced IL-6 and IL-8 production in Caco-2 intestinal epithelial cells through inhibition of p38 mitogen-activated protein kinase and NF-kappaB pathways. Cytokine 23: 31–40.

39. Hsieh SC, Tsai CY, Sun KH, Tsai YY, Tsai ST, et al. (1995) Defective spontaneous and bacterial lipopolysaccharide-stimulated production of interleukin-1 receptor antagonist by polymorphonuclear neutrophils of patients with active systemic lupus erythematosus. Br J Rheumatol 34: 107–112.

40. Danis VA, Millington M, Hyland VJ, Grennan D (1995) Cytokine production by normal human monocytes: inter-subject variation and relationship to an IL-1 receptor antagonist (IL-1Ra) gene polymorphism. Clin Exp Immunol 99: 303–310.

41. Santtila S, Savinainen K, Hurme M (1998) Presence of the IL-1RA allele 2 (IL1RN*2) is associated with enhanced IL-1beta production in vitro. Scand - J Immunol 47: 195–198.

42. Vamvakopoulos J, Green C, Metcalfe S (2002) Genetic control of IL-1beta bioactivity through differential regulation of the IL-1 receptor antagonist. Eur J Immunol 32: 2988–2996.

43. Tarlow JK, Blakemore AI, Lennard A, Solari R, Hughes HN, et al. (1993) Polymorphism in human IL-1 receptor antagonist gene intron 2 is caused by variable numbers of an 86-bp tandem repeat. Hum Genet 91: 403–404.

44. Korthagen NM, van Moorsel CH, Kazemier KM, Ruven HJ, Grutters JC (2012) IL1RN genetic variations and risk of IPF: a meta-analysis and mRNA expression study. Immunogenetics 64: 371–377.

45. Nilsson N, Carlsten H (1994) Estrogen induces suppression of natural killer cell cytotoxicity and augmentation of polyclonal B cell activation. Cell Immunol 158: 131–139.

46. Kanda N, Tsuchida T, Tamaki K (1999) Estrogen enhancement of anti-double-stranded DNA antibody and immunoglobulin G production in peripheral blood mononuclear cells from patients with systemic lupus erythematosus. Arthritis Rheum 42: 328–337.

47. Paharkova-Vatchkova V, Maldonado R, Kovats S (2004) Estrogen preferentially promotes the differentiation of CD11c+ CD11b(intermediate) dendritic cells from bone marrow precursors. J Immunol 172: 1426–1436.

48. Suzuki T, Shimizu T, Yu HP, Hsieh YC, Choudhry MA, et al. (2007) Salutary effects of 17beta-estradiol on T-cell signaling and cytokine production after trauma-hemorrhage are mediated primarily via estrogen receptor-alpha. Am J Physiol Cell Physiol 292: C2103–2111.

49. Cohen JH, Danel L, Cordier G, Saez S, Revillard JP (1983) Sex steroid receptors in peripheral T cells: absence of androgen receptors and restriction of estrogen receptors to OKT8-positive cells. J Immunol 131: 2767–2771.

50. Speirs V, Kerin MJ, Newton CJ, Walton DS, Green AR, et al. (1999) Evidence for transcriptional activation of ERalpha by IL-1beta in breast cancer cells. Int J Oncol 15: 1251–1254.

51. Bouman A, Moes H, Heineman MJ, de Leij LF, Faas MM (2001) The immune response during the luteal phase of the ovarian cycle: increasing sensitivity of human monocytes to endotoxin. Fertil Steril 76: 555–559.

52. Cannon JG, Dinarello CA (1985) Increased plasma interleukin-1 activity in women after ovulation. Science 227: 1247–1249.

53. Polan ML, Loukides JA, Honig J (1994) Interleukin-1 in human ovarian cells and in peripheral blood monocytes increases during the luteal phase: evidence for a midcycle surge in the human. Am J Obstet Gynecol 170: 1000–1006; discussion 1006–1007.

54. Herrington DM, Howard TD, Brosnihan KB, McDonnell DP, Li X, et al. (2002) Common estrogen receptor polymorphism augments effects of hormone replacement therapy on E-selectin but not C-reactive protein. Circulation 105: 1879–1882.

55. Liu ZH, Cheng ZH, Gong RJ, Liu H, Liu D, et al. (2002) Sex differences in estrogen receptor gene polymorphism and its association with lupus nephritis in Chinese. Nephron 90: 174–180.

Dysregulated Cytokine Production by Dendritic Cells Modulates B Cell Responses in the NZM2410 Mouse Model of Lupus

Allison Sang[1], Ying-Yi Zheng[1], Yiming Yin[1], Igor Dozmorov[2], Hao Li[3], Hui-Chen Hsu[3], John D. Mountz[3], Laurence Morel[1]*

1 Department of Pathology, Immunology, and Laboratory Medicine, University of Florida, Gainesville, Florida, United States of America, 2 Department of Immunology, University of Texas Southwestern Medical Center, Dallas, Texas, United States of America, 3 Clinical Immunology and Rheumatology, Department of Medicine, University of Alabama at Birmingham, Birmingham, Alabama, United States of America

Abstract

The breakdown in tolerance of autoreactive B cells in the lupus-prone NZM2410-derived B6.*Sle1.Sle2.Sle3* (TC) mice results in the secretion of autoantibodies. TC dendritic cells (DCs) enhance B cell proliferation and antibody secretion in a cytokine-dependent manner. However, the specific cytokine milieu by which TC DCs activate B cells was not known. In this study, we compared TC and C57BL/6 (B6) control for the distribution of DC subsets and for their production of cytokines affecting B cell responses. We show that TC DCs enhanced B cell proliferation through the production of IL-6 and IFN-γ, while antibody secretion was only dependent on IL-6. Pre-disease TC mice showed an expanded PDCA1+ cells prior to disease onset that was localized to the marginal zone and further expanded with age. The presence of PDCA1+ cells in the marginal zone correlated with a Type I Interferon (IFN) signature in marginal zone B cells, and this response was higher in TC than B6 mice. *In vivo* administration of anti-chromatin immune complexes upregulated IL-6 and IFN-γ production by splenic DCs from TC but not B6 mice. The production of BAFF and APRIL was decreased upon TC DC stimulation both *in vitro* and *in vivo*, indicating that these B cell survival factors do not play a role in B cell modulation by TC DCs. Finally, TC B cells were defective at downregulating IL-6 expression in response to anti-inflammatory apoptotic cell exposure. Overall, these results show that the TC autoimmune genetic background induces the production of B cell-modulating inflammatory cytokines by DCs, which are regulated by the microenvironment as well as the interplay between DC.

Editor: Marc S. Horwitz, University of British Columbia, Canada

Funding: JDM is supported by VA Merit Review Grant (1I01BX000600-01), National Institutes of Health/National Institute of Allergy and Infectious Diseases (1AI 071110), and Rheumatology Education Foundation. HCH is supported by NIH/NIAID (1RO1AI083705) and Lupus Research Institute. The funders had no role in study design, data collection and analysis, decision to publish, or preparation of the manuscript.

Competing Interests: The authors have declared that no competing interests exist.

* Email: morel@ufl.edu

Introduction

Systemic lupus erythematosus (SLE) is an autoimmune disease characterized by the loss of tolerance to self-antigens by B cells, resulting in the production of pathogenic autoantibodies (autoAbs). Dendritic cells (DC) can be classified into two main categories, classical DCs (cDC) and plasmacytoid DCs (pDC). Both pDCs and cDCs promote autoAb secretion by B cells. pDCs produce type I IFN in response to apoptotic cell autoantigens, and cDCs activated either by type I IFN or T cells secrete IL-6. Furthermore, both type I IFN and IL-6 can contribute directly or indirectly to autoAb production [1]. We have used the NZM2410-derived B6.*Sle1.-Sle2.Sle3* (TC) lupus-prone mouse to investigate how DCs contribute to B cell dysfunction. TC mice are C57BL/6 (B6) congenic mice that express the three lupus susceptibility loci (*Sle1, Sle2, Sle3*) that are necessary and sufficient to induce a full clinical disease similar to that of NZM2410. The TC autoimmune phenotypes include early pre-disease lymphocyte activation, the production of high titers of anti-dsDNA IgG by 5 month of age, and lupus nephritis by 7 month of age [2].

We have previously shown that anti-CD40 stimulated bone-marrow derived DCs (BMDC) from TC mice secreted high levels of IL-6 and induced B cell proliferation and Ab production [3]. IL-6 is an essential cytokine for B cell proliferation and plasma cell differentiation [4,5]. In SLE patients, IL-6 levels correlate with disease activity [6,7]. Blocking IL-6 signaling in murine models of lupus ameliorated disease and suppressed the production of anti-dsDNA autoAbs [8,9]. However, the inability of IL-6 antagonists to block DC-mediated B cell proliferation indicates that additional cytokines produced by TC DCs regulate B cell functions.

pDCs selectively express TLR7 and TLR9 which recognize RNA or DNA [10]. The activation of pDCs by apoptotic cell debris results in the production of large amounts of type I IFNs that have pleiotropic effects on B cells, including enhanced activation, survival, Ab and cytokine secretion [11]. A type I IFN signature has been recognized as a hallmark of lupus pathogenesis [12], and a recent study has identified a type I IFN signature in both cDCs and pDCs from TC mice that preceded disease onset, suggesting a causative role in pathogenesis [13].

Depletion of both cDCs and pDCs ameliorated lupus patho-genesis in the MRL/*lpr* model, including a decreased plasmablast numbers and autoAb production, suggesting a direct effect on B cells [14]. DCs can contribute to B cell-related pathogenesis both by the production of inflammatory cytokines and B cell survival factors. Cell-to-cell contact between activated DCs and B cells was not required to induce proliferation, which further confirmed the importance of DC-derived cytokines in lupus pathology [3]. Since there is no correlation between elevated DC numbers and autoimmunity [15], functional differences, including increased production of inflammatory cytokines, are most likely responsible for the role DCs play in lupus. The expression of CD86 is elevated on DCs from SLE patients, indicating that DCs have an activated phenotype during active disease [16]. Recent work has shown that DC-specific ablation of *Shp1*, a phosphatase highly expressed by DCs, led to a lupus-like phenotype with significantly elevated secretion of inflammatory cytokines by DCs [17]. Overall, these studies suggest that defects in DC regulation create an environ-ment that fosters the activation of self-reactive B cells into Ab-producing cells.

In this study, we explore the effects of DCs from lupus-prone TC mice on B cell function. Our results show that anti-CD40 activated BMDCs from TC lupus-prone mice induce a greater B cell proliferation in an IL-6 and IFN-γ dependent manner. In addition, IL-6, but not IFN-γ produced by DCs, enhances the secretion of IgM by B cells. Confirming these results, splenic DCs from TC mice produce elevated levels of IL-6 and IFN-γ in the presence of anti-chromatin ICs. Total splenic DCs from TC mice have an expanded pDC population that is largely concentrated in the marginal zone (MZ). This expansion correlated with a type I IFN signature in TC MZ B cells, suggesting an interaction between pDCs and MZ B cells in the lupus mice. Finally, MZ B cells from TC mice maintained a higher IL-6 secretion in response to anti-inflammatory apoptotic cells than MZ B cells from B6 mice. Overall, these results demonstrate that the dysregulation of cytokine networks in DCs from lupus mice, in which IL-6 and both type I and II IFNs play a major role, contribute to the activation of pathogenic B cells.

Materials and Methods

Mice

The B6.NZM-*Sle1*$^{NZM2410/Aeg}$ *Sle2*$^{NZM2410/Aeg}$ *Sle3*$^{NZM2410/Aeg}$/LmoJ (TC in this paper) congenic strain has been previously described [18]. Age-matched C57BL/6J (B6) mice were used for all experiments. Only female mice were used in this study at the age indicated for each experiment. All mice were bred and maintained at the University of Florida in specific pathogen-free conditions.

Ethic statement

Experiments using mice reported here were approved by the Institutional Animal Care and Use Committee of the University of Florida (UF #201303860).

Flow Cytometry

Single cell suspensions of splenocytes were treated with 155 mM of NH_4Cl for 5 min to lyse red blood cells and were passed through a pre-separation filter (Miltenyi Biotec) to remove debris. Cells were blocked on ice for 30 min with 10% rabbit serum and anti-CD16/32 (2.4G2) in staining buffer (2.5% FBS, 0.05% sodium azide in PBS). Cells were then stained for 30 min on ice with pre-determined amounts of the following fluorophore-conjugated or biotinylated Abs: CD21 (4E3), CD23 (B3B4), IgM

(II/41), CD11c (HL3), CD8 (53-6.7), DCIR2 (33D1), DEC205 (205yekta), PDCA-1 (927), IFNγ (XMG1.2), all purchased from either eBiosciences or BD Biosciences. Dead cells were gated out with the Fixable Viability Dye eFluor 780. Intracellular staining for IFN-γ was performed on cells fixed and permeabilized with eBiosciences reagents. Stained cells were processed on a CyAn flow cytometer (Beckman Coulter) and at least 100,000 cells were acquired per sample. Flow cytometry data sets were analyzed with the FCS Express software (De Novo).

Generation of BMDCs and BMDC/B Cell Co-Cultures

Bone marrow (BM)-derived DCs (BMDCs) were differentiated with 10 ng/ml GM-CSF (Peprotech) and 5 ng/ml IL-4 (Pepro-tech), then purified with anti-CD11c beads (Miltenyi Biotec), as previously described [3]. CD43$^-$ B cells were isolated from B6 splenocytes by negative selection (Miltenyi Biotec). For BMDC-B cell co-cultures, 2×10^4 BMDCs from either TC or B6 mice were cultured for 5 d with 10^5 B cells and 10 ug/ml anti-CD40 Ab (1C10) (eBioscience) in duplicate as previously described [3]. The effect of cytokine inhibition on B cell proliferation was studied by adding 10 ug/ml of anti-IL-6 (MP5-20F3) (BD Biosciences) and/or anti-IFN-γ (XMG1.2) (eBioscience) to the co-cultures. To quantify cytokine secretion by activated BMDCs, 2×10^4 BMDCs were cultured with 10 ug/ml anti-CD40 Ab for 24 h, after which RNA was extracted for qRT-PCR and gene array analyses, and supernatants were collected from the cultures for ELISA. IFN-γ was also quantified by intracellular flow cytometry, and BMDCs stimulated with either IL-12 (5 ng/ml) or IL-18 (20 ng/ml) were used as positive controls. Mice used in these experiments were 2–3 months of age.

In Vivo Cytokine Production

Two month old mice were first injected i.p. with 250 ul of pristane (Sigma) on d0 and d7. On d10, they were injected with 10^7 cells from the PL2-8 hybridoma (anti-chromatin IgG2b) [19] or from the C4010 hybridoma (anti-TNP IgG2a^b) [20], or with PBS, then sacrificed on d17. DCs from mice that received the hybridoma cells or controls were isolated from collagenase (Roche) -digested spleens by positive selection with anti-CD11c magnetic beads as previously described [21].

Cytokine and Gene Expression Quantification

Gene expression was quantified by qPCR from RNA extracted from BMDCs, splenic DCs or from sorted MZ/FO B cells using Sybr Green (Applied Biosystems) as previously described [22]. *Gapdh* was used as internal control. The results were normalized to the average unstimulated or 2 month old B6 values. The primers used are listed in Table 1. In addition, a Taqman Gene Expression Assay (Applied Biosystems) was used to measure *Irf7* (Mm00516788_m1) expression relative to *Ppia* (Mm02342429_g1) endogenous control. ELISA kits were used to quantify IL-6, IL-10, IFN-γ (BD Biosciences), and BAFF (R&D Systems) from the culture supernatants. Additional cytokines from culture supernatants were assessed using the Mouse Autoimmune Response Multi-Analyte ELISArray Kit (Qiagen), all according to the manufacturers' instructions. Microarray gene expression profiling was performed from B6 B cells cultured for 5 d with the supernatant of anti-CD40-activated BMDCs from either B6 or TC mice (N = 4 in each group), as previously described [3]. cDNAs from the B6 B cells was synthesized and labeled with the Ovation Biotin RNA Amplification and Labeling System (NuGEN Technologies, Inc.) before hybridization to Affymetrix Mouse Genome 430 2.0 arrays. The analysis was conducted as previously described [23]. Functional analysis of identified genes was performed with Ingenuity Pathway Analysis (IPA; Ingenuity Systems, Redwood City, CA). In this paper, we focused on the IFN-γ inducible genes that were differentially expressed between the B cells stimulated with supernatant from either TC or B6 BMDCs with at least a 2 fold difference and a p value≤0.01 for 2-tailed t tests.

Confocal Imaging and Quantitation

Spleens from 2 and 7 month old B6 and TC mice were snap-frozen in Tissue TeK freezing medium (Fisher). Seven micrometer thick frozen sections were fixed to slides in ice-cold acetone for 15 min, air dried for 30 sec and blocked with 1.5% BSA in PBS for 30 min at room temperature. The sections were then stained for 30 min at room temperature in a humidified chamber with purified rat anti mouse PDCA-1 antibody (rat IgG2b; Miltenyi Biotec) and followed by Alexa 555–conjugated goat anti-rat IgG (Life Technologies) for another 30 min. Sections stained only with fluorescence labeled secondary antibody were used as control. All tissue sections were mounted in ProLong Gold Antifade Reagent (Life Technologies) and viewed with a Leica DM IRBE inverted Nomarski/epifluorescence microscope outfitted with Leica TCS NT laser confocal optics. Imaging quantitation was performed with MetaMorph 7.5, image analysis (Molecular Devices, Downingtown, PA, USA). The number of PDCA-1$^+$ cells was computed for the whole splenic section as well as for the marginal zone.

Apoptotic Cell Cultures

To generate apoptotic cells, thymocytes were cultured with 1 uM Dexamethasone (Sigma) for 4 h at 37°C. Staining with 7AAD and Annexin V (BD Biosciences) determined that this treatment typically resulted in 45% of Annexin V$^+$ apoptotic thymocytes and in 1% of 7AAD$^+$ Annexin V$^-$ necrotic thymocytes. Marginal zone and follicular B cells were sorted from purified splenic CD43$^-$ B cells as IgM$^+$CD21$^+$CD23$^-$ for MZ B cells and IgM$^+$CD21$^-$CD23$^+$ for FO B cells, using a FACS Aria-II cell sorter (BD Biosciences). Post-sorting purity of either subset was greater than 90%. The sorted MZ or FO B cells were co-cultured at a 1:7 ratio with apoptotic thymocytes and 1 ug/ml CpG-B (Invivogen) for 3 d at 37°C. Cytokines were quantified from extracted RNA and culture supernatant by qPCR and ELISA, respectively.

Statistical Analysis

Data analysis was performed with GraphPad Prism 6.0 software. Unless indicated, graphs show means and standard errors of the mean (SEM). Statistical significance between strains was determined by two-tailed Mann-Whitney tests or t tests (paired when appropriate) if the data was normally distributed. Multiple comparison test corrections were applied when needed. When indicated, results were normalized to average values for control B6 samples. Significance levels in figures were labeled as * for p<0.05, ** for p<0.01, and *** for p<0.001.

Results

BMDCs from TC lupus-prone mice enhance B cell proliferation through IL-6 and IFN-γ

To compare the effect of T-cell activated DCs on B cells between lupus-prone TC and B6 mice, we used co-cultures of anti-CD40 activated BMDCs from either strain and B6 B cells [3]. Without Flt3L, BMDCs have been shown to mainly correspond to cDCs [24]. Anti-CD40-activated BMDCs obtained from TC mice resulted in a greater number of live B6 B cells than B6 BMDCs *in vitro* (Fig. 1A), confirming our previous results [3]. No difference was observed in the number of dead cells (data not shown). As previously reported, CD40 stimulation in B cells in the absence of BMDCs resulted in similar low levels of proliferation in both strains, indicating that the primary target of anti-CD40 activation in the co-cultures are the DCs. In addition, unstimulated DCs from either strain were not able to support B cell proliferation. Since cell-to-cell contact was not required between TC DCs and B cells to enhance B cell proliferation [3], we compared cytokine secretion between unstimulated and anti-CD40 stimulated B6 and TC BMDCs. As reported previously [3,25], anti-CD40 stimulated TC BMDCs secreted significantly more IL-6 than B6 BMDCs, and no IL-6 was secreted from unstimulated BMDCs in either strain (Fig. 1B). In addition, *Il6* message expression was higher in anti-CD40 stimulated TC than B6 BMDCs although no difference was seen in the absence of stimulation (Fig. 1C).

Quantification of B cell survival factors APRIL and BAFF showed that unstimulated TC BMDCs had higher expression than B6 BMDCs for both cytokines (Fig. 1D–E), which confirms previous studies reporting higher levels of BAFF in these mice [26]. Anti-CD40 stimulation significantly decreased APRIL and BAFF expression in TC BMDCs but not B6 BMDCs. BAFF secretion could not be detected in the culture supernatant of either stimulated or unstimulated DCs (data not shown). This suggests that the enhanced B cell proliferation mediated by anti-CD40 stimulated TC-BMDCs does not result from an increased B cell survival induced by either of these two cytokines. A recent study has shown that the transcriptional repressor Blimp-1 has a

Table 1. Primer sequences for qPCR.

Gene	Forward Primer	Reverse Primer
IL-6	ACCAGAGGAAATTTTCAATAGGC	TGATGCACTTGCAGAAAACA
IL-10	TGTCAAATTCATTCATGGCCT	ATCGATTTCTCCCCTGTGAA
IFN-γ	GAGCTCATTGAATGCTTGGC	GCGTCATTGAATACACACCTG
BAFF	TGCCTTGGAGGAGAAAGAGA	GGCAGTGTTTTGGGCATATT
APRIL	CAGTCCTGCATCTTGTTCCA	GCAGATAAATTCCAGTGTCCC
Blimp-1	GCCAACCAGGAACTTCTTGTGT	AGGATAAACCACCCGAGGGT
Isg-15	GAGCTAGAGCCTGCAGCAAT	TAAGACCGTCCTGGAGCACT
Mx1	GATCCGACTTCACTTCCAGATGG	CATCTCAGTGGTAGTCAACCC
Gapdh	AGCTTGTCATCAACGGGAAG	GTGGTTCACACCCATCACAA

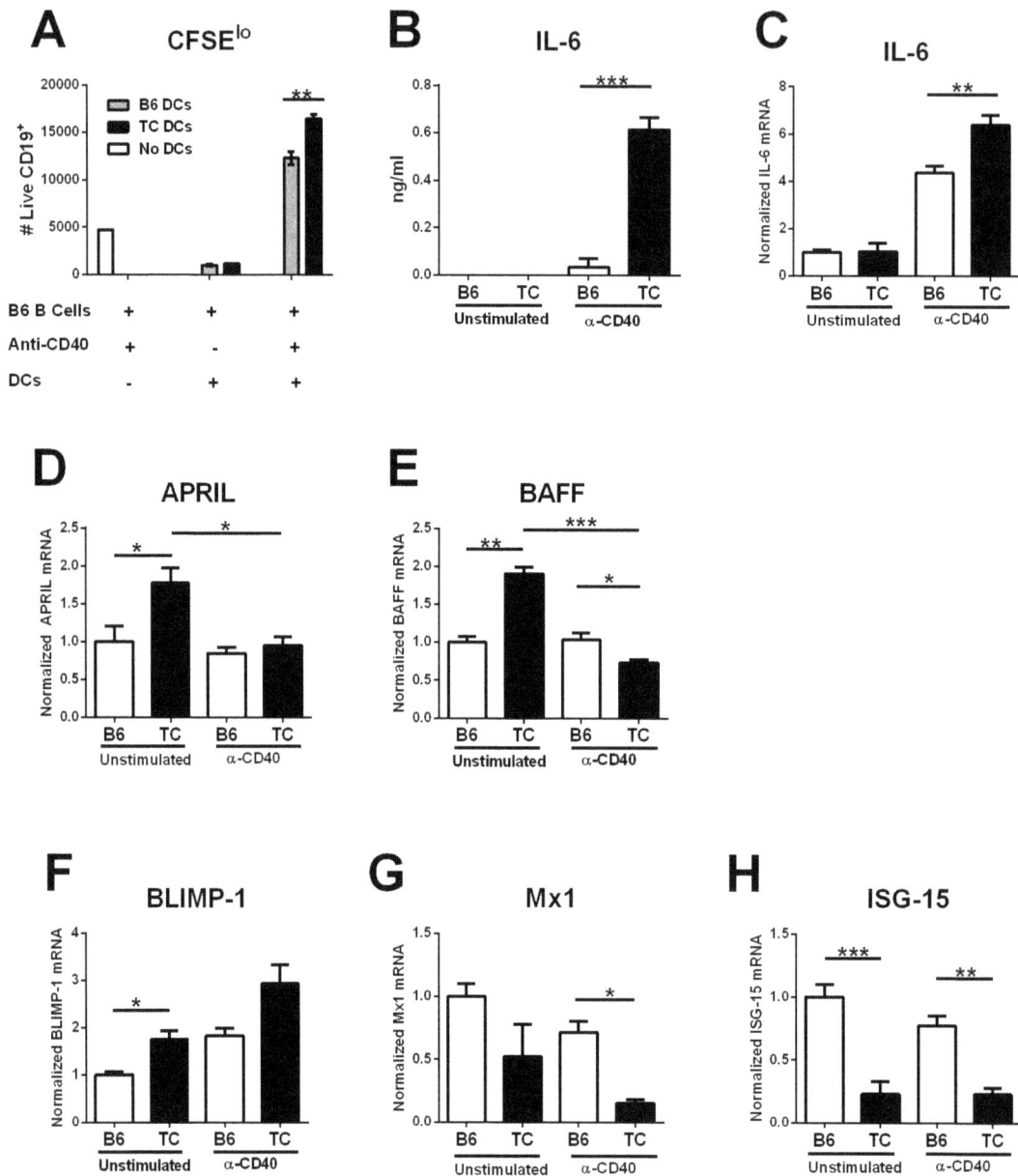

Figure 1. Anti-CD40 activated TC-derived BMDCs secrete high levels of IL-6. A. 10^5 B6 B cells were co-cultured with 2×10^4 TC or B6 BMDCs for 5 d in the presence of anti-CD40 Ab to activate the BMDCs. As controls, B cells were cultured alone with anti-CD40, and DCs were co-cultured with B cells in the absence of anti-CD40. B cell proliferation was measured as the number of live CD19$^+$ CFSE^{lo} cells. Data are representative from two independent experiments. **B.** IL-6 production in the supernatant from 2×10^4 BMDCs stimulated or not with anti-CD40 Ab for 24 h. **C-H.** IL-6, APRIL, BAFF, BLIMP-1, *Mx1*, and *Isg-15* gene expression in BMDCs stimulated or not with anti-CD40 Ab for 24 h. Message expression was normalized to *Gapdh* and expressed relative to the mean values for unstimulated B6 BMDCs for each gene. Significance levels of Bonferroni's multiple comparisons test are shown (N=3 mice per strain per experiment).

tolerogenic function in DCs, and Blimp-1-deficient DCs over-express IL-6, which lead to the development of lupus-like autoAbs [27]. However, Blimp-1 expression was increased in unstimulated and there was a trend for stimulated TC BMDCS as compared to B6 (Fig. 1F). This result demonstrates that the increased IL-6 production by activated TC DCs is not due to a decreased *Prdm1* (encoding for Blimp-1) expression. We also compared the expression of type 1 IFN inducible genes that have been reported to be increased in DCs from young TC mice [13]. Contrary to this previous study, however, we found that TC BMDCs express

significantly lower levels of both *Mx1* and *Isg-15* than B6 BMDCs (Fig. 1G-H).

IFN-γ expression was similar between unstimulated BMDCs from the two strains, but it was significantly higher in TC than B6 BMDCs after anti-CD40 stimulation (Fig. 2A). This difference of expression was confirmed by intracellular flow-cytometry (Fig. 2B), and anti-CD40 stimulation induced a similar IFN-γ production in TC BMDCs than either IL-12p70 or IL-18 (Fig. 2C), two cytokines that have been reported to induce IFN-γ production in DCs [28]. In addition, either IL-12 or IL-18 induced a higher production of IFN-γ by TC than B6 BMDCs

(MFI: 30.51 ± 3.18 vs. $21.47\pm.71$ for IL-12; 27.24 ± 2.32 vs. 19.78 ± 1.10 for IL-18; $p<0.05$). To determine the mechanisms by which TC DC-produced cytokines regulated B cell functions, we compared the gene expression in B6 B cells that had been stimulated with the supernatant of either B6 or TC anti-CD40-stimulated BMDCs. As previously shown [3], the TC-produced supernatant induced a greater percentage of B cells to proliferate than the B6-produced supernatant (Fig. 2D). The B cells stimulated by TC-produced supernatant showed a significant activation of the IFN-γ pathway (Fig. S1), with 19 differentially expressed IFN-γ inducible genes that were found at least a two-fold higher level than in B cells stimulated with B6-procuded supernatant (Fig. 2E). No IFN-γ inducible gene was found at a significantly lower level in B cells stimulated with TC-produced supernatant (data not shown). These results show that anti-CD40 stimulates IFN-γ production in TC DCs, which in turn activates a transcription program in B cells. Interestingly, the array analysis also showed an increase in *Il17a* message expression in B cells exposed to TC-produced supernatant (235.50 ± 68.56 vs. 40.75 ± 1.80, $p=0.03$), as well as in the expression of genes induced by *Il17a* (Fig. S1). IL-6 is a major inducer of IL-17 expression in T cells [29], although IL-6- and RORγt-independent Il-17 programming can be induced by in B cells by *Trypanosoma* [30]. Our data suggest that IL-6 produced by activated TC BMDCs induce IL-17 expression in B cells. Overall, our results showed that IL-6 and IFN-γ are the two major cytokines that are over-expressed in T cell-activated TC BMDCs, and suggest that they may be responsible for the functional changes that we have described in TC DC-stimulated B cells.

IL-6 is a critical cytokine secreted by DCs that induces immunoglobulin production from B cells [31,32]. Accordingly, blocking IL-6 in the DC/B cell co-cultures significantly decreased IgM production induced by either B6 or TC BMDCs (Fig. 3A and B). However, blocking of IL-6 was not sufficient to significantly reduced B cell proliferation induced by either B6 or TC BMDCs (Fig. 3C). Similarly, blocking IFN-γ, the other cytokine produced at higher levels by activated TC BMDCS has little effect on B cell proliferation (Fig. 3C), and had no effect on IgM secretion (data not shown). However, dual inhibition of IL-6 and IFN-γ significantly reduced B cell proliferation induced by both TC and B6 BMDCs, and reduced the effect of TC BMDCS to that of untreated B6 BMDCs. This significant reduction in B cell numbers obtained with the blocking antibodies did not result from increased cell death in the TC BMDC co-cultures as the number of dead B cells in the culture was equal in the B6 and TC BMDC co-cultures (data not shown). Therefore, TC DC-derived IL-6 and IFN-γ in combination increase B cell proliferation and, in addition, DC-derived IL-6 increases IgM production.

Plasmacytoid DCs are expanded in TC mice at a young age

We characterized splenic cDC and pDC subsets in young TC and B6 mice to assess whether the differences observed between B6 and TC BMDCs precede disease onset *in vivo*. The cDC subset can be subdivided into migratory CD8- myeloid DCs and CD8+ resident lymphoid DCs [33,34]. Two month old TC and B6 mice had similar percentages of both myeloid (CD11c+ CD8-) and lymphoid (CD11c+ CD8+) splenic DCs (Fig. 4A-C). Since previous results showed that aged TC mice have elevated numbers of myeloid DCs [25], this suggests that the expansion of that myeloid DCs is age-dependent and may be secondary to disease onset. Thus given that the BMDCs in our cultures are mainly cDCs, as pDCs require Flt3L for differentiation [24], elevated levels of IL-6 and IFN-γ are produced by activated TC cDCs that are expanded

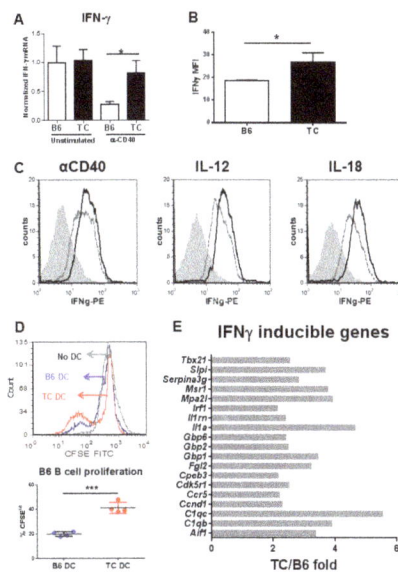

Figure 2. Anti-CD40 activated TC-derived BMDCs secrete IFN-γ.
A. IFN-γ gene expression in BMDCs stimulated or not with anti-CD40 Ab for 24 h. Message expression was normalized to *Gapdh* and expressed relative to the mean values for unstimulated B6 BMDCs for each gene. (N=7 per group). **B**. Intracellular IFN-γ expression expressed as mean fluorescence intensity (MFI) in BMDCs stimulated or not with anti-CD40 Ab for 24 h (N=4 per strain). **C**. Representative FACS plots showing intracellular IFN-γ staining in CD11c^hi viability dye-negative anti-CD40 stimulated BMDCs (corresponding to the graph in B). The middle and right-side overlays shown BMDCs stimulated with IL-12p70 and IL-18 as controls. The solid black lines correspond to TC DCs and the broken lines correspond to B6 DCs. The filled gray histograms show the isotype control. **D**. B6 B cell proliferation measured as CSFE dilution in response to anti-CD40-activated TC BMDC (red) or B6 BMDC (blue) supernatant. The profile of B cell alone is shown as control. Representative FACS overlays and quantitation. **E**. Differential expression of IFN-γ-inducible genes in the B cells shown in D. The graph shows the TC over B6 fold expression for all the IFN-γ-inducible genes that are expressed as a $p<0.01$ different level between the B cells activated with the two different types on activated BMDCs.

after disease onset. We also evaluated a subset of MZ-localized DCIR2+ DEC205- DCs that have been shown to play a role in the activation of extrafollicular B cells [35]. However, young TC and B6 mice showed similar percentage of DCIR2+ (Fig. 4D-E), or DEC205+ splenic DCs (data not shown). This indicated that this recently described DC subset is not involved in the TC model.

Importantly, the percentage of CD11c^mid PDCA-1+ pDCs was significantly higher in young TC mice than in B6 (Fig. 4F, G). It is interesting that while the young B6 mice had a very consistent percentage of pDCs (about 1% splenocytes), the distribution of the TC values was much more variable ($F=51.39$, $p=0.001$), suggesting that this variable rate of expansion of pDCs may be related to the variation in disease onset that is typically observed in these mice [2]. The pDC expansion documented by flow cytometry was confirmed by histology, which showed that the abundance of pDCs in TC spleens was greater than in B6 spleens (Fig. 5A–C). Furthermore, PDCA-1 staining in the spleen showed that pDCs were largely confined to the MZ in both strains (Fig. 5A). The percentage of pDCs in the MZ was higher in TC mice both at 2 month (pre-disease) and at 6 month of age (ongoing autoimmune disease) than in B6 mice. Moreover, the MZ pDCs expanded with age in TC mice, but not in B6 mice (Fig. 5C).

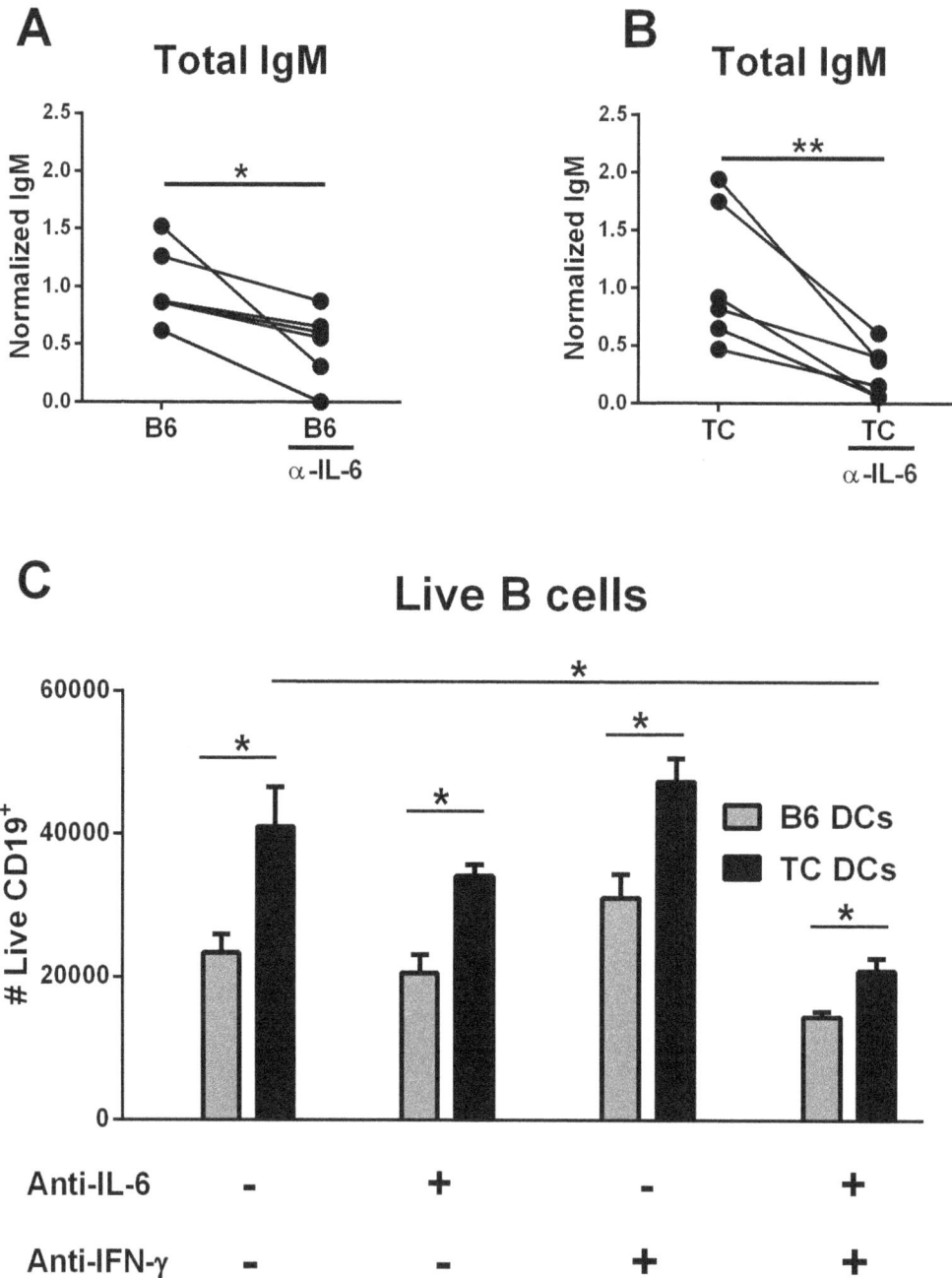

Figure 3. Enhanced B cell proliferation by TC BMDCs is IL-6 and IFN-γ dependent. 2×10^4 BMDCs were co-cultured with 10^5 B cells with anti-CD40 Ab for 5 d. Blocking Abs for IL-6 and/or IFN-γ were added to the co-culture. Blocking IL-6 significantly decreased IgM secretion in co-cultures with either B6 (**A**) or TC (**B**) BMDCs. The significant reduction of the B cell numbers in the TC BMDC co-cultures required the combined blocking of IL-6 and IFN-γ (**C**). Significance was determined by two-tailed paired tests.

pDCs are known for their capacity to secrete high levels of Type I IFNs [10]. TC splenic B cells express a Type I IFN signature prior to disease onset [13]. The preferential localization of pDCs in the MZ of TC mice suggested that the IFN response in B cells was dependent on their location. To test this hypothesis, RNA was extracted from sorted MZ or follicular (FO) B cells that were cultured with CpG-B, a TLR9 ligand with a full phosphorothioate backbone that strongly activates B cells but stimulates weakly IFN-α secretion. *Irf7* and *Isg-15* are two Type I IFN stimulated genes that are expressed at high levels in splenic B cells from young TC mice as compared to B6 [13]. Consistent with our finding that

pDCs are largely located in the MZ, *Irf7* and *Isg-15* expression was higher in MZB than in FOB cells from both strains (Fig. 5D-E). In addition, *Irf7* expression tended to be higher (p = 0.059) in TC than in B6 MZ B cells (Fig. 5D), but *Isg-15* expression was similar between B6 and TC MZ B cells (Fig. 5E). Meanwhile, *Mx1* expression, a commonly used indicator of the Type I IFN signature, could not be detected in either MZ or FO B cells (data not shown), which confirms a recent study showing low expression of *Mx1* by splenic B cells [13]. These results indicate that prior to disease onset, the TC lupus-prone background leads to an

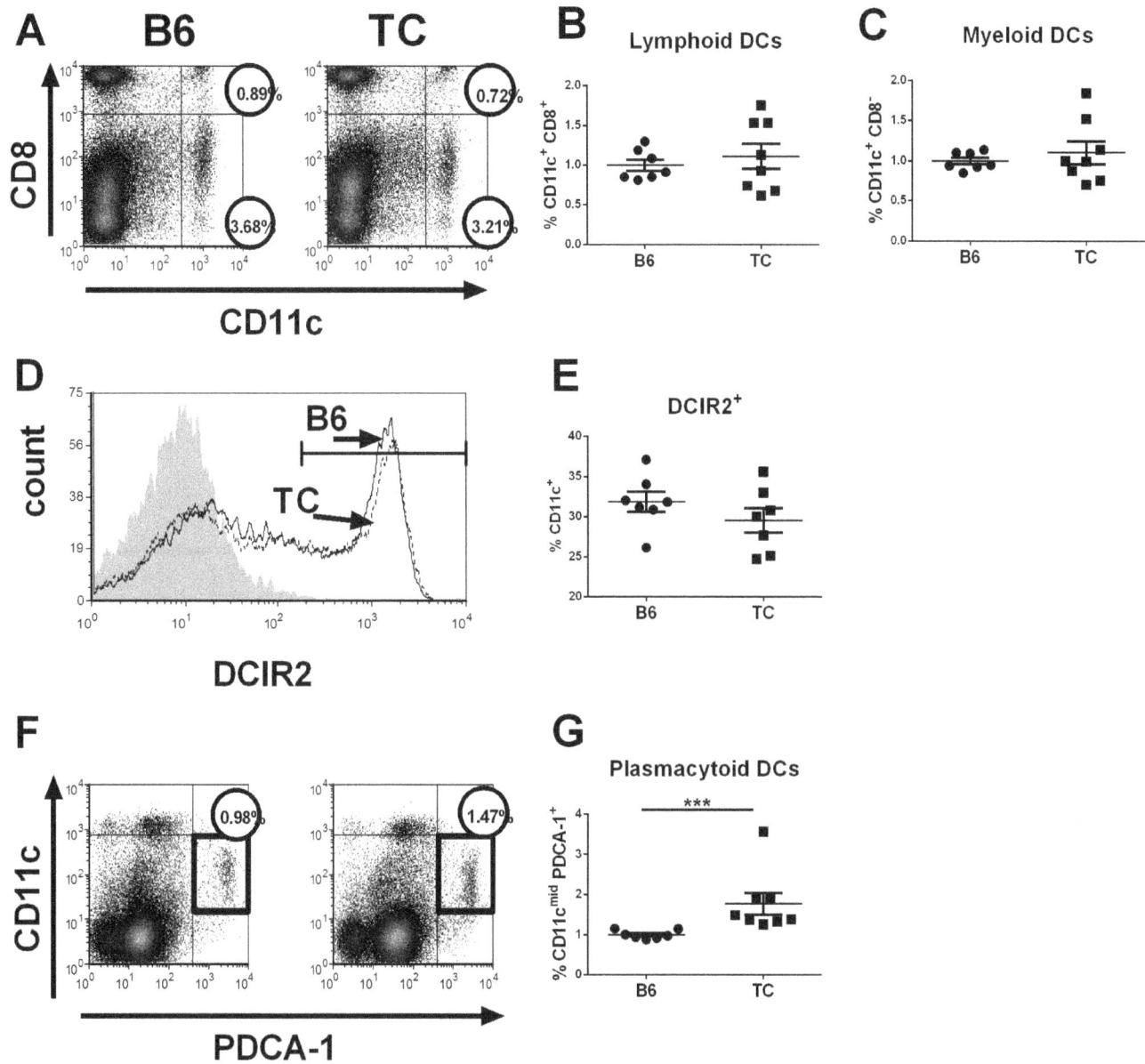

Figure 4. The plasmacytoid DC subset is expanded in young TC mice. Splenic DCs were isolated from 2-3 month old TC and B6 mice. **A.** Representative FACS plots showing the percentage of (**B**) myeloid DCs (CD11c$^+$ CD8$^-$) and (**C**) lymphoid DCs (CD11c$^+$ CD8$^+$). **D.** Representative histogram of DCIR2$^+$ expression on CD11c$^+$ splenic DCs in B6 (black line) and TC (dotted line) mice. The shaded histogram shows the isotype control and the horizontal line the gate for DCIR2$^+$ DCs. The percentage of splenic CD11c$^+$ DCs expressing DCIR2 in each strain is shown in (**E**). **F–G.** Plasmacytoid DCs were identified as CD11c^{mid} PDCA-1$^+$. Graphs show data from two experiments that were normalized to B6 means. Significance levels of two-tailed Mann-Whitney tests are shown.

Chromatin ICs induce IL-6 and IFN-γ secretion in splenic DCs

In addition to Type I IFNs, splenic DCs produce various cytokines in response to TLR7/TLR9 stimulation by anti-chromatin immune complexes (IC) [36], which are a driving factor of lupus pathology [37]. It was of interest to study the DC cytokine response to TLR7/TLR9 ligation *in vivo*, given that TLR7 and TLR9 are expressed at high levels in pDCs [38], a population expanded prior to disease onset in TC mice. To determine the effect of chromatin ICs on the cytokine production

by splenic DCs, we treated young B6 and TC mice with PL2-8 hybridoma cells, which secrete IgG2b anti-chromatin Abs that bind endogenous chromatin to form anti-chromatin IgG2b ICs [39]. Mice were pre-treated with pristane to allow for hybridoma cell survival and sacrificed one week after the hybridoma immunization [19], when cytokine levels were quantified from purified splenic DCs (Fig. 6A).

Anti-chromatin ICs increased the production of IL-6 and IFN-γ in both B6 and TC DCs as compared to mice treated with pristane alone or with a hybridoma that does not produce ICs (Fig. 6B–C). IL-6 and IFN-γ production was significantly higher in TC than in B6 DCs. These results showed that anti-chromatin ICs induced a greater production of IL-6 and IFN-γ expression in TC splenic

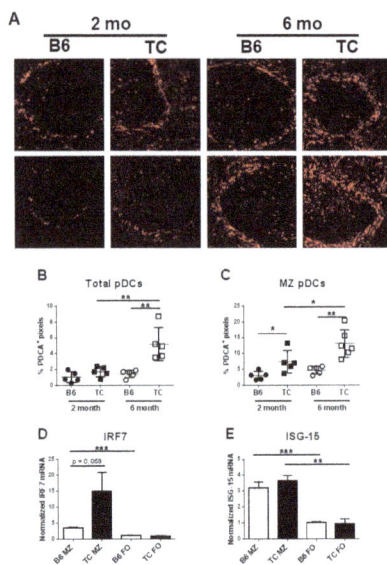

Figure 5. pDCs accumulation in the MZ of TC mice is correlated with a Type I IFN response in MZ B cells. A. Representative splenic sections stained with PDCA-PE showing localization of pDCs in representative 2 month or 6 month old B6 and TC mice. PDCA-1 staining is shown in red (Magnification at 20× dry objective with zooming at 1024*1024; The final magnification is approximately 14.47×20). The percentage of pDCs in total (**B**) and in the MZ (**C**) per splenic section. The location of the marginal zone was determined by the simultaneous presence of IgM⁺ B cells and SIGN-R1⁺ MZ macrophages (data not shown). Data includes 2–3 splenic sections per mouse from two mice per strain per age group. RNAs from sorted MZ or FO B cells cultured with CpG-B for 3 d were assayed for *Irf7* (**D**) and *Isg-15* (**E**) expression by qRT-PCR. Message expression was normalized to *Gapdh*. Significance levels of two-tailed t tests are shown.

DCs. We also examined the effect of hybridoma immunization on BAFF and APRIL levels. While BAFF expression was undetectable in the splenic DCs from immunized mice, APRIL levels were equal between the two strains (Fig. 6D), confirming the results obtained *in vitro* with stimulated BMDCs. Meanwhile, *Isg-15* has been shown to be expressed at higher levels in B6 pDCs than in TC pDCs [13]. Hybridoma immunization resulted in the same trend, with higher *Isg-15* expression in B6 than in TC splenic DCs (Fig. 6E), which could be due to the fact that anti-chromatin ICs expand the pDC population.

We also compared cytokine expression by splenic DCs from untreated TC and B6 mice. Two-month old TC mice produce very little anti-chromatin IgG, while 6-month old TC mice have produced large amounts of these autoantibodies for at least 2 months. The comparison of the cytokines produced by DCs from these two untreated age groups as well as from age-matched B6 controls therefore provided additional information about TC intrinsic determinants vs. anti-chromatin IC determinants. DCs from the older untreated TC mice showed elevated IL-6 levels (Fig. 6F) but decreased IFN-γ as compared to untreated B6, while there was no difference in the younger mice (Fig. 6G). As the levels of IFN-γ declined with age *in vivo* in TC mice, it is possible that the majority of IFN-γ is secreted by a small subset of DCs whose effects are dependent on location rather than size, but their effect is magnified under strong stimulatory conditions. BAFF expression (Fig. 6H) increased with age in DCs from untreated TC mice, and there was a trend toward a greater expression in older TC than B6 DCs. APRIL levels (Fig. 6I) were lower in untreated TC than B6

DCs and remained unchanged with age. Finally, consistent with the results obtained with anti-chromatin IC immunization, there was a lower mRNA expression of *Isg-15* in untreated older TC mice compared to age-matched B6 (Fig. 6J), which could also be due to the relative expansion of pDCs. These results together suggest that *in vivo* chronic self-antigen or IC stimulation of DCs mainly induced IL-6 in TC mice.

Apoptotic cells preferentially reduce IL-6 secretion in B6 MZ B cells

Anti-chromatin ICs also have the potential to elicit a direct response from B cells given that they also express TLR7 and TLR9. Furthermore, TLR9 signaling is essential for the production of the anti-inflammatory cytokine IL-10 by B cells when exposed to apoptotic cells [40]. We hypothesized that the production of inflammatory cytokines by DCs from TC mice impaired the anti-inflammatory response of B cells in response to apoptotic cells. We tested this hypothesis by comparing the downregulation of IL-6 and up-regulation of IL-10 expression by B6 and TC B cells in response to apoptotic cells. Expression of IL-10 can be induced at high levels in MZ, but not FO, B cells cocultured with apoptotic cells and this upregulation was associated with the maintenance of tolerance in normal mice [40]. Therefore, splenic B cells from B6 and TC mice were sorted into FO and MZ B cells and co-cultured with B6 apoptotic cells. This resulted, as expected, by the production of IL-10 by MZ, but not FO, B cells (Fig. 7A). B6 and TC MZ B cells had similar levels of IL-10 mRNA following induction. Interestingly the increased IL-10 levels coincided with significantly decreased IL-6 levels in B6 but the difference was not significant for TC MZ B cells (Fig. 7B).

To further understand if the IL-6 down-regulation in the presence of IL-10 is impaired in the B cells from lupus-prone TC mice, we measured the cytokine levels in the culture supernatants. Confirming the qPCR results, IL-10 levels were equal between B6 and TC MZ B cells cultured with apoptotic cells (Fig. 7C). However, TC MZ B cells secreted significantly more IL-6 than B6 MZ B cells (Fig. 7D). Therefore, the IL-10 to IL-6 ratio was higher in B6 MZ B cells (Fig. 7E). This indicates that the TC lupus-prone B cells are less responsive to anti-inflammatory conditions, resulting in the inefficient down-regulation of the inflammatory cytokine IL-6.

Discussion

B cell tolerance is dysregulated in SLE resulting in the secretion of pathogenic autoAbs. Cytokines play an important role in both promoting and regulating immune responses. We have previously shown that activated DCs promote B cell proliferation and Ab secretion without direct cell to cell interaction via the secretion of cytokines [3]. Furthermore, TC DCs elicit a stronger B cell response than B6 DCs. Here we show that both IL-6 and IFN-γ are required for the TC DC-mediated enhancement of B cell proliferation. However, IL-6 and IFN-γ can compensate for each other as dual inhibition was necessary to restore proliferation to normal levels. Meanwhile, inhibition studies showed that IL-6, but not IFN-γ, was essential for inducing IgM secretion in both B6 and TC mice.

TC DCs did not promote B cell proliferation through the secretion of B cell survival factors as BAFF and APRIL secretion was not elevated in anti-CD40 activated TC DCs. Although unstimulated TC BMDCs produce significantly more BAFF and APRIL than B6 BMDCS, anti-CD40 stimulation eliminated this difference. Given that similar results were obtained after *in vivo* TLR stimulation with anti-chromatin ICs, this suggests that DC-

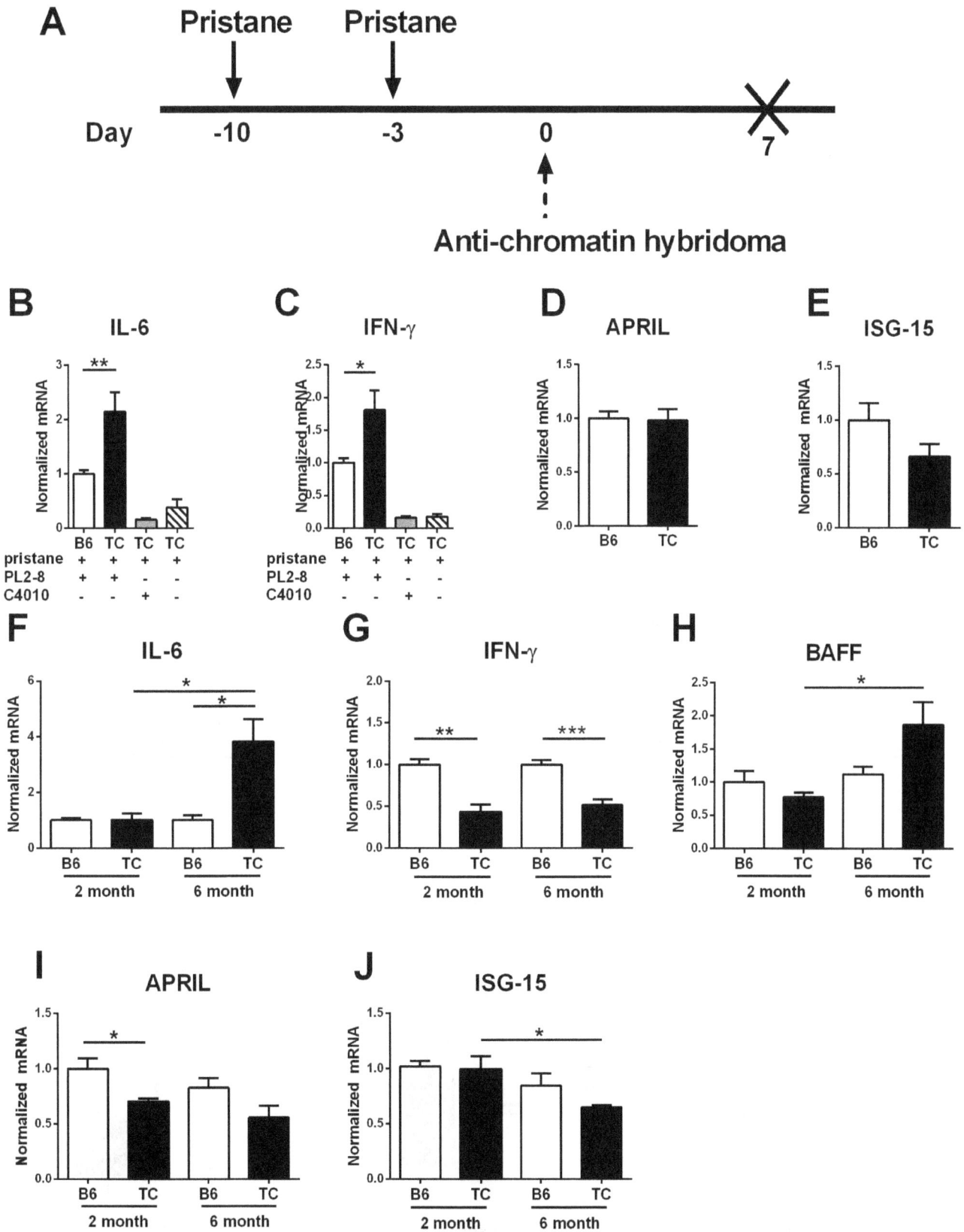

Figure 6. Anti-chromatin ICs induce inflammatory cytokine secretion by splenic DCs in TC mice. A–E. Two month old TC and B6 mice were pre-treated with pristane on days -10 and -3 (solid arrows) followed by immunization with an IgG2b anti-chromatin secreting hybridoma (dashed line) on day 0. Anti- anti-TNP IgG2a[b] C4010 immunization or pristane alone were used as controls. Splenic DCs were isolated on day 7 as shown in **A**, and cytokine expression was quantified by qPCR. Results show the relative mRNA levels of IL-6 (**B**), IFN-γ (**C**), APRIL (**D**), and *Isg-15* (**E**) in these treated mice. **F–J**. splenic DCs were obtained from untreated 2 or 6 month old TC or B6 mice and expression levels of IL-6 (**F**), IFN-γ (**G**), BAFF

(**H**), APRIL (**I**), and *Isg*-15 (**J**) were quantified by qRT-PCR. Cytokine expression was normalized to *Gapdh* and expressed relative to the mean values for B6 DCs (**B–E**) and 2 month old B6 DCs (**F–G**). Results are shown as mean and SEM per group (n = 6 per strain). Significance levels of two-tailed t tests are shown.

derived BAFF and APRIL do not play a significant role in the dysregulation of TC B cells in inflammatory conditions. Since BAFF levels are elevated in NZM2410 mice [26] and in SLE patients [41], it is possible that BMDCs before they are activated in the periphery by T cells or nucleic acid-containing ICs or other cell types are responsible for regulating B cells via the secretion of BAFF and APRIL survival factors. Therefore, activated TC DCs promote B cell proliferation and Ab secretion exclusively by the secretion of pro-inflammatory cytokines.

The recent report showing that Blimp-1 deficiency in DCs resulted in a lupus phenotype that was dependent on IL-6 production [27] led us to investigate whether the high level of IL-6 production by TC DCs was due to a Blimp-1 deficiency. Moreover, PRDM1/BLIMP-1 polymorphisms have been associated with SLE susceptibility in genome-wide association studies [42]. Our results showed, however, a significantly higher Blimp-1 expression in TC BMDCs than in B6, which remained higher

after anti-CD40 stimulation. Blimp-1 negatively regulates DC development but positively regulate DC maturation [43]. More specifically, Blimp-1 expression increases in DCs after TLR activation in a p38 MAPK and NF-kB-dependent manner. Therefore, the increase in Blimp-1 expression in TC DCs fits with their increased level of activation and function [25]. Our results showed, however, that the increased IL-6 production occurs in spite of high Blimp-1 level in B6.TC mice.

pDCs have been a main focus of DC studies in SLE given their high secretion of Type-I IFNs after TLR7/TLR9 stimulation [10]. A previous study showed that both pDCs and myeloid DCs are expanded in aged TC mice [25]. Furthermore, TC DCs express a Type I IFN signature prior to disease onset [13]. We have not been able to reproduce this finding for BMDCs from young mice, and at this time it is not clear whether different environmental conditions for the mice or experimental conditions for the DCs are responsible for this discrepancy. However, we showed that TC

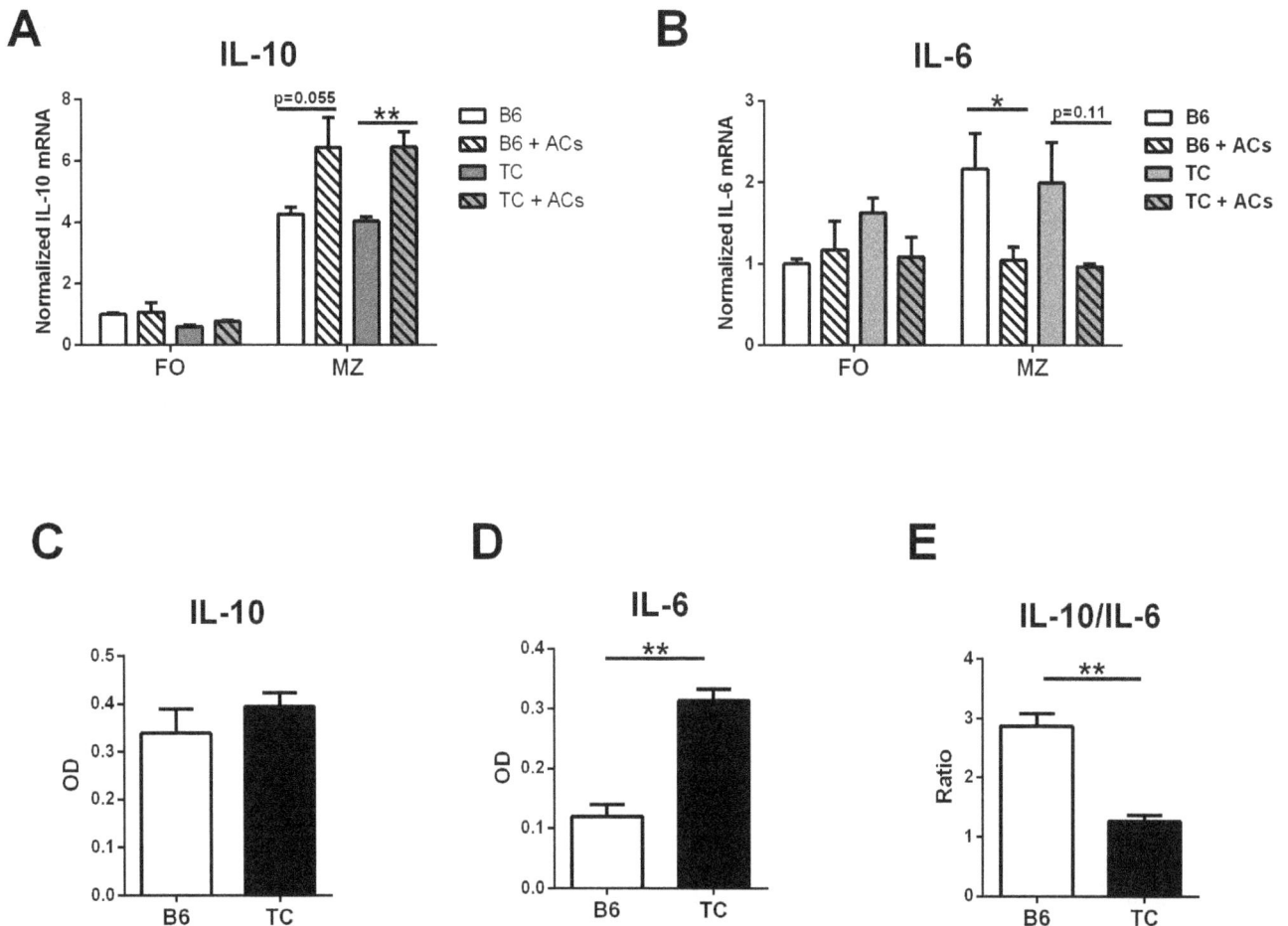

Figure 7. Apoptotic cells preferentially reduce IL-6 secretion by B6 but not TC MZ B cells. Sorted FO and MZ B cells (N = 3 per strain from 2 different sorts) were cultured for 3 d with CpG in the presence or absence of apoptotic cells. IL-10 (**A**) and IL-6 (**B**) mRNA levels in MZ and FO B cells were quantified by qRT-PCR. Message expression was normalized to *Gapdh* and expressed relative to B6 FO B cells. Data from three independent experiments are shown. Culture supernatant from TC and B6 MZ B cells cultured with apoptotic cells was assayed for IL-10 (**C**) and IL-6 (**D**) by ELISA. **E**. Ratio of IL-10 to IL-6 production of MZ B cells cultured with apoptotic cells. Results show mean and SEM value. Significance levels of two-tailed t-tests are shown.

mice have an expanded pDC population prior to disease onset while the myeloid and lymphoid subsets increase with disease progression. Interestingly, we found that the pDCs were enriched in the MZ in both B6 and TC mice, but this expansion does not overlap with the DCIR2+ subset that has been recently reported in the MZ [35]. pDCs expansion and localization to the MZ has been previously reported after CpG treatment [44], Toxoplasma infection [45], as well as primary cutaneous marginal zone lymphomas [46]. Our study is the first, to our knowledge, to report a naturally occurring concentration of pDCs in the MZ that expands with age in autoimmune mice. Accordingly, MZB cells displayed an enhanced type I IFN signature as compared to FO B cells, and there was a significant difference between the TC and B6 mice. We have shown that type I IFN-activated MZB cells promote autoantigen transport and induce T cell activation in BXD2 lupus-prone mice [47,48]. Our present results suggest that the local activation of MZB cells by pDCs is likely a critical event that occurs in lupus pathogenesis.

The TLR7/TLR9 signaling pathway is complex and results in the secretion of different pro-inflammatory cytokines depending on the structure and location of the TLR ligands [49,50]. Therefore, TLR7/TLR9 signaling can also affect pathology in a Type-I IFN independent manner. DCs that lacked the TLR-adaptor protein MyD88 showed an overall decrease in the levels of inflammatory cytokines in the spleen after TLR9 stimulation with CpG [36,51]. Furthermore, TLR signaling by DCs also affects B cell function as MyD88 deficient DCs had significantly lower levels of IgG2a anti-nucleosome autoAbs [52]. In addition, human pDCs stimulated with ICs isolated from SLE patients induced greater levels of inflammatory cytokines, including IL-6 and IFN-γ, in a TLR-9 dependent manner [53]. Here we showed that *in vivo* exogenous administration of anti-chromatin ICs resulted in elevated production of IL-6 and IFN-γ by splenic DCs of TC mice. Thus TLR7/9 stimulation promoted secretion of pro-inflammatory cytokines in lupus prone mice, potentially as a result on the expansion MZ pDCs.

Given the high levels of pro-inflammatory cytokines found in the TC lupus background, it is difficult to determine if the expression of anti-inflammatory cytokines is altered in these mice. We focused on the expression of IL-10, an anti-inflammatory cytokine that has been proposed to both contribute to and protect from SLE. SLE patients present elevated levels of serum IL-10 that correlate with disease activity [54], and polymorphisms in the IL-10 gene have been associated with SLE susceptibility [55,56], with the risk allele associated with an increased expression [57]. On the other hand, IL-10 overexpression on the TC background reduced total IgM and delayed the production of ANAs [58]. Furthermore, IL-10 has suppressive effects when produced by regulatory B cells (Breg) [59], and the loss of IL-10 production by these B cells results in systemic autoimmunity [60]. Finally, the clearance of apoptotic

cells requires the production of IL-10 to prevent the induction of autoimmunity [61]. Following the experimental protocol by Miles et al [62], we induced IL-10 secretion in MZ B cells co-cultured with apoptotic cells Under these conditions TC MZ B cells expressed equal mRNA levels of IL-10 than B6 MZ B cells and in both strains this treatments resulted in decreased levels of IL-6. Interestingly, cytokine quantification from the culture supernatant showed that TC mice still had significantly higher expression of IL-6 under anti-inflammatory conditions and thus the IL-10 to IL-6 ratio for these mice was lower than for B6. These results indicate that although IL-10 secretion is equally induced in both strains, the lupus-prone TC mice do not effectively reduce IL-6 levels under anti-inflammatory conditions.

In summary, the cytokine milieu in TC lupus background favors the production of pro-inflammatory cytokines capable of modulating B cell responses. In particular, IL-6 and IFN-γ secretion by TC DCs enhances B cell proliferation. TC mice have an expanded pDC population that localizes to the MZ and correlates with an elevated Type I IFN response in MZ but not FO B cells. In addition, TLR7/TLR9 stimulation resulted in the secretion of higher levels of IL-6 and IFN-γ by splenic DCs. However, under anti-inflammatory conditions the TC lupus background cannot efficiently repress production of IL-6 by MZ B cells. Taken together, dysregulations in cytokine networks are present in the lupus-prone TC mice and aid in the breakdown of B cell tolerance.

Supporting Information

Figure S1   Pathway analysis of gene expression in B6 B cells cultured with supernatant from anti-CD40 stimulated BMDCS from either B6 or TC mice. Green and red symbols show genes significantly over-expressed in B cells exposed to B6 and TC-produced BMDC supernatant, respectively. White symbols show genes that represent functional intermediates in the pathways.

Acknowledgments

We thank Neal Benson from the University of Florida ICBR Cellomic Core for cell sorting, Nathalie Kanda for outstanding mouse husbandry, and Dr. Zhiwei Xu for technical advice. We also thank Sindhu Arivazhagan, Yuan Xu, Dr. Michael Clare-Salzler, and Dr. Westley Reeves (all from the University of Florida) for reagents. Confocal imaging data acquisition was carried out at the UAB Rheumatic Diseases Core Center-Analytic Imaging and Immunoreagents Core (P30 AR048311).

Author Contributions

Conceived and designed the experiments: HCH JDM LM. Performed the experiments: AS YYZ HL HCH. Analyzed the data: AS YYZ ID HL HCH LM. Wrote the paper: AS HCH JDM LM.

References

1. Jego G, Pascual V, Palucka AK, Banchereau J (2005) Dendritic cells control B cell growth and differentiation. Curr Dir Autoimmun 8: 124–139.

2. Morel L, Croker BP, Blenman KR, Mohan C, Huang G, et al. (2000) Genetic reconstitution of systemic lupus erythematosus immunopathology with poly-congenic murine strains. Proc Natl Acad Sci USA 97: 6670–6675.

3. Wan S, Zhou Z, Duan B, Morel L (2008) Direct B cell stimulation by dendritic cells in a mouse model of lupus. Arthritis Rheum 58: 1741–1750.

4. Cassese G, Arce S, Hauser AE, Lehnert K, Moewes B, et al. (2003) Plasma cell survival is mediated by synergistic effects of cytokines and adhesion-dependent signals. J Immunol 171: 1684–1690.

5. Hirano T, Kishimoto T (1989) Interleukin 6 and plasma cell neoplasias. Prog Growth Factor Res 1: 133–142.

6. Esposito P, Balletta MM, Procino A, Postiglione L, Memoli B (2009) Interleukin-6 release from peripheral mononuclear cells is associated to disease activity and treatment response in patients with lupus nephritis. Lupus 18: 1329–1330.

7. Linker-Israeli M, Deans RJ, Wallace DJ, Prehn J, Ozeri-Chen T, et al. (1991) Elevated levels of endogenous IL-6 in systemic lupus erythematosus. A putative role in pathogenesis. J Immunol 147: 117–123.

8. Finck BK, Chan B, Wofsy D (1994) Interleukin 6 promotes murine lupus in NZB/NZW F1 mice. J Clin Invest 94: 585–591.

9. Mihara M, Takagi N, Takeda Y, Ohsugi Y (1998) IL-6 receptor blockage inhibits the onset of autoimmune kidney disease in NZB/W F1 mice. Clin Exp Immunol 112: 397–402.

10. Lande R, Gilliet M (2010) Plasmacytoid dendritic cells: key players in the initiation and regulation of immune responses. Ann N Y Acad Sci 1183: 89–103.

11. Kiefer K, Oropallo MA, Cancro MP, Marshak-Rothstein A (2012) Role of type I interferons in the activation of autoreactive B cells. Immunol Cell Biol 90: 498–504.

12. Elkon KB, Wiedeman A (2012) Type I IFN system in the development and manifestations of SLE. Curr Opin Rheumatol 24: 499–505.
13. Sriram U, Varghese L, Bennett HL, Jog NR, Shivers DK, et al. (2012) Myeloid dendritic cells from B6.NZM Sle1/Sle2/Sle3 lupus-prone mice express an IFN signature that precedes disease onset. J Immunol 189: 80–91.
14. Teichmann LL, Ols ML, Kashgarian M, Reizis B, Kaplan DH, et al. (2010) Dendritic cells in lupus are not required for activation of T and B cells but promote their expansion, resulting in tissue damage. Immunity 33: 967–978.
15. Ganguly D, Haak S, Sisirak V, Reizis B (2013) The role of dendritic cells in autoimmunity. Nat Rev Immunol 13: 566–577.
16. Gerl V, Lischka A, Panne D, Grossmann P, Berthold R, et al. (2010) Blood dendritic cells in systemic lupus erythematosus exhibit altered activation state and chemokine receptor function. Ann Rheum Dis 69: 1370–1377.
17. Kaneko T, Saito Y, Kotani T, Okazawa H, Iwamura H, et al. (2012) Dendritic cell-specific ablation of the protein tyrosine phosphatase Shp1 promotes Th1 cell differentiation and induces autoimmunity. J Immunol 188: 5397–5407.
18. Morel L, Croker BP, Blenman KR, Mohan C, Huang G, et al. (2000) Genetic reconstitution of systemic lupus erythematosus immunopathology with poly-congenic murine strains. Proc Natl Acad Sci U S A 97: 6670–6675.
19. Herlands R, William J, Hershberg U, Shlomchik M (2007) Anti-chromatin antibodies drive in vivo antigen-specific activation and somatic hypermutation of rheumatoid factor B cells at extrafollicular sites. Eur J Immunol 37: 3339–3351.
20. Hannum LG, Ni D, Haberman AM, Weigert MG, Shlomchik MJ (1996) A disease-related rheumatoid factor autoantibody is not tolerized in a normal mouse: implications for the origins of autoantibodies in autoimmune disease. J Exp Med 184: 1269–1278.
21. Xu Z, Vallurupalli A, Fuhrman C, Ostrov D, Morel L (2011) An NZB-derived locus suppresses chronic graft versus host disease and autoantibody production through non-lymphoid bone-marrow derived cells. J Immunol 186: 4130–4139.
22. Lantow M, Sivakumar R, Zeumer L, Wasserfall C, Zheng YY, et al. (2013) The granulocyte colony stimulating factor pathway regulates autoantibody produc-tion in a murine induced model of systemic lupus erythematosus. Arthritis Res Ther 15: R49.
23. Cuda CM, Li S, Liang S, Yin Y, Potula HH, et al. (2012) Pre-B cell leukemia homeobox 1 is associated with lupus susceptibility in mice and humans. J Immunol 188: 604–614.
24. Brawand P, Fitzpatrick DR, Greenfield BW, Brasel K, Maliszewski CR, et al. (2002) Murine plasmacytoid pre-dendritic cells generated from Flt3 ligand-supplemented bone marrow cultures are immature APCs. J Immunol 169: 6711–6719.
25. Wan S, Xia C, Morel L (2007) IL-6 produced by dendritic cells from lupus-prone mice inhibits CD4+CD25+ T cell regulatory functions. J Immunol 178: 271–279.
26. Ramanujam M, Bethunaickan R, Huang W, Tao H, Madaio M, et al. (2010) Selective blockade of BAFF for the prevention and treatment of systemic lupus erythematosus nephritis in NZM2410 mice. Arthritis Rheum 62: 1457–1468.
27. Kim SJ, Zou YR, Goldstein J, Reizis B, Diamond B (2011) Tolerogenic function of Blimp-1 in dendritic cells. J Exp Med 208: 2193–2199.
28. Vremec D, O'Keeffe M, Hochrein H, Fuchsberger M, Caminschi I, et al. (2007) Production of interferons by dendritic cells, plasmacytoid cells, natural killer cells, and interferon-producing killer dendritic cells. Blood 109: 1165–1173.
29. Kimura A, Kishimoto T (2010) IL-6: Regulator of Treg/Th17 balance. Eur J Immunol 40: 1830–1835.
30. Bermejo DA, Jackson SW, Gorosito-Serran M, Acosta-Rodriguez EV, Amezcua-Vesely MC, et al. (2013) Trypanosoma cruzi trans-sialidase initiates a program independent of the transcription factors ROR[gamma]t and Ahr that leads to IL-17 production by activated B cells. Nat Immunol 14: 514–522.
31. Dubois B, Massacrier C, Vanbervliet B, Fayette J, Briere F, et al. (1998) Critical role of IL-12 in dendritic cell-induced differentiation of naive B lymphocytes. J Immunol 161: 2223–2231.
32. G J, AK P, JP B, C C, V P, et al. (2003) Plasmacytoid dendritic cells induce plasma cell differentiation through type I interferon and interleukin 6. Immunity 19: 225.
33. Satpathy AT, Wu X, Albring JC, Murphy KM (2012) Re(de)fining the dendritic cell lineage. Nat Immunol 13: 1145–1154.
34. Merad M, Sathe P, Helft J, Miller J, Mortha A (2013) The dendritic cell lineage: ontogeny and function of dendritic cells and their subsets in the steady state and the inflamed setting. Annu Rev Immunol 31: 563–604.
35. Chappell CP, Draves KE, Giltiay NV, Clark EA (2012) Extrafollicular B cell activation by marginal zone dendritic cells drives T cell-dependent antibody responses. J Exp Med 209: 1825–1840.
36. Boulé M, Broughton C, Mackay F, Akira S, Marshak-Rothstein A, et al. (2004) Toll-like receptor 9-dependent and -independent dendritic cell activation by chromatin-immunoglobulin G complexes. J Exp Med 199: 1631–1640.
37. Marshak-Rothstein A, Rifkin IR (2007) Immunologically active autoantigens: the role of toll-like receptors in the development of chronic inflammatory disease. Annu Rev Immunol 25: 419–441.
38. Kadowaki N, Ho S, Antonenko S, Malefyt RW, Kastelein RA, et al. (2001) Subsets of human dendritic cell precursors express different toll-like receptors and respond to different microbial antigens. J Exp Med 194: 863–869.
39. Losman MJ, Fasy TM, Novick KE, Monestier M (1992) Monoclonal autoantibodies to subnucleosomes from a MRL/Mp(-)+/+ mouse. Oligoclon-ality of the antibody response and recognition of a determinant composed of histones H2A, H2B, and DNA. The J Immunol 148: 1561–1569.
40. Miles K, Heaney J, Sibinska Z, Salter D, Savill J, et al. (2012) A tolerogenic role for Toll-like receptor 9 is revealed by B-cell interaction with DNA complexes expressed on apoptotic cells. Proc Natl Acad Sci U S A 109: 887–892.
41. Petri M, Stohl W, Chatham W, McCune WJ, Chevrier M, et al. (2008) Association of plasma B lymphocyte stimulator levels and disease activity in systemic lupus erythematosus. Arthritis Rheum 58: 2453–2459.
42. Gateva V, Sandling JK, Hom G, Taylor KE, Chung SA, et al. (2009) A large-scale replication study identifies TNIP1, PRDM1, JAZF1, UHRF1BP1 and IL10 as risk loci for systemic lupus erythematosus. Nat Genet 41: 1228–1233.
43. Chan YH, Chiang MF, Tsai YC, Su ST, Chen MH, et al. (2009) Absence of the transcriptional repressor Blimp-1 in hematopoietic lineages reveals its role in dendritic cell homeostatic development and function. J Immunol 183: 7039–7046.
44. Asselin-Paturel C, Brizard G, Chemin K, Boonstra A, O'Garra A, et al. (2005) Type I interferon dependence of plasmacytoid dendritic cell activation and migration. J Exp Med 201: 1157–1167.
45. Bierly AL, Shufesky WJ, Sukhumavasi W, Morelli AE, Denkers EY (2008) Dendritic cells expressing plasmacytoid marker PDCA-1 are Trojan horses during Toxoplasma gondii infection. J Immunol 181: 8485–8491.
46. Kutzner H, Kerl H, Pfaltz MC, Kempf W (2009) CD123-positive plasmacytoid dendritic cells in primary cutaneous marginal zone B-cell lymphoma: diagnostic and pathogenetic implications. Am J Surg Pathol 33: 1307–1313.
47. Wang JH, Li J, Wu Q, Yang P, et al. (2010) Marginal zone precursor B cells as cellular agents for type I IFN-promoted antigen transport in autoimmunity. J Immunol 184: 442–451.
48. Wang JH, Wu Q, Yang P, Li H, Li J, et al. (2011) Type I interferon-dependent CD86(high) marginal zone precursor B cells are potent T cell costimulators in mice. Arthritis Rheum 63: 1054–1064.
49. Honda K, Ohba Y, Yanai H, Negishi H, Mizutani T, et al. (2005) Spatiotemporal regulation of MyD88-IRF-7 signalling for robust type-I interferon induction. Nature 434: 1035–1040.
50. Negishi H, Ohba Y, Yanai H, Takaoka A, Honma K, et al. (2005) Negative regulation of Toll-like-receptor signaling by IRF-4. Proc Natl Acad Sci U S A 102: 15989–15994.
51. Hou B, Reizis B, DeFranco AL (2008) Toll-like receptors activate innate and adaptive immunity by using dendritic cell-intrinsic and -extrinsic mechanisms. Immunity 29: 272–282.
52. Teichmann LL, Schenten D, Medzhitov R, Kashgarian M, Shlomchik MJ (2013) Signals via the adaptor MyD88 in B cells and DCs make distinct and synergistic contributions to immune activation and tissue damage in lupus. Immunity 38: 528–540.
53. Means TK, Latz E, Hayashi F, Murali MR, Golenbock DT, et al. (2005) Human lupus autoantibody-DNA complexes activate DCs through cooperation of CD32 and TLR9. J Clin Invest 115: 407–417.
54. Hofmann SR, Rösen-Wolff A, Tsokos GC, Hedrich CM (2012) Biological properties and regulation of IL-10 related cytokines and their contribution to autoimmune disease and tissue injury. Clin Immunol 143: 116–127.
55. Wang B, Zhu J-M, Fan Y-G, Xu W-D, Cen H, et al. (2013) Association of the − 1082G/A polymorphism in the interleukin-10 gene with systemic lupus erythematosus: A meta-analysis. Gene 519: 209–216.
56. Liu P, Song J, Su H, Li L, Lu N, et al. (2013) IL-10 gene polymorphisms and susceptibility to systemic lupus erythematosus: a meta-analysis. PLoS One 8: e69547.
57. Sakurai D, Zhao J, Deng Y, Kelly JA, Brown EE, et al. (2013) Preferential binding to Elk-1 by SLE-associated IL10 risk allele upregulates IL10 expression. PLoS Genet 9: e1003870.
58. Blenman KR, Duan B, Xu Z, Wan S, Atkinson MA, et al. (2006) IL-10 regulation of lupus in the NZM2410 murine model. Lab Invest 86: 1136–1148.
59. Mauri C, Blair PA (2010) Regulatory B cells in autoimmunity: developments and controversies. Nat Rev Rheumatol 6: 636–643.
60. Xiao S, Brooks CR, Zhu C, Wu C, Sweere JM, et al. (2012) Defect in regulatory B-cell function and development of systemic autoimmunity in T-cell Ig mucin 1 (Tim-1) mucin domain-mutant mice. Proc Natl Acad Sci U S A 109: 12105–12110.
61. Ling G-S, Cook HT, Botto M, Lau Y-L, Huang F-P (2011) An essential protective role of IL-10 in the immunological mechanism underlying resistance vs susceptibility to lupus induction by dendritic cells and dying cells. Rheumatology 51: 1773–1784.
62. Mohan C, Alas E, Morel L, Yang P, Wakeland E (1998) Genetic dissection of SLE pathogenesis. Sle1 on murine chromosome 1 leads to a selective loss of tolerance to H2A/H2B/DNA subnucleosomes. J Clin Invest 101: 1362–1372.

Lupus-Prone Mice Fail to Raise Antigen-Specific T Cell Responses to Intracellular Infection

Linda A. Lieberman, George C. Tsokos*

Division of Rheumatology, Department of Medicine, Beth Israel Deaconess Medical Center, Harvard Medical School, Boston, Massachusetts, United States of America

Abstract

Systemic lupus erythematosus (SLE) is characterized by multiple cellular abnormalities culminating in the production of autoantibodies and immune complexes, resulting in tissue inflammation and organ damage. Besides active disease, the main cause of morbidity and mortality in SLE patients is infections, including those from opportunistic pathogens. To understand the failure of the immune system to fend off infections in systemic autoimmunity, we infected the lupus-prone murine strains B6.*lpr* and BXSB with the intracellular parasite *Toxoplasma gondii* and survival was monitored. Furthermore, mice were sacrificed days post infection and parasite burden and cellular immune responses such as cytokine production and cell activation were assessed. Mice from both strains succumbed to infection acutely and we observed greater susceptibility to infection in older mice. Increased parasite burden and a defective antigen-specific IFN-gamma response were observed in the lupus-prone mice. Furthermore, T cell:dendritic cell co-cultures established the presence of an intrinsic T cell defect responsible for the decreased antigen-specific response. An antigen-specific defect in IFN- gamma production prevents lupus-prone mice from clearing infection effectively. This study reveals the first cellular insight into the origin of increased susceptibility to infections in SLE disease and may guide therapeutic approaches.

Editor: Laurel L. Lenz, University of Colorado School of Medicine, United States of America

Funding: This work was supported by National Institutes of Health - NIH AI049954. The funders had no role in study design, data collection and analysis, decision to publish, or preparation of the manuscript.

Competing Interests: The authors have declared that no competing interests exist.

* Email: gtsokos@bidmc.harvard.edu

Introduction

Systemic lupus erythematosus (SLE) is a debilitating disease, primarily affecting women, and presents with manifestations in most organs [1]. Aside from active disease, infections represent the major cause of morbidity and mortality [2,3]. In fact, it has been reported 20–55% of all deaths of SLE patients result from infections [3]. Notwithstanding the fact that immunosuppressive drugs, routinely used in the treatment of patients with SLE, contribute to the increased rates of infections, inherent defects in the innate and acquired immune responses play an important role in susceptibility. For example, although T cells provide excessive help to B cells to produce autoantibodies, they are unable to raise proper cytotoxic responses [4] and they produce decreased levels of IL-2 [5]. Furthermore, autoantibodies against various cell components likely contribute to the increased incidence of infection in these patients [6,7]. The mechanism of increased susceptibility to infection by SLE patients has not been well examined and this paper begins to unravel this phenomenon.

In addition to common infections, patients with SLE suffer from infections with opportunistic pathogens such as *Listeria monocytogenes*, *Cryptococcus neoformans*, *Pneumocystis carinii* and *Toxoplasma gondii* [8]. *T. gondii* is an intracellular parasite that often results in asymptomatic infection in healthy individuals as the parasite develops strategies to coexist with host cells [9]. Immunity to *T. gondii* is driven by IFN-gamma production [10]. SLE patients have higher titers of antibodies against *T. gondii* as

compared to healthy controls [11] and a diagnosis of toxoplasmosis can easily be missed as the symptoms are similar to that of lupus cerebritis [12]. As with other CNS infections in SLE patients, *T. gondii* presents difficult diagnostic and therapeutic decisions.

To better understand the proclivity of SLE patients to suffer infections, we infected lupus-prone mice with *T. gondii*. Because individual lupus-prone murine strains do not epitomize the full spectrum of human disease, we infected two genetically-diverse lupus-prone murine strains (B6.*lpr*, BXSB) with this parasite and observed survival as well as elements of the cellular immune response. We report here that lupus-prone mice succumbed during the acute stage of infection due to increased parasite burden, independent of elevated systemic IFN-gamma levels in the serum. We found that *T. gondii*-infected mice display a severely depressed antigen-specific T cell IFN-gamma response that likely accounts for the increased mortality. This information sheds new light on the origin of increased susceptibility to infections in systemic autoimmunity and suggests the need for new approaches to mitigate infection-related morbidity and mortality.

Materials and Methods

Mice

Two strains of lupus-prone mice and appropriate controls were purchased for these studies. Female C57BL/6 mice were age and sex matched with B6.*lpr* mice and the lupus-prone male BXSB mice were age matched with female BXSB littermates (Jackson Laboratories, Bar Harbor, ME). Mice were randomly assigned to control or experimental group. Three to six mice per group were used for each experiment and replicated multiple times as indicated in the figure legend. CBA (Jackson Laboratories, Bar Harbor, ME) and Swiss Webster (Taconic, Germantown, NY) mice were used for *in vivo* maintenance of parasites. Mice were group housed in the barrier facility in the Center for Life Science at Beth Israel Deaconess Medical Center with a twelve-hour light/dark cycle.

Parasites

The Me49 strain of *T. gondii* was used for these studies (ATCC, Manassas, VA). Parasites were maintained and passaged *in vivo* in Swiss Webster or CBA mice. Parasites were also maintained *in vitro* in HS27 human foreskin fibroblast cells (ATCC, Manassas, VA). Parasites were prepared from mouse brain isolates and diluted in phosphate buffered saline for injections.

Survival Curves

Lupus-prone mice and appropriate controls were infected intraperitoneally with the Me49 strain of *T. gondii*. Infected mice were monitored daily for signs of lethargy, ruffling, and abnormal ambulation. If mice displayed any one of these criteria, they were then monitored twice daily. Mice were sacrificed by gas cylinder CO_2 when they became moribund and that day post infection was considered the survival endpoint.

ELISA, serum collection, urine collection, antibody treatment

Splenocytes from infected animals were stimulated *in vitro* with 5 ng/ml of IL-12 or 20 ug/ml of STAg for 72 h and supernatants were assayed for IFN-gamma by ELISA (eBiosciences, San Diego, CA). IFN-gamma and other cytokines were measured from serum collected from the tail vein by a multiplex bead assay (Bio-Rad, Hercules, CA). Anti-dsDNA was measured by ELISA from murine serum monthly to assess autoimmune status (Alpha Diagnostic International, San Antonio, TX). Urine was collected overnight in metabolic cages once a month and proteinuria was measured to monitor lupus-disease progression. Anti-PD-L1 (gift from Gordon Freeman Dana Farber Research Institute, Boston, MA) was administered intraperitoneally at 200 mg starting at day −1 before infection and every third day thereafter.

Flow cytometry

Splenocytes or peritoneal exudate cells were surface stained with the following markers (CD3, CD4, CD8, NK1.1, B220, CD5, CD11-b, GR-1, CD11c, F4/80, IA/IE, H-2k, CD44, CD62L, CD80, CD86, PD-1, PD-L1, Tim-3, Ly6G, CD21, CD23, CD38, CD25, Fas, FoxP3; Biolegend, San Diego, CA) and cells were collected on an LSRII flow cytometer (Becton Dickinson, CA). Data was analyzed using FlowJo software (Treestar, Ashland, OR).

Recall response

Spleens were removed from mice following sacrifice 7 days post-infection. Splenocytes were isolated and plated at 4×10^5 cells/well in 96 well plates. Cells were stimulated with the parasite antigen STAg and/or IL-12 for 72 hours. STAg was prepared as previously described [13]. IFN-gamma production was measured by ELISA.

Non-specific TCR stimulation

$CD3^+$ T cells were purified from spleens of naïve B6.*lpr* and BXSB mice by negative selection (Pan T cell isolation kit II, Miltenyi, Auburn, CA) and stimulated with anti-CD3 (0.5ug/ml; eBiosceinces) and anti-CD28 (1 ug/ml; Biolegend) for 3 days. Supernatants were assayed for IFN-gamma production by ELISA.

Parasite Burden

Cells were collected by peritoneal lavage with 5 ml cold PBS following the sacrifice of the mice and cytospins were prepared to determine parasite burden. Slides were stained with Hema3 Stain (Biochemical Sciences, Swedesboro, NJ) and sealed with mounting medium (Richard Allan Scientific, Kalamazoo, MI). Parasite burden was assessed by counting a minimum of 500 cells per cytospin in a blinded manner.

T cell:DC mixing experiment

Lupus-prone and control mice were infected with *T. gondii* and 7 days later spleens were removed and splenocytes were prepared. $CD11c^+$ cells were isolated by magnetic separation using positive selection ($CD11c^+$ isolation kit, Miltenyi, Auburn, CA). The flow-through was collected and $CD3^+$ cells were isolated by negative selection from the same animal (Pan T cell isolation kit II, Miltenyi, Auburn, CA). Cells were plated in 96 well plates at a ratio of 5 T cells to 1 dendritic cell (T-3×10^5: DC-6×10^4). Antigen was added to the wells (STAg 20 ug/ml) and the plate was incubated for 72 hours at 37°C, 5% CO_2. Supernatants were assayed for IFN-gamma production by ELISA (eBioscience, San Diego, CA).

Statistical analysis

Unpaired two-tailed Student t tests were calculated using PRISM software (GraphPad). A p value of <0.05 was considered significant.

Ethics Statement

All murine work was reviewed and approved by the IACUC at Beth Israel Deaconess Medical Center. Beth Israel Deaconess Medical Center is AAALAC accredited and complies with all federal, state, and local laws. These studies were carried out under IACUC protocols 101–2009 and 069–2012.

Results

Lupus-prone mice are susceptible to infection with *T. gondii*

We used a model of *T. gondii* infection to investigate whether inherent immune dysfunction in lupus-prone mice leads to increased susceptibility to infection. Because none of the commonly used lupus-prone murine strains perfectly mimic human SLE disease, we decided to study two different mouse strains. The mice we chose to investigate were B6.*lpr* (mutated lymphoproliferation (*lpr*) gene), and the BXSB strain (male mice have the Y chromosome linked autoimmune accelerator gene (*Yaa*)). The B6.*lpr* mice are defective in Fas-mediated signaling [14], while the BXSB mice overexpress *Tlr7* [15]. The onset of lupus disease in these mice occurs at different time points, therefore we infected mice 1–3 months before the onset of the disease to ensure that the results would not be complicated by immune abnormalities and organ damage imposed by disease activity. Accordingly, the mice studied had increased levels of anti-dsDNA antibodies but they had not yet developed proteinuria.

First we infected B6.*lpr* mice intraperitoneally with *T. gondii* at 20 weeks of age as they displayed a significant increase in circulating anti-dsDNA antibodies as compared to wild type controls, but they did not exhibit any proteinuria. Similarly, BXSB mice were infected at 14 weeks of age. We found that although they are genetically different, both SLE-prone mice rapidly succumbed to acute infection within twelve days post-infection (Figure 1A). This differs from previously published data in which NZBWF1 mice were orally infected with *T. gondii*, resulting in a chronic infection [16]. This variance may have to do with the different genetic background of those mice and/or the route of infection as peroral infection often results in chronic disease.

Additionally, we infected younger mice to determine whether susceptibility to infection is affected by age as mice develop more autoimmune manifestations with age. B6.*lpr* mice were infected at 14 weeks of age and BXSB mice were infected at 8 weeks of age. We found that mice expressing lower levels of anti-dsDNA (therefore less autoimmunity) were less susceptible to infection compared to older mice suggesting immunosuppression increases with disease progression (Figure 1B). All of the following studies were conducted on B6.*lpr* mice at 20 weeks of age and BXSB mice at 14 weeks of age.

Lupus-prone mice display an increased parasite burden following infection

Previous studies have established that many immunocompromised mice succumb to acute *T. gondii* infection when they are unable to control parasite replication, an event linked to defects in cytokine production or function. We measured parasite burden in the peritoneum of infected mice and in B6.*lpr* we found a significantly higher parasite burden in mice 9 days post infection (p = 0.001) (Figure 2A). An increased parasite burden was observed 7 days post infection in the BXSB mice (p<0.0001) (Figure 2B). These data indicate that lupus-prone mice are unable to effectively control parasite replication.

Systemic IFN-gamma does not sufficiently protect against *T. gondii* infection

The major route of resistance to *T. gondii* infection is IL-12 driven IFN-gamma production. Increased parasite burden is often associated with decreased IFN-gamma production [17]. We examined serum cytokine levels at the peak of IFN-gamma production, 7 days after infection, and found no significant difference in the systemic levels of IFN-gamma in B6.*lpr* mice (Figure 3A). In fact, the levels of IFN-gamma in the B6.*lpr* mice after infection tended to be higher than that of wild type mice, though this difference did not reach significance. Conversely, IFN-gamma levels in BXSB mice were significantly decreased

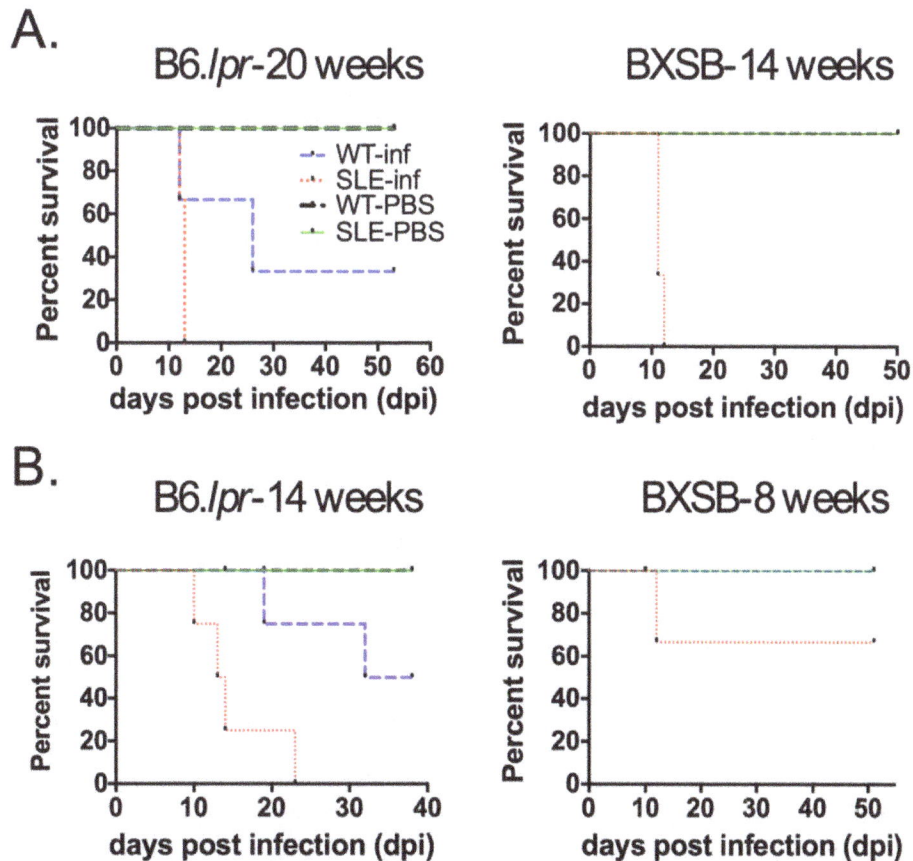

Figure 1. Lupus-prone mice succumb to acute infection with *T. gondii*. (A) Two strains of SLE-prone mice exhibiting exacerbated autoimmune markers but no lupus pathology were infected with 20 Me49 i.p. and survival was monitored. B6.*lpr* mice were age and sex matched with C57BL/6 mice. Male BXSB mice were age-matched with females of the colony who do not develop lupus-like disease. All lupus-prone mice succumbed to infection within the first 12 days of infection. (B) Younger mice were infected for the above strains and it was observed that they had increased survival. Each survival curve represents at least two replicates of 3–6 mice per group.

A.   B6.*lpr*

B.   BXSB

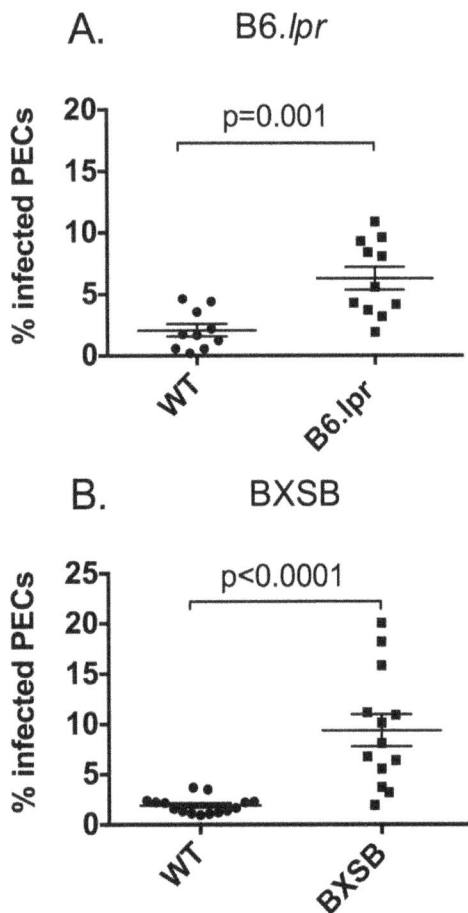

Figure 2. Parasite burden is increased in lupus-prone mice. Mice were sacrificed 7–10 days following infection and peritoneal lavage was performed. A cytospin was prepared from each mouse and then the percent of infected cells was quantified. (A) B6.*lpr* mice showed a significant increase in parasite burden 9 dpi. (B) BXSB mice had significantly increased parasite burden 7 dpi. Each experiment was carried out 2–3 times with 3–6 mice per group.

A.

B.

Figure 3. Systemic IFN-gamma does not sufficiently protect lupus-prone mice. IFN-gamma levels were measured in the serum of lupus-prone mice 7 days post infection (dpi) by multiplex. No significant differences were found between infected B6.*lpr* mice and infected WT controls (A). BXSB mice had reduced levels of systemic IFN-gamma (B). B6.*lpr* mice were 20 weeks of age and BXSB mice were 14 weeks of age. Each experiment was carried out at least 3 times with 3–6 mice per group.

(Figure 3B). This suggests IL-12 levels may also be decreased, but we found no defect in systemic IL-12 (data not shown).

T cell antigen specific IFN-gamma production is decreased in lupus-prone mice following *T. gondii* infection

We examined activation markers on various cell types from the spleen and the peritoneum of infected (and uninfected) lupus-prone mice but found no significant differences in distribution or activation markers as compared to wild type mice (data not shown). Since T cell activation appeared normal as evidenced by no significant differences in the percentage of $CD3^+CD4^+$ $CD44^{hi}CD62L^{lo}$ or $CD3^+CD8^+CD44^{hi}CD62L^{lo}$ cells, we asked whether T cells from lupus-prone mice were functionally competent. To address this question, we assessed the ability of these cells to respond to specific antigen stimulation. We stimulated splenocytes from infected mice with *T. gondii*-specific antigen (STAg) for 3 days *in vitro* and measured IFN-gamma production in the culture supernatants. We found that cells from infected B6.*lpr* (Figure 4A) and BXSB mice (Figure 4B) produced

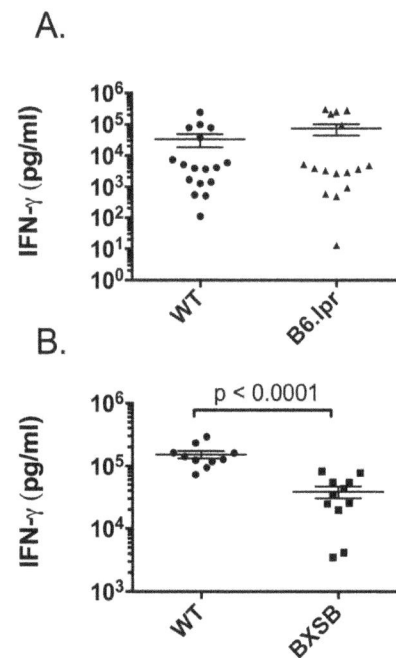

greatly reduced levels of antigen-specific IFN-gamma indicating a defective antigen recall response.

To ensure that this response was indeed antigen specific and not due to a non-specific T cell defect in these mice, $CD3^+$ T cells were purified from spleens of naïve B6.*lpr* and BXSB mice and stimulated with anti-CD3 and anti-CD28 for 3 days. Supernatants were assayed for IFN-gamma production and we did not find any defect in the ability of these cells to respond to non-specific TCR stimuli (Figure 5). In fact, in both B6.*lpr* and BXSB mice, we observed an increased IFN-gamma response as compared to the wild type controls. Similarly, an increased IFN-gamma response has been reported following TCR stimulation of peripheral T cells from SLE patients [18].

An intrinsic T cell defect leads to decreased antigen-specific response

The decreased antigen-specific response observed in lupus-prone mice is due to decreased IFN-gamma production by T cells. To investigate whether this is due to an intrinsic T cell defect or the result of defective antigen presentation, we purified T cells and dendritic cells (DCs) from spleens of infected wild type or lupus-prone mice and mixed them *in vitro* in the presence or absence of *T. gondii* antigen. There was a baseline level of IFN-gamma produced in the absence of STAg (Figure 6 lower portion) and this is to be expected since the parasite is present in the splenocyte cultures isolated from infected animals. We found that T cells from lupus-prone mice mixed with DCs from wild type mice produced less IFN-gamma as compared to wild type T cells mixed with DCs from lupus-prone mice which produced similar levels of IFN-gamma as wild type T cells mixed with wild type DCs (Figure 6

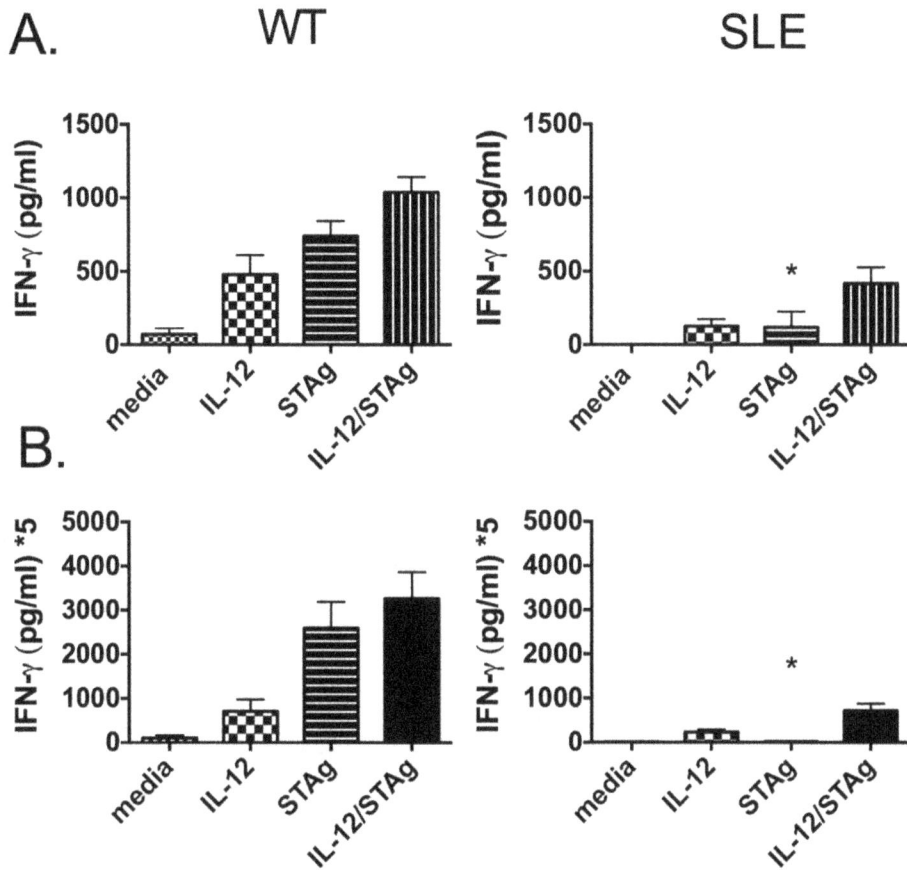

Figure 4. Antigen-specific response is defective in lupus-prone mice. Splenocytes were collected from infected mice 7 dpi and were stimulated 3 days in vitro with either IL-12 (5ng/ml), STAg (20 ug/ml), or IL-12+ STAg. Supernatants were assayed by ELISA for IFN-gamma production. A significant decrease in antigen-specific IFN-gamma was observed (*). (A) B6.*lpr* (B) BXSB. B6.*lpr* mice were 20 weeks of age and BXSB mice were 14 weeks of age. This experiment is representative of 2–3 individual experiments with 3–4 mice per group.

upper portion). Therefore, we conclude that antigen presentation is intact in the lupus-prone mice, but these mice harbor an intrinsic T cell defect leading to decreased IFN-gamma production.

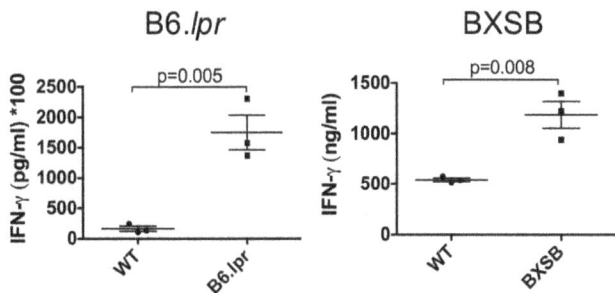

Figure 5. TCR-stimulation is not defective in lupus-prone mice. T cells were isolated from splenocytes of either B6.*lpr* or BXSB mice and the appropriate controls. Cells were stimulated with anti-CD3/anti-CD28 for 72 hours and supernatants were assayed for IFN-gamma production by ELISA. The IFN-gamma response to non-specific TCR stimulation was intact in these mice. B6.*lpr* mice were 20 weeks of age and BXSB mice were 14 weeks of age. This experiment is representative of two individual experiments.

Discussion

One of the leading causes of morbidity and mortality in SLE patients is infection. It is well known that the immune system of SLE patients is dysregulated but there has been little insight as to how it responds to challenge with infectious organisms. The use of steroids and other immunosuppressive drugs in SLE patients complicates the ability to separate the effects of the drugs from the natural dysregulation of the immune response triggered by disease. Lupus-prone mice allow us to parse the immune response to infectious agents in the context of autoimmunity. We show in this study that lupus-prone mice display increased susceptibility to infection which is accentuated as disease progresses. To our surprise, lupus-prone mice succumbed acutely to infection with the prototypic Th1-inducing pathogen *T. gondii*; this occurred in both B6.*lpr* mice and BXSB mice. We observed decreased systemic IFN-gamma production in the BXSB mice therefore it was not surprising that there was a decreased ability to control parasite burden as it has been well established that IFN-gamma is necessary for control of this parasite. Furthermore, it has previously been reported that BXSB mice are susceptible to acute infection with the intracellular parasite *Trypanosoma cruzi* [19]. Conversely, the B6.*lpr* mice did not have decreased systemic IFN-gamma, therefore the dichotomy between the increased levels of IFN-gamma in the serum of B6.*lpr* mice following infection (similar to what is seen in wild type mice), and the inability to

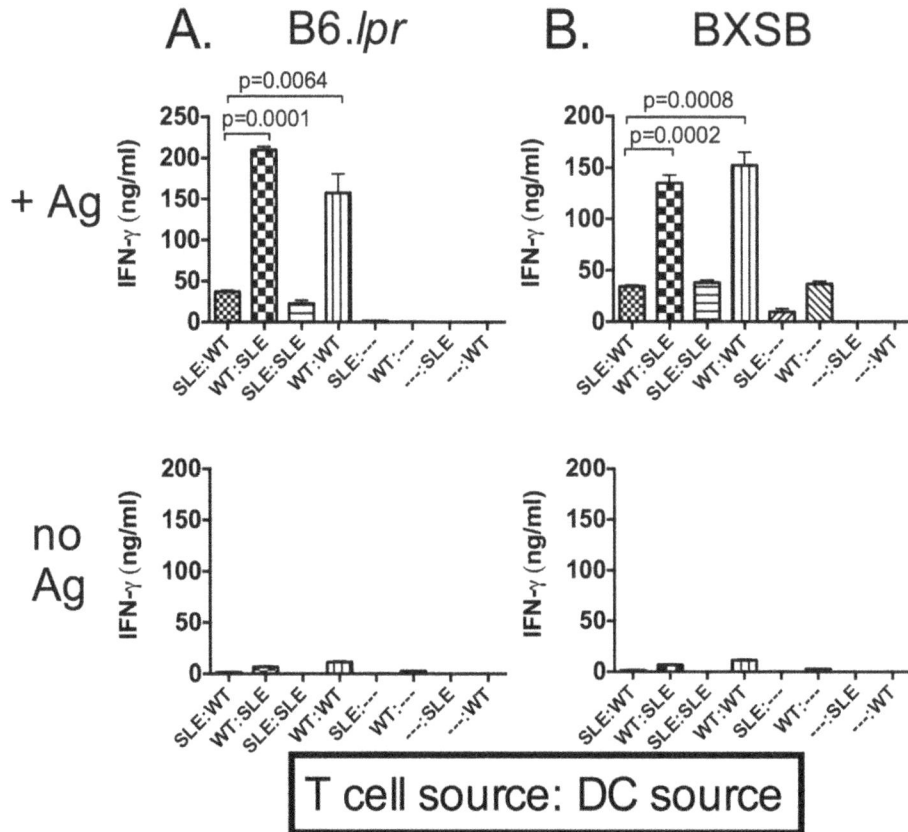

Figure 6. An intrinsic T cell defect is responsible for the decrease in antigen-specific IFN-gamma production. CD3[+] T cells and CD11c[+] DCs were isolated from splenocytes of infected mice 7 dpi. Cells were mixed at a ratio of 5:1 (T:DC) and incubated for 72 hours +/− STAg. IFN-gamma was measured from supernatants by ELISA. (A) B6.*lpr*; (B) BXSB; each assay was performed 3 times in triplicate. B6.*lpr* mice were 20 weeks of age and BXSB mice were 14 weeks of age.

contain parasite replication, was unexpected. This may be explained by considering the sources of IFN-gamma during *T. gondii* infection. During early infection, systemic IFN-gamma comes from multiple cellular sources with NK cells being a major producer of IFN-gamma. While this IFN-gamma will be protective, it does not provide sufficient protection for the mice to survive beyond acute infection (approximately two weeks in wild type mice) [20]. Antigen-specific IFN-gamma production from T cells is necessary for protection against this pathogen [21].

Interestingly, patients with SLE are susceptible to infection with other Th1 pathogens such as *Salmonella spp.* [6] though they have elevated levels of IFN-gamma [22,23]. This may be explained by a decreased ability of IFN-gamma to bind the IFN-gamma receptor or perhaps a defect in signaling through this receptor. It has been reported by one group that polymorphisms in the IFN-gammaR may increase the likelihood of SLE development and it has been shown that these polymorphisms can lead to an alteration in receptor function, resulting in a decreased response to IFN-gamma [24,25]. Conversely, another group concluded these polymorphisms are not associated with SLE in a different patient population [26].

The significantly decreased production of antigen-specific IFN-gamma in response to infection was unexpected. The expression of autoimmunity has been found to be dependent on the presence of IFN-gamma particularly during late stages of disease. Elevated IFN-gamma levels contribute to tissue damage and it has been reported that lupus-prone mice in which IFN-gamma or IFN-

gammaR has been deleted display reduced disease and mortality [27]. From our studies, it appears that non-specific IFN-gamma production found in lupus-prone mice is not sufficient to provide defense against infectious agents; survival may depend on antigen-specific IFN-gamma. As shown in Figure 1B, mice that have not yet developed significant autoimmunity survive longer than mice that have established autoimmune disease. We questioned if this increased protection was reliant on antigen-specific IFN-gamma production. Interestingly, recall responses from splenocytes of infected 14-week old B6.*lpr* mice or 8-week old BXSB mice displayed no defect in antigen specific IFN-gamma production (data not shown) suggesting this T cell function is integral to a successful immune response to *T. gondii*.

Upon observation that IFN-gamma was decreased in recall cultures, we wanted to know if this was due to a defect in antigen presentation or if it was a result of T cell dysfunction. We found that T cells are directly responsible for the defect in antigen specific IFN-gamma production as T:DC co-cultures revealed that antigen presentation is intact in these lupus-prone mice. Studies from our group and others have identified various defects in T cell signaling in SLE T cells and this may contribute in part to the observations made in these studies [28]. It should be considered that though the same number of T cells were added to the mixing cultures from either wild type or lupus-prone mice, the ratio of parasite-specific cells to other T cells present may be different between mouse strains. The lupus-prone mice may not increase their number of *T. gondii*-specific T cells as robustly as wild type mice. New tools may allow us to identify the percentage of antigen-specific T cell clones in the future.

During this study we found that lupus-prone mice trended towards increased expression of PD-1 on CD4$^+$ T cells from infected mice as compared to T cells from infected wild type mice (data not shown). We considered that T cells had become refractive to stimulation due to the increased levels of PD-1, a molecule known to be upregulated on functionally exhausted T cells [29]. Furthermore, it has been reported that the PD-1:PD-L1 pathway plays a role in inhibiting the functionality of CD8$^+$ T cells during chronic *T. gondii* infection [30]. We indirectly blocked PD-1 signaling by injecting anti-PD-L1 into B6.*lpr* mice prior to and following infection with *T. gondii*. Though it has been reported that infecting PD-L1$^{-/-}$ mice results in better outcomes for some infections, we found that blocking PD-L1 did not affect survival of lupus-prone mice. Similarly, it has been reported that blocking PD-L1 during acute *L. monocytogenes* infection does not enhance the immune response [31]. We concluded that the defect we observed in the lupus-prone mice was not likely due to functional exhaustion, though it should be noted that we did not block secondary ligands to PD-1, such as PD-L2 or PD-L3.

Our data present novel insight into the cellular immune events that account for increased susceptibility of lupus-prone mice to infection. At the translational level, our data suggest that in addition to antibiotics, the correction of failing T cell function in SLE patients should produce more favorable clinical outcomes following infections.

Acknowledgments

I would like to thank Robin Bossé, Poonam Rani and Jessica Beltran for technical help with these experiments and Katalin Kis-Toth for helpful scientific discussions.

Author Contributions

Conceived and designed the experiments: LAL GCT. Performed the experiments: LAL. Analyzed the data: LAL. Contributed to the writing of the manuscript: LAL GCT.

References

1. Tsokos GC (2011) Systemic lupus erythematosus. NEJM 365: 2110–2121.
2. Cervera R, Khamashta MA, Font J, Sebastiani GD, Gil A, et al. (2003) Morbidity and mortality in systemic lupus erythematosus during a 10-year period: a comparison of early and late manifestations in a cohort of 1,000 patients. Medicine (Baltimore) 82: 299–308.
3. Goldblatt F, Chambers S, Rahman A, Isenberg DA (2009) Serious infections in British patients with systemic lupus erythematosus: hospitalisations and mortality. Lupus 18: 682–689.
4. Mok CC, Lau CS (2003) Pathogenesis of systemic lupus erythematosus. J Clin Pathol 56: 481–490.
5. Lieberman LA, Tsokos GC (2010) The IL-2 defect in systemic lupus erythematosus disease has an expansive effect on host immunity. J Biomed Biotechnol 2010: 740619.
6. Iliopoulos AG, Tsokos GC (1996) Immunopathogenesis and spectrum of infections in systemic lupus erythematosus. Semin Arthritis Rheum 25: 318–336.
7. Maddur MS, Vani J, Lacroix-Desmazes S, Kaveri S, Bayry J (2010) Autoimmunity as a predisposition for infectious diseases. PLoS Pathog 6: e1001077.
8. Doria A, Canova M, Tonon M, Zen M, Rampudda E, et al. (2008) Infections as triggers and complications of systemic lupus erythematosus. Autoimmun Rev 8: 24–28.
9. Hunter CA, Sibley LD (2012) Modulation of innate immunity by *Toxoplasma gondii* virulence effectors. Nat Rev Microbiol 10: 766–778.
10. Dupont CD, Christian DA, Hunter CA (2012) Immune response and immunopathology during toxoplasmosis. Semin Immunopathol 34: 793–813.
11. Wilcox MH, Powell RJ, Pugh SF, Balfour AH (1990) Toxoplasmosis and systemic lupus erythematosus. Ann Rheum Dis 49: 254–257.
12. Zamir D, Amar M, Groisman G, Weiner P (1999) *Toxoplasma* infection in systemic lupus erythematosus mimicking lupus cerebritis. Mayo Clin Proc 74: 575–578.
13. Sharma SD, Mullenax J, Araujo FG, Erlich HA, Remington JS (1983) Western Blot analysis of the antigens of *Toxoplasma gondii* recognized by human IgM and IgG antibodies. J Immunol 131: 977–983.
14. Watanabe-Fukunaga R, Brannan CI, Copeland NG, Jenkins NA, Nagata S (1992) Lymphoproliferation disorder in mice explained by defects in Fas antigen that mediates apoptosis. Nature 356: 314–317.
15. Subramanian S, Tus K, Li QZ, Wang A, Tian XH, et al. (2006) A Tlr7 translocation accelerates systemic autoimmunity in murine lupus. PNAS 103: 9970–9975.
16. Chen M, Aosai F, Norose K, Mun HS, Ishikura H, et al. (2004) *Toxoplasma gondii* infection inhibits the development of lupus-like syndrome in autoimmune (New Zealand Black x New Zealand White) F1 mice. Int Immunol 16: 937–946.
17. Lieberman LA, Cardillo F, Owyang AM, Rennick DM, Cua DJ, et al. (2004) IL-23 provides a limited mechanism of resistance to acute toxoplasmosis in the absence of IL-12. J Immunol 173: 1887–1893.
18. Harigai M, Kawamoto M, Hara M, Kubota T, Kamatani N, et al. (2008) Excessive production of IFN-gamma in patients with systemic lupus erythematosus and its contribution to induction of B lymphocyte stimulator/B cell-activating factor/TNF ligand superfamily-13B. J Immunol 181: 2211–2219.
19. Nickell SP, Hoff R, Boyer MH (1985) Susceptibility to acute *Trypanosoma cruzi* infection in autoimmune strains of mice. Parasite Immunol 7: 377–386.
20. Hunter CA, Subauste CS, Van Cleave VH, Remington JS (1994) Production of gamma interferon by natural killer cells from *Toxoplasma gondii*-infected SCID mice: regulation by interleukin-10, interleukin-12, and tumor necrosis factor alpha. Infect Immun 62: 2818–2824.
21. Gazzinelli R, Xu Y, Hieny S, Cheever A, Sher A (1992) Simultaneous depletion of CD4+ and CD8+ T lymphocytes is required to reactivate chronic infection with *Toxoplasma gondii*. J Immunol 149: 175–180.
22. Viallard JF, Pellegrin JL, Ranchin V, Schaeverbeke T, Dehais J, et al. (1999) Th1 (IL-2, interferon-gamma (IFN-gamma)) and Th2 (IL-10, IL-4) cytokine production by peripheral blood mononuclear cells (PBMC) from patients with systemic lupus erythematosus (SLE). Clin Exp Immunol 115: 189–195.
23. Tucci M, Lombardi L, Richards HB, Dammacco F, Silvestris F (2008) Overexpression of interleukin-12 and T helper 1 predominance in lupus nephritis. Clin Exp Immunol 154: 247–254.
24. Nakashima H, Inoue H, Akahoshi M, Tanaka Y, Yamaoka K, et al. (1999) The combination of polymorphisms within interferon-gamma receptor 1 and receptor 2 associated with the risk of systemic lupus erythematosus. FEBS Lett 453: 187–190.
25. Tanaka Y, Nakashima H, Hisano C, Kohsaka T, Nemoto Y, et al. (1999) Association of the interferon-gamma receptor variant (Val14Met) with systemic lupus erythematosus. Immunogenetics 49: 266–271.
26. Yao X, Chen ZQ, Gong JQ, Chen M, Li AS, et al. (2007) The interferon-gamma receptor gene polymorphisms (Val14Met and Gln64Arg) are not associated with systemic lupus erythematosus in Chinese patients. Arch Dermatol Res 299: 367–371.
27. Theofilopoulos AN, Koundouris S, Kono DH, Lawson BR (2001) The role of IFN-gamma in systemic lupus erythematosus: a challenge to the Th1/Th2 paradigm in autoimmunity. Arthritis Res 3: 136–141.
28. Moulton VR, Tsokos GC (2011) Abnormalities of T cell signaling in systemic lupus erythematosus. Arthritis Res Ther 13: 207.
29. Francisco LM, Sage PT, Sharpe AH (2010) The PD-1 pathway in tolerance and autoimmunity. Immunol Rev 236: 219–242.
30. Bhadra R, Gigley JP, Weiss LM, Khan IA (2011) Control of *Toxoplasma* reactivation by rescue of dysfunctional CD8+ T-cell response via PD-1-PDL-1 blockade. Proc Natl Acad Sci U S A 108: 9196–9201.
31. Rowe JH, Johanns TM, Ertelt JM, Way SS (2008) PDL-1 blockade impedes T cell expansion and protective immunity primed by attenuated *Listeria monocytogenes*. J Immunol 180: 7553–7557.

Permissions

All chapters in this book were first published in PLOS ONE, by The Public Library of Science; hereby published with permission under the Creative Commons Attribution License or equivalent. Every chapter published in this book has been scrutinized by our experts. Their significance has been extensively debated. The topics covered herein carry significant findings which will fuel the growth of the discipline. They may even be implemented as practical applications or may be referred to as a beginning point for another development.

The contributors of this book come from diverse backgrounds, making this book a truly international effort. This book will bring forth new frontiers with its revolutionizing research information and detailed analysis of the nascent developments around the world.

We would like to thank all the contributing authors for lending their expertise to make the book truly unique. They have played a crucial role in the development of this book. Without their invaluable contributions this book wouldn't have been possible. They have made vital efforts to compile up to date information on the varied aspects of this subject to make this book a valuable addition to the collection of many professionals and students.

This book was conceptualized with the vision of imparting up-to-date information and advanced data in this field. To ensure the same, a matchless editorial board was set up. Every individual on the board went through rigorous rounds of assessment to prove their worth. After which they invested a large part of their time researching and compiling the most relevant data for our readers.

The editorial board has been involved in producing this book since its inception. They have spent rigorous hours researching and exploring the diverse topics which have resulted in the successful publishing of this book. They have passed on their knowledge of decades through this book. To expedite this challenging task, the publisher supported the team at every step. A small team of assistant editors was also appointed to further simplify the editing procedure and attain best results for the readers.

Apart from the editorial board, the designing team has also invested a significant amount of their time in understanding the subject and creating the most relevant covers. They scrutinized every image to scout for the most suitable representation of the subject and create an appropriate cover for the book.

The publishing team has been an ardent support to the editorial, designing and production team. Their endless efforts to recruit the best for this project, has resulted in the accomplishment of this book. They are a veteran in the field of academics and their pool of knowledge is as vast as their experience in printing. Their expertise and guidance has proved useful at every step. Their uncompromising quality standards have made this book an exceptional effort. Their encouragement from time to time has been an inspiration for everyone.

The publisher and the editorial board hope that this book will prove to be a valuable piece of knowledge for researchers, students, practitioners and scholars across the globe.

List of Contributors

Edmund A. Rossi, Chien-Hsing Chang and David M. Goldenberg
Immunomedics, Inc., Morris Plains, New Jersey, United States of America
IBC Pharmaceuticals, Inc., Morris Plains, New Jersey, United States of America

David M. Goldenberg
Center for Molecular Medicine and Immunology, Morris Plains, New Jersey, United States of America

Zhenke Wen, Lin Xu and Sidong Xiongs
Institute for Immunobiology, Shanghai Medical College of Fudan University, Shanghai, China

Wei Xu, Zhinan Yin, Xiaoming Gao and Sidong Xiong
Jiangsu Key Laboratory of Infection and Immunity, Institutes of Biology and Medical Sciences, Soochow University, Suzhou, Jiangsu Province, China

Rui-Xue Leng, Wei Wang, Han Cen, Mo Zhou, Chen-Chen Feng, Yan Zhu, Xiao-Ke Yang, Mei Yang, Yu Zhai, Bao-Zhu Li, Xiao-Song Wang, Rui Li, Gui-Mei Chen, Hong Chen, Hai- Feng Pan and Dong-Qing Ye
Department of Epidemiology and Biostatistics, School of Public Health, Anhui Medical University, Hefei, Anhui, People's Republic of China
Anhui Provincial Laboratory of Population Health and Major Disease Screening and Diagnosis, Anhui Medical University, Hefei, Anhui, People's Republic of China

Christian Lood, Helena Tydén, Gunnar Sturfelt, Andreas Jönsen and Anders A. Bengtsson
Department of Clinical Sciences Lund, Section of Rheumatology, Lund University and Ska°ne University Hospital, Lund, Sweden

Birgitta Gullstrand and Lennart Truedssons
Department of Laboratory Medicine Lund, Section of Microbiology, Immunology and Glycobiology, Lund University, Lund, Sweden

Vojislav Jovanović, Nurhuda Abdul Aziz, Yan Ting Lim, Amanda Ng Ai Poh, Sherlynn Jin Hui Chan, Eliza Ho Xin Pei, Fei Chuin Lew, Michael D. Kemeny and Paul A. MacAry
Immunology Programme and Department of Microbiology, National University of Singapore, Singapore

Eoin F. McKinney, Paul A. Lyons and Kenneth G. C. Smith
Cambridge Institute for Medical Research, Cambridge, United Kingdom
Department of Medicine, University of Cambridge, School of Clinical Medicine, Addenbrooke's Hospital, Cambridge, United Kingdom

Guanghou Shui, Li Bowen and Markus R. Wenk
Department of Biochemistry, National University of Singapore, Singapore

Andrew M. Jenner
School of Biological Sciences, Illawara Health and Medical Research Institute, University of Wollongong, Australia

Hiroshi Furukawa, Shomi Oka, Akiko Komiya, Naoshi Fukui, Naoyuki Tsuchiya and Shigeto Tohma
Clinical Research Center for Allergy and Rheumatology, Sagamihara Hospital, National Hospital Organization, Sagamihara, Japan

Kota Shimada and Shoji Sugii
Department of Rheumatology, Tokyo Metropolitan Tama Medical Center, Fuchu, Japan

Atsushi Hashimoto
Department of Rheumatology, Sagamihara Hospital, National Hospital Organization, Sagamihara, Japan

Tatsuo Nagai and Shunsei Hirohata
Department of Rheumatology and Infectious Disease, Kitasato University School of Medicine, Sagamihara, Japan

Keigo Setoguchi
Allergy and Immunological Diseases, Tokyo Metropolitan Cancer and Infectious Diseases Center Komagome Hospital, Tokyo, Japan

Akira Okamoto
Department of Rheumatology, Himeji Medical Center, National Hospital Organization, Himeji, Japan

Noriyuki Chiba
Department of Rheumatology, Morioka Hospital, National Hospital Organization, Morioka, Japan

Eiichi Suematsu
Department of Internal Medicine and Rheumatology, Clinical Research Institute, National Hospital Organization, Kyushu Medical Center, Fukuoka, Japan

Taiichiro Miyashita and Kiyoshi Migita
Nagasaki Medical Center, National Hospital Organization, Omura, Japan

Akiko Suda and Shouhei Nagaoka
Department of Rheumatology, Yokohama Minami Kyosai Hospital, Yokohama, Japan

Naoyuki Tsuchiya
Molecular and Genetic Epidemiology Laboratory, Faculty of Medicine, University of Tsukuba, Tsukuba, Japan

Zev Sthoeger, Heidy Zinger, Amir Sharabi and Edna Mozes
Department of Immunology, The Weizmann Institute of Science, Rehovot, Israel

Zev Sthoeger and Ilan Asher
Department of Internal Medicine B and Clinical Immunology, Kaplan Medical Center, Rehovot, Israel

Rajalingham Sakthiswary and Azman Ali Raymond
Department of Medicine, Universiti Kebangsaan Malaysia Medical Centre, Cheras, Kuala Lumpur, Malaysia

Lina-Marcela Diaz-Gallo, Elena Sànchez and Javier Martin
Cellular Biology and Immunology Department, Instituto de Parasitologíay Biomedicina "López-Neyra", Consejo Superior de Investigaciones Científicas (IPBLN- Consejo Superior de Investigaciones Científicas), Granada, Spain

Norberto Ortego-Centeno
Department of Internal Medicine, Hospital Clínico San Cecilio, Granada, Spain

Jose Mario Sabio
Department of Internal Medicine, Hospital Virgen de las Nieves, Granada, Spain

Francisco J. García-Hernández
Department of Internal Medicine, Hospital Virgen del Rocío, Sevilla, Spain

Enrique de Ramón
Department of Internal Medicine, Hospital Carlos Haya, Málaga, Spain

Miguel A. González-Gay
Department of Rheumatology, Instituto de Formación e Investigación Marqués de Valdecilla, Hospital Universitario Marqués de Valdecilla, Santander, Spain

Torsten Witte
Department of Clinical Immunology and Rheumatology, Hannover Medical School, Hannover, Germany

Hans-Joachim Anders
Medical department and policlinic IV, Klinikum der Universität, München, Munich, Germany

María F. González-Escribano
Department of Immunology, Hospital Virgen del Rocío, Sevilla, Spain

Laia Vilà, Miguel Baena and Emma Barroso
Department of Pharmacology and Therapeutic Chemistry, School of Pharmacy, University of Barcelona, Barcelona, Spain

Núria Roglans, Marta Alegret, Manuel Merlos and Juan C. Laguna
Institute of Biomedicine, University of Barcelona, Barcelona, Spain

Núria Roglans, Marta Alegret, Manuel Merlos and Juan C. Laguna
CIBER (Centro de Investigación Biomédica en Red) of Physiopathology of Obesity and Nutrition, Barcelona, Spain

Su-li Wang and Liang-jing Lu
Department of Rheumatology, Ren Ji Hospital, School of Medicine, Shanghai Jiao Tong University, Shanghai, China

Bin Wu
Clinical Outcomes and Economics Group, Department of pharmacy, Ren Ji Hospital, School of Medicine, Shanghai Jiao Tong University, Shanghai, China

Li-an Zhu, Lin Leng and Richard Bucala
Department of Medicine, Section of Rheumatology, Yale University School of Medicine, The Anlyan Center, New Haven, Connecticut, United States of America

Masahiro Moritoki and Masakazu Kohno
Department of Cardiorenal and Cerebrovascular Medicine, Faculty of Medicine, Kagawa University, Kagawa, Japan

Takeshi Kadowaki, Toshiro Niki and Mitsuomi Hirashima
Department of Immunology and Immunopathology, Faculty of Medicine, Kagawa University, Kagawa, Japan

Takeshi Kadowaki and Genichiro Soma
Department of Holistic Immunology, Kagawa University, Kagawa, Japan

Daisuke Nakano
Department of Pharmacology, Faculty of Medicine, Kagawa University, Kagawa, Japan

Hirohito Mori, Hideki Kobara, Tsutomu Masaki and Mitsuomi Hirashima
Department of Gastroenterology and Neurology, Faculty of Medicine, Kagawa University, Kagawa, Japan

Anna M. Timofeeva, Valentina N. Buneva and Georgy A. Nevinsky
Institute of Chemical Biology and Fundamental Medicine, Siberian Division of Russian Academy of Sciences, Novosibirsk, Russia

Pavel S. Dmitrenok
Pacific Institute of Bioorganic Chemistry, Far East Division, Russian Academy of Sciences, Vladivostok, Russia

Ludmila P. Konenkova
Institute of Clinical Immunology, Siberian Division of Russian Medical Academy of Sciences, Novosibirsk, Russia

Valentina N. Buneva and Georgy A. Nevinsky
Novosibirsk State University, Novosibirsk, Russia

Desmond Y. H. Yap, Susan Yung, Qing Zhang, Colin Tang and Tak Mao Chan
Division of Nephrology, Department of Medicine, Queen Mary Hospital, The University of Hong Kong, Hong Kong

Liliane Fossati-Jimack, Guang Sheng Ling, Andrea Cortini, Marta Szajna, Talat H. Malik, Matthew C. Pickering, H. Terence Cook and Marina Botto
Centre for Complement and Inflammation Research, Division of Immunology and Inflammation, Department of Medicine, Imperial College, London, United Kingdom

Jacqueline U. McDonald and Philip R. Taylors
Cardiff Institute of Infection and Immunity, Cardiff University School of Medicine, Cardiff, United Kingdom

Fabrizio Conti, Fulvia Ceccarelli, Carlo Perricone, Francesca Miranda, Simona Truglia, Laura Massaro, Viviana Antonella Pacucci, Virginia Conti, Izabella Bartosiewicz, Francesca Romana Spinelli, Cristiano Alessandri and Guido Valesini
Lupus Clinic, Reumatologia, Dipartimento di Medicina Interna e Specialità Mediche, Sapienza Università di Roma, Rome, Italy

Yanxing Cai, Weijuan Zhang and Sidong Xiong
Department of Immunology and Institute for Immunobiology, Shanghai Medical College, Fudan University, Shanghai, People's Republic of China

Sidong Xiong
Institutes of Biology and Medical Sciences, Soochow University, Suzhou, People's Republic of China

Adriana Rojas-Villarraga
Center for Autoimmune Diseases Research (CREA), School of medicine and health sciences, Universidad del Rosario, Bogotá, Colombia

July-Vianneth Torres-Gonzalez
Medical social service provision mandatory, research assistant in partnership with the School of Medicine and Health Sciences, Universidad del Rosario, Bogotá, Colombia

Ángela-María Ruiz-Sternberg
Departamento de investigación Grupo Investigación Clínica, School of Medicine and Health Sciences, Universidad del Rosario, Bogotá, Colombia

Te-Chun Shen, Chia-Hung Chen, Chih-Yen Tu, Te-Chun Hsia, Chuen-Ming Shih and Wu-Huei Hsu
Division of Pulmonary and Critical Care Medicine, Department of Internal Medicine, China Medical University Hospital and China Medical University, Taichung, Taiwan

Te-Chun Shen
Division of Pulmonary and Critical Care Medicine, Department of Internal Medicine, Chu Shang Show Chwan Hospital, Nantou, Taiwan

Cheng-Li Lin
Department of Public Health, China Medical University, Taichung, Taiwan

Cheng-Li Lin
Management Office for Health Data, China Medical University Hospital, Taichung, Taiwan

Yen-Jung Chang
Department of Health Promotion and Health Education, National Taiwan Normal University, Taipei, Taiwan

Christie Fitch-Rogalsky, Whitney Steber, Terri Lupton, Liam Martin, Susan G. Barr, Dianne P. Mosher, James Wick and Marvin J. Fritzler
Faculty of Medicine, University of Calgary, Calgary, Alberta, Canada

Michael Mahler
INOVA Diagnostics Inc., San Diego, California, United States of America

Elisa Lazzari, Joan NíGabhann, Siobhán Smith and Caroline A. Jefferies
Molecular and Cellular Therapeutics, Research Institute, Royal College of Surgeons in Ireland, Dublin, Ireland

Justyna Korczeniewska and Betsy J. Barnes
Department of Biochemistry and Molecular Biology, Rutgers Biomedical and Health Sciences, Newark, New Jersey, United States of America, Rutgers Biomedical and Health Sciences, New Jersey Medical School- Cancer Center, Newark, New Jersey, United States of America

Xinghong Ding
Analysis and Testing Center, Zhejiang Chinese Medical University, Hangzhou, China

Jinbo Hu
College of Pharmaceutical Science, Zhejiang Chinese Medical University, Hangzhou, China

Chengping Wen and Yongsheng Fan
College of Basic Medicine, Zhejiang Chinese Medical University, Hangzhou, China

Zhishan Ding
College of Life Science, Zhejiang Chinese Medical University, Hangzhou, China

Li Cai, Xing-xin Xue, Jia-jia Wang, Shai-di Tang, Shao-wen Tang and Yun Zhang
Department of Epidemiology and Biostatistics, School of Public Health, Nanjing Medical University, Jiangning District, Nanjing, Jiangsu, China

Jin-wei Zhang
Department of Anesthesiology, Affiliated Drum Tower Hospital of Medical College of Nanjing University, Gulou District, Nanjing, Jiangsu, China

Zhi-gang Wang and Xian Xia
Department of Nosocomial Infection Control, General Hospital of Beijing Military Region, Dongcheng District, Beijing, China

Jie Wang
State Key Laboratory of Reproductive Medicine, Nanjing Medical University, Jiangning District, Nanjing, Jiangsu, China
Department of General Practice, Kangda College, Nanjing Medical University, Jiangning District, Nanjing, Jiangsu, China

Yun Zhang
Institute of Epidemiology and Microbiology, Huadong Research Institute for Medicine and Biotechnics, Nanjing, Jiangsu, China

Allison Sang, Ying-Yi Zheng, Yiming Yin and Laurence Morel
Department of Pathology, Immunology, and Laboratory Medicine, University of Florida, Gainesville, Florida, United States of America

Igor Dozmorov
Department of Immunology, University of Texas Southwestern Medical Center, Dallas, Texas, United States of America

Hao Li, Hui-Chen Hsu and John D. Mountz
Clinical Immunology and Rheumatology, Department of Medicine, University of Alabama at Birmingham, Birmingham, Alabama, United States of America

Linda A. Lieberman and George C. Tsokos
Division of Rheumatology, Department of Medicine, Beth Israel Deaconess Medical Center, Harvard Medical School, Boston, Massachusetts, United States of America

Index

A

Angina Pectoris, 26, 30, 71

Anti-cardiolipin, 25-29, 32-33, 36, 39, 41

Anti-lipid Antibody, 35

Anti-phospholipid Antibodies, 25, 32-33, 39

Antibody-mediated Thrombosis, 25, 32

Antinuclear Antibodies, 72, 164, 170-171

Autoimmune Disease, 1-2, 9, 18-19, 23, 35, 42, 58, 70-71, 80, 83, 88, 96, 111, 155, 158-159, 163, 166-167, 171-172, 179, 182, 193, 203, 207, 214, 220

B

B-cell Depletion, 1-2, 4-7

C

Cardiolipin, 33, 36, 39, 41

Celiac Disease, 66, 70

Chemokines, 9, 15, 138

Chronic Obstructive Pulmonary Disease, 158, 162

Criterion Validity, 83, 85, 87

Cytokine, 1, 9, 18, 23, 52-53, 57-59, 71, 76, 80, 82, 89, 118-122, 125-128, 138-139, 142, 144, 146, 181, 198, 201-205, 207, 209-213, 215, 217, 221

D

Dysregulated Cytokine, 203

E

Encephalytogenic Oligopeptides, 98

Epratuzumab, 1-8

Erythematosus, 1, 7-9, 18-20, 23-25, 29, 31, 33-36, 42-45, 50-52, 58-61, 65-66, 70-71, 76, 87-88, 110-111, 118-119, 132-136, 149, 151, 154-158, 166, 181-182, 201-203, 221

F

Flare, 36-39, 41-42, 53, 59, 111-113, 117, 130-134, 147

Fluorescence Microscopy, 4-5

G

Galectin, 88, 90, 96-97

Gene Expression, 52-59, 70, 138-139, 144, 146, 175, 178-179, 181, 201, 204, 206-207, 213

Gene-sex Interaction, 21-22

Genotyping, 22-24, 46, 67, 194, 200

Glomerular Injury, 9, 11

H

Hepatic Triglyceride, 74, 78

Hormonal Replacement Therapy, 147, 149-151

Human Leukocyte Antigen, 44, 51

Hydroxycholesterol, 35-36, 41

Hyperglycemia, 30

Hypertension, 26, 30, 51, 60-61, 63, 72, 82, 156, 159-160, 162, 182

I

Inflammation, 9, 15, 18, 23, 25, 34-35, 71, 77, 80, 82, 88, 96-98, 117-120, 124, 127-128, 136, 145-146, 148, 156, 158, 160, 163, 181, 187, 191-192, 198, 215

Inflammatory Diseases, 26, 33, 35, 165

Interferon, 19, 21-23, 34, 42, 52-53, 59, 61, 126, 128, 172, 175, 180-181, 192, 200, 203, 214, 221

Interleukin, 9, 18, 23, 59, 76, 126, 128-129, 156, 181, 193-194, 196, 198, 201-202, 213-214, 221

J

Jieduquyuziyin, 182, 191-192

L

Liquid Chromatography, 37, 39, 182-183, 192

Lupus, 1-2, 7-11, 13-27, 29, 31, 33-37, 39, 42-45, 50-62, 65-66, 70-71, 76, 80-85, 87-90, 92-98, 110-115, 122, 126-137, 149, 151, 154-158, 166, 180-183, 201-206, 212-221

Lupus Erythematosus, 1, 7-9, 18-20, 23-25, 29, 31, 33-36, 42-45, 50-52, 58-61, 65-66, 76, 82-84, 96-98, 118-119, 132-136, 149, 151, 154-158, 166, 181-182, 201-203, 221

Lupus Nephritis, 8-11, 13-18, 39, 43, 71, 80-82, 88-89, 93, 96, 111-115, 117-118, 129, 136-137, 139, 141, 143-146, 156, 170, 191, 201-203, 213

Lymphocytes, 3-4, 8, 35, 53-54, 58-59, 74, 76, 97, 160, 214, 221

M

Macrophage Polarization, 136, 139, 142, 146

Mannose-binding Lectin, 136-137, 145-146

Mass Spectrometry, 37, 39, 103, 105, 109, 182-183, 192

Metabolic Syndrome, 71, 77, 82, 156

Monocytes, 2, 4-5, 8, 36, 119-122, 124-129, 146, 157, 179-180, 191, 202

Mononuclear Cells, 1, 15, 36, 52, 58-59, 172-173, 201-202, 213, 221

Murine, 10-11, 15, 18, 52-53, 55-59, 71-72, 80-82, 88, 95, 97, 120-121, 128-129, 136-140, 142, 145-146, 148, 155-156, 180-181, 192, 203, 213-216, 221

Murine Model, 52-53, 59, 71, 80, 136-137, 139-140, 142, 156, 180, 192, 214

Myelin Basic Protein, 98-99, 105, 110

Myocardial Infarction, 26, 29-31, 33, 71

N
Neutropenia, 119

O
Obesity, 30, 71-72, 82
Oligopeptides, 98-101, 105, 107, 110
Oral Contraceptives, 134, 147, 149-150, 154-156
Oxidized Phosphatidylcholine, 35-36, 39, 41

P
Peptide, 15, 18, 45-46, 51-59, 89, 96, 100-101, 103, 110
Peripheral Blood, 1, 15, 18, 36, 52, 59, 67, 120, 172-173, 181, 202, 221
Phagocytosis, 119-122, 124, 126-128
Phosphatidylcholine, 35-36, 39, 41, 182, 191
Plasma Cell Apoptosis, 88, 93, 95-96
Plasmid, 137, 174, 178
Platelet Activation, 25-29, 32-34, 191
Platelets, 25-34, 154, 191-192
Polymorphisms, 19, 21-23, 51, 61, 65-68, 140, 145-146, 172, 176, 179, 193-194, 197-198, 200-201, 212-214, 220-221
Proinflammatory Cytokines, 180

Q
Quality of Life, 83, 87, 191

R
Rapid Resolution, 182-183
Rheumatoid Arthritis, 2, 8, 15, 18, 25-26, 29-31, 33, 44-48, 51, 66, 70, 96, 98, 100, 129, 146, 154, 156, 159, 162, 165-166, 170-171, 201
Rheumatology, 8, 18, 22, 24-27, 33-34, 39, 42-45, 51, 58, 65-67, 70, 83-84, 87, 128, 130-131, 134-135, 145-146, 148, 151, 156, 163-167, 171, 181, 191, 194, 201, 203, 214-215
Ribonucleoprotein, 44-45, 165, 167, 181
Rituximab, 1-8, 97

S
Splenocytes, 9, 52, 54, 74-76, 80, 89, 137, 145, 204, 207, 216, 218-220
Systemic Lupus Erythematosus, 1, 7-9, 18-20, 23-25, 29, 31, 33-36, 50-52, 65-66, 76, 82-84, 96-98, 118-119, 132-136, 149, 151, 154-158, 166, 170-172, 191-194, 201-203, 221

T
T Cell Apoptosis, 52
T Cell Ubiquitin, 66
Thrombosis, 25, 30, 32
Tolerogenic Peptide, 52, 55-56, 58-59
Trogocytosis, 1-2, 4-8

V
Veltuzumab, 1-8
Vitamin D, 60-65

www.ingramcontent.com/pod-product-compliance
Lightning Source LLC
Chambersburg PA
CBHW080528200326
41458CB00012B/4372